Iserson's Getting Into A Residency

Iserson's Getting Into A Residency

A GUIDE FOR MEDICAL STUDENTS

Eighth Edition

Kenneth V. Iserson
M.D., MBA, FACEP, FAAEM

Galen Press LTD • Tucson, Arizona

First Published 1988
Second Edition 1990
Third Edition 1993
Fourth Edition 1996
Fifth Edition 2000
Sixth Edition 2003
Seventh Edition 2006
Eighth Edition, 2013

Bulk purchase terms are available. Please contact our special sales department.

GALEN PRESS, Ltd.
P.O. BOX 64400
TUCSON, AZ 85728-4400
PHONE (520) 577-8363   FAX (520) 529-6459
Orders (U.S. & Canada) 1-800-442-5369
Sales@galenpress.com
www.galenpress.com

ISBN-13: 978-1-883620-36-3 (softcover)
ISBN-13: 978-1-883620-37-0 (e-book)

KENNETH V. ISERSON, M.D., MBA, FACEP, FAAEM
Professor Emeritus of Emergency Medicine
University of Arizona College of Medicine, Tucson, AZ

FREIDA is a registered trademark of the American Medical Association.
Windows is a registered trademark of Microsoft, Inc.

Library of Congress Cataloging-in-Publication Data

Iserson, Kenneth V.
   Iserson's getting into a residency : a guide for medical students / Kenneth
V. Iserson. – 8th ed.
      p. ; cm.
   Rev. ed. of: Getting into a residency / Kenneth V. Iserson. 7th ed. 2006.
   Includes bibliographical references and index.
   ISBN-13: 1-883620-36-3 (pbk.)
      1. Residents (Medicine)–Selection and appointment–United States. 2. Medical
   education–United States. I. Title: Getting into a residency. II. Iserson, Kenneth V.
   Getting into a residency. III. Title.
      [DNLM: 1. Internship and Residency–United States. 2. Education, Medical,
   Graduate–United States. W 20 I78i 2013]
   RA972 .I74 2013
   610'.71"550973–dc2

Printed in the United States of America.
10 9 8 7 6 5 4 3 2 1

Contents

List of Figures

Acknowledgments

Those having torches will pass them on to others.

Plato, *The Republic*

Of the making of books,
there is no end.

Ecclesiastes, 12

THIS BOOK WOULD NOT EXIST but for the significant help I received from others. First and foremost is the fantastic assistance and support from my wife, Mary Lou Iserson, C.P.A. Acting as both a skilled and persistent editor, and the resident computer whiz, she has midwifed every edition.

I greatly appreciate the help of the many students and physicians who took time to add to the book's content by sending me letters and e-mails containing comments and suggestions (some of which are quoted in this edition).

As always, I owe a debt of gratitude to my friends at the University of Arizona Health Sciences Library, who continue to amaze me by finding sources of information in inscrutable ways. I am especially grateful to Nga T. Nguyen, B.A., B.S., Senior Library Specialist, and Ms. Hannah Fisher, R.N., M.L.S., AHIP, who helped to update important details, such as organization addresses and bibliographic references. Also thanks to an ingenious and always reliable researcher, Robert Fisher, M.L.S, Tucson, AZ.

Special thanks also goes to Donald Witzke, Ph.D., now at the University of Kentucky Medical Center, Lexington, who has strongly supported this book's concept and has acted as a superb content reviewer for many editions.

A variety of people at the organizations mentioned in this book helped supply valuable updated information for this edition. These include Douglas Perry, Executive Director, San Francisco Matching Program; James W. Tysinger, Ph.D., Department of Family and Community Medicine, University of Texas Health Sciences Center at San Antonio; Mona M. Singer, Executive Director, National Residency Matching Program; Walter "Waldo" Wentz, Assistant Director, National Residency Matching Program; George V. Richard, Ph.D., Director, and his staff, Careers in Medicine Program, Association of American Medical Colleges; Various staff members, American Medical Women's Association; Joyce L. Obradovic, American Osteopathic Association; and Janett Forte, MSW, LCSW, IWH Program Director, the Virginia Commonwealth University Women's Health Institute.

Numerous staff members associated with the following departments within the American Medical Association also provided invaluable assistance: the Center for Health Policy Research, the Medical Student Section, *FREIDA*, the Department of Marketing & Strategic Analysis; and the AMA Alliance.

Aside from our Library's reference staff, those from the University of Arizona College of Medicine who assisted in updating this book included Chris Leadem, Ph.D., Sr. Associate Dean, Admissions & Student Affairs; Pat Oltman, Coordinator, Office of Student Affairs; and James M. Woolfenden, M.D., Professor of Nuclear Medicine.

My special appreciation goes to George H. Zimny, Ph.D., for graciously allowing a markedly abbreviated version of his Medical Specialty Preference Inventory to be included in this text.

I would be remiss if I did not also thank the people at Galen Press, especially my editor, Jennifer Gilbert, who helped immensely by verifying and clarifying the many changes in this edition. Mary Lou Sherk, also at Galen Press, has been wonderful in supporting this project and helping make it the success it has been. Part of that success is due to Sarah Hinman of Stornetta Publications, who gave the book its wonderful design.

Finally, I wish to thank Dr. Louis Olsen, M.D., of Baltimore, Maryland. One of the few ideal physicians I know, this Family Physician suffered the strain of acting as my mentor throughout medical school—for which I will be ever grateful. It is to him that I owe much of what I am as a clinician and teacher.

A Little History

SITTING ON A BOOKSHELF ABOVE my desk is the slim, 317-page first edition of *Getting Into A Residency*. Published in 1988, it recalls a time of typewriters, and mailed program information and applications. "Computer searches" didn't appear in the book until the third edition in 1993; and they were usually done by the library staff! Things have changed, although not always for the better.

While some parts of the specialty selection/USMLE testing/information gathering/residency application systems have improved, others remain unnecessarily confusing, costly, and stressful. Hopefully, this latest edition of the book will clarify such areas and guide readers through the process.

A huge change in all our lives has been the advent of e-books. This text, for the first time, is now available electronically, as well as in hard copy.

System changes affecting *all applicants* since the first edition, with the newest changes in this edition, include:

- *FREIDA* and Internet sites that contain specialty-specific information.
- On-line specialty and career counseling through both the Association of American Medical Colleges (AAMC) and the Glaxo Pathway Evaluation Program.
- Widespread participation in the Electronic Residency Applications Service (ERAS), which eliminates most paper applications to individual programs.
- On-line debt/money management information and counseling provided by the AAMC.
- USMLE and COMLEX-USA have both added on-site exams that use simulated patients.
- The "Scramble" for unmatched applicants has been replaced with the much more civilized SOAP system, operated through ERAS and the National Residency Matching Program.

For *Osteopathic students*, huge changes have occurred, including:
- Much more transparency about which postgraduate positions are actually available and funded.
- An increase in the number of residency programs that are approved by both American Osteopathic Association (AOA) and ACGME (M.D.).
- The AOA has made it much easier to get ACGME training approved to qualify for medical licensure.
- More specialties now offer AOA training, often with the first year integrated into the entire program.
- There are many more Osteopathic graduates than in the past.

Women may have seen the biggest changes:
- Women's numbers within medicine have increased dramatically.
- Women are represented in virtually all specialties and subspecialties.

International Medical Graduates have also seen changes:
* The number of IMGs has increased.
* The English-language tests have been incorporated into USMLE Step 3CS, which must be taken in the United States.
* The ECFMG has become more user-friendly.
* States now require U.S. postgraduate trainees to be licensed.
* Visas have become more difficult to obtain.

Many of these changes have helped applicants. Yet the system has become too costly and unnecessarily complex. My suggestions to *make the entire process a bit more user-friendly* include:

1. *Programs should limit the number of applicant interviews*, especially for those outside a one-day (non-flight) travel radius. Residency program faculty have no right to ask marginal applicants to pay exorbitant amounts for travel, board and lodging to interview at programs where they have little chance of matching.
2. *Eliminate USMLE Step 2CS and COMLEX Part 2CS.* These tests have virtually 100% pass rates for medical students at U.S. schools. Instead, make passing a uniform OSCE (Objective-Structured Clinical Exam) at their medical school mandatory for graduation. For IMGs, offer an equivalent test at strategic sites around the world that are more accessible and less expensive to get to.
3. *For both M.D. and D.O. postgraduate programs, all specialties should agree to participate in both ERAS and the NRMP.* Ideally, this would eliminate the bizarre "early matches" that force applicants to select a specialty much earlier than they would otherwise. It would also allow more students to participate in couples matching, and generally make life easier for everyone. Other than historical precedent, there is no reason not to do this.
4. *Eliminate the bizarre terms that only serve to confuse applicants.* For example, why does the ECFMG use "token" instead of password? Why does the NRMP have applicants "certify" rather than approve their Rank-Order Lists? And, couldn't there have been a term for the replacement for the Scramble other than "SOAP," which is the common term for ward and clinic notes? There are lots of other examples. Let's remember, and implement, the KISS principle: Keep It Simple, Stupid!

This book originally was written to help medical students and other applicants traverse what seemed to be a complex process. That many generations of students and physicians have benefitted warms my heart. I hope that this edition continues in that tradition.

Kenneth V. Iserson, M.D., 2013

Preface to the First Edition

Knowing how to get a job is as important as knowing how to do a job.
Robert Half

OVER THE YEARS, MANY STUDENTS have come to me seeking career advice. In some cases the advice was about my own specialty. But often it concerned the mechanics of finding a personal niche in medicine and assuring that the individual was able to get a training position in his or her area of interest. Sadly, most of these medical students had not spent enough time investigating all the choices available. Many believed that since they had chosen medicine as a career, and since they had achieved the long-sought-after goal of entering medical school, the significant choices were behind them. Nothing could be further from the truth.

Medicine is a diverse and complicated profession. The physician practicing Pathology is in a different world from the Family Practitioner or Physiatrist. The Radiologist's practice has little in common with that of the Anesthesiologist. Unfortunately, these differences are not as obvious as they might be in many medical school settings.

While students know, or will know, something about the practices of the Internist, Family Physician, General Surgeon, Pediatrician, Obstetrician, and Psychiatrist from their required third-year rotations, even here their knowledge may be skewed toward picturing the individuals only in the hospital setting. Rarely does this setting constitute the majority of the clinician's practice. This is insufficient knowledge upon which to base a career. In addition, most medical students are unaware of their many training options. (Many haven't even heard the term "Physiatrist" before. This is a specialist in Physical and Rehabilitation Medicine.)

The first part of this book briefly describes the specialty choices available to you. It also provides you with a method of analyzing your own interests to compare them with those of physicians practicing in various medical fields.

Even if you do make a career decision, how do you use your medical school experience to optimize your chances of getting into the specialty and program that you finally decide upon? The basic medical school wisdom is that an industrious student will get his or her just rewards. Not necessarily! There is so much to do and so little time in which to accomplish it. You need to know how to maximize your efforts. The second part of the book encompasses this.

And then, how do you know where to interview, how to get an interview, and how to interview? Although students in other professions are given basic information on how to get their first job, this information is not generally passed on to medical students. You need this knowledge as you prepare to get your first job in medicine. You will find it in the third part of the book.

Finally, how to best utilize the Matching systems? What pitfalls must you avoid? What opportunities can you take advantage of? The last part of the book deals with these questions.

This text, in concert with your mentor and Dean of Students, is designed to guide you through the process of selecting a specialty field, helping you to maximize your efforts toward getting into your chosen specialty and program, selecting programs that meet your personal needs, getting interviews at these programs, doing well at the interviews, and ultimately matching with these programs.

This book is intended to serve as a guide for the student who wants to be a winner—who is actively participating in taking those steps necessary to get into the residency he or she wants. Different parts of the book will be relevant to different students with diverse goals in mind. To make this book work for you, you should read it all, charting the course to your goal. This can be done by *checking* or *flagging* those items relevant to *your* goal and what you must do to achieve it. After you have charted your course, you can then use this as a plan for action. As you complete each activity, check it off. Write in the book, highlight what is relevant and make it work for you.

If you are reading this book, it means that you are willing to put forth a little effort in preparing for your upcoming major career step. Just owning the book will not be sufficient. You must read it and apply the information diligently. Success can be yours if you expend the energy.

If any part of this book particularly helps you, or you find errors or omissions, please let me know. You can be assured that any insights you share will be considered for the future editions of this book.

Best of luck in your exciting life in medicine!

K. V. Iserson, M.D.
December, 1987

1

The Big Picture

Luck is a crossroad where preparation and opportunity meet.

Anonymous

Your Problem

IF YOUR RICH RELATIVE JUST DONATED $15 million to endow a desperately needed chair of advanced biohypergraphics (or to help hire a new football coach) at the institution you would like to attend, you may not have much of a problem securing a residency slot there. Unfortunately, most of us are not in this position. Residencies are getting picky about their selections, because it costs about $174,800 per year (2012 dollars) to educate a resident. And, with the rapidly decreasing number of quality residency positions, even the endowment ploy may not guarantee you entrance—although helping to hire the football coach probably would.

In recent years, about 8% of the U.S. medical students attempting to find a residency position through the National Residents Matching Program (NRMP) did not match. Not exactly the kind of odds you would choose! And the odds are even worse in some of the specialties that do not use the NRMP. That does not mean you should settle for a residency in a specialty and career that you don't love. In Lewis Carroll's *Alice's Adventures in Wonderland*, the Queen provided excellent advice:

> Alice laughed: 'There's no use trying,' she said; 'one can't believe impossible things.'
> 'I daresay you haven't had much practice,' said the Queen. 'When I was your age, I always did it for half an hour a day. Why, sometimes I've believed as many as six impossible things before breakfast.'

Getting a residency in the specialty you desire, at the institution you crave, is a **COMPETITION**. It has **RULES**, which you may not know unless you have been out in the working world as a professional before entering medical school. These rules correspond in many ways to those used to get executive positions in business. They also approximate the rules you will follow to get a job after residency—assuming that you, like most of your colleagues, join a group practice.

In many ways, resident-selection rules are arcane—having been derived from the ancient art of choosing an apprentice. One thing is certain: just as in the days of yore, choice apprenticeship positions are few and far between.

A physician from the Philippines related a horrifying story of his experiences not many years ago. As now, the Philippines had very good quality medical schools. They taught from American texts and used the same curriculum. But they produced more medical graduates than there were spaces available for residency training. Since physicians were required to have advanced training to get a medical license, many medical school graduates ended up doing odd jobs (this individual drove a taxi) until they could get residency positions in the United States. That situation is now being duplicated in many other countries.

These events happened when we had a severe shortage of doctors in this country, and physicians graduating from U.S. medical schools could get into almost any specialty that they desired. The only real question was where.

Today, the increasing numbers of graduating medical students represent the hope of preventing a looming physician shortage. In 2008, there were 252 physicians per 100,000 population (one physician per 396 persons). According to the AAMC's Center for Workforce Studies, if current conditions remain fairly constant, the U.S. physician workforce will increase by about 11%, from 773,809 in 2010 to 869,900 in 2025. Still, the United States will have fewer physicians than necessary. That is not surprising, since 25% of practicing physicians are at least 60-years-old; one-third are at least 55-years-old. But the shortfall also stems from physicians working fewer hours than in prior years, male physicians retiring at a younger age, an increasing elderly population that will need more healthcare, and continuing geographic misdistribution of physicians.

In 2012, international medical graduates (IMGs) (27.5%) and Osteopathic physicians (D.O.s) (6.8%) comprised a steadily increasing percentage of all residents, while the percentage of Canadians (<1%) remained constant and that of U.S. medical graduates (65.4%) decreased. There were over 24,000 PGY-1 *positions* available to students, which is about the same number as existed in

1994. The number of residency and fellowship *programs*, however, increased from 7,435 in 1994 to more than 8,500 in 2012.

By 2013, the expansion of existing M.D.- and D.O.-granting medical schools and a plethora of new schools will augment first-year enrollment by 21%, increasing competition for residency positions. Yet, partly due to Medicare's cap on residency training reimbursement, the number of graduate medical education (residency and fellowship) slots is expanding much more slowly than the increase in medical school graduates. In 2011, there were approximately 100,000 residency and fellowship positions approved by the Accreditation Council for Graduate Medical Education (ACGME). This was essentially the same number as in 1993–94. In 2011, two subspecialties had no training programs and seven subspecialties had only one program. While the number of U.S. residents and fellows has increased 95% since 1970, their percentage in relation to the total physician population has decreased from 15.3% in 1970 to 12% in 2012.

Applicants already overwhelm the most sought-after residency programs and institutions; in the future, competition will increase. But don't despair. This book will show you how to get the residency that you long for. Basically, success comes from applying the **three golden rules:**

1. **Be Assertive!** No one can look out for your interests better than you. Determine what you want and need, then go after it. This means that you should get a mentor/adviser, research opportunities, special externships or rotations, or additional career counseling and information. Remember—the course of *your entire professional life* depends on whether you get a good residency in your chosen field!

2. **Time It Right!** Nothing is worse than doing all the right things— but at the wrong time. This includes getting started. As you will learn from this book, if you are just beginning the process as a senior medical student, you are probably already behind the eight ball. If you are a third-year student, you have more time to get your act together—but you had better work fast. The essence of timing is to *start early*, *apply early*, and *interview late*. While "the early bird gets the worm" is a trite expression, it is worth heeding—at least until you schedule your interviews (*see* Chapter 16).

3. **Go for the Gold!** Most medical students I know tend to "put down" both themselves and the training they received from their medical school. "It's only a state school" or "I wasn't AOA," they

moan. This negative attitude makes them aim much lower than they should, both in the specialty they seek and in the institutional slots they pursue. My father was a professional salesman. His advice for success was, *"Sell yourself—no one will do it for you."* While you compete for your goal, keep these words close to your heart. Remember, it's your life and your career!

The Process

Performing well in medical school is hard enough, but then, to obtain a residency position, you must learn the arcane language, processes, and alternatives associated with the licensing tests, gathering residency program information, submitting applications, and dealing with the matching programs. Even those U.S. students going into mainline specialties such as Internal Medicine or Family Medicine must learn the lingo to succeed. Those entering Neurology, Ophthalmology, Neurological Surgery, Otolaryngology, or Urology must contend with more complex systems. The system is extremely complicated for Osteopathic medical students and physicians, as well as for international medical graduates (IMGs), who first must decide which of the multiple pathways they should follow.

Figure 1.1 is an overview of the routes and procedures for residency application. Note that some elements pertain only to Osteopaths; others pertain only to IMGs. Each of these steps is discussed in greater detail later in this book.

Figure 1.1
Getting Into a Residency—The Component Parts

EXAMS

M.D. Students/Graduates

USMLE
- Most M.D. students must pass Steps 1, 2CK, and 2CS to get a residency position.
- M.D.s must pass all three Steps to obtain a medical license.

D.O. Students/Graduates

COMLEX (D.O.s only)
- Most D.O. residencies require passing Levels 1, 2PE, and 2CE.
- Completion of all three Levels required for licensure.

USMLE
- D.O.s may also use this exam in most states.

RESIDENCY PROGRAM INFORMATION

M.D. Students/Graduates

- *FREIDA*
- AMA *Graduate Medical Education Directory* (the "Green Book")

D.O. Students/Graduates

- AOA-net (*Opportunities*)

Information from individual programs' websites and printed materials.
Information from specialty websites and on-line residency catalogues.

APPLICATION SUBMISSION

M.D. Students/Graduates

Electronic Residency Application Service (ERAS)
- Used by most M.D. residency programs.

Centralized Application Service (CAS)
- Used by M.D. "Advanced" programs in the San Francisco Matching Program.

D.O. Students/Graduates

Electronic Residence Application Service (ERAS)
- Used by most D.O. internships (students only)

Individual Program Applications (often, Universal Application)
- Used by some M.D. and all D.O. training programs, and many subspecialty fellowships.

Figure 1.1 (continued)

MATCHING PROGRAMS

M.D. Students/Graduates	*D.O. Students/Graduates*
• National Resident Matching Program (NRMP)	• AOA Intern/Resident Registration (National Matching Service)
• NRMP Specialty Matching Program	
• San Francisco Matching Program	
• Urology Match	

Military Match

No Matching Program

• Used by "off-cycle" applicants, D.O. residencies, and many fellowship programs.

INTERNATIONAL MEDICAL GRADUATES

ECFMG Certificate Required	*Fifth Pathway*
USMLE	• An alternative to ECFMG certification for U.S. citizen IMGs from selected schools.
• Must pass Steps 1, 2CK, and 2CS for ECFMG certification.	
	• This program no longer exists. However, the ECFMG will continue to act as the Dean's Office for those who have successfully completed this program.
VISA	
• Required for non-U.S. citizens/ permanent residents.	

2

The Specialties

If you don't know where you are going, you won't know when you get there.

Anonymous

The Choices

IN GOING THROUGH THE PROCESS of tentatively selecting a specialty—because a tentative selection is all you should make if you are reading this during your preclinical or early clinical years—*make sure to choose for yourself*. Don't select a specialty based on:

- **What your parents want you to do.** "You're going to be a Surgeon, just like your old man," your father has said since you were in preschool.

- **What your spouse wants you to do.** "Make sure that you go into something where you will be home nights and weekends."

- **The specialty that your lab partner selected.** Did you forget that while your partner was dissecting those tiny little nerves in Anatomy you had trouble finding the biceps muscle?

- **Mental images from the books and television shows that first attracted you to medicine.** Do you really think Emergency Physicians see only crises interspersed with sexual escapades, as *ER* and *Grey's Anatomy* depict?

"Knowing" The Specialty You Will Enter

Many students begin medical school "knowing" the specialty they will enter; most of them are wrong. Studies suggest that more than one-third of medical students make a specialty selection before medical school (although it often subsequently changes), about the same number decide during their third-year clerkships, and fewer decide either during their basic science years or after their basic clerkships.

Overall, only 20% of students who "know" what field they want to practice upon entering medical school actually pursue that field for residency training. More than one-third of those entering medical school who are interested in

Obstetrics/Gynecology, Psychiatry, Family Medicine, or Emergency Medicine ultimately pursue those fields. In general, older students are more likely to commit to a career path early in medical school. But the likelihood is that you will change your mind as you experience new and exciting adventures during your medical education journey.

Even in my student days, decades past, we knew that our specialty choices would probably not last out the first year. My anatomy partner, for example, foolishly blurted out during our first day of medical school that he would be a Pediatric Surgeon. Okay, so he was good at dissection, but no one believed that he would really follow through with that goal. Of course, he was the exception. We now send e-mail to him at the Section of Pediatric Surgery.

A Medical Career?

An uncomfortable question needs to be raised before selecting a career path in medicine. That is, do you really want to be a physician? Of course you have already spent a great deal of time pursuing this goal. But is it still what you want? You now know a lot more about medicine and, hopefully, about yourself than when you started this trek toward a medical career. Now is the time to reflect upon whether this choice is still right for you.

An American Medical Association survey yielded disturbing results—*39% of practicing physicians probably or definitely would not go to medical school,* if they had known as much about a career in medicine when entering as they know now. If you also feel that way, now would be an appropriate time to consider jumping ship. Yes, this could deal a large blow to your self-esteem. And you might feel that you have failed the relatives and friends who have been cheering you on. But the bottom line is to do a personal assessment to determine whether your goals and desires will still be met by a medical career.

Medicine's Opportunities

Before you do anything too hastily, however, consider that medicine has more options for its practitioners than any other profession (Figures 2.7, 2.8, and 2.9). Many of those who say that they are not happy in medicine may only be dissatisfied with their specialty. If you choose your specialty wisely, you stand the best chance of being fulfilled by your medical career (Figure 2.1).

Figure 2.1
Essentials of Specialty Selection

1. Keep an open mind about your career direction in medicine. Most students enter medical school with a limited view of the range of exciting career opportunities in medicine, even (or especially) if their parents are physicians.

2. Be open to the many new possibilities and experiences that medical school offers.

3. Know that even the largest medical centers and extensive medical school curricula do not expose students to the entire scope of available medical careers.

4. Aggressively seek new, interesting career opportunities—wherever you find them.

5. Remember what excites you about a medical career.

Choose a specialty that fits your own needs, wants, and interests. Medical students considering which specialty to enter say that they give consideration to: the time they will have for their family and personal life (81%); their professional autonomy within the specialty (53%); potential income (29%); risk of malpractice (29%); and risk of contracting AIDS (10%). In assessing your own needs, consider the presence of a family in your future. You may also realize that given the increase in managed care organizations, professional autonomy is an illusion for many physicians. The debt you owe, however, is real and current.

Don't let your financial burden unduly influence your decision. Don't choose a specialty just for the big bucks. Unfortunately, that is how some of your classmates may decide upon their future direction. But forty or more years of misery in a specialty that does not interest you is not worth it. The happiest physicians are those who enjoy their work. Between 60% and 75% of medical students change their specialty choice during medical school; 20% of residents in training switch to unrelated areas; and 16% of physicians in practice change their specialty identification. Try to figure out which area of medicine you will enjoy for your entire professional life. It will be worth the time you spend doing it.

Figure 2.2
The Process of Choosing a Specialty

Adapted from: *New Physician*. July-August 1986:19.

Specialty Choice

The process of choosing a specialty is complex and involves multiple steps (Figure 2.2). Initially you must assess your own strengths and weaknesses and likes and dislikes. The process has been described as "trying on possible selves" (i.e., projecting oneself into hypothetical career and personal roles). Medical students must make specialty choices that fit with their own personalities, so that they are compatible with other practitioners in the specialty and are able to master the specialty's content and skills. As students go through medical school, they make these choices in three ways:

1. They confirm that a pre-existing specialty choice meets their needs.
2. They select a specialty that includes many of the areas they find interesting.
3. They eliminate specialties as they discover things about themselves and the specialties that are not compatible.

The biggest decision for most students in their specialty selection is whether to enter a surgical or a non-surgical specialty. After looking over the available specialties, make a tentative choice. Then gather enough information, both by reading and through experience, to confirm that you have made the correct selection. With this commitment, you will experience some relief and stability. But making this decision can also lead to anxiety. Such anxiety is a normal part of making a major decision and is termed "post-purchase dissonance." If your anxiety is more severe than this (more than the feeling that you get after you have signed the papers on a new car or an expensive computer system), your career decision should be investigated further—and perhaps changed.

Figure 2.3 lists the significance of factors that students consider when choosing a residency program. Their importance may vary by specialty.

Once you make a career decision, expect to hear negative comments about your chosen specialty as you rotate through clinical clerkships. This behavior is typical of medical practitioners. Physicians, as well as other professionals, often believe that the "holy grail" is whatever professional area they chose, and that everyone else does less important work, works less hard, makes too much money for what they do, or is incompetent. Whether this is a way to bolster their self-esteem or reinforce their career choice, or results from their interactions with other practitioners and their patients is uncertain. However, just as professional baseball pitchers cannot allow themselves to be affected by catcalls from the stands, medical students allow these comments to influence their career decisions only at their own peril.

Jobs—The Ultimate Goal

Completing medical school and residency seems pointless if you cannot ultimately get a position in your specialty. You need to take a realistic look at the specialties. Some fields are already crowded; others, according to the best estimates, soon will be. Over the past decade, some graduates, especially in Anesthesiology, Plastic Surgery, and Pathology, have had trouble finding jobs, although in the current health care market, the situation seems to change annually. In response, many residency programs have reduced the number of training positions.

Those programs that have lost the most positions include Family Medicine, Internal Medicine, Pathology, and Pediatrics. Twice as many residency directors in university-based programs anticipate losing positions as do those in university-affiliated and community-based programs. This will dramatically increase the competition for university-based positions. However, positions have recently been added at many residencies in Anesthesiology, Emergency Medicine, and Radiation Oncology.

Residency directors foresee an increase in job opportunities for residency graduates in Anesthesiology (due to decreasing numbers of graduates to fill the positions opened by retiring anesthesiologists), Family Medicine, Internal Medicine, and Pediatrics. They believe fewer jobs will be available for new Ophthalmologists, Orthopedic Surgeons, Radiologists, and Pathologists.

Despite these predictions, any specialty that you really like, whether or not it is populated by a horde of other physicians, will most likely suit you the best.

So where do all these physicians practice? The U.S. regions with the most physicians per capita are New England (CT, ME, MA, NH, RI, VT) with one physician for every 221 people and the Middle Atlantic (PA, NJ, NY) with one physician for every 254 people. The regions with the fewest physicians per capita are: the East South Central (KY, AL, MS, TN) and the Mountain (AZ, CO, ID, MT, NV, NM, UT, WY) with one physician per 385 and 391 people, respectively, and the West South Central (AR, LA, OK, TX) with only one physician per 415 people.

The states with the highest physician-to-population ratios are listed in Figure 2.4.

Figure 2.3
Factors Important to Students When Selecting a Residency Program

Very Important
- Quality of training program
- Current resident satisfaction
- General impression of the program gained during the interview
- Diversity of training experience
- Geographic location
- Resident quality/makeup
- Faculty/staff quality
- Your personal fit with program/ personalities

Important
- Conference/didactic teaching
- High level of resident responsibility for patients
- Opportunities for post-residency training
- High patient volume
- Program's prestige
- Family considerations

Less Important
- Department and faculty's prestige
- Program director's qualities
- Extent of staff supervision
- Program's flexibility
- Lifestyle factors
- Manageable caseload
- Size of resident staff
- Call schedules
- Elective availability
- Physical plant
- Opportunity to conduct research
- Salary/Benefits
- Cost of living

Not Important
- Management opportunities
- Affiliation with VA hospital
- Availability of support services
- Opportunity to treat AIDS patients
- Absence of AIDS from patient population
- Training only in one hospital

Figure 2.4
States with the Most Physicians per Capita
(Ratio of persons per each physician)

1. District of Columbia	113	6. Connecticut	234
2. Massachusetts	192	7. Rhode Island	236
3. Maryland	212	8. Hawaii	273
4. Vermont	225	9. New Jersey	283
5. New York	229	10. Pennsylvania	285

Adapted from American Medical Association: *Physician Characteristics and Distribution in the U.S., 2010*. Chicago, IL: American Medical Association, 2010, p. 456, Table 6.17.

Medicine's Future

I hope you will have a long career in medicine, during which you will see many changes, not only in the science and art of medicine, but also in health care delivery systems. Your choice of specialty will, in part, determine how well you weather these changes. At present, three important factors appear to be influencing the course of health care delivery: the role of primary care versus specialist physicians, the role of managed care delivery systems, and the number of physicians in each specialty compared to those that are needed to provide adequate care for the population. While these factors are clearly interrelated, I will attempt to provide you with a brief overview of the individual elements.

Primary Care

Before looking at individual specialties, you should know what is meant by the term "primary care"—a hot topic among health planners, politicians, and medical school deans.

Primary care is ideally the point at which patients enter the health treatment system. Primary care practitioners, now also referred to as "Generalists," should be able to diagnose and treat 80% or more of their patients, oversee the activities of any specialists involved in their patient's care, and provide continuity of care. Whether many practitioners actually do all these activities is questionable. It is especially difficult to provide continuity of care, since patients frequently switch their managed care plans (HMOs, PPOs, IPAs, etc.).

What specialties are considered "primary care"? Certainly, the term encompasses General Internal Medicine, Family Medicine, and General Pediatrics. Does it also include Obstetrics and Gynecology, Emergency

Medicine, Psychiatry, Internal Medicine subspecialties, Dermatology, and Neurology? All have been proposed as being "primary care." In some cases their practitioners do exactly what the definition implies—sometimes better than those in the three generalist specialties. But, why all this fuss?

The answer is, for money and survival. You may have noticed that many senior faculty members extol the virtues of primary care. Perhaps this is because national groups and legislators have recently been reviewing medical schools performance. A key measure of a medical school's performance, especially at state-financed schools, is the percentage of their graduates practice medicine in rural or underserved urban environments. The thought is that primary care physicians are more likely to practice in these underserved locales. With more than one-third of U.S. medical schools having an explicit mission to produce primary care physicians, the folks who control the purse strings now carefully review whether they are meeting this goal.

Medical schools have been only marginally successful in promoting primary care specialties. Although the number of graduates planning a career in Family Medicine, General Internal Medicine, Internal Medicine/Pediatrics, or General Pediatrics grew from 14.6% of 1992's graduating class to about 33% in 2012, this number is misleading, since 73% of them say they plan on training in a subspecialty. This is particularly true for those entering Internal Medicine. Even Osteopathic medical school graduates, most of whom entered the primary care specialties in the past, now have less interest in primary care, since opportunities in other specialties have opened up for them.

For several decades, the federal government's regulatory and funding arms have attempted to limit the number of non-primary care residency and fellowship (except Geriatrics) positions. A primary care designation has helped some specialties attract money and residents.

Multiple groups continue to advocate for more primary care residency positions, although it has become clear that there may be enough primary care practitioners—they just are not distributed adequately. About 90% of all primary care physicians practice in metropolitan areas, and about 73% of those who still do patient care are office based. General Practitioners (84%) and Family Practitioners (79%) most commonly have office-based practices; only 67% of Internists are office-based.

Over the past three decades, the number of physicians in primary care increased 110%. Among them, General Internists comprise 38% of all primary care physicians; Family Practitioners, 28%; Obstetrician/Gynecologists, 13%; General Pediatricians, 19%; and General Practitioners, 3%. (General Practitioners are usually physicians who practice general medicine and do not hold Board certification; nearly two-thirds are at least 55-years-old.) The subspecialists in these fields also increased, with the largest increase occurring in Pediatric subspecialties.

States with the highest ratio of primary care physicians to all physicians are Illinois (34%); New Jersey (31%); Michigan (33%); and Texas, California, and Ohio (32% each). Thirty-seven percent of all IMGs practice in primary care, as do 30% of U.S. medical graduates and 24% of Canadian medical graduates practicing in the United States.

Nearly three-fourths (71%) of all U.S. physicians are Board-certified, which is similar to the percentage (67%) of those practicing primary care. The highest percentage of those with primary care Board certification is in Family Medicine (72%), while Board certification among Pediatricians is 74%; Obstetrician/Gynecologists, 78%; and General Internists, 64%. About 88% of primary care subspecialists have their Boards.

Based on current residency trends, the AMA believes that the future non-specialist primary care workforce will include mostly women, IMGs, and D.O.s. Which students choose to enter primary care, especially Family Medicine? The largest percentage are women, who comprise almost half (49%) of primary care residents. The second largest group is IMGs; about 43% of Family Medicine residents now are IMGs (as opposed to about 22% in 1999).

Studies of U.S. medical students suggest that they are strongly influenced by many factors, but perhaps the most important is whether they entered medical school thinking that they would be a Family Physician. Students are more likely to enter Family Medicine if they have a rural background; have low income expectations and little debt; are Hispanic, married, or older; and are not concerned about having control of their work hours. (Additional factors are listed in Figure 2.5.) One study also suggested that students who were less Machiavellian tended to go into primary care. (Heh! Heh! Heh! Were you saying you wanted to subspecialize?)

One warning, however. A recent survey showed that 40% of America's primary care physicians would choose another career if they could start over. According to the researchers, the most dissatisfied primary care physicians had originally entered medicine for the intellectual challenge and stimulation. They are often unhappy due to boredom and infrequent therapeutic success. Those who entered the medicine primarily to "help people" were still satisfied with the choice they had made. They derive most of their satisfaction from social interactions with their patients.

No one really knows how many primary care practitioners we need. However, we don't seem to have enough and, with the aging population, the situation will inevitably get worse. Specialists, rather than primary care physicians, provide most of the care for one in five Americans, with most

Figure 2.5
Reasons Why Students Choose Primary Care/
Non-Primary Care Specialties

Factors important to students when selecting a primary care specialty:
1. Good match with personal interests.
2. Long-term relationship with patients.
3. Broad practice area.
4. Caring for ambulatory patients.
5. Preventive interventions.
6. Diverse patient populations.
7. Enhanced patient interactions.
8. Breadth of clinical activities and content.
9. Influence of role models and mentors.

Factors important when selecting a non-primary care specialty:
1. Good match with personal interests.
2. Lifestyle and quality of life.
3. Higher income.
4. Narrow practice area.
5. Seeing immediate results of interventions.
6. Doing procedures and having technical skills.
7. Caring for critical patients.
8. Intellectual challenge.
9. Pace of practice.
10. Specific setting: ED, OR, ICU.

Adapted from: Garibaldi RA, Popkave C, Bylsma W: Career plans for trainees in internal medicine residency programs. *Acad Med.* 2005;80(5):507-12; and Burack JH, Irby DM, Carline JD, et al.: A study of medical students' specialty-choice pathways: trying on possible selves. *Acad Med.* 1997;72(6):534-41.

of these patients being elderly. Mid-level providers, (e.g., Physician Assistants and Nurse Practitioners) also care for a large number of patients that were once under the care of primary care physicians. Because of these changes, one must wonder if the era of the primary care practitioner may have passed. Yet bureaucrats with little grasp of the big picture will most likely determine the future availability of training positions.

At present, residency graduates intending to practice primary care are doing very well; they report that they get more than fifty recruitment offers during their residency (IMGs get fewer). Their salary expectations are also rising, although whether they will get what they hope for remains to be seen.

Federal Healthcare Mandates & the Managed Care Environment

As this book goes to press, it remains unclear how drastically the Health Care and Education Reconciliation Act of 2010 will affect patient access (the number of healthcare providers needed). It appears, however, that a large number of previously under-insured Americans will have the ability to pay for healthcare services. That may significantly increase the need for physician services.

Over the past decades, managed care organizations have spearheaded the changes in healthcare delivery, and they may play an even bigger role as government attempts to rein in costs. "Managed care" includes a wide variety of organizational structures, from large group practices relying on salaried physicians and their own hospitals to every other imaginable permutation of physicians, insurance companies, and hospitals. What they have in common is that rather than emphasizing quality medical care or the physician-patient relationship (some may still have these), they emphasize cost-effectiveness. With the runaway cost of medical care and the increasing availability of high technology, high-cost diagnostic and treatment modalities, such a change was inevitable. As can be seen in Figure 2.6, physicians now commonly participate in managed care.

A wag once commented that if we treated medicine like agriculture and paid every unneeded licensed physician $100,000 to not practice medicine, we could balance the federal budget. Indeed, the more practicing physicians we have, the more medical tests and procedures are ordered and the more costs increase. Specialists do far more tests and procedures than primary care practitioners; hospitalized patients get the most tests and the most procedures. Managed care organizations, therefore, profit by keeping as many patients as possible away from specialists and hospitals. They have been very successful at doing this in many parts of the country. You can see the effects of this in the many hospitals that have closed or been forced to merge, the specialists who wish to retrain into primary care, the new specialty graduates who cannot get jobs in locales they desire, and the specialty societies that plan to close residency and fellowship programs.

Among the key skills needed to be a successful practitioner within the managed care environment are the ability to diagnose and treat a wide variety of common illnesses, the ability to recognize when you are beyond your depth clinically, an ability and willingness to see many patients quickly, an ability to work with many other physicians and non-physician health care providers, an understanding of how to effectively use information systems (computers), and a willingness to tolerate the unwieldy clinical and financial maze of managed care organizations. These are skills that, for the most part, can and should be learned during medical school and residency. An optimal place to learn such skills is to work within a managed care framework, gaining experience either by dealing with such organizations from the outside or, better yet, by spending some time working in managed care groups. Unfortunately, only 20% of teaching hospitals use such facilities for residency training, and the amount of education in managed care settings varies by specialty.

While managed care is the current buzzword in health care delivery, the caveat when charting your future career is to always plan for the next system— and perhaps for the system after that. For example, the emerging buzz phrase is "quality-based reimbursement." (Of course, the problems are how "quality" is defined and who does the defining.)

The "Right" Number of Physicians

Medicine and medical care delivery systems are changing so fast that no one can predict exactly how many physicians we will need or what will be the optimal balance of specialties over the course of your career—or even for the next ten years. Figure 5.5 provides an educated guess of how many physicians will be in the various specialties in the future. Whether these numbers represent too many or too few physicians is, at present, unclear. Some pessimistic studies suggest that about 40% of all medical specialists could be unnecessary by the end of this decade.

Economic necessity is pushing the health care system to encourage more non-physicians (Nurse Practitioners, Nurse-Anesthetists, Nurse- and lay-midwives, Physician Assistants, Optometrists, Clinical Psychologists, Pharmacists, and others) to practice medicine. In some cases, they are decreasing the need for specialist physicians (Anesthesiologists, Ophthalmologists) while in other cases, such as in the primary care specialties, their numbers have not reduced the need for practitioners.

When considering what specialty to enter, you will hear conflicting opinions about the future need for physicians in various specialties. As the truism goes, "There are liars, damn liars, and statisticians." Worse yet are those who interpret those statistics, often incompletely or incorrectly, to make their points. Take all these prognostications (including those in this book) with a grain of salt.

Your best course of action is to use all the factors you trust to be valid, including estimations of the potential job markets. Next, assess which specialty best fits your needs, your interests, and your personality. Then pursue your specialty choice with all of your determination.

The future will come, no matter what you do. Therefore, your best strategy is to prepare yourself to *enjoy* your medical career.

Figure 2.6
Percentage of Specialty Physicians in Practices
with Managed Care Contracts

Specialty	Any Managed Care Contract	Private	Medicare	Medicaid
Obstetrics/Gynecology	98%	6%	71%	68%
Otolaryngology	98	98	72	73
Cardiology	96	94	85	65
Pediatrics	96	92	20	78
Radiology	96	92	74	72
Anesthesiology	95	92	76	76
General Surgery	93	95	75	71
Family Medicine Practice	91	88	58	61
ALL PHYSICIANS	**91**	**87**	**62**	**62**
Gen Internal Med	90	86	67	58
Dermatology	90	85	57	34
Pathology	86	82	64	59
Emergency Med.	82	72	66	66
Psychiatry	74	67	41	37

Adapted from: American Medical Association. *Physician Socioeconomic Statistics 2000–2002.* Chicago, IL: AMA, 2001. Available information suggests that the data in this figure continues to represent the current situation in 2010.

Figure 2.7
American Board of Medical Specialties (M.D.)-Approved Specialty Boards,
Certifications, and Special Qualification Categories

American Board	Certification	Subspecialty
Allergy & Immunology	Allergy & Immunology	
Anesthesiology	Anesthesiology	Critical Care Medicine Hospice & Palliative Medicine Pain Medicine
Colon & Rectal Surgery	Colon & Rectal Surgery	
Dermatology	Dermatology	Dermatopathology Pediatric Dermatology
Emergency Medicine	Emergency Medicine	Emergency Medical Services Hospice & Palliative Med Medical Toxicology Pediatric Emergency Med Sports Medicine Undersea & Hyperbaric Med
Family Medicine	Family Medicine	Adolescent Medicine Geriatric Medicine Hospice & Palliative Medicine Sleep Medicine Sports Medicine
Internal Medicine	Internal Medicine	Adolescent Medicine Adv Heart Fail & Transp Cardiology Cardiovascular Disease Clin Cardiac Electrophysiology Critical Care Medicine Endocrinology, Diabetes & Metab Gastroenterology Geriatric Medicine Hematology Hospice & Palliative Medicine Infectious Diseases Interventional Cardiology Medical Oncology Nephrology Pulmonary Disease Rheumatology Sleep Medicine Sports Medicine Transplant Hepatology
Medical Genetics	Clin Biochemical Genetics Clin Cytogenetics Clin Molecular Genetics Clin Genetics (M.D. only)	Medical Biochem Genetics Molecular Genetic Pathology

Figure 2.7 (continued)

American Board	Certification	Subspecialty
Neurological Surgery	Neurological Surgery	
Nuclear Medicine	Nuclear Medicine	
Obstetrics & Gynecology	Obstetrics & Gynecology	Critical Care Medicine Gynecologic Oncology Hospice & Palliative Medicine Maternal & Fetal Medicine Reproductive Endocrinology/Infertility
Ophthalmology	Ophthalmology	
Orthopedic Surgery	Orthopedic Surgery	Orthopedic Sports Medicine Surgery of the Hand
Otolaryngology	Otolaryngology	Neurotology Sleep Medicine
Pathology	Anatomic & Clin Pathology Anatomic Pathology Clinical Pathology	Blood Bank/Transfusion Med Chemical Pathology Clinical Informatics Cytopathology Dermatopathology Forensic Pathology Hematology Medical Microbiology Molecular Genetic Pathology Neuropathology Pediatric Pathology
Pediatrics	Pediatrics	Adolescent Medicine Child Abuse Pediatrics Developmental-Behavioral Peds Hospice & Palliative Medicine Medical Toxicology Neonatal-Perinatal Med Neurodevelopmental Disabilities Pediatric Cardiology Pediatric Critical Care Med Pediatric Emergency Med Pediatric Endocrinology Pediatric Gastroenterology Pediatric Hematology-Oncology Pediatric Infectious Diseases Pediatric Nephrology Pediatric Pulmonology Pediatric Rheumatology Pediatric Sports Medicine Pediatric Transplant Hepatology Sleep Medicine

(continued)

Figure 2.7 (continued)

American Board	Certification	Subspecialty
Physical Medicine & Rehabilitation	Physical Medicine & Rehabilitation	Brain Injury Medicine Hospice & Palliative Medicine Neuromuscular Medicine Pain Medicine Pediatric Rehabilitation Med Spinal Cord Injury Med Sports Medicine
Plastic Surgery	Plastic Surgery	Plastic Surgery within the Head & Neck Surgery of the Hand
Preventive Medicine	Aerospace Medicine Occupational Medicine Public Health & General Preventive Med	Medical Toxicology Undersea & Hyperbaric Medicine
Psychiatry & Neurology	Neurology Neurology with Special Qualifications in Child Neurology Psychiatry	Addiction Psychiatry Brain Injury Medicine Child & Adolescent Psychiatry Clinical Neurophysiology Epilepsy Forensic Psychiatry Geriatric Psychiatry Hospice & Palliative Medicine Neurodevelopmental Disabilities Pain Medicine Psychosomatic Medicine Sleep Medicine Vascular Neurology
Radiology	Diagnostic Radiology Radiation Oncology Radiological Physics	Diagnostic Medical Physics Hospice & Palliative Medicine Nuclear Medical Physics Nuclear Radiology Pediatric Radiology Therapeutic Medical Physics Vascular/Interventional Radiology
Surgery	Surgery Vascular Surgery	General Surgical Oncology Hospice & Palliative Medicine Pediatric Surgery Surgery of the Hand Surgical Critical Care
Thoracic Surgery	Thoracic Surgery	Congenital Cardiac Surgery
Urology	Urology	

Information from the American Board of Medical Specialties.

**Figure 2.8
Approved Specialty Boards, Certification, and
Special Qualification Categories (D.O.)#**

American Osteopathic Board	Primary Certification	Certification of Special Qualifications†	Certification of Added Qualifications††
Anesthesiology	Anesthesiology		Critical Care Med Pain Management
Dermatology	Dermatology		Dermatopathology MOHS-Micrographic Surg
Emergency Medicine	Emergency Medicine		Emergency Med Svcs Medical Toxicology* Sports Med
Family Physicians	Family Practice (& Osteopathic Manipulative Treatment)		Adolescent/Young Geriatric Med Hospice & Palliative Med Sleep Med Sports Med Undersea & Hyperbaric Med
Internal Medicine	Internal Medicine	Allergy/Immunology Cardiology Endocrinology Gastroenterology Hematology Infectious Disease Nephrology Oncology Pulmonary Dis Rheumatology	Addiction Med Clin Cardiac Electrophysiology Critical Care Med Geriatric Med Hospice & Palliative Med Interventional Cardiology Sleep Med Sports Med Undersea & Hyperbaric Med
Neurology & Psychiatry	Neurology Psychiatry	Child & Adolescent Child/Adolescent Neurology Psychiatry	Addiction Med Geriatric Psychiatry Hospice & Palliative Med Neurophysiology Sleep Medicine
Neuromusculo-skeletal Medicine	Neuromusculoskeletal Med & Osteopathic Manipulative Medicine		Sports Medicine
Nuclear Medicine			
Obstetrics & Gynecology	Obstetrics & Gynecology	Gynecologic Oncology Maternal/Fetal Med Reproductive Endocrinology	

(continued)

Figure 2.8 (continued)

Ophthalmology & Otolaryngology	Ophthalmology Otolaryngology Otolaryngology/Facial Plastic Surg		Otolaryngic Allergy Sleep Medicine
Orthopedic Surgery	Orthopedic Surgery		Hand Surgery
Pathology	Anatomic Pathology Anatomic Pathology & Lab Med Laboratory Medicine	Forensic Pathology	Blood Banking/ Transfusion Dermatopathology
Pediatrics	Pediatrics	Adolescent/Young Adult Med Neonatology Ped. Allergy/ Immunol Ped Endocrinology	Sports Medicine
Physical Medicine & Rehabilitation	Physical Medicine & Rehabilitation		Hospice & Palliative Med Sports Medicine
Preventive Medicine	Preventive Med/ Aerospace Med Preventive Med/ Occupational- Environmental Med Preventive Med/ Public Health		Occupational Med Undersea & Hyperbaric Med
Proctology	Proctology		
Radiology	Diagnostic Radiology Radiation Oncology		Angiography & Interventional Radiology Diagnostic Ultrasound Nuclear Radiology Pediatric Radiology
Surgery	General Vascular Surg Neurological Surg Plastic & Reconstructive Surg Surgery (General) Thoracic Cardiovascular Surg Urological Surg		Surg Critical Care

Osteopathic training programs do not exist in most approved specialties and subspecialties.

* Also available to diplomates of other AOA Boards.

† (Requires General Certification—Equivalent to "Subspecialty")

†† (Requires General Certification or Certification of Special Qualifications—Equivalent to "Subspecialty")

Adapted from information on the AOA website (www.osteopathic.org), April 2012.

Figure 2.9
M.D. and D.O. Physicians in Practice by Specialty

Specialty	M.D. Physicians*	Osteopathic Physicians**	% Of All Practicing Physicians***
Allergy & Immunology	4,259	122	0.5
Anesthesiology	42,230	2,668	5.3
Cardiovascular Disease	22,723	757	2.8
Colon & Rectal Surgery	1,412	27	0.2
Dermatology	11,034	496	1.4
Emergency Medicine	31,722	3,673	4.2
Family Medicine	85,392	14,945	11.8
Gastroenterology	12,722	440	1.5
General Practice	9,564	2,956	1.5
General Surgery	37,977	1,171	4.6
Internal Medicine, General	160,107	7,061	19.7
Medical Genetics	570	8	0.1
Neurological Surgery	5,508	85	0.7
Neurology	15,212	702	1.9
Nuclear Medicine	1,474	45	0.2
Obstetrics & Gynecology	42,635	2,283	5.3
Ophthalmology	18,217	406	2.2
Orthopedic Surgery	24,822	1,273	3.1
Otolaryngology	9,417	381	1.2
Pathology, Anat/Clin	19,125	451	2.3
Pediatrics, General	75,129	2,805	9.2
Pediatric Cardiology	1,966	21	0.2
Plastic Surgery	7,216	90	0.9
Physical Med & Rehab	8,533	1,197	1.1
Psychiatry	40,904	1,508	5.0
Pulmonary Diseases	10,704	459	1.3
Radiology (All)	34,503	1,206	4.2
Thoracic Surgery	4,622	68	0.6
Urology	10,493	208	1.3
Other Specialties	8,708	333	1.1
Others in Practice	50,347	4,003**	6.4
Total	**851,096**	**41,849**	***

* Adapted from: American Medical Association: *Physician Characteristics and Distribution in the U.S.* Chicago, IL: AMA, 2011, Tables 5.2, 5.3, 5.4, 6.2, 6.3.

** Includes physicians in Osteopathic Manipulative Medicine. Data from AOA.

*** Does not add up to 100% due to rounding.

3

Specialty Descriptions

The specialist learns more and more about less and less until, finally,
he knows everything about nothing; while the generalist learns less and less
about more and more until, finally, he knows nothing about everything.

Donsen's Law

BEFORE YOU JUMP INTO A SPECIALTY DECISION, first look at the wide range of medical specialties that are available. You may be surprised at the diversity within the house of medicine. There are probably many specialties listed here that you have never heard of; there definitely are many that you will have no contact with during medical school. You may have encountered others only peripherally. But they all are options for you. Most of these specialties provide certification—either primarily, such as Pediatrics and Surgery, or as a subspecialty, such as Forensic Pathology and Hematology. Some, such as Acute Care (Trauma) Surgery and Hospitalist, are gradually being accepted as distinct subspecialties by the medical community, but do not yet have subspecialty examinations or certifications.

Nearly three-fourths (73%) of all U.S. physicians hold specialty or subspecialty board certification. Overall, the majority of physicians who do get board certified have done better in medical school and residency than their counterparts who don't. Most physicians must now pass an initial exam to become certified, with future periodic recertifications to assess their clinical performance.

Read these descriptions to open your mind to the scope of available career choices. There is no point in leaping ahead until you know what lies before you.

The ease of acquiring a residency position in each specialty varies, and has changed markedly in recent years. Nearly all specialties have become more difficult to enter: An additional 2,840 U.S. citizens participated in the NRMP Match between 2008 and 2012 (+18%) without a significant increase in postgraduate positions. Nevertheless, the difficulty of obtaining a training position in each specialty can be expressed by assigning each specialty a relative difficulty factor, just as in competitive diving. While it is impossible to give exact numbers, an approximation is possible. Beside each specialty's name in the descriptions below, the difficulty factor is indicated by using a one (*) to five (*****) asterisk scale. *In specialties with one asterisk you should have the*

*least difficulty getting a residency position (or into the field, if there is no residency);
and in those with five asterisks, the most difficulty.* Remember, though, that even
the easiest specialties to enter have some very competitive programs, and even
the most difficult to enter have some less competitive programs. So, only use
the asterisk system as *a general guide, not as an absolute truth.*

Some specialties are entered through the completion of Fellowship
training, which is obtained after first finishing a prerequisite residency. These
specialties are designated by "(F)". The terminology PGY-1, PGY-2, etc. (or,
occasionally, OGME-1, OGME-2, etc., for Osteopaths), equates to the specified
"postgraduate year."

Some specialties have programs that accept new residents other than
in July. The number of programs offering these slots is listed. The specific
programs, as well as those that offer part-time (shared-schedule) positions, can
be found by selecting "optional criteria" in *FREIDA.*

The figures in Chapter 23 contain additional information that may guide
you when making a decision. This includes the prerequisites for training in
the various specialties, the total number of programs in each specialty, and the
approximate number of entry-level positions open each year. Figure 2.9 lists
the total number of physicians currently practicing in each specialty. A visual
description of the length of specialty training for both M.D. and Osteopathic
(D.O.) physicians can be found in Figures 3.1 and 3.2 at the end of this chapter.
Figure 3.3 ranks most specialties and subspecialties by physicians' satisfaction
with their career and gives the hours per week spent doing patient care. Figure
14.6 lists the number of programs in each specialty that have part-time/shared-
schedule positions available.

After you have looked through this chapter, use an evaluation tool
such as the Pathway Evaluation Program (http://medweb.usc.edu/pathways/
intro.htm) or the AAMC's Careers in Medicine (http://services.aamc.org/
careersinmedicine/), as well as the Personal Trait Analysis in Chapter 4, to
compare your likes and dislikes in medical practice to those of practitioners in
most of the major specialties.

For clarification, "ACGME" stands for Accreditation Council for Graduate
Medical Education, the body that approves M.D. residencies. "AOA" in
"AOA-Approved Programs" stands for American Osteopathic Association, the
body that approves D.O. residencies. "NRMP" stands for National Residency
Matching Program, used by most medical students to obtain a residency
position. It is described in detail in Chapter 23. (For M.D.s, "AOA" also stands
for a prestigious medical school honorary society.)

Legend for Specialty Descriptions

*	Entry into a training program is **Very Easy**
**	Entry into a training program is **Easy**
***	Entry into a training program is **Difficult**
****	Entry into a training program is **Very Difficult**
*****	Entry into a training program is **Extremely Difficult**

(F) **Fellowship** training following completion of an initial residency.

(I) **Integrated** program: training at one site for residency and subspecialty following completion of medical school. It often shortens the time needed to complete subspecialty training.

(C) **Categorical**

(P) **Preliminary**

(CR) **Combined Residency**

The Osteopathic listings are only for funded programs and positions.

In the boxes listing the positions for each specialty, the terms mean:

"ACGME-Approved Programs"—Programs approved for M.D.s

"AOA-Approved Programs"—Programs approved for D.O.s

"1st-Yr. Spots"—PGY-1 (Intern) Positions

"Adv. Spots Avail. to M.D. Students"—Positions (PGY-2 or above) with which M.D. students can match

"Funded Entry-Level D.O. Spots"—All funded beginning positions in AOA-approved residency programs. These only accept D.O.s unless they are jointly accredited by both the AOA and ACGME.

"All Entry-Level M.D. Spots"—All beginning positions in ACGME-approved specialty training programs. These spots may also be available to D.O.s, depending upon the program and institution's policies.

"Programs with childcare"—Programs with *on-site* childcare available

"N/A"—no data available

Information in the tables reflects the available data for that specialty from 2012. Some specialties provide only limited data.

Aerospace Medicine ***

Specialty Overview: Aerospace Medicine is a specialty within Preventive Medicine. Practitioners are responsible for the medical care and safety of individuals involved in military and civilian aviation and space travel. This includes crew members and ground personnel. The Federal Aviation Administration, NASA, the military, and the aerospace industry employ most flight surgeons and aviation medical examiners. They are usually engaged in clinical medicine, research and development, or administration. Medical certification of pilots for flight duty often constitutes a large part of their clinical practice, and most physicians in this field are pilots.

Training: Two years of training are required after internship. One of these years must be spent obtaining an advanced degree in a relevant area, usually a master's degree in Public Health. The second residency year devotes more time to clinical Aerospace Medicine. A fourth year of training, teaching, practice, or research is required to take the Board examination. There are two military Aerospace Medicine programs (Brooks Air Force Base, Texas, and Pensacola Naval Air Station, Florida) and two civilian programs (Wright State University, Ohio, and University of Texas at Galveston-NASA).

Match: To be eligible for the military programs, an individual must already be in the military and practicing as a Flight Surgeon.

Aerospace Medicine

ACGME-Approved Programs	4	AOA-Approved Programs	0
Adv. Spots Avail. to M.D. Students	0	All Entry-Level D.O. Spots	0
All Entry-Level M.D. Spots	45		

For more information, contact:

- Aerospace Medical Association, (703) 739-2240; www.asma.org.
- American College of Preventive Medicine, (202) 466-2044; www.acpm.org/residency.htm.
- American Osteopathic College of Occupational and Preventive Medicine, (800) 558-8686; www.aocopm.org.

Allergy And Immunology (F) **

Specialty Overview: Allergy and Immunology is a subspecialty of both Internal Medicine and Pediatrics devoted to the diagnosis and treatment of allergic, asthmatic, and immunologic diseases. There is a great deal of art, as well as science, in the Allergist-Immunologist's practice. The patients they see most frequently have asthma and chronic or seasonal allergies. Practitioners get most of their patients through referrals. There is usually very little emergency or night call. Practice opportunities are more restricted than in the past, due to an increasing number of physicians in other fields who do allergy testing and treatment. Allergist-Immunologists are mainly office-based and are concentrated in metropolitan areas. Research opportunities in this field are growing dramatically because of the increasing recognition of the role of immunologic factors in diseases. Allergist-Immunologists average 53 hours per week doing patient care.

Training: Training is two years after completing either a Pediatric or an Internal Medicine residency. It includes experiences in both pediatric and adult diseases. Fellows are expected to participate in research.

Match: About 60% of Allergy and Immunology programs are in the Specialties Match run by the NRMP, with about 95% of applicants matching. Match results are announced in May.

Allergy and Immunology

ACGME-Approved Programs	73	AOA-Approved Programs	0
1st-Yr. Spots for M.D. Students	0	Funded Entry-Level D.O. Spots	0
Adv. Spots Avail. to M.D. Students	0	% IMG Residents	14
All Entry-Level M.D. Spots	151	Avg. Res. Work Hours/Week	45
% Women Residents	54	Programs with Childcare	32
Avg. Ratio of Full-Time Physician Faculty to Fellows	2.7	Programs offering a "Primary Care Track"	1
% Training in Hospital Outpatient Clinics	55	Programs offering Multiple Start Dates	8
% Training in Non-Hospital Community Ambulatory Clinics	13	Programs allowing Moonlighting	49

For more information, contact:

- American Academy of Allergy, Asthma, & Immunology, (414) 272-6071; www.aaaai.org.
- American Association of Immunologists, (301) 530-7178; www.aai.org.
- American College of Allergy, Asthma, & Immunology, (847) 427-1200; www.acaai.org.
- American Osteopathic College of Allergy and Immunology, 16128 E. Kingstree Blvd., Fountain Hills, AZ 95268; (480) 585-1580.

Anesthesiology ****

Specialty Overview: Anesthesiologists give general and regional anesthesia during surgical, obstetric, diagnostic, and therapeutic procedures; function as Critical Care physicians; and give anesthetic blocks in conjunction with pain clinics. Surgical anesthesia is often described as "59 minutes of boredom and 1 minute of terror," to illustrate the drama that can occur at any point in a case. Anesthesiologists often specialize in Pediatric, Neurosurgical, Obstetric, Cardiothoracic, or Ambulatory Anesthesia, although Critical Care (*see* Critical Care), Hospice and Palliative Medicine, and Pain Medicine (*see* Pain Medicine) are the only formal subspecialties. Anesthesiology remains primarily a hospital-based specialty with frequent night call for most practitioners, although the rapid expansion of outpatient surgery has changed this a little. Research continues to push the practice of Anesthesiology into an ever more elegant and scientific realm. The growing use of less-expensive Nurse-Anesthetists and a declining number of surgeries has decreased the need for Anesthesiologists, although the number of Anesthesiologists has increased by about one-third in the past decade. Over the past decades, Anesthesiology's popularity as a specialty selection has varied tremendously. At present, it is again very popular. Anesthesiologists average 45 hours per week doing patient care.

Training: Training consists of a "base" year, essentially a Transitional, Preliminary, or Categorical internship in a clinical specialty, followed by three years of training in Clinical Anesthesiology. Residency programs in Anesthesiology start at either the first (PGY-1) or the second (PGY-2) postgraduate year. The training is essentially the same for Osteopathic physicians. Training in the subspecialties of Adult Cardiothoracic Anesthesiology (128 positions), Anesthesia Critical Care Medicine (91 positions) or Pediatric Anesthesiology (173 positions) takes a minimum of one year after completing an Anesthesiology residency. (In 2007, all ACGME-accredited Pain Medicine programs under Anesthesiology, Neurology, Physical Medicine & Rehabilitation, and Psychiatry were combined into a multidisciplinary Pain Medicine subspecialty.)

Match: In recent years, about 97% of the available PGY-1 positions filled through the NRMP Match. Of the PGY-2 positions available through the NRMP Match, about 95% filled in the Match. Some PGY-4 positions are available in specialty areas (Pediatric, Neurosurgical, etc.) and can be applied for separately from normal Anesthesiology programs.

Other Useful Information: Anesthesiology residencies tend to look both for good performance in preclinical Physiology and Pharmacology courses and for how well students have done in their Internal Medicine and Anesthesiology clerkships. Those going into the field are detail-oriented, dislike long-term patient relationships, and can remain calm in the face of clinical schedules over which they often have little control. Since working with a team is vital, great importance is given to the applicant's interview.

Anesthesiology

ACGME-Approved Programs	191	AOA-Approved Programs	11
1st-Yr. Spots for M.D. Students	919	Funded Entry-Level D.O. Spots	26
Adv. Spots Avail. to M.D. Students	577	% IMG Residents	15
All Entry-Level M.D. Spots	1,476	Avg. Res. Work Hours/Week	61
% Women Residents	36	Programs with Childcare	49
Avg. Ratio of Full-Time Physician Faculty to Residents/Fellows	1.3	Programs offering a "Primary Care Track"	1
% Training in Hospital Outpatient Clinics	12	Programs offering Multiple Start Dates	39
% Training in Non-Hospital Community Ambulatory Clinics	5	Programs allowing Moonlighting	67

For more information, contact:

- American Academy of Pain Medicine, (847) 375-4731; www.painmed.org.
- American Osteopathic College of Anesthesiologists, (517) 339-0919; www.aocaonline.org.
- American Society of Anesthesiologists, (847) 825-5586; www.asahq.org.

Cardiology (F) **

Specialty Overview: Cardiologists (the specialty is officially known as "Cardiovascular Disease") primarily deal with adult patients who have diseases of the heart and circulatory system. They are involved in both the diagnosis and the medical treatment of these diseases. The core of the specialty is the medical history and physical diagnosis augmented by the latest medical technology and medications. Cardiologists are divided by the nature of their practices into invasive and non-invasive specialists. Invasive Cardiologists perform angiography (catheters in arteries) to visualize and treat vascular obstructions, primarily of the coronary arteries. This is an evolving, expanding, and quite lucrative area of the specialty. Cardiologists are generally office-based, but spend about one-third of their professional time in hospitals. This frequently includes long hours and significant night call.

There is a projected deficit of, in particular, general and interventional cardiologists by 2025 due to, in part, an aging population, rising obesity and type 2 diabetes, and an increase in heart disease with a decrease in cardiovascular mortality. About 30% of cardiologists are IMGs, while only 12% of general cardiologists and less than 10% of interventional cardiologists are women. (Pediatric cardiology is the exception, with 30%.) Cardiologists average 47 hours per week doing patient care.

Training: Training is currently a three-year fellowship following completion of an Internal Medicine or a Pediatric residency. One year (or in a few 4-year programs, two years) is devoted to research. Specialty certification in Cardiology is time-limited, and requires periodic recertification. An additional year of training is necessary for certification in Cardiac Electrophysiology or Interventional Cardiology. Post-fellowship training is also available in Nuclear Cardiology. For Osteopathic physicians, training follows internship and two years of Internal Medicine residency.

Match: About 95% of ACGME-approved programs and positions in adult Cardiovascular Disease are available through the NRMP Medical Specialties Match Program and 94% in Pediatric Cardiology are available through the NRMP Pediatric Specialties Spring Match. Match results are announced in June, one year before the applicant starts specialty training. About 99% of available Adult Cardiology positions filled in the Match, as did 84% of those in Pediatric Cardiology.

Cardiology (Internal Medicine)**

ACGME-Approved Programs	181	AOA-Approved Programs	15
1st-Yr. Spots for M.D. Students	0	Funded Entry-Level D.O. Spots	65
Adv. Spots Avail. to M.D. Students	0	% IMG Residents	39
All Entry-Level M.D. Spots	2,465	Avg. Res. Work Hours/Week	54
% Women Residents	20	% Training in Hospital Outpatient Clinics	15
Avg. Ratio of Full-Time Physician Faculty to Fellows	1.7	% Training in Non-Hospital Community Ambulatory Clinics	11

Pediatric Cardiology***

ACGME-Approved Programs	50	AOA-Approved Programs	0
1st-Yr. Spots for M.D. Students	0	Funded Entry-Level D.O. Spots	0
Adv. Spots Avail. to M.D. Students	0	% IMG Residents	27
All Entry-Level M.D. Spots	362	Avg. Res. Work Hours/Week	57
% Women Residents	40	% Training in Non-Hospital Community Ambulatory Clinics	9
Avg. Ratio of Full-Time Physician Faculty to Fellows	1.7		
% Training in Hospital Outpatient Clinics	16		

For more information, contact:

- American College of Cardiology, (202) 375-6000; www.cardiosource.org.
- American College of Osteopathic Internists, (301) 656-8877; www.acoi.org.
- American Academy of Pediatrics, (847) 434-4000; www.aap.org.

Child And Adolescent Psychiatry (F) ***

Specialty Overview: Child and Adolescent Psychiatrists diagnose and treat mental, emotional, and behavioral disorders in children, adolescents, and their families. Child Psychiatrists work in concert with Pediatricians, courts, schools, and social service agencies. Averaging 35 hours per week doing patient care, they often have both inpatient and outpatient practices, frequently working as part of a multidisciplinary team. The shortage of Child and Adolescent Psychiatrists has reached crisis levels: in 2009 there were fewer than 7,500 practitioners in the United States to serve a population of almost 74 million children and adolescents, about 20% of whom have a mental disorder with some functional impairment.

Training: Fellowships for both M.D.s and D.O.s consist of two years of Child and Adolescent Psychiatry in addition to at least two years (following internship) of General Psychiatry. Child and Adolescent Psychiatry training can start any time after the internship year, but generally begins after the PGY-2 year in Psychiatry. There are also nine programs with five years of training combining Pediatrics, Psychiatry, and Child and Adolescent Psychiatry. These programs consist of two years of Pediatrics, one-and-a-half years of adult Psychiatry, and one-and-a-half years of Child and Adolescent Psychiatry, making trainees eligible for Board certification in all three specialties. For information about this training, see the list at www.aacap.org/training/tbtpd.htm and contact the individual programs. Combined programs are more difficult to match with than programs in either Pediatrics or Psychiatry.

Match: About 88% of ACGME-approved programs and positions in Child and Adolescent Psychiatry are available through the NRMP Medical Specialties Match. Match results are announced the January before the applicant starts specialty training. In recent years, about 91% of applicants found positions through the Match. About 85% of available positions fill in the Match. There were 17 positions combining Pediatrics, Psychiatry, and Child and Adolescent Psychiatry available to medical students through the NRMP PGY-1 Match.

Child and Adolescent Psychiatry

ACGME-Approved Programs	124	AOA-Approved Programs	1
1st-Yr. Spots for M.D. Students	0	Funded Entry-Level D.O. Spots	1
Adv. Spots Avail. to M.D. Students	0	% IMG Residents	29
All Entry-Level M.D. Spots	452	Avg. Res. Work Hours/Week	44
% Women Residents	57	% Training in Non-Hospital	18
Avg. Ratio of Full-Time Physician Faculty to Fellows	1.8	Community Ambulatory Clinics	
% Training in Hospital Outpatient Clinics	32		

For more information, contact:

- American Academy of Child & Adolescent Psychiatry, (202) 966-7300; www.aacap.org.
- American College of Osteopathic Neurologists and Psychiatrists, 28595 Orchard Lake Rd., Ste. 200, Farmington Hills, MI 48334; (248) 553-0010, ext. 295.

Child Neurology *

Specialty Overview: Child Neurologists diagnose and manage neurological disorders of the infant, child, and adolescent. They treat diseases of the brain, spinal cord, and neuromuscular system. Many such problems are congenital or developmental in nature. Practitioners, most often based at academic medical centers, usually see patients in consultation for primary care physicians. The profession is not heavily based on procedures, but performing and interpreting EEGs is common. Child Neurologists average 40 hours per week doing patient care.

Training: Before entering a Child Neurology program, applicants must have completed either: (1) at least two years of an approved Pediatric residency, (2) a PGY-1 year acceptable for Neurology training (broad-based clinical experience, primarily in Internal Medicine) and a year of Pediatrics, or (3) a year of Pediatrics and a year of basic neuroscience training. Training in Child Neurology is an additional three years: one year in clinical adult Neurology and one year in clinical Child Neurology. The third year is devoted to studying Electrodiagnostic Neurology, Neuropathology, Neuroradiology, Neuro-Ophthalmology, Child & Adolescent Psychiatry, and the basic neurosciences. Trainees are eligible to take the American Board of Pediatrics examination after their second year of Child Neurology training.

Match: Child Neurology joined the NRMP Match in 2012. They offered PGY-1 and PGY-2 positions. There is a non-refundable $100 registration fee. The Match is for PGY-3 positions and occurs in January, before the NRMP Match. Applicants must register with both the NRMP and the CNMP, even if they will be entering an "integrated" program that arranges the first two years of training. Open positions are often available and can be accessed through the CNMP website.

Child Neurology

ACGME-Approved Programs	71	AOA-Approved Programs	0
1st-Yr. Spots for M.D. Students	99	Funded Entry-Level D.O. Spots	0
Adv. Spots Avail. to M.D. Students	47	% IMG Residents	34
All Entry-Level M.D. Spots	146	Avg. Res. Work Hours/Week	58
% Women Residents	62	% Training in Non-Hospital Community Ambulatory Clinics	12
Avg. Ratio of Full-Time Physician Faculty to Fellows	7.0		
% Training in Hospital Outpatient Clinics	29		

For more information, contact:

- American Academy of Neurology, (651) 695-2717; www.aan.com.
- American College of Osteopathic Neurologists and Psychiatrists, 28595 Orchard Lake Rd., Ste. 200, Farmington Hills, MI 48334; (248) 553-0010, ext. 295.
- The Child Neurology Society, (651) 486-9447; www.childneurologysociety.org.

Colon And Rectal Surgery (F) ***

Specialty Overview: Colon and Rectal Surgeons diagnose and treat disorders of the intestinal tract, rectum, anal canal, and perianal areas that are amenable to surgical treatment. They are involved not only in operative treatment but also in diagnostic procedures, including colonoscopy. Most practitioners in this specialty are located in medium to large cities and get the majority of their patients by referral from other physicians. Colon and Rectal Surgeons average 54 hours per week doing patient care. A small specialty, the field grew by 42% between 1990 and 2005, while graduate trainee numbers rose 35% and the number of DOs who are colorectal surgeons grew 100% between 2004 and 2008.

Training: The training consists of a complete residency in General Surgery followed by a one-year fellowship in Colon and Rectal Surgery. While there are no Osteopathic training programs in this specialty, they have the more limited specialty of Proctology, consisting of two years of training after internship.

Match: Nearly all positions are listed in the NRMP Specialties Match. Results of the Match for positions beginning in July are released in November of the prior year. In recent years, 67% of applicants matched and 97% of available positions filled in the Match.

Colon and Rectal Surgery

ACGME-Approved Programs	49	AOA-Approved Programs	0
1st-Yr. Spots for M.D. Students	0	Funded Entry-Level D.O. Spots	0
Adv. Spots Avail. to M.D. Students	0	% IMG Residents	27
All Entry-Level M.D. Spots	84	Avg. Res. Work Hours/Week	52
% Women Residents	35	Programs with Childcare	12
Avg. Ratio of Full-Time Physician Faculty to Fellows	1.6	Programs offering a "Primary Care Track"	2
% Training in Hospital Outpatient Clinics	27	Programs offering Multiple Start Dates	1
% Training in Non-Hospital Community Ambulatory Clinics	23	Programs allowing Moonlighting	5

Proctology (Osteopathic only)

AOA-Approved Programs	1	All entry-level D.O. Spots	2

For more information, contact:

- American Osteopathic College of Proctology, (765) 342-3686; www.aocpr.org.
- American Society of Colon & Rectal Surgeons, (847) 290-9184; www.fascrs.org.

Complementary And Alternative Medicine *

Specialty Overview: Complementary and Alternative Medicine (CAM), also known as Integrative or Holistic Medicine, uses medical therapies not generally considered part of conventional Western medicine. These often include mind-body medicine (acupuncture, yoga, meditation, hypnotherapy, music therapy, aromatherapy, therapeutic touch), manipulative and body-based practices (spinal manipulation, massage, reflexology), "natural product treatments" (herbs, vitamins, homeopathy), movement therapies, energy (magnet and light therapy), and traditional medical practices. Practitioners can use these methods alone, but often combine them with standard therapies. About 40% of Americans may use CAM each year, and there is increasing pressure on insurance companies to pay for this therapy.

While complementary and conventional therapies are often used simultaneously to reduce side effects and to increase well-being, alternative therapies are employed in place of conventional medicine to cure disease. Many physicians who are CAM practitioners have not completed extensive training in these areas. As insurance companies begin paying for more CAM procedures, this will change.

Training: Most Family Medicine programs and about half of all Internal Medicine Programs offer some training in CAM. However, most of this training consists only of a single rotation, an elective, or a short survey course. Some programs in other specialties offer similar experiences. Relatively few residencies offer fully integrated CAM training. While fellowships exist, both in general CAM and in specialized areas, most are within Family Medicine and Internal Medicine departments.

Match: Students can match into residencies with CAM training. The American Medical Students Association (AMSA) website maintains the ICAM (Integrative, Complementary and Alternative Medicine) Resource Center, which includes a list of university Integrative Medicine centers and a database of CAM courses, electives, internships, and programs searchable by institution or type of program. Also, the Consortium of Academic Health Centers for Integrative Medicine website features a list of clinically-oriented training opportunities at its 44 participating U.S. and Canadian medical centers. Once such programs are identified, go to their website or contact them to ascertain whether the amount of CAM training they offer meets your needs. Fellowships must be contacted individually.

Other Useful Information: This area is being driven by public demand. With its own research funding institute at NIH and the likelihood of widespread insurance payments for such therapy, this specialty will certainly grow over the coming decade.

For more information, contact:

- AMSA, Humanistic Medicine committee; http://www.amsa.org/AMSA/Homepage/About/Committees/HumanisticMedicine.aspx.
- Consortium of Academic Health Centers for Integrative Medicine, (612) 624-9166; http://www.imconsortium.org.
- National Center for Complementary and Alternative Medicine, National Institutes of Health, http://nccam.nih.gov/training/opportunities/.

Critical Care (F) ***

Specialty Overview: Critical Care physicians work in hospital intensive care units managing the overall care of critically ill medical and surgical patients. The practice requires both a broad knowledge of serious medical and surgical conditions and a specialized knowledge of respiratory, fluid, and cardiovascular management. Many Critical Care physicians alternate their duties in the critical care unit with practice in their primary specialty. The majority of Critical Care physicians in adult units are Internists, most commonly specialists in Pulmonary Diseases. Night call for or night duty in the intensive care unit is common. Most individuals in this specialty are located in large cities. Critical Care physicians average 66 hours (Anesthesia), 64 hours (Surgeons), 51 hours (Pediatricians), or 48 hours (Internists) per week doing patient care.

　　Training: At present, positions leading to certificates of special competence are offered in Critical Care from the American Boards of Internal Medicine (1 to 3 years after residency), Anesthesiology (1 year), and Surgery (1 year). Pediatrics offers Critical Care as a subspecialty (3 years after residency). Other Boards may offer a similar certification in the future. Internal Medicine offers two routes to certification: either a one-year fellowship following completion of subspecialty training, or a two-year fellowship following residency. A common program design is to incorporate Critical Care into a three-year Pulmonary Diseases fellowship, leading to dual subspecialty certification (see *Pulmonary Diseases*).

　　Match: Virtually all adult Critical Care programs combined with Pulmonary Disease training (Internal Medicine), those in Pediatric Critical Care, and those in Surgical Critical Care are in the NRMP Fellowship Match. For other Critical Care training, contact the individual programs, which are listed in *FREIDA*.

Adult Critical Care (Anesthesiology)

ACGME-Approved Programs	46	AOA-Approved Programs	0
1st-Yr. Spots for M.D. Students	0	Funded Entry-Level D.O. Spots	0
Adv. Spots Avail. to M.D. Students	0	% IMG Residents	24
All Entry-Level M.D. Spots	91	Avg. Res. Work Hours/Week	60
% Women Residents	29	% Training in Non-Hospital Community Ambulatory Clinics	10
Avg. Ratio of Full-Time Physician Faculty to Fellows	8.5		
% Training in Hospital Outpatient Clinics	43		

Adult Critical Care (Internal Medicine)

ACGME-Approved Programs	33	AOA-Approved Programs	3
1st-Yr. Spots for M.D. Students	0	Funded Entry-Level D.O. Spots	5
Adv. Spots Avail. to M.D. Students	0	% IMG Residents	61
All Entry-Level M.D. Spots	179	Avg. Res. Work Hours/Week	55
% Women Residents	19	% Training in Non-Hospital Community Ambulatory Clinics	10
Avg. Ratio of Full-Time Physician Faculty to Fellows	6.2		
% Training in Hospital Outpatient Clinics	10		

Adult Pulmonary Disease/Critical Care (Internal Medicine)

ACGME-Approved Programs	97	AOA-Approved Programs	4
1st-Yr. Spots for M.D. Students	0	Funded Entry-Level D.O. Spots	10
Adv. Spots Avail. to M.D. Students	0	% IMG Residents	49
All Entry-Level M.D. Spots	344	Avg. Res. Work Hours/Week	54
% Women Residents	27	% Training in Non-Hospital Community Ambulatory Clinics	7
Avg. Ratio of Full-Time Physician Faculty to Fellows	1.8		
% Training in Hospital Outpatient Clinics	17		

Adult Critical Care (Surgery)****

ACGME-Approved Programs	97	AOA-Approved Programs	1
1st-Yr. Spots for M.D. Students	0	Funded Entry-Level D.O. Spots	1
Adv. Spots Avail. to M.D. Students	0	% IMG Residents	13
All Entry-Level M.D. Spots	196	Avg. Res. Work Hours/Week	61
% Women Residents	27	% Training in Non-Hospital Community Ambulatory Clinics	30
Avg. Ratio of Full-Time Physician Faculty to Fellows	7.8		
% Training in Hospital Outpatient Clinics	23		

Pediatric Critical Care*

ACGME-Approved Programs	60	AOA-Approved Programs	0
1st-Yr. Spots for M.D. Students	0	Funded Entry-Level D.O. Spots	0
Adv. Spots Avail. to M.D. Students	0	% IMG Residents	28
All Entry-Level M.D. Spots	119	Avg. Res. Work Hours/Week	65
% Women Residents	46	% Training in Non-Hospital	0
Avg. Ratio of Full-Time Physician Faculty to Fellows	2.8	Community Ambulatory Clinics	
% Training in Hospital Outpatient Clinics	5		

For more information, contact:

- American College of Osteopathic Internists, (301) 656-8877; www.acoi.org.
- Society of Critical Care Medicine, (847) 827-6869; www.sccm.org.

Dermatology *****

Specialty Overview: Dermatologists deal with patients who have both acute and chronic skin disorders. They diagnose skin lesions and use both chemotherapy and surgery to affect cures. Dermatologists get referrals from other physicians and see patients who refer themselves. There is little night call and very rarely an inpatient service associated with a Dermatology practice. While still the smallest surgical specialty, Dermatologic Surgeons increased by 118% and residents by 39% in recent years. The number of women in training and practice has increased by 66% and 190%, respectively. Dermatologists average 33 hours per week doing patient care.

Following Dermatology training, fellowships are available in Procedural Dermatology, Mohs Micrographic Surgery, and Dermatopathology. Mohs Micrographic Surgery treats skin cancers, with the physician acting as surgeon, pathologist and reconstructive surgeon. Dermatopathology is a subspecialty of both Pathology and Dermatology. Emphasis is placed on the diagnosis of skin disorders using appropriate microscopic techniques including light and electron microscopy, immunopathology, histochemistry, and aspects of cutaneous mycology, bacteriology, and entomology. Dermatopathologists average 52 hours per week doing patient care.

Training: Dermatology residencies are three years following initial training. There are 23 PGY-1 positions in four-year programs. Dermatopathology training consists of a one-year fellowship. It is designed for either a research or a clinical practice. At least six months of the training must be in either clinical Dermatology for those trained in Pathology, or Anatomic Pathology for those trained in Dermatology.

Match: Nearly all positions that begin at the PGY-2 level are available to medical students through the NRMP Advanced Match. Most applicants must arrange their own internship. Several programs require the prior completion of a residency in another specialty. Entrance to the specialty is very competitive. In recent years, 99% of the positions offered through the NRMP Match filled.

Dermatology

ACGME-Approved Programs	115	AOA-Approved Programs	18
1st-Yr. Spots for M.D. Students	23	Funded Entry-Level D.O. Spots	21
Adv. Spots Avail. to M.D. Students	340	% IMG Residents	4
All Entry-Level M.D. Spots	363	Avg. Res. Work Hours/Week	45
% Women Residents	62	Programs with Childcare	35
Avg. Ratio of Full-Time Physician Faculty to Residents	1.3	Programs offering a "Primary Care Track"	3
% Training in Hospital Outpatient Clinics	79	Programs offering Multiple Start Dates	10
% Training in Non-Hospital Community Ambulatory Clinics	17	Programs allowing Moonlighting	47

Dermatopathology (F)

ACGME-Approved Programs	54	AOA-Approved Programs	0
1st-Yr. Spots for M.D. Students	0	Funded Entry-Level D.O. Spots	0
Adv. Spots Avail. to M.D. Students	0	% IMG Residents	16
All Entry-Level M.D. Spots	91	Avg. Res. Work Hours/Week	40
% Women Residents	45	% Training in Non-Hospital Community Ambulatory Clinics	30
Avg. Ratio of Full-Time Physician Faculty to Fellows	9.3		
% Training in Hospital Outpatient Clinics	43		

For more information, contact:

- American Academy of Dermatology, (866) 503-7546; www.aad.org.
- American Osteopathic College of Dermatology, (800) 449-2623; www.aocd.org.
- American Society for Dermatologic Surgery, (847) 956-0900; www.asds-net.
- American Society of Dermatology, (561) 873-8335; www.asd.org/.

Emergency Medicine ****

Specialty Overview: Emergency Physicians are mainly hospital-based and deal with the entire spectrum of acute illness and injury in all age groups. Hands-on physical diagnosis and the use of both medical and surgical therapeutic modalities are an integral part of the specialty. Emergency Physicians are trained to stabilize patients with acute injuries and deal with life-threatening conditions. They now also handle a quarter of the nation's acute care patient visits and increasingly care for large numbers of patients who need hospital admission but for whom no inpatient bed is available. Hours are long, but schedules are fixed in advance. There is rarely a call schedule outside of assigned working hours in this specialty. Most practitioners in the specialty work in medium to large cities. Many new Emergency Medicine opportunities are available at academic centers and in research. All sources agree that there will still be a shortage of Emergency Physicians in the year 2025, since the number of emergency department visits continues to climb dramatically as people have less access to primary care physicians. Less than 1% of Emergency Physicians leave the field each year. Emergency Physicians average 29 hours per week doing patient care. In the last 15 years, there was an 87% increase in the number of Emergency Physicians.

Training: Training is three to four years in length. Programs also exist combining Emergency Medicine with Internal Medicine, Pediatrics, or Family Medicine. These programs are five years long and lead to dual certification. Osteopathic physicians have the option of combining Emergency Medicine with training in Family Medicine.

Fellowships following residency leading to subspecialty certification are offered in Medical Toxicology (25 programs), Pediatric Emergency Medicine (through both Emergency Medicine [19 programs] and Pediatrics [46 programs]), Sports Medicine (5 programs), and Emergency Medical Service Administration. Some Critical Care programs accept Emergency Medicine residency graduates. Fellowships are also available in Research, Hospice & Palliative Medicine, Undersea & Hyperbaric Medicine, Medical Education, Medical Information Services, and International Medicine.

Match: Most programs begin in the first year and are available through the NRMP PGY-1 Match. Those that begin at the PGY-2 level require at least one year of prior training in a Transitional internship or an Internal Medicine, Surgery, or Family Medicine residency, and are available through the NRMP Advanced Match. Students can also enter the five-year combined programs in Emergency Medicine–Internal Medicine and Emergency Medicine–Pediatrics.

Nearly all fellowship positions in Pediatric Emergency Medicine are available through the NRMP Fellowship Match. In recent years, of those positions available through the Fellowship Match, 74% filled and 79% of applicants obtained positions. Match day is in December, the year before the fellowship begins.

Other Useful Information: Residency programs look for high USMLE scores, research experience, election to AOA (honorary), and outstanding performance on Emergency Medicine clerkships. In recent years, 99% of the available PGY-1 positions filled through the NRMP Match. Of the PGY-2 positions available through the NRMP Match, 100% filled in the Match.

Emergency Medicine****

ACGME-Approved Programs	153	AOA-Approved Programs	36
1st-Yr. Spots for M.D. Students	1,668	Funded Entry-Level D.O. Spots	210
Adv. Spots Avail. to M.D. Students	19	% IMG Residents	8
All Entry-Level M.D. Spots	1,668	Avg. Res. Work Hours/Week	55
% Women Residents	39	Programs offering a "Primary Care Track"	8
Avg. Ratio of Full-Time Physician Faculty to Residents/Fellows	0.9		
% Training in Hospital Outpatient Clinics	13	Programs offering Multiple Start Dates	14
		Programs with Childcare	47
% Training in Non-Hospital Community Ambulatory Clinics	6	Programs allowing Moonlighting	87

Emergency Medicine–Pediatrics (CR)**

ACGME-Approved Programs	3	AOA-Approved Programs	1
1st-Yr. Spots for M.D. Students	7	Funded Entry-Level D.O. Spots	0
Adv. Spots Avail. to M.D. Students	0	% IMG Residents	0
All Entry-Level M.D. Spots	7	Avg. Res. Work Hours/Week	66
% Women Residents	58	% Training in Non-Hospital Community Ambulatory Clinics	2
Avg. Ratio of Full-Time Physician Faculty to Residents	15.5		
% Training in Hospital Outpatient Clinics	18		

Emergency Medicine–Internal Medicine (CR)**

ACGME-Approved Programs	11	AOA-Approved Programs	13
1st-Yr. Spots for M.D. Students	26	Funded Entry-Level D.O. Spots	23
Adv. Spots Avail. to M.D. Students	0	% IMG Residents	7
All Entry-Level M.D. Spots	26	Avg. Res. Work Hours/Week	59
% Women Residents	33	% Training in Non-Hospital Community Ambulatory Clinics	2
Avg. Ratio of Full-Time Physician Faculty to Residents	10.7	Programs with Childcare	4
% Training in Hospital Outpatient Clinics	22		

Pediatric Emergency Medicine (F) *****

ACGME-Approved Programs	48	AOA-Approved Programs	0
1st-Yr. Spots for M.D. Students	0	Funded Entry-Level D.O. Spots	0
Adv. Spots Avail. to M.D. Students	0	% IMG Residents	14
All Entry-Level M.D. Spots	99	Avg. Res. Work Hours/Week	42
% Women Residents	60	% Training in Non-Hospital Community Ambulatory Clinics	6
Avg. Ratio of Full-Time Physician Faculty to Fellows	3.3		
% Training in Hospital Outpatient Clinics	35		

Emergency Medicine–Family Medicine

ACGME-Approved Programs	2	AOA-Approved Programs	9
1st-Yr. Spots for M.D. Students	4	Funded Entry-Level D.O. Spots	8

For more information, contact:

- American Academy of Emergency Medicine, (800) 884-2236; www.aaem.org/.
- American Academy of Emergency Medicine Resident and Student Association; www.aaemrsa.org/.
- American College of Emergency Physicians, (800) 798-1822; www.acep.org.
- American College of Osteopathic Emergency Physicians, (800) 521-3709; www.acoep.org.
- Emergency Medicine Residents Association, (866) 566-2942; www.emra.org.
- Society for Academic Emergency Medicine, (847) 813-9823; www.saem.org.

Endocrinology, Diabetes And Metabolism (F) *

Specialty Overview: Endocrinologists treat patients with diseases of the endocrine (glandular) system and with a wide variety of hormonal abnormalities. The most common endocrine diseases include diabetes mellitus, obesity, high lipid (blood fats or cholesterol) levels, and thyroid disorders. Patients are often referred to Endocrinologists for failure to grow, early or late puberty, excess hair growth, metabolic syndrome, high calcium levels, osteoporosis, pituitary tumors, or reproductive problems. Endocrinologists also consult in the rapidly growing area of Nutrition & Metabolism. This includes helping provide postoperative and chronic-disease patients with nutritional support. Many Endocrinologists also participate in clinical or basic-science research. Given the epidemic levels of obesity and an aging population, the number of endocrinologists will continue to be inadequate in the foreseeable future. At present, for example, the ratio of obese children to Pediatric Endocrinologists is about 17,000 to one. Endocrinologists average 45 hours per week (Internists) and 35 hours per week (Pediatricians) doing patient care.

Training: Training is two years following an Internal Medicine residency or three years following a Pediatric residency. For Osteopathic physicians, training follows internship and two years of Internal Medicine residency.

Match: About 93% of programs participate in the NRMP Medical Specialties Matching Program, and in recent years, about 92% of the positions filled.

Endocrinology, Diabetes and Metabolism (Internal Medicine)

ACGME-Approved Programs	125	AOA-Approved Programs	1
1st-Yr. Spots for M.D. Students	0	Funded Entry-Level D.O. Spots	1
Adv. Spots Avail. to M.D. Students	0	% IMG Residents	40
All Entry-Level M.D. Spots	607	Avg. Res. Work Hours/Week	46
% Women Residents	66	% Training in Non-Hospital Community Ambulatory Clinics	14
Avg. Ratio of Full-Time Physician Faculty to Fellows	2.5		
% Training in Hospital Outpatient Clinics	51		

Pediatric Endocrinology

ACGME-Approved Programs	67	AOA-Approved Programs	0
1st-Yr. Spots for M.D. Students	0	Funded Entry-Level D.O. Spots	0
Adv. Spots Avail. to M.D. Students	0	% IMG Residents	38
All Entry-Level M.D. Spots	99	Avg. Res. Work Hours/Week	45
% Women Residents	81	% Training in Non-Hospital Community Ambulatory Clinics	18
Avg. Ratio of Full-Time Physician Faculty to Fellows	2.3		
% Training in Hospital Outpatient Clinics	52		

For more information, contact:

- American College of Osteopathic Internists, (301) 656-8877; www.acoi.org.
- Endocrine Society, (301) 941-0200; www.endo-society.org.
- American Academy of Pediatrics, (847) 434-4000; www.aap.org.

Family Medicine *

Specialty Overview: Family Physicians treat entire families, as did the General Practitioners of the past. They spend more than 90% of their time in direct patient care. The spectrum of their practice varies with the extent of their training, their interests, the area of the country, the number of other medical practitioners in the area, and their local hospital's rules. Family Physicians practice mostly in an outpatient setting. They provide primary care to a diverse population, unlimited by the patient's age, sex, organ system affected, or disease. They usually have a significant number of pediatric and geriatric patients. Delivering babies, although always a part of their training, is not always a part of the practice. Due to the rising cost of professional liability insurance, the irregular hours involved, and other factors, many Family Physicians severely limit this aspect of their practices. Dealing with the behavioral aspects of medicine, including family life-cycle events (birth, stress, grief) and delivering other psychological services are a large part of Family Medicine.

Most Family Physicians enter group practices, and most participate in some type of managed health care delivery system (HMO, PPO, IPA). Many have assumed the often-uncomfortable role of "gatekeeper" or "case manager" within these systems and end up allocating services to patients. The average Family Physician works 51 hours per week, with two-thirds of the time spent on office visits and the balance spent on hospital rounds, on other patient visits, and doing surgical or manipulative procedures.

There is a shortage of Family Physicians aggravated by an increased demand in managed care systems and rural areas. A 2009 report called for 39,000 more Family Physicians by 2020 in order that all Americans have access to a primary care physician. Part of the reason for this shortage is that the specialty suffers from a lack of recognition, both publicly and professionally, which discourages new physicians from entering this field. And, while many Family Physicians work longer hours than their colleagues and often must know how to treat a broader range of medical problems, their remuneration is one of the lowest in medicine. Physicians in this field get satisfaction from providing continuity of care to patients, within the context of their entire family, throughout the various stages of life.

Training: Training is three years in length. Residencies combining Family Medicine and Internal Medicine last four years; those combining Family Medicine and Psychiatry are five years long. Osteopathic residencies are generally two years in length following internship and one program exists combining Family Practice with Osteopathic Manipulative Medicine. Family Medicine faculty rely heavily on applicant interviews and performance on clinical rotations to select residents. About 10% of Family Physicians specialize. Family Medicine residency graduates (M.D.s) can take one-year Adolescent Medicine, Geriatric Medicine (72 positions) or Sports Medicine (165 positions) fellowships.

Osteopaths can take a two-year Geriatrics fellowship after their first year of Family Practice residency or a two-year Osteopathic Manipulative Medicine fellowship after completing their residency.

Match: In recent years, about 91% of the available PGY-1 positions filled through the NRMP Match.

Family Medicine

ACGME-Approved Programs	457	AOA-Approved Programs	144
1st-Yr. Spots for M.D. Students	2,740	Funded Entry-Level D.O. Spots	661
Adv. Spots Avail. to M.D. Students	0	% IMG Residents	43
All Entry-Level M.D. Spots	2,740	Avg. Res. Work Hours/Week	64
% Women Residents	54	Programs offering a "Primary Care Track"	199
Avg. Ratio of Full-Time Physician Faculty to Residents	0.7		
% Training in Hospital Outpatient Clinics	21	Programs offering Multiple Start Dates	147
		Programs allowing Moonlighting	286
% Training in Non-Hospital Community Ambulatory Clinics	16	Programs with Women's track	90
		Programs with Hospitalist track	43
Programs with Childcare	126		

Family Medicine–Internal Medicine (CR)**

ACGME-Approved Programs	2	AOA-Approved Programs	0
1st-Yr. Spots for M.D. Students	4	Funded Entry-Level D.O. Spots	0
Adv. Spots Avail. to M.D. Students	0	% IMG Residents	10
All Entry-Level M.D. Spots	4	Avg. Res. Work Hours/Week	64
% Women Residents	44	% Training in Non-Hospital Community Ambulatory Clinics	11
Avg. Ratio of Full-Time Physician Faculty to Residents	7.3		
% Training in Hospital Outpatient Clinics	19	Programs with Childcare	0
		Programs offering a "Primary Care Track"	1

Family Medicine–Psychiatry (CR)**

ACGME-Approved Programs	8	AOA-Approved Programs	0
1st-Yr. Spots for M.D. Students	12	Funded Entry-Level D.O. Spots	0
Adv. Spots Avail. to M.D. Students	0	% IMG Residents	5
All Entry-Level M.D. Spots	12	Avg. Res. Work Hours/Week	57
% Women Residents	43	% Training in Non-Hospital Community Ambulatory Clinics	15
Avg. Ratio of Full-Time Physician Faculty to Residents/Fellows	10.0		
% Training in Hospital Outpatient Clinics	21		

Family Practice with OMM, OMT, or Neuromuscular Medicine (D.O.s only)

AOA-Approved Programs	5	Funded Entry-Level D.O. Spots	10

For more information, contact:

- American Academy of Family Physicians, (800) 274-2237; www.aafp.org.
- American College of Osteopathic Family Physicians, (800) 323-0794; www.acofp.org.

Gastroenterology (F) ***

Specialty Overview: Gastroenterologists are Internists and Pediatricians who diagnose and treat diseases of the esophagus, stomach, small and large intestines, liver, pancreas, and gallbladder. A large number of their patients have ulcer disease or chronic diseases of the liver, intestinal tract, or pancreas. Recent advances in endoscopy (esophagogastroduodenoscopy, colonoscopy, and endoscopic retrograde cholangiopancreatography) have increased the number of procedures that Gastroenterologists perform. Gastroenterologists are predominantly office-based. They take some night call and many have active inpatient services. Gastroenterologists average 47 hours per week (Internists) and 50 hours per week (Pediatricians) doing patient care. Advanced training in areas such as clinical genetics, obesity and nutrition, women's health, geriatrics, GI malignancies, hepatology, and global health will have increasing importance in years to come.

Training: As a subspecialty of Internal Medicine, training consists of a three-year fellowship following completion of an Internal Medicine residency. Pediatric Gastroenterology fellowships last three years after a Pediatric residency. For Osteopathic physicians, training follows internship and two years of Internal Medicine residency.

Match: Because many programs have fall application deadlines, it is best to contact them at least two years before your expected start date. In recent years, about 91% of participating Gastroenterology programs and 96% of positions filled in NRMP's Medical Specialties Matching Program, while about 95% of Pediatric Gastroenterology programs participated in NRMP's Pediatric Specialties Spring Match, with 86% of positions filled through the Match. Match results are announced in June.

Gastroenterology (Internal Medicine)

ACGME-Approved Programs	159	AOA-Approved Programs	7
1st-Yr. Spots for M.D. Students	0	Funded Entry-Level D.O. Spots	6
Adv. Spots Avail. to M.D. Students	0	% IMG Residents	29
All Entry-Level M.D. Spots	446	Avg. Res. Work Hours/Week	52
% Women Residents	30	% Training in Non-Hospital Community Ambulatory Clinics	5
Avg. Ratio of Full-Time Physician Faculty to Fellows	1.1		
% Training in Hospital Outpatient Clinics	23		

Pediatric Gastroenterology **

ACGME-Approved Programs	51	AOA-Approved Programs	0
1st-Yr. Spots for M.D. Students	0	Funded Entry-Level D.O. Spots	0
Adv. Spots Avail. to M.D. Students	0	% IMG Residents	32
All Entry-Level M.D. Spots	69	Avg. Res. Work Hours/Week	46
% Women Residents	48	% Training in Non-Hospital Community Ambulatory Clinics	1
Avg. Ratio of Full-Time Physician Faculty to Fellows	1.2		
% Training in Hospital Outpatient Clinics	33		

For more information, contact:

- American College of Gastroenterology, (301) 263-9000; http://gi.org.
- American College of Osteopathic Internists, (301) 656-8877; www.acoi.org.
- American Gastroenterological Association, (301) 654-2055; www.gastro.org.
- American Academy of Pediatrics, (847) 434-4000; www.aap.org.
- North American Society for Pediatric Gastroenterology, Hepatology & Nutrition, (215) 233-0808; www.naspghan.org.

Geriatric Medicine (F) *

Specialty Overview: Geriatric Medicine is a primary-care subspecialty that deals with the complex medical and psychosocial problems of older adults. About 20,000 Geriatric clinicians are currently needed and the demand for physicians with special skills in Geriatric Medicine is rapidly increasing. By 2030, 20% of all Americans will be older than 65 and the United States will need more than 36,000 Geriatricians. People aged 85 and older are the fastest growing segment of the population, with expected growth from 4 million people today to 19 million by 2050. Currently, there are just over 7,000 certified Geriatricians and 1,700 Geriatric Psychiatrists, but these numbers are expected to decline as practicing Geriatricians retire.

While one-third of all patients seen by Internists are over 65-years-old, nearly half of Geriatricians' patients are over 75 years-old. Geriatricians average 48 hours per week doing patient care.

Opportunities exist in academic medicine and research, corporate (HMO) medicine, community medicine, long-term care, and private practice. Geriatricians generally earn less than their primary care colleagues despite their additional training, in part because of lower Medicare reimbursement rates. However, a recent trend has led to more competitive salaries for hospital-based Geriatricians. Geriatricians must be able to work within a multi-specialty team of both medical and non-medical personnel.

Training: Most Geriatricians complete a three-year residency training in Family Medicine and Internal Medicine or a four-year residency in Psychiatry before entering a one-year fellowship. Some of the programs operate jointly, with both the Internal Medicine and Family Medicine programs participating. Psychiatry has its own programs. Osteopathic fellowships are available for those completing one or two years of any other residency.

Match: There is no matching program for any Geriatric fellowship, so contact the programs directly. *FREIDA* has a list of programs.

Geriatric Medicine (Family Medicine)*

ACGME-Approved Programs	42	AOA-Approved Programs	5
1st-Yr. Spots for M.D. Students	0	Funded Entry-Level D.O. Spots	9
Adv. Spots Avail. to M.D. Students	0	% IMG Residents	59
All Entry-Level M.D. Spots	72	Avg. Res. Work Hours/Week	41
% Women Residents	42	% Training in Non-Hospital Community Ambulatory Clinics	26
Avg. Ratio of Full-Time Physician Faculty to Fellows	3.7		
% Training in Hospital Outpatient Clinics	32		

Geriatric Medicine (Internal Medicine)*

ACGME-Approved Programs	107	AOA-Approved Programs	1
1st-Yr. Spots for M.D. Students	0	Funded Entry-Level D.O. Spots	1
Adv. Spots Avail. to M.D. Students	0	% IMG Residents	66
All Entry-Level M.D. Spots	301	Avg. Res. Work Hours/Week	44
% Women Residents	57	% Training in Non-Hospital Community Ambulatory Clinics	19
Avg. Ratio of Full-Time Physician Faculty to Fellows	4.9		
% Training in Hospital Outpatient Clinics	35		

Geriatric Psychiatry*

ACGME-Approved Programs	54	AOA-Approved Programs	0
1st-Yr. Spots for M.D. Students	0	Funded Entry-Level D.O. Spots	0
Adv. Spots Avail. to M.D. Students	0	% IMG Residents	55
All Entry-Level M.D. Spots	84	Avg. Res. Work Hours/Week	39
% Women Residents	52	% Training in Non-Hospital Community Ambulatory Clinics	14
Avg. Ratio of Full-Time Physician Faculty to Fellows	8.5		
% Training in Hospital Outpatient Clinics	42		

For more information, contact:
- American Academy of Family Physicians, (913) 906-6000; www.aafp.org.
- American College of Osteopathic Internists, (301) 656-8877; www.acoi.org.
- American Geriatrics Society, (212) 308-1414; www.americangeriatrics.org.
- American Association for Geriatric Psychiatry, (301) 654-7850; www.aagpgpa.org.

Hand Surgery (F) ***

Specialty Overview: Hand surgeons primarily treat diseases of and injuries to the hand and forearm. Nearly all have training in either Orthopedic Surgery or Plastic Surgery. Advances in the specialty have come with development of new microsurgical techniques. Some Hand Surgeons do reimplantation surgery after traumatic amputations. This surgery normally requires a specialized center. One benefit to Hand Surgery is that it is usually done sitting down. Much of the surgery is now done on outpatients. Hand Surgeons average 59 hours per week doing patient care.

Training: Fellowship training in Hand Surgery lasts one year after a residency in Orthopedic Surgery, Plastic Surgery, or General Surgery.

Match: Most Hand Surgery positions (the majority through Orthopedic Surgery) fill through the Specialty Match run by the NRMP Combined Musculoskeletal Matching Program. Match results are announced in May.

Hand Surgery (Orthopedic Surgery)*****

ACGME-Approved Programs	55	AOA-Approved Programs	0
1st-Yr. Spots for M.D. Students	0	Funded Entry-Level D.O. Spots	0
Adv. Spots Avail. to M.D. Students	0	% IMG Residents	11
All Entry-Level M.D. Spots	132	Avg. Res. Work Hours/Week	54
% Women Residents	19	% Training in Non-Hospital Community Ambulatory Clinics	26
Avg. Ratio of Full-Time Physician Faculty to Fellows	3.2		
% Training in Hospital Outpatient Clinics	26		

Hand Surgery (Plastic Surgery)***

ACGME-Approved Programs	13	AOA-Approved Programs	0
1st-Yr. Spots for M.D. Students	0	Funded Entry-Level D.O. Spots	0
Adv. Spots Avail. to M.D. Students	0	% IMG Residents	21
All Entry-Level M.D. Spots	21	Avg. Res. Work Hours/Week	54
% Women Residents	14	% Training in Non-Hospital Community Ambulatory Clinics	15
Avg. Ratio of Full-Time Physician Faculty to Fellows	4.7		
% Training in Hospital Outpatient Clinics	21		

Hand Surgery (General Surgery)***

ACGME-Approved Programs	1	AOA-Approved Programs	0
1st-Yr. Spots for M.D. Students	0	Funded Entry-Level D.O. Spots	0
Adv. Spots Avail. to M.D. Students	0	% IMG Residents	43
All Entry-Level M.D. Spots	8	Avg. Res. Work Hours/Week	60
% Women Residents	14	% Training in Non-Hospital Community Ambulatory Clinics	45
Avg. Ratio of Full-Time Physician Faculty to Fellows	1.8		
% Training in Hospital Outpatient Clinics	10		

For more information, contact:

- American Academy of Orthopaedic Surgeons, (847) 823-7186; www.aaos.org.
- The American Orthopaedic Association, (847) 318-7330; www.aoassn.org/.
- American Osteopathic Academy of Orthopedics, (800) 741-2626; www.aoao.org.
- American Association for Hand Surgery, (800) 333-8835; www.handsurgery.org.
- American Society for Surgery of the Hand, (847) 384-8300; www.assh.org.

Hematology–Oncology (F) ***

Specialty Overview: Although separate specialties, Hematology (the diagnosis and treatment of diseases of the blood) and Oncology (the diagnosis and treatment of patients with cancer) are often combined in both training and practice. The specialty is predominantly office-based, but practitioners often have a large primary or consultative inpatient service. Night call and emergencies can be frequent. Most specialists in this field work in medium to large cities. Hematologists and Oncologists are drawn from the specialties of Pediatrics and Internal Medicine. Hematologist-Oncologists average 47 hours per week (Internists) and 39 hours per week (Pediatricians) doing patient care. Hematologist-Pathologists average 45 hours per week doing patient care. Oncologist-Internists average 40 hours per week doing patient care. More than 11,000 physicians currently practice Hematology, Oncology, or both. By 2020, oncology visits are projected to increase by 48%, in part due to an aging population, while the supply of oncologists is projected to increase by only 14%.

Training: Training in either Hematology or Oncology is usually a two-year fellowship, but many programs combine the two specialties into three-year fellowships. A one-year fellowship in Hematology can follow completion of an Internal Medicine or a Pediatric residency, or three years of a Pathology residency. For Osteopathic physicians, training follows internship and two years of Internal Medicine residency.

Match: The NRMP runs the Hematology and Hematology-Oncology Matches through their Medical Specialties Matching Program, with 100% and 93% of programs participating, respectively, and 100% and 90% of positions filling in recent years. Match results are announced in June. They also run the Pediatric Hematology/Oncology Fellowship Match, with 87% of programs participating and 90% of positions filled. Match day is in May, a year before the program starts.

Hematology (Internal Medicine)

ACGME-Approved Programs	6	AOA-Approved Programs	0
1st-Yr. Spots for M.D. Students	0	Funded Entry-Level D.O. Spots	0
Adv. Spots Avail. to M.D. Students	0	% IMG Residents	59
All Entry-Level M.D. Spots	35	Avg. Res. Work Hours/Week	54
% Women Residents	28	% Training in Non-Hospital Community Ambulatory Clinics	10
Avg. Ratio of Full-Time Physician Faculty to Fellows	2.2		
% Training in Hospital Outpatient Clinics	28		

Hematology (Pathology)

ACGME-Approved Programs	81	AOA-Approved Programs	0
1st-Yr. Spots for M.D. Students	0	Funded Entry-Level D.O. Spots	0
Adv. Spots Avail. to M.D. Students	0	% IMG Residents	28
All Entry-Level M.D. Spots	127	Avg. Res. Work Hours/Week	46
% Women Residents	50	% Training in Non-Hospital Community Ambulatory Clinics	5
Avg. Ratio of Full-Time Physician Faculty to Fellows	5.4		
% Training in Hospital Outpatient Clinics	13		

Oncology (Internal Medicine)

ACGME-Approved Programs	16	AOA-Approved Programs	1
1st-Yr. Spots for M.D. Students	0	Funded Entry-Level D.O. Spots	1
Adv. Spots Avail. to M.D. Students	0	% IMG Residents	64
All Entry-Level M.D. Spots	57	Avg. Res. Work Hours/Week	50
% Women Residents	36	% Training in Non-Hospital Community Ambulatory Clinics	25
Avg. Ratio of Full-Time Physician Faculty to Fellows	2.2		
% Training in Hospital Outpatient Clinics	49		

Hematology–Oncology (Internal Medicine)*

ACGME-Approved Programs	132	AOA-Approved Programs	1
1st-Yr. Spots for M.D. Students	0	Funded Entry-Level D.O. Spots	2
Adv. Spots Avail. to M.D. Students	0	% IMG Residents	47
All Entry-Level M.D. Spots	475	Avg. Res. Work Hours/Week	52
% Women Residents	43	% Training in Non-Hospital Community Ambulatory Clinics	18
Avg. Ratio of Full-Time Physician Faculty to Fellows	2.1		
% Training in Hospital Outpatient Clinics	35		

Pediatric Hematology–Oncology*****

ACGME-Approved Programs	68	AOA-Approved Programs	0
1st-Yr. Spots for M.D. Students	0	Funded Entry-Level D.O. Spots	0
Adv. Spots Avail. to M.D. Students	0	% IMG Residents	34
All Entry-Level M.D. Spots	151	Avg. Res. Work Hours/Week	55
% Women Residents	58	% Training in Non-Hospital Community Ambulatory Clinics	3
Avg. Ratio of Full-Time Physician Faculty to Fellows	3.0		
% Training in Hospital Outpatient Clinics	32		

For more information, contact:

- American College of Osteopathic Internists, (301) 656-8877; www.acoi.org.
- American Society of Clinical Oncology, (571) 483-1300; www.asco.org.
- American Society of Hematology, (202) 776-0544; www.hematology.org.

Hospice & Palliative Medicine *

Specialty Overview: This subspecialty addresses the medical component of palliative care by supporting the patient's quality of life throughout the course of a terminal illness, and managing factors that contribute to suffering of the patient and their family. Clinical skills include using an interdisciplinary team approach to assess and manage the physical, psychological and spiritual suffering of patients with life-threatening illnesses.

Training: Training consists of a one-year fellowship following completion of an ACGME-accredited program in Anesthesiology, Emergency Medicine, Family Medicine, Internal Medicine, Neurology, Obstetrics & Gynecology, Pediatrics, Physical Medicine & Rehabilitation, Psychiatry, Radiation Oncology, or Surgery.

Match: Because many programs have fall application deadlines, it is best to contact them individually at least two years before your expected start date.

Hospice & Palliative Medicine

ACGME-Approved Programs	67	AOA-Approved Programs	5
1st-Yr. Spots for M.D. Students	0	Funded Entry-Level D.O. Spots	9
Adv. Spots Avail. to M.D. Students	0	% IMG Residents	30
All Entry-Level M.D. Spots	190	% Training in Non-Hospital Community Ambulatory Clinics	12
% Training in Hospital Outpatient Clinics	15		

For more information, contact:

- American Academy of Hospice & Palliative Medicine, (847) 375-4712; www.aahpm.org.

Hospitalist *

Specialty Overview: Under current definitions, physicians are hospitalists if they spend 25% or more of their time caring for patients admitted or transferred to the hospital by their primary doctors. Their practice has been described as "caring for horizontal patients"; when patients are discharged, office-based physicians take over their care. This is the fastest growing specialty in the history of American medicine: this has been encouraged by managed care organizations that want their office-based physicians primarily to see outpatients while streamlining the treatment given to inpatients, i.e., to reduce lengths of stay and costs. Having Hospitalists see all inpatients saves the time required for other physicians to do rounds and may help alleviate the stress from decreased numbers of resident physicians.

Hospitalists must balance the demands of patients, families, primary physicians, hospitals, and insurers. They seem to be doing this well, and are currently in 5,000 institutions. Although the original description of Hospitalists raised the question of whether these physicians would suffer "burnout" more than others, recent studies demonstrate that their burnout rate is no greater than physicians in Emergency Medicine or Critical Care. Of the estimated 28,000 Hospitalists, about 75% are Internists, 11% are Pediatricians, and 3% are Family Physicians. It is estimated that there will be about 50,000 Hospitalists by 2020. At some academic centers, Hospitalists do most of the inpatient teaching to residents and students. Two benefits of being a Hospitalist are having set work hours and receiving a salary 30% higher than General Internists.

It is unlikely that Hospitalist will become an official specialty in the near future. That would push managed care groups and hospitals to require such certification for all primary care physicians caring for hospitalized patients—a situation no one wants.

Training: Currently, training generally consists of completing an Internal Medicine, Pediatrics, or Family Medicine residency. About 151 residency programs have special tracks to train Hospitalists. These programs, most of which are in Internal Medicine and Family Medicine, as well as the 62 Hospitalist Fellowships can be located by checking the "Optional Criteria" button when searching *FREIDA*. These fellowships are one or two years long. Most of these programs include special training dealing with end-of-life care, interaction with other specialists (especially surgeons), managed care, quality improvement and patient safety, teamwork, hospital systems and infrastructure, care available outside the hospital, and business and communication skills.

For more information, contact:

- Society of Hospital Medicine, (800) 843-3360; www.hospitalmedicine.org/.

Infectious Diseases (F) *

Specialty Overview: Infectious Diseases specialists diagnose and treat contagious diseases. At the onset of the antibiotic era the specialty was thought to be on the edge of extinction; it made an impressive comeback due to the great diversity of drug-resistant bacteria, the AIDS epidemic, the fear of bioterrorism, and the threat of a worldwide flu pandemic. Infectious Diseases specialists act as consultants to other physicians. Many are also involved in research and most work in major medical centers. With the increased importance of nosocomial infections, many Infectious Diseases specialists work part-time as hospital infection control officers. Physicians in this subspecialty generally receive lower salaries than those specialists who are more procedure-oriented. Many Infectious Diseases specialists also practice General Internal Medicine. The nation's 8,000 Infectious Diseases Internists average 43 hours per week doing patient care.

Training: Training consists of either a two-year fellowship following completion of an Internal Medicine residency or a three-year fellowship after a Pediatric residency. For Osteopathic physicians, training follows internship and two years of an Internal Medicine residency.

Match: Applicants match with Infectious Diseases fellowships by using the NRMP Medical Specialties Matching Program. About 89% of programs participate in the Match and 89% of the positions were filled in recent years. Match day is in June, a year before the program begins. Pediatric Infectious Diseases programs can be found in *FREIDA* and should be directly contacted.

Infectious Diseases (Internal Medicine)

ACGME-Approved Programs	145	AOA-Approved Programs	2
1st-Yr. Spots for M.D. Students	0	Funded Entry-Level D.O. Spots	4
Adv. Spots Avail. to M.D. Students	0	% IMG Residents	50
All Entry-Level M.D. Spots	366	Avg. Res. Work Hours/Week	52
% Women Residents	50	% Training in Non-Hospital Community Ambulatory Clinics	9
Avg. Ratio of Full-Time Physician Faculty to Fellows	2.7		
% Training in Hospital Outpatient Clinics	17		

Pediatric Infectious Diseases

ACGME-Approved Programs	62	AOA-Approved Programs	0
1st-Yr. Spots for M.D. Students	0	Funded Entry-Level D.O. Spots	0
Adv. Spots Avail. to M.D. Students	0	% IMG Residents	37
All Entry-Level M.D. Spots	74	Avg. Res. Work Hours/Week	48
% Women Residents	65	% Training in Non-Hospital	17
Avg. Ratio of Full-Time Physician Faculty to Fellows	3.2	Community Ambulatory Clinics	
% Training in Hospital Outpatient Clinics	16		

For more information, contact:

- American College of Osteopathic Internists, (301) 656-8877; www.acoi.org.
- Infectious Diseases Society of America, (703) 299-0200; www.idsociety.org.

Internal Medicine ** to ***

Specialty Overview: Internists (specialists in Internal Medicine, not to be confused with "interns") are divided into General Internists and subspecialists in Internal Medicine (see the subspecialties listed under "Internal Medicine" in Figures 2.7 and 2.8). The General Internist provides longitudinal care to adult patients with both acute and chronic diseases. In rural areas, the General Internist often acts as a consultant to other practitioners on complex medical cases. In suburban and urban areas, however, other primary care practitioners usually consult with Internal Medicine subspecialists; surgical specialists consult with both General and subspecialty Internists. Urban General Internists provide primary health care and treat non-surgical diseases such as diabetes, hypertension, and congestive heart failure on both an inpatient and an outpatient basis. They are also very active in managed care plans such as HMOs.

Students attracted to General Internal Medicine seek an intellectual challenge, have an interest in primary care, and often had a positive experience during their third-year Internal Medicine rotation. General Internal Medicine, however, has been less popular among students and housestaff in recent years. This trend may be due to several factors, including: an income lower than that of either the average physician or the Internal Medicine subspecialist, General Internal Medicine's relatively low prestige, the perception that caring for chronically ill patients is burdensome, and the increasing hassles of practice. Many students avoid Internal Medicine because they perceive that the housestaff and attendings they work with are overworked, unhappy, and under-rewarded. Studies show that General Internists are less satisfied with their jobs than are either Family Physicians or Internal Medicine subspecialists. However, the growth of managed care plans and societal pressure to have more primary care physicians have led to increased job opportunities for General Internists. Approximately 25% of Internal Medicine Residents plan to be General Internists because they prefer to care for ambulatory patients, believe it offers them an opportunity to have long-term relationships with patients, and does not involve caring for critically ill patients.

Internal Medicine is often described as "less procedural and more cerebral" than other specialties. While this may be true for General Internists, it is not true of the procedure-oriented subspecialists in Gastroenterology, Critical Care, Pulmonary Disease, and Cardiology. The average Internist (General and subspecialty) has a 54-hour work week (49 hours doing patient care), with 47% of the time spent in office visits, 18% on hospital rounds, 27% on other patient care activities, and 3% doing surgical/manipulative procedures. In some areas of the country, the amount of hospital time is decreasing as Hospitalists assume inpatient tasks.

Training: Training in Internal Medicine is three years in length. Programs that combine Internal Medicine with Family Medicine (*see* Family Medicine–Internal Medicine), Pediatrics (*see* below), Preventive Medicine, or Nuclear Medicine are four years long. Programs combining Internal Medicine with Emergency Medicine (*see* Emergency Medicine–Internal Medicine), Medical Genetics, Neurology, Physical Medicine & Rehabilitation, or Psychiatry are each five years long. These combined programs qualify graduates for board examinations in both specialties. If an Osteopathic graduate enters an Internal Medicine "specialty-track" internship, the Internal Medicine training time is shortened by one year.

One of the advantages of Internal Medicine training is the number of options available following residency. More than two-thirds of Internal Medicine residency graduates go on to subspecialize. However, individuals completing Internal Medicine residencies in markets with high managed care penetration are less likely to subspecialize than are those training in areas with less managed care impact. Many physicians do not finalize their decision to practice as either General Internists or subspecialists until well into their residency. Following residency, fellowships are available in: Cardiovascular Disease; Clinical Cardiac Electrophysiology; Critical Care Medicine; Endocrinology, Diabetes & Metabolism; Gastroenterology; Geriatric Medicine; Hematology; Hematology & Oncology; Hospice & Palliative Medicine; Infectious Disease; Interventional Cardiology; Oncology; Nephrology; Pulmonary Disease; Pulmonary Disease and Critical Care Medicine; Rheumatology; Sleep Medicine; Sports Medicine and Transplant Hepatology.

FREIDA lists some positions as "Internal Medicine" and some as "Medicine-Primary." The difference between the two types of programs is that there is more, but often only slightly more, time spent in an ambulatory clinic and a continuity clinic in the latter type. Graduates of both programs take the same Board examination. Some programs, labeled "Primary Care Internal Medicine," emphasize outpatient clinic training, although they seldom have more clinic hours than inpatient training. These come closer than the usual residency programs to mimicking the actual practice of a General Internist, although all Internal Medicine programs have increased the amount of time spent in ambulatory settings over the past few years.

Match: Virtually all ACGME-approved positions in Internal Medicine are listed in the NRMP PGY-1 Match. In recent years, 99% of the available PGY-1 Categorical (three-year) positions filled through the NRMP Match, with 27% of the positions taken by foreign graduates. About 1,800 Internal Medicine positions are listed as "Preliminary" and are for only one year of training (before beginning training in other specialties). U.S. graduates filled 77% of these positions in 2012.

Other Useful Information: Internal Medicine led the way in postgraduate education reform and their training programs have more experience with the requirement that limits the number of hours residents work to 80 hours per week, averaged over four weeks. Residents at all levels of training have, on average, at least one day per week free of hospital duties. They also must spend at least 25% of their three-year training in ambulatory settings. Not all programs, though, comply with these requirements.

Internal Medicine (C)**; (P)***

ACGME-Approved Programs	389	AOA-Approved Programs	66
1st-Yr. Spots for M.D. Students (C)	5,277	Funded Entry-Level D.O. Spots	415
1st-Yr. Spots for M.D. Students (P)	1,661	% IMG Residents	44
Adv. Spots Avail. to M.D. Students	0	Avg. Res. Work Hours/Week	65
All Entry-Level M.D. Spots	7,138	Programs offering a "Primary Care Track"	114
% Women Residents	44		
Avg. Ratio of Full-Time Physician Faculty to Residents	0.9	Programs offering Multiple Start Dates	60
% Training in Hospital Outpatient Clinics	22	Programs allowing Moonlighting	235
% Training in Non-Hospital Community Ambulatory Clinics	8	Programs offering a Women's Track	22
Programs with Childcare	139	Programs offering a Hospitalist Track	50

Internal Medicine–Neurology (CR) *

ACGME-Approved Programs	2	AOA-Approved Programs	0
1st-Yr. Spots for M.D. Students	2	Funded Entry-Level D.O. Spots	0
Adv. Spots Avail. to M.D. Students	0	% IMG Residents	32
All Entry-Level M.D. Spots	2	Avg. Res. Work Hours/Week	56
% Women Residents	37	% Training in Non-Hospital Community Ambulatory Clinics	6
Avg. Ratio of Full-Time Physician Faculty to Residents	43.6		
% Training in Hospital Outpatient Clinics	26		

Internal Medicine–Preventive Medicine (CR) *

ACGME-Approved Programs	6	AOA-Approved Programs	0
1st-Yr. Spots for M.D. Students	5	Funded Entry-Level D.O. Spots	0
Adv. Spots Avail. to M.D. Students	0	% IMG Residents	51
All Entry-Level M.D. Spots	5	Avg. Res. Work Hours/Week	55
% Women Residents	51	% Training in Non-Hospital Community Ambulatory Clinics	20
Avg. Ratio of Full-Time Physician Faculty to Residents	6.7		
% Training in Hospital Outpatient Clinics	29		

Internal Medicine, Primary **

ACGME-Approved Programs	56	AOA-Approved Programs	0
1st-Yr. Spots for M.D. Students	311	Funded Entry-Level D.O. Spots	0
Adv. Spots Avail. to M.D. Students	0		
All Entry-Level M.D. Spots	290		

Internal Medicine–Psychiatry (CR) **

ACGME-Approved Programs	10	AOA-Approved Programs	0
1st-Yr. Spots for M.D. Students	20	Funded Entry-Level D.O. Spots	0
Adv. Spots Avail. to M.D. Students	0	% IMG Residents	25
All Entry-Level M.D. Spots	20	Avg. Res. Work Hours/Week	58
% Women Residents	41	% Training in Non-Hospital Community Ambulatory Clinics	7
Avg. Ratio of Full-Time Physician Faculty to Residents	36.0		
% Training in Hospital Outpatient Clinics	23		

For more information, contact:

- American College of Osteopathic Internists, (301) 656-8877; www.acoi.org.
- American College of Physicians–American Society of Internal Medicine, (800) 523-1546; www.acponline.org.
- Society of General Internal Medicine, (800) 822-3060; www.sgim.org.

Internal Medicine–Pediatrics ***

Specialty Overview: Combined Internal Medicine–Pediatrics training programs are designed for individuals who wish to have a primary care practice for families without offering obstetric and surgical services. About 80% of these programs' graduates see both adults and children in their practice, and about 20% work in rural or underserved areas.

Graduates of these combined training programs report that they feel as comfortable as other Pediatricians handling infant, child, and adolescent cases, but less comfortable than Family Physicians treating adolescent health problems. Although they are more comfortable than Family Physicians dealing with complex Internal Medicine patients, they report being less comfortable than other Internists treating intensive care and geriatric patients. Internist-Pediatricians average 51 hours per week doing patient care.

Completion of combined programs makes the individual eligible to take the specialty Board examination in both Pediatrics and Internal Medicine. The combined programs are not reviewed by the certifying bodies (Residency Review Committees) as a whole program. Rather, the Internal Medicine and Pediatrics programs are each reviewed and approved separately. The number of combined programs is growing. A listing can be found both on *FREIDA* and in the "Green Book's" Appendices.

Training: Training is four years in length, with a minimum of twenty months of Internal Medicine. The programs are, for the most part, integrated. Trainees take blocks of Internal Medicine and then blocks of Pediatrics. This often leads to spending nearly two years at the intern level of training. More than 90% of Internal Medicine-Pediatrics residents complete the program, and about 20% go on to subspecialize. Most graduates feel that they needed to spend more time in the ambulatory setting and less in intensive care.

Match: In recent years, about 95% of the available PGY-1 positions filled through the NRMP Match.

Internal Medicine–Pediatrics

ACGME-Approved Programs	77	AOA-Approved Programs	2
1st-Yr. Spots for M.D. Students	362	Funded Entry-Level D.O. Spots	4
Adv. Spots Avail. to M.D. Students	0	% IMG Residents	20
All Entry-Level M.D. Spots	362	Avg. Res. Work Hours/Week	66
% Women Residents	54	Programs with Childcare	36
Avg. Ratio of Full-Time Physician Faculty to Residents	14.1	Programs offering a "Primary Care Track"	19
% Training in Hospital Outpatient Clinics	29	Programs offering Multiple Start Dates	21
% Training in Non-Hospital Community Ambulatory Clinics	13	Programs allowing Moonlighting	65

For more information, contact:

- American College of Physicians–American Society of Internal Medicine, (800) 523-1546; www.acponline.org.
- American Academy of Pediatrics, (847) 434-4000; www.aap.org.

Medical Genetics *

Specialty Overview: Medical Genetics is the newest ABMS-recognized medical specialty. Clinical geneticists provide diagnostic, management and genetic counseling for genetically influenced health issues. Medical Genetics physicians also coordinate screening programs for inborn errors of metabolism, hemogloinopathies, chromosome abnormalities, neural tube defects, and other genetic conditions. Currently, more than 2,200 physicians have been certified in M.D. Clinical Genetics. Most come from the specialties of Pediatrics, Obstetrics & Gynecology, or Internal Medicine. As genetic factors underlying many diseases become better understood, Clinical Geneticists will be increasingly called on to manage complex care across a variety of specialties.

Training: Two years of training in another medical specialty is required before admission to a two-year Medical Genetics program. Some programs offer all four years of training. Fourteen programs combine training in Medical Genetics with Pediatrics and four programs combine Medical Genetics with Internal Medicine in five-year residency programs. It is also possible to combine a Maternal Fetal Medicine fellowship and a Medical Genetics residency.

Match: Nearly all Medical Genetics programs are listed in *FREIDA*. Programs must be contacted directly before participation in the NRMP Match. Match results are announced in December.

Medical Genetics

ACGME-Approved Programs	51	AOA-Approved Programs	0
1st-Yr. Spots for M.D. Students	1	Funded Entry-Level D.O. Spots	0
Adv. Spots Avail. to M.D. Students	0	% IMG Residents	43
All Entry-Level M.D. Spots	84	Avg. Res. Work Hours/Week	44
% Women Residents	61	Programs with Childcare	17
Avg. Ratio of Full-Time Physician Faculty to Fellows	6.2	Programs offering a "Primary Care Track"	4
% Training in Hospital Outpatient Clinics	62	Programs offering Multiple Start Dates	28
% Training in Non-Hospital Community Ambulatory Clinics	17	Programs allowing Moonlighting	29

For more information, contact:

- American College of Medical Genetics, (301) 718-9603; www.acmg.net.
- The American Society of Human Genetics, www.ashg.org.
- American Board of Medical Genetics, (301) 634-7315; www.abmg.org/.

Medical Management/Administration *

Specialty Overview: Medical managers have existed almost as long as the profession. (As soon as there were two physicians, one was assuredly the administrator.) Recently, Medical Management has come into its own with the increasing complexity of Byzantine government rules, the maze of managed care organizations, and the constantly changing patient and payer demands. Also called "Medical Administration," these specialists compete with non-physicians who also try to manage health care systems.

Since managing physicians is somewhat like herding cats, it is often a thankless job. Yet many physicians try it at various stages of their careers—especially in the decade before they retire. Many such positions are available in hospitals, group practices, clinics, insurance companies, and corporations.

Closely linked to Medical Management is "Managed Care Medicine." Those taking courses in this area also intend to manage other physicians, but often with the more defined goal of working within managed care. According to the *New England Journal of Medicine* [1999;341(25):1945-8], the inherent conflicts in the medical director's role are "satisfying the desires of patients and physicians, on the one hand, and the financial profit or survival of the organization, on the other, and between the unlimited demands of individual patients and the limited resources of society."

Training: Courses are available through the American College of Physician Executives, the National Association of Managed Care Physicians, and various MBA and MPH programs.

For more information, contact:

- National Association of Managed Care Physicians, (804) 527-1905; namcp.org.
- American College of Physician Executives, (800) 562-8088; www.acpe.org.
- American Medical Directors Association, (800) 876-2632; www.amda.com.

Medical Toxicology (F) *

Specialty Overview: Medical Toxicologists diagnose, treat, and consult on a wide variety of intentional, accidental, and industrial poisonings. Toxicology is a subspecialty of Emergency Medicine, Pediatrics, and Preventive Medicine, although no Pediatrics-based programs exist.

Training: Training programs are usually two years following the primary residency. A current list is on *FREIDA*.

Match: Fellowships, usually within Emergency Medicine or Preventive Medicine departments, are obtained by contacting each program directly.

Medical Toxicology (all)			
ACGME-Approved Programs	30	AOA-Approved Programs	0
1st-Yr. Spots for M.D. Students	0	Funded Entry-Level D.O. Spots	0
Adv. Spots Avail. to M.D. Students	0	% IMG Residents	15
All Entry-Level M.D. Spots	68	Avg. Res. Work Hours/Week	41
% Women Residents	30	Avg. Ratio of Full-Time Physician Faculty to Fellows	2.5

For more information, contact:

- American Academy of Pediatrics, (847) 434-4000; www.aap.org.
- American College of Emergency Physicians, (800) 798-1822; www.acep.org.
- American College of Occupational and Environmental Medicine, (847) 818-1800; www.acoem.org.
- Society for Academic Emergency Medicine, (847) 813-9823; www.saem.org.
- Society of Toxicology, (703) 438-3115; www.toxicology.org.

Neonatal–Perinatal Medicine (F) ***

Specialty Overview: Neonatologists treat the problems associated with premature births. Their practice centers on the neonatal intensive care unit. They are critical care Pediatricians for those neonates who do not yet have the capacity to live without medical assistance. As with other critical care specialists, they must be able to skillfully perform procedures—but they must work on *very* small babies. The size of the infants they work with has progressively decreased. Neonatologists work closely with a specialized team of nurses, social workers, and respiratory therapists. They also work closely with families to sort out both medical and ethical issues of care. The nation's 5,000 Neonatologists average 53 hours per week doing patient care.

Training: Fellowships are two years in length following a residency in Pediatrics.

Match: In recent years, about 95% of programs participated in the NRMP Neonatal-Perinatal Fellowship Match, with 76% of the positions filled and 92% of applicants matching. Match results are announced in September.

Neonatal–Perinatal Medicine

ACGME-Approved Programs	91	AOA-Approved Programs	0
1st-Yr. Spots for M.D. Students	0	Funded Entry-Level D.O. Spots	0
Adv. Spots Avail. to M.D. Students	0	% IMG Residents	42
All Entry-Level M.D. Spots	221	Avg. Res. Work Hours/Week	58
% Women Residents	60	% Training in Non-Hospital Community Ambulatory Clinics	5
Avg. Ratio of Full-Time Physician Faculty to Fellows	2.2		
% Training in Hospital Outpatient Clinics	7		

For more information, contact:

- Section on Perinatal Pediatrics, American Academy of Pediatrics, (847) 434-4000; www.aap.org/perinatal.
- American College of Osteopathic Pediatricians, (800) 621-1773; www.acopeds.org/.

Nephrology (F) *

Specialty Overview: Nephrologists diagnose and (non-surgically) treat diseases of the kidney and the urinary system. Most of their patients have chronic diseases requiring long-term care. Managing dialysis and the treatment of dialysis and renal transplant patients are large parts of most Nephrologists' practices. The specialty is predominantly office-based. However, practitioners may have large primary or consultative inpatient services. Night call can be frequent. Nephrologists average 55 hours (Internists) or 42 hours (Pediatricians) per week doing patient care. Although the number of Nephrology fellows roughly doubled in the past twenty years, a workforce shortage is predicted due to the dramatic rise in chronic kidney disease and end state renal disease combined with fewer USMGs opting for Internal Medicine residencies. IMGs make up nearly half of all nephrology fellows. There are about 7,500 Nephrologists in the United States.

Training: Training is generally a two-year fellowship following the completion of an Internal Medicine residency or three years after a Pediatric residency. For Osteopathic physicians, training follows internship and two years of an Internal Medicine residency.

Match: Nephorology applicants use the NRMP Medical Specialties Matching Program; in recent years, about 94% of positions were filled through the match. All Pediatric Nephrology programs participated in the NRMP Pediatric Specialties Spring Match, with about 62% of positions filled. Match results are announced in June.

Nephrology (Internal Medicine)

ACGME-Approved Programs	151	AOA-Approved Programs	6
1st-Yr. Spots for M.D. Students	0	Funded Entry-Level D.O. Spots	11
Adv. Spots Avail. to M.D. Students	0	% IMG Residents	58
All Entry-Level M.D. Spots	374	Avg. Res. Work Hours/Week	54
% Women Residents	36	% Training in Non-Hospital	14
Avg. Ratio of Full-Time Physician Faculty to Fellows	1.9	Community Ambulatory Clinics	
% Training in Hospital Outpatient Clinics	23		

**Pediatric Nephrology **

ACGME-Approved Programs	39	AOA-Approved Programs	0
1st-Yr. Spots for M.D. Students	0	Funded Entry-Level D.O. Spots	0
Adv. Spots Avail. to M.D. Students	0	% IMG Residents	43
All Entry-Level M.D. Spots	50	Avg. Res. Work Hours/Week	44
% Women Residents	65	% Training in Non-Hospital Community Ambulatory Clinics	17
Avg. Ratio of Full-Time Physician Faculty to Fellows	2.5		
% Training in Hospital Outpatient Clinics	44		

For more information, contact:

- American College of Osteopathic Internists, (301) 656-8877; www.acoi.org.
- American Society of Nephrology, (202) 659-0599; www.asn-online.org.
- Renal Physicians Association, (301) 468-3515; www.renalmd.org.

Neurological Surgery *****

Specialty Overview: Neurosurgeons provide operative and non-operative management of lesions of the brain, spinal cord, peripheral nerves, and their supporting structures (skull, spine, meninges, CNS blood supply). Many are also involved in pain management. This requires much manual dexterity and a willingness to accept both dramatic successes and long-term failures in patient care. New developments in autologous and fetal tissue/stem cell transplantation and in stereotactic surgery for epilepsy, Parkinson's Disease, and tumors may increase the need for Neurosurgeons during the next decade. Patients range in age from neonates to the elderly. Night call and emergency surgery are frequent parts of Neurosurgical practice. The nation's 3,500 Neurosurgeons average 52 hours per week doing patient care. Recent Neurosurgery trainees rose slightly (10%), while female trainees increased by 17% and IMG trainees increased by 41%.

Training: Residency training lasts 6 years following one year of General Surgery. Trainees must spend a minimum of 36 months in clinical Neurological Surgery and 3 months in clinical Neurology. The balance of time can be spent studying relevant basic sciences, such as Neuropathology and Neuroradiology, or related fields, such as Pediatric Neurosurgery and Spinal Surgery. The specific areas covered during these extra months are the key differences among this specialty's training programs.

Match: All civilian residency programs are in the NRMP's Match. (The Neurosurgery Fellowship Match (NSMP), with 20 programs, goes through www.sfmatch.org.) About 99% of positions filled in the NRMP Match. Rank-order lists are due in December and results are distributed in late January.

Neurological Surgery			
ACGME-Approved Programs	98	AOA-Approved Programs	9
1st-Yr. Spots for M.D. Students	196	Funded Entry-Level D.O. Spots	15
Adv. Spots Avail. to M.D. Students	0	% IMG Residents	13
All Entry-Level M.D. Spots	196	Avg. Res. Work Hours/Week	77
% Women Residents	12	Programs with Childcare	35
Avg. Ratio of Full-Time Physician Faculty to Residents	1.2	Programs offering a "Primary Care Track"	3
% Training in Hospital Outpatient Clinics	18	Programs offering Multiple Start Dates	12
% Training in Non-Hospital Community Ambulatory Clinics	17	Programs allowing Moonlighting	9

For more information, contact:

• American Association of Neurological Surgeons, (888) 566-2267; www.aans.org.
• American College of Osteopathic Surgeons, (800) 888-1312; www.facos.org.

Neurology (I)**

Specialty Overview: Neurologists diagnose and non-surgically treat patients with diseases of the brain, spinal cord, peripheral nerves, and neuromuscular system. Many of these patients have headaches, strokes, or seizure disorders. Neurologists follow not only these patients but also those with chronic neuromuscular diseases. Many of their patients are referred from other clinicians. It is anticipated that the need for Neurologists will increase as the population ages. While the specialty is predominantly office-based, Neurologists may have large primary or consultative inpatient services. Night call can be frequent, especially in solo or small group practices. Neurologists average 54 hours per week doing patient care.

Training: Training is three years after a general PGY-1 year, most often in Internal Medicine, Pediatrics, or a Transitional program. Some Neurology programs have their own PGY-1 year, and so are four years long. Combined programs, which take five years to complete, exist in Internal Medicine–Neurology (*see* Internal Medicine), Neurology–Nuclear Medicine, and Neurology–Physical Medicine & Rehabilitation. Two programs that are seven years long combine Neurology, Diagnostic Radiology, and Neuroradiology. Eight programs combine Neurology and Psychiatry. Post-residency fellowships exist in Child Neurology (69 programs, See "Child Neurology"), Epilepsy (17 programs; 1 to 2 years), Neurodevelopmental Disabilities (9 programs; 4 years), Clinical Neurophysiology (91 programs; 3 years), Endovascular Surgical Neuroradiology (1 program; 1 year), Neuromuscular Medicine (24 programs; 1 year), and Vascular Neurology (65 programs; 1 year). Basic Neurology training programs are similar for Osteopathic physicians. (In 2007, all ACGME-accredited pain medicine programs under Anesthesiology, Neurology, Physical Medicine & Rehabilitation, and Psychiatry were combined into a multidisciplinary Pain Medicine subspecialty.)

Match: ACGME-approved programs generally match through the NRMP Match. Most positions are filled a year ahead of time (matching for the year after internship). However, positions not previously filled are offered for the same year to those who have finished at least an internship. When applying to a Neurology program, simultaneously apply for a PGY-1 position through the NRMP. Even if the Neurology program has a first year built into it (i.e., integrated program), you need to apply for their PGY-1 position as your top choice. Other Neurology programs require you to locate a PGY-1 position independently through the NRMP Match. Positions in programs combining Neurology with another specialty, such as Psychiatry or Internal Medicine, generally must be obtained through the NRMP Match or negotiated directly with the program. In recent years, 100% of PGY-1 applicants matched.

Neurology

ACGME-Approved Programs	142	AOA-Approved Programs	6
1st-Yr. Spots for M.D. Students	292	Funded Entry-Level D.O. Spots	8
Adv. Spots Avail. to M.D. Students	346	% IMG Residents	37
All Entry-Level M.D. Spots	638	Avg. Res. Work Hours/Week	64
% Women Residents	44	Programs offering a "Primary Care Track"	11
Avg. Ratio of Full-Time Physician Faculty to Residents	1.5		
		Programs offering Multiple Start Dates	26
% Training in Hospital Outpatient Clinics	25		
		Programs allowing Moonlighting	61
% Training in Non-Hospital Community Ambulatory Clinics	3	Programs offering a Women's Track	8
Programs with Childcare	44		

For more information, contact:

- American Academy of Neurology, (800) 879-1960; www.aan.com.
- American Association of Electrodiagnostic Medicine, (800) 884-2236; www.aaem.net.
- American College of Osteopathic Neurologists and Psychiatrists, 28595 Orchard Lake Rd, Ste. 200, Farmington Hills, MI 48334; (248) 553-0010, ext. 295.
- American Neurological Association, (952) 545-6284; www.aneuroa.org.

Nuclear Medicine *

Specialty Overview: Specialists in Nuclear Medicine use radioactive materials both to diagnose and to treat diseases by imaging the body's physiologic functions. The field combines medical practice with certain aspects of the physical sciences, including physics, mathematics, statistics, computer science, chemistry, and radiation biology. Specialists in Nuclear Medicine, unlike those in Radiation Oncology, use radioactive materials that are "unsealed" (i.e., free in the bloodstream) for their diagnostic studies and treatments. At some institutions, they also perform radioimmunoassay tests. Practitioners in the specialty have no primary patient-care responsibility and little night call. Many individuals who are currently practicing Nuclear Medicine have not been formally trained or certified in the specialty. However, anyone newly entering the field is expected to have been fully trained. The future of the specialty may be either very dynamic or rather static, depending upon how rapidly some currently innovative techniques, especially those related to PET scanning, become widely available. Nuclear Medicine physicians average 56 hours per week doing patient care. The number of physicians in the field has only increased 10% in the past 15 years.

Training: Training consists of two years of Nuclear Medicine following, interspersed with, or, in a few cases, preceding two years of initial training in another clinical specialty, most commonly Radiology, Internal Medicine, or Pathology. Other fields of clinical training have also been rather freely accepted. Osteopathic programs also accept two years of initial training in Family Medicine. Radiology residents doing a year of training in Nuclear Radiology occupy some of the positions that exist for training in Nuclear Medicine. Note, however, that Nuclear Medicine is a specialty distinct from Nuclear Radiology.

Match: Nearly all positions are obtained by negotiating with individual programs. Except for the few programs in the NRMP Advanced Match, contact the programs directly.

Nuclear Medicine

ACGME-Approved Programs	56	AOA-Approved Programs	0
1st-Yr. Spots for M.D. Students	98	Funded Entry-Level D.O. Spots	0
Adv. Spots Avail. to M.D. Students	4	% IMG Residents	60
All Entry-Level M.D. Spots	102	Avg. Res. Work Hours/Week	47
% Women Residents	39	Programs with Childcare	16
Avg. Ratio of Full-Time Physician Faculty to Residents/Fellows	2.3	Programs offering a "Primary Care Track"	2
% Training in Hospital Outpatient Clinics	62	Programs offering Multiple Start Dates	23
% Training in Non-Hospital Community Ambulatory Clinics	10	Programs allowing Moonlighting	26

For more information, contact:

- American College of Nuclear Medicine, (703) 326-1190; www.acnmonline.org.
- SNM (Society of Nuclear Medicine), (703)708-9000; http:/interactive.snm.org.
- American Osteopathic Board of Nuclear Medicine, (800) 621-1773; www.aobnm.org.

Obstetrics And Gynecology ***

Specialty Overview: Obstetricians deal with pregnancy in women. Gynecologists deal with medical and surgical diseases of the female reproductive tract and with infertility. While some specialists in this field work primarily in one area or the other, most work in both Obstetrics and Gynecology. This is the only surgical specialty that is considered "Primary Care."

Obstetric practice has been greatly affected by the rising cost of medical liability insurance and the increasing propensity to sue physicians. Because of this, Obstetricians are, in increasing numbers, eliminating deliveries from their practices or reducing the provision of care for patients who have or are likely to have high-risk pregnancies. As the population ages and there is a greater awareness of women's health care needs, there will be a need for more Gynecologists.

The specialty combines both surgical and non-surgical approaches to disease, and is increasingly using endoscopic surgical techniques (minimally invasive surgery). The average Obstetrician-Gynecologist, in a 58-hour work week, spends about 50% of the time seeing patients in the office and 33% in surgery or in the delivery room.

The field of Obstetrics and Gynecology is primarily office-based, but frequently has a sizable inpatient load. A busy Obstetrics practice consists of considerable emergency and night call. An increasing number of women are entering this field. In general, the smaller the training program and the fewer patients they see, the less competitive it is. This field has experienced the greatest percentage increase in female residents over recent years; about 58% of residents in 1996 and 80% in 2009 were women.

Training: The basic training program in Obstetrics and Gynecology consists of four years of training following medical school. If Osteopathic graduates enter an Obstetrics/Gynecology "specialty-track" internship, their Obstetrics and Gynecology training time is shortened by one year. The malpractice climate has had an adverse effect on some training programs, leading to Obstetrics residents not being given an opportunity to exercise a level of responsibility appropriate to their level of training. (Along with General Surgeons, Obstetricians have the highest incidence of malpractice claims.) Following residency, physicians can take subspecialty fellowships in Reproductive Endocrinology (more commonly known as Infertility); Gynecologic Oncology, which requires extra surgical training; Maternal-Fetal Medicine, in which physicians treat the developing child *in utero*; and Female Pelvic Medicine and Reconstructive Surgery. The AAMC's Center for Workforce Studies projects a shortage of between 2,500 and 4,000 medical and gynecologic oncologists by 2020.

Match: In recent years, 100% of the available PGY-1 positions filled through the NRMP Match. Most positions in Gynecologic Oncology (39 programs), Maternal-Fetal Medicine (69 programs), and Reproductive Endocrinology (38 programs) go through the NRMP Obstetric/Gynecology Specialty Match, with rank lists due in early October and matching in late October the year before the July start date. Female Pelvic Medicine & Reconstructive Surgery (182 programs) applicants register with NRMP's FPRS Fellowship Match, overseen by the American Boards of OB-GYN and Urology.

Obstetrics and Gynecology

ACGME-Approved Programs	251	AOA-Approved Programs	31
1st-Yr. Spots for M.D. Students	1,240	Funded Entry-Level D.O. Spots	64
Adv. Spots Avail. to M.D. Students	0	% IMG Residents	24
All Entry-Level M.D. Spots	1,240	Avg. Res. Work Hours/Week	73
% Women Residents	76	Programs offering a "Primary	62
Avg. Ratio of Full-Time Physician Faculty to Residents	1.2	Care Track"	
		Programs offering Multiple Start Dates	20
% Training in Hospital Outpatient Clinics	29		
		Programs allowing Moonlighting	49
% Training in Non-Hospital Community Ambulatory Clinics	13	Programs offering a Women's Track	101
Programs with Childcare	98	Programs offering a Hospitalist Track	9

For more information, contact:

- American Congress of Obstetricians & Gynecologists, (202) 638-5577; www.acog.org.
- American College of Osteopathic Obstetricians & Gynecologists, (800) 875-6360; www.acoog.com.
- American Society for Reproductive Medicine, www.asrm.org.
- Association of Professors of Gynecology & Obstetrics, www.apgo.org.

Occupational Medicine *

Specialty Overview: Occupational Medicine, one of Preventive Medicine's specialties, focuses on the work environment's health effects and ways to protect workers. Residency training includes epidemiology and disease surveillance, toxicology, biostatistics, and health services administration. Occupational physicians investigate suspected clusters of work-related illness or outbreaks of environmental disease, evaluate injury causation, determine fitness for work, and apply health and safety regulations in the workplace. They also often direct preventive programs that promote worker health and reduce workplace hazards. Occupational physicians work in industry, teaching hospitals, government, or occupational health clinics. As the positions in industry decrease, private occupational health clinics have become a burgeoning area for those in the field. In these clinics, they often treat work-related injuries and evaluate patients with work-related disabilities. Specialists rarely take night call or have inpatient responsibilities.

Training: Training consists of two or three years following internship. Part of the time is used to get a graduate degree in an appropriate area, usually a Master of Public Health. To take the Board examination, a fourth year of training, teaching, practice, and/or research is required. Osteopathic physicians can specialize in Preventive Medicine–Occupational Medicine–Environmental Medicine.

Match: Contact individual programs directly.

Occupational Medicine

ACGME-Approved Programs	33	AOA-Approved Programs	0
1st-Yr. Spots for M.D. Students	0	Funded Entry-Level D.O. Spots	0
Adv. Spots Avail. to M.D. Students	0	% IMG Residents	n/a
All Entry-Level M.D. Spots	108	Programs offering Multiple Start Dates	15
Programs with Childcare	9		
Programs offering a "Primary Care Track"	6	Programs allowing Moonlighting	18

For more information, contact:

- American College of Occupational and Environmental Medicine, (847) 818-1800; www.acoem.org.
- American College of Preventive Medicine, (202) 466-2044; www.acpm.org.
- American Osteopathic College of Occupational and Preventive Medicine, (800) 558-8686; www.aocopm.org.

Ophthalmology *****

Specialty Overview: Ophthalmologists prevent, diagnose, and treat the diseases and abnormalities of the eye and periocular structures. A combination of office-based medical practice and surgical treatment of diseases makes this a popular specialty. Ophthalmologists treat patients of all ages, often using high-technology equipment in both diagnosis and therapy. Patients are usually seen as outpatients. Many Ophthalmologists take some night call, but they rarely have to go into the hospital after-hours. Inpatient services represent a small proportion of the care they deliver. With Optometrists performing many of the functions once reserved for Ophthalmologists, the field is rapidly becoming over-staffed; in recent years, the workforce has contracted. During the same period, however, women in practice and in training increased by 16% and 17%, respectively; the number of DOs in the field grew by 12%. Ophthalmologists average 52 hours per week doing patient care.

Training: The training consists of three years following an internship. Residency programs place great emphasis on high class standing and research experience. They try to officially limit each student to one "audition elective," but this has had varying success. Over the past decade, entering Ophthalmology has become slightly less difficult, although it remains a "difficult-to-enter" specialty.

Match: Matching is through the Ophthalmology Matching Program sponsored by the Association of University Professors of Ophthalmology and run by the San Francisco Matching Program, www.sfmatch.org. There is a non-refundable $100 registration fee. They also run the Centralized Application Service (CAS) for all civilian Ophthalmology applicants. Fellowship applicants for Neuro-Opthalmology and Ophthalmic Pathology subspecialties must register for the Match and contact those programs directly. Rank order lists for PGY-2 positions are submitted in December and matching occurs in January for positions beginning 18 months later. Individuals usually arrange their own internships through the NRMP PGY-1 Match. The Ophthalmology Matching Program also runs a Vacancy Information System, available through their website. In recent years, 73% of applicants matched.

Fellowship positions, except for Ophthalmic Plastic & Reconstructive Surgery (Oculoplastics), are offered through the Ophthalmology Fellowship Matching Program run by the San Francisco Matching Program. There is a non-refundable $275 fee. In recent years, the following percentage of positions were filled for these subspecialties: Cornea/External Disease, 92%; Glaucoma, 99%; Pediatric Ophthalmology, 82%; Retina, 92%; and Uveitis, 100%. The Fellowship Match is held in May, one year before the July starting date. Oculoplastic fellowships are matched through the NRMP Specialty Matching Program; fewer than half the applicants find a position.

Ophthalmology

ACGME-Approved Programs	118	AOA-Approved Programs	9
1st-Yr. Spots for M.D. Students	0	Funded Entry-Level D.O. Spots	11
Adv. Spots Avail. to M.D. Students	458	% IMG Residents	7
All Entry-Level M.D. Spots	458	Avg. Res. Work Hours/Week	52
% Women Residents	41	Programs with Childcare	35
Avg. Ratio of Full-Time Physician Faculty to Residents	2.0	Programs offering a "Primary Care Track"	9
% Training in Hospital Outpatient Clinics	89	Programs offering Multiple Start Dates	4
% Training in Non-Hospital Community Ambulatory Clinics	12	Programs allowing Moonlighting	28

For more information, contact:

- American Academy of Ophthalmology, (415) 561-8500; www.aao.org.
- American Osteopathic Colleges of Ophthalmology, (800) 455-9404; www.aocoohns.org.

Orthopedic Surgery *****

Specialty Overview: Orthopedic Surgeons treat diseases and injuries of the spine, pelvic bones and extremities. Using surgery, medications, and physical therapy, their goal is to preserve maximal function of the musculoskeletal system. Much Orthopedic Surgery that was once performed on an inpatient basis is now done as ambulatory surgery. Individuals who like to work with their hands go into this specialty. Many have hobbies such as woodworking that emphasize this, and the majority are sports-oriented. Many Orthopedic Surgeons take night and emergency call during their entire career.

Orthopedic Surgeons average 61 hours per week doing patient care. Among subspecialists, Adult Reconstructive Orthopedic Surgeons average 53 hours per week doing patient care; Orthopedic Spinal Surgeons, 53 hours; Orthopedic Sports Medicine physicians, 55 hours; and Pediatric Orthopedic Surgeons, 56 hours. In recent years, Orthopedic Surgery trainees increased only slightly, by 5%, while the number of female and IMG trainees grew by 33% and 11%, respectively.

Training: Training consists of one year in a broad medical specialty followed by four years of Orthopedics. Orthopedic Surgery is one of the most competitive specialties. Programs look for high USMLE scores, research experience, election to AOA (honorary), and successful "audition clerkships." Both subspecialty training and certification are available in Hand Surgery (*see* Hand Surgery). One-year fellowship positions also exist in Musculoskeletal Oncology (10 programs), Adult Reconstructive Orthopedics (21 programs), Foot and Ankle Orthopedics (10 programs), Orthopedic Sports Medicine (*see* Sports Medicine), Pediatric Orthopedics (23 programs), Orthopedic Trauma (10 programs), and Orthopedic Surgery of the Spine (16 programs).

Match: In recent years, virtually all of the available PGY-1 positions filled through the NRMP Match. Orthopedic fellowship positions are arranged individually with most training programs. Orthopedic Hand Surgery uses the NRMP's Combined Musculoskeletal Match, while Spine Surgery goes through the San Francisco Matching Program. In recent years, 83% of applicants matched.

Orthopedic Surgery

ACGME-Approved Programs	161	AOA-Approved Programs	30
1st-Yr. Spots for M.D. Students	682	Funded Entry-Level D.O. Spots	85
Adv. Spots Avail. to M.D. Students	51	% IMG Residents	3
All Entry-Level M.D. Spots	733	Avg. Res. Work Hours/Week	71
% Women Residents	12	Programs with Childcare	52
Avg. Ratio of Full-Time Physician Faculty to Residents	0.8	Programs offering a "Primary Care Track"	8
% Training in Hospital Outpatient Clinics	33	Programs offering Multiple Start Dates	6
% Training in Non-Hospital Community Ambulatory Clinics	13	Programs allowing Moonlighting	34

Adult Reconstructive Orthopedics (F)

ACGME-Approved Programs	21	AOA-Approved Programs	0
1st-Yr. Spots for M.D. Students	0	Funded Entry-Level D.O. Spots	0
Adv. Spots Avail. to M.D. Students	0	% IMG Residents	38
All Entry-Level M.D. Spots	36	Avg. Res. Work Hours/Week	53
% Women Residents	0	% Training in Hospital Outpatient Clinics	38
Avg. Ratio of Full-Time Physician Faculty to Fellows	2.4		
		% Training in Non-Hospital Community Ambulatory Clinics	20

Musculoskeletal Oncology (F)

ACGME-Approved Programs	10	AOA-Approved Programs	0
1st-Yr. Spots for M.D. Students	0	Funded Entry-Level D.O. Spots	0
Adv. Spots Avail. to M.D. Students	0	% IMG Residents	21
All Entry-Level M.D. Spots	14	Avg. Res. Work Hours/Week	54
% Women Residents	21	% Training in Non-Hospital Community Ambulatory Clinics	1
Avg. Ratio of Full-Time Physician Faculty to Fellows	2.3		
% Training in Hospital Outpatient Clinics	26		

Orthopedic Spine Surgery (F)

ACGME-Approved Programs	16	AOA-Approved Programs	0
1st-Yr. Spots for M.D. Students	0	Funded Entry-Level D.O. Spots	0
Adv. Spots Avail. to M.D. Students	0	% IMG Residents	25
All Entry-Level M.D. Spots	27	Avg. Res. Work Hours/Week	54
% Women Residents	12	% Training in Non-Hospital Community Ambulatory Clinics	30
Avg. Ratio of Full-Time Physician Faculty to Fellows	5.0	Programs offering Multiple Start Dates	2
% Training in Hospital Outpatient Clinics	25		

Pediatric Orthopedics (F)

ACGME-Approved Programs	23	AOA-Approved Programs	0
1st-Yr. Spots for M.D. Students	0	Funded Entry-Level D.O. Spots	0
Adv. Spots Avail. to M.D. Students	0	% IMG Residents	19
All Entry-Level M.D. Spots	33	Avg. Res. Work Hours/Week	42
% Women Residents	19	% Training in Non-Hospital Community Ambulatory Clinics	12
Avg. Ratio of Full-Time Physician Faculty to Fellows	5.1	Programs offering Multiple Start Dates	4
% Training in Hospital Outpatient Clinics	42		

For more information, contact:

- American Academy of Orthopaedic Surgeons, (847) 823-7186; www.aaos.org.
- American Osteopathic Academy of Orthopedics, (800) 741-2626; www.aoao.org.

Otolaryngology *****

Specialty Overview: Otolaryngologists, or Head and Neck Surgeons, specialize in the evaluation and treatment of medical and surgical problems of the head and neck region, including disorders of the ears, upper respiratory tract, and upper GI tract. The specialty is frequently referred to as ENT (Ear, Nose, & Throat). Practitioners have substantial office practices with varying amounts of surgery, which is mostly performed in an ambulatory setting. Most practitioners have few inpatients. Since managed care organizations have targeted some of this specialty's common procedures, such as tympanotomies, for decreased use, the field may become over-staffed. Otolaryngological Surgery has experienced relatively flat growth in recent years, and a decline in trainees. Women in training, however, grew by 45%, and by 25% in practice over the past several years, while IMG trainees increased by 46%—but declined in practice by 15%. Otolaryngologists spend an average 52 hours per week doing patient care.

Training: Training consists of one or two years of General Surgery followed by three or four years of ENT training. Two-year fellowships and certification are available in Laryngology (24 programs), Neurotology (9 programs), Pediatric Otolaryngology (22 programs). Additional fellowships are available in Facial Plastic & Reconstructive Surgery (42 programs) and in Head & Neck Cancer Surgery. About 25% of all residency graduates take additional fellowship training.

Most Osteopathic physicians train in the combined specialty of Otolaryngology/Facial Plastic Surgery. One approved program exists for D.O.s in Otolaryngic Allergy. Osteopathic residents who take a "specialty-track" internship in the specialty can shorten their training by one year.

Match: All ENT programs go through the NRMP Match. Internship positions are obtained through the NRMP PGY-1 Match. In recent years, nearly 99% of applicants matched. The Pediatric Otolaryngology, Neurotology, and Facial Plastic & Reconstructive Surgery subspecialty fellowships use the San Francisco Matching Program, www.sfmatch.org; there is a $50 application fee, and applicants should contact programs directly.

Otolaryngology

ACGME-Approved Programs	107	AOA-Approved Programs	0
1st-Yr. Spots for M.D. Students	285	Funded Entry-Level D.O. Spots	0
Adv. Spots Avail. to M.D. Students	0	% IMG Residents	3
All Entry-Level M.D. Spots	285	Avg. Res. Work Hours/Week	67
% Women Residents	29	Programs with Childcare	40
Avg. Ratio of Full-Time Physician Faculty to Residents	1.2	Programs offering a "Primary Care Track"	6
% Training in Hospital Outpatient Clinics	40	Programs offering Multiple Start Dates	2
% Training in Non-Hospital Community Ambulatory Clinics	10	Programs allowing Moonlighting	19

Otolaryngology/Facial Plastic Surgery (D.O.s only)

AOA-Approved Programs	18	Funded entry-level D.O. positions	16

For more information, contact:

- American Academy of Otolaryngology–Head and Neck Surgery, (703) 836-4444; www.entnet.org.
- American Osteopathic Colleges of Ophthalmology, (800) 455-9404; www.aocoohns.org.
- American Laryngological Association, (615) 509-5525; www.alahns.org.

Pain Medicine (F) *

Specialty Overview: Pain Medicine, previously called "Pain Management," is concerned with the study of pain, the prevention of pain, and the evaluation, treatment, and rehabilitation of persons with acute, chronic or cancer pain. A Pain Medicine physician serves as a consultant to other physicians but is often the principal treating physician. In recognition that pain control is an integral component of patient care, all ACGME-accredited Pain Medicine programs in the specialties of Anesthesiology, Neurology, Physical Medicine & Rehabilitation, and Psychiatry were combined into a multidisciplinary Pain Medicine subspecialty in 2007. Specialists work in hospitals and independent pain control clinics, and use a variety of pain management techniques. Pain Medicine practitioners average 55 hours per week doing patient care.

   Training: Pain Medicine fellowships are one year following the completion of a core residency in one of the sponsoring specialties.

   Match: Contact programs directly. They are listed in *FREIDA*.

Pain Medicine

ACGME-Approved Programs	94	AOA-Approved Programs	1
1st-Yr. Spots for M.D. Students	0	Funded Entry-Level D.O. Spots	1
Adv. Spots Avail. to M.D. Students	0	% IMG Residents	22
All Entry-Level M.D. Spots	312	Avg. Res. Work Hours/Week	45
% Women Residents	20	% Training in Non-Hospital Community Ambulatory Clinics	7
Avg. Ratio of Full-Time Physician Faculty to Fellows	2.6	Programs offering Multiple Start Dates	7
% Training in Hospital Outpatient Clinics	77		

For more information, contact:

* American Academy of Pain Medicine, (847) 375-4731; www.painmed.org.
* American College of Osteopathic Pain Management & Sclerotherapy, Inc., (302) 376-8080; www.acopms.com.

Pathology *

Specialty Overview: Pathologists are laboratory-based physicians who are often said to be the "doctor's doctor." They act as consultants for other physicians, helping them to determine the nature of disease in tissue, body fluids, or the entire organism. They apply the methods of the basic sciences to the detection of disease, but generally have little or no direct contact with (live) patients; they interact with other physicians. Pathologists' lives are generally low-key and there is little or no in-hospital night call.

The field is divided into the areas of *Anatomic Pathology*, i.e., autopsies, Cytopathology, and Surgical Pathology (gross and microscopic pathology); and *Clinical Pathology*, i.e., Hematology, Microbiology, Clinical Chemistry, and Blood Banking/Transfusion Medicine. Eighty percent of Pathologists, especially Anatomic Pathologists, are hospital-based. About 15% of Pathologists also function as researchers and teachers in university medical centers or medical schools—frequently while also maintaining an active Pathology practice. In the past, the income has been very generous, especially for Clinical Pathology. However, changes in reimbursement have decreased Pathologists' income. Pathologists average 44 hours per week doing clinical work. Among subspecialists, Blood Banking/Transfusion Pathologists average 40 hours per week, Cytopathologists average 44 hours per week, and Forensic Pathologists average 47 hours per week doing clinical work. The number of physicians going into Pathology has only increased 13% in the past 15 years.

Training: A residency can be taken separately in either Clinical Pathology or Anatomic Pathology (three years), or the two can be combined (four years). A "credentialing year," usually taken before beginning a Pathology residency, is required prior to taking the Board examination. It can consist of a clinical year, clinical experience, or clinically related research. Subspecialty training following the initial residency is available in Neuropathology (33 programs), which requires two years; and in Forensic Pathology (37 programs), Dermatopathology (*see* Dermatology), Blood Banking/Transfusion Medicine (46 programs), Chemical Pathology (2 programs), Pediatric Pathology (22 programs), Hematology (*see* Hematology), Selective Pathology (57 programs), Cytopathology (87 programs), or Medical Microbiology (12 programs), each requiring one year. Ninety percent of current pathology residents intend to apply for fellowship training.

Match: In recent years, about 96% of the available PGY-1 positions filled through the NRMP Match; 14% were filled by foreign graduates. For subspecialty positions, contact the programs directly.

Pathology, Anatomic & Clinical

ACGME-Approved Programs	148	AOA-Approved Programs	0
1st-Yr. Spots for M.D. Students	521	Funded Entry-Level D.O. Spots	0
Adv. Spots Avail. to M.D. Students	0	% IMG Residents	35
All Entry-Level M.D. Spots	521	Avg. Res. Work Hours/Week	50
% Women Residents	53	Programs offering a "Primary Care Track"	5
Avg. Ratio of Full-Time Physician Faculty to Residents	1.7		
% Training in Hospital Outpatient Clinics	9	Programs offering Multiple Start Dates	56
		Programs allowing Moonlighting	64
% Training in Non-Hospital Community Ambulatory Clinics	6	Programs offering a Women's Track	5
Programs with Childcare	67		

For more information, contact:

- American Osteopathic College of Pathologists, (312) 202-8197; www.doaocp.org.
- American Society of Clinical Pathologists, (800) 267-2727; www.ascp.org.
- College of American Pathologists, (800) 323-4040; www.cap.org.
- InterSociety Council for Pathology Information, (301) 634-7200; www.pathologytraining.org.

Pediatric Surgery (F) *****

Specialty Overview: Pediatric Surgeons diagnose and treat surgical diseases in children. Depending upon their training, they deal with abdominal, urologic, and thoracic problems, as well as multiple trauma. Because a high volume of patients is needed to support such a specialized practice, most Pediatric Surgeons live in moderate- or large-size cities, and are associated with major medical centers. Since this is a subspecialty of General Surgery, applicants must first complete a General Surgery residency. In recent years, the number of Pediatric General and subspecialty surgeon trainees increased by 35% and 15% respectively. Pediatric Surgeons work very hard, averaging 73 hours per week doing patient care.

Training: Training in Pediatric Surgery is two years in length.

Match: Almost all programs use the NRMP Pediatric Surgery Fellowship Match. In recent years, nearly 100% of the available positions filled, but only 51% of applicants matched. Rank-order lists are due in April; results are available in May, 14 months before the July starting date.

Other Useful Information: Fellowship directors look for individuals who work well with others, do well in interviews, and have been favorably recommended by practicing Pediatric Surgeons who the directors know. In recent years, the number of women in Pediatric Surgical Specialties grew by 36%, versus a 20% growth in Pediatric General Surgery. The number of IMGs in Pediatric Surgical Specialties rose by 29%, while their numbers declined by 12% for Pediatric General Surgery.

Pediatric Surgery

ACGME-Approved Programs	35	AOA-Approved Programs	0
1st-Yr. Spots for M.D. Students	0	Funded Entry-Level D.O. Spots	0
Adv. Spots Avail. to M.D. Students	0	% IMG Residents	6
All Entry-Level M.D. Spots	35	Avg. Res. Work Hours/Week	74
% Women Residents	29	% Training in Non-Hospital Community Ambulatory Clinics	13
Avg. Ratio of Full-Time Physician Faculty to Fellows	4.1		
% Training in Hospital Outpatient Clinics	16		

For more information, contact:

• American Pediatric Surgical Association, (847) 480-9576; www.eapsa.org.

Pediatrics * to ***

Specialty Overview: Pediatricians take care of pediatric patients. While that may sound circular, it is the only way to describe many Pediatric practices. Pediatricians may at one time have dealt primarily with children, but they have now expanded the scope of their practice to include adolescents and young adults. In some cases, Pediatricians continue to care for their patients into adulthood, especially those with illnesses like cystic fibrosis that used to be uniformly fatal during childhood. Pediatricians do a great deal of well-child and preventive care. More recently, they are being asked to fill the often uncomfortable role of "gatekeeper" or "case manager" for prepaid health plans. In this position, they determine their patients' access to care.

Progressively fewer Pediatricians are opting for solo private practice, with two-thirds working in group practices. Much of the intensive exposure to ill children seen by residents and medical students during their training does not exist for the practicing General Pediatrician. Office-based for the most part, Pediatricians rarely utilize surgical techniques such as suturing or fracture reduction. The average Pediatrician, in a 50-hour work week, spends more than half of the time on office visits and the rest on non-clinical care activities, hospital rounds, and additional clinical activities. Pediatrics is one of the lowest paying medical specialties. Most Pediatricians choose this field because they love working with children. The field has grown 68% in the past 15 years, in part because the number of subspecialty fellowships increased by 56%. Except for neonatology, however, every pediatric specialty was experiencing shortages in 2010. More women and fewer IMGs are entering this field than in previous years.

Training: Initial Pediatric residency training is three years. The *NRMP Directory* lists 65 positions as "Pediatrics–Primary." These positions are integrated into normal Pediatric programs, but offer slightly more outpatient and continuity clinic experience. Graduates of both types of programs take the same Board examination. There are also four-year residencies combining Pediatrics with Internal Medicine. Some five-year programs combine Pediatrics with Dermatology, Emergency Medicine, Psychiatry/Child Psychiatry, Medical Genetics, or Physical Medicine & Rehabilitation. (*See* listings under Internal Medicine, Emergency Medicine, and Child/Adolescent Psychiatry for additional information.) Osteopathic residents who take a "specialty-track" internship in Pediatrics can shorten their training by one year.

Following initial Pediatric residency training, more than one-third of all graduates specialize. Subspecialty training (each is two to three years long) following the initial residency is available in: Developmental & Behavioral Pediatrics (37 programs), Neonatal–Perinatal Medicine (97 programs), Pediatric Cardiology (50 programs), Pediatric Critical Care Medicine (60 programs), Pediatric Emergency Medicine (48 programs), Pediatric Endocrinology (67 programs), Pediatric Gastroenterology (54 programs), Pediatric Hematology–Oncology (68 programs), Pediatric Nephrology (39 programs), Pediatric Pulmonology (48 programs), and Sports Medicine (9 programs).

Fellowships are also possible in Adolescent Medicine (26 programs), Pediatric Dermatology (15 programs), Pediatric Transplant Hepatology (4 programs), Pediatric Infectious Diseases (62 programs), and Pediatric Rheumatology (28 programs). Child Neurology (69 programs; *see* "Child Neurology") training can be started after two years of a Pediatrics residency.

Match: In recent years, about 98% of the available PGY-1 positions filled through the NRMP Match; about 12% of the positions were filled by international medical graduates. Fellowships in Developmental & Behavioral Pediatrics, Pediatric Critical Care Medicine, Pediatric Emergency Medicine, and Pediatric Rheumatology go through the NRMP Pediatric Specialties Fall Match, with Match results announced in December. Fellowships in Pediatric Cardiology, Pediatric Gastroenterology, Pediatric Nephrology and Pediatric Pulmonology go through the NRMP Pediatric Specialties Spring Match with Match results announced in June. Pediatric Hematology–Oncology goes through the NRMP Specialty Match with Match results announced in May.

Pediatrics (C) ***; (P) ***; (Primary) *

ACGME-Approved Programs	190	AOA-Approved Programs	15
1st-Yr. Spots for M.D. Students	2,475	Funded Entry-Level D.O. Spots	62
Adv. Spots Avail. to M.D. Students	0	% IMG Residents	24
All Entry-Level M.D. Spots	2,475	Avg. Res. Work Hours/Week	67
% Women Residents	72	Programs offering a "Primary	57
Avg. Ratio of Full-Time Physician Faculty to Residents	2.2	Care Track"	
		Programs offering Multiple Start	49
% Training in Hospital Outpatient Clinics	35	Dates	
		Programs allowing Moonlighting	119
% Training in Non-Hospital Community Ambulatory Clinics	12	Programs offering a Hospitalist Track	7
Programs with Childcare	80		

For more information, contact:

- American Academy of Pediatrics, (847) 434-4000; www.aap.org.
- American College of Osteopathic Pediatricians, www.acopeds.org.

Physical Medicine And Rehabilitation **

Specialty Overview: Physiatrists (specialists in Physical Medicine & Rehabilitation, or PM&R) deal with the diagnosis, evaluation, and treatment of patients with impairments or disabilities that involve musculoskeletal, neurologic, cardiovascular, or other body systems. Physiatrists diagnose and treat patients of all ages with: (1) musculoskeletal pain syndromes, industrial and sports injuries, degenerative arthritis, or lower back pain; and (2) severe impairments amenable to rehabilitation from strokes, spinal cord and brain injuries, amputations, and multiple trauma. They perform electrodiagnosis (i.e., EMG, nerve conduction, somatosensory evoked potentials). The Physiatrist's goal is to maximize the patient's physical, psychosocial, and job-related recovery, as well as to alleviate pain. Depending upon their practice, they may have frequent or no night call. Physiatrists average 48 hours per week doing patient care. Many more PM&R positions are available than there are residency graduates to fill them.

Training: Residency training is four years. This can be either three years following at least one year of prior training or a straight four-year program. Program details are listed on *FREIDA*. There is one combined program in Pediatrics–PM&R (6 programs). Following residency, fellowship training is available in Hospice & Palliative Medicine (8 programs); Musculoskeletal Rehabilitation (53 programs); Neuromuscular Medicine (7 programs); Pediatric Rehabilitation Medicine (15 programs); Spine Rehabilitation Medicine (47 ·

programs); Spinal Cord Injury Medicine (19 programs); EMG (8 programs); Brain Injury Rehabilitation (8 programs); Informatics (9 programs); Research (11 programs); Sports Medicine (47 programs); and Pain Medicine (40 programs). (In 2007, all ACGME-accredited pain medicine programs under Anesthesiology, Neurology, Physical Medicine & Rehabilitation, and Psychiatry were combined into a multidisciplinary Pain Medicine subspecialty.)

Osteopathic physicians can also take training in Neuromuscular Medicine or take an extra year ("+1") of Osteopathic Manipulative Medicine (OMM) after an AOA-approved residency. Many D.O.s with advanced training in these techniques have the "problem" of too many patients seeking their services. Some programs allow M.D.s to apply.

Match: In recent years, about 95% of the available PGY-1 positions filled through the NRMP Match. Of the PGY-2 positions available through the NRMP Match, about 97% filled.

Physical Medicine & Rehabilitation

ACGME-Approved Programs	26	AOA-Approved Programs	3
1st-Yr. Spots for M.D. Students	86	Funded Entry-Level D.O. Spots	5
Adv. Spots Avail. to M.D. Students	281	% IMG Residents	20
All Entry-Level M.D. Spots	367	Avg. Res. Work Hours/Week	54
% Women Residents	40	Programs with Childcare	28
Avg. Ratio of Full-Time Physician Faculty to Residents	1.1	Programs offering a "Primary Care Track"	3
% Training in Hospital Outpatient Clinics	27	Programs offering Multiple Start Dates	11
% Training in Non-Hospital Community Ambulatory Clinics	12	Programs allowing Moonlighting	41

Family Practice-OMM (D.O. only)

AOA-Approved Programs	7	Funded Entry-Level D.O. Spots	23

Neuromuscular Medicine (D.O. only)

AOA-Approved Programs	15	Funded Entry-Level D.O. Spots	43

For more information, contact:

- American Academy of Physical Medicine & Rehabilitation, (847) 737-6000; www.aapmr.org.
- American Osteopathic Board of Neuromusculoskeletal Medicine; (317) 879-1881; aobnmm.org.
- American Osteopathic College of Physical Medicine and Rehabilitation, (908) 329-0270; www.aocpmr.org.
- Association of Academic Physiatrists, (410) 712-7120; www.physiatry.org.

Plastic Surgery (I) (F) *****

Specialty Overview: Plastic Surgeons operatively treat disfigurements of the body, whether they are congenital, traumatically induced, or caused by aging. This area of Surgery is as much an art as a science, and an artist's vision is said to be necessary to excel in the field. Microsurgery and liposuction are two of the field's newer techniques. There is a large amount of night call to the emergency room, especially early in a practitioner's career. Much of Plastic Surgery is done on an ambulatory basis. While the number of plastic surgeons grew slightly in recent years by about 5%, the number of applicants declined 8%. Women in Plastic Surgery, however, increased in both practice (25%) and training (15%). Plastic Surgeons average 52 hours per week doing patient care.

Training: Plastic Surgery offers two routes for training as of 2010. The "integrated" route is aimed at senior medical students who match at the PGY-1 level. These programs, which use the NRMP Match and Electronic Residency Application Service (ERAS), accept medical students into six-year Plastic Surgery programs. The "independent" route is for those who first complete at least three years in a General Surgery program; complete a Neurological Surgery, Otolaryngology, Orthopedic Surgery, or Urology residency; or complete a program in Oral and Maxillofacial Surgery. They then have at least two, and often three, years of Plastic Surgery training. These "independent" programs use the San Francisco Match and the Centralized Application Service (CAS).

Applicants must ascertain the minimum requirements by contacting each program and obtaining the "Resident Registration and Evaluation of Training" form from the American Board of Plastic Surgery (www.abplsurg.org). This form must be completed prior to applying for residencies. Individuals with more training have a better chance of getting a position. Applicants should visit the website of the Association of Academic Chairmen of Plastic Surgery for more details.

Postgraduate fellowships and certification are available in Hand Surgery (13 programs). Additional training in Plastic Surgery and fellowships in Craniofacial Surgery (5 programs), Microsurgery (31 programs), and Burn Surgery are also available following completion of the primary Plastic Surgery residency. Osteopathic physicians can also train in Otolaryngology/Facial Plastic Surgery (*see* Otolaryngology).

Match: About 33% of entry-level positions are available to medical students through the NRMP Match. The rest, 51 programs and 101 positions, with a 73% match rate in recent years, are reserved for residents already in or about to complete their surgical training, and are available through the Plastic Surgery Residency Match, www.sfmatch.org.

Plastic Surgery

ACGME-Approved Programs	57	Funded Entry-Level D.O. Spots	5
1st-Yr. Spots for M.D. Students	101	% IMG Residents	5
Adv. Spots Avail. to M.D. Students	20	Avg. Res. Work Hours/Week	64
All Entry-Level M.D. Spots	221	Programs with Childcare	27
% Women Residents	23	Programs offering a "Primary Care Track"	4
Avg. Ratio of Full-Time Physician Faculty to Residents/Fellows	1.6		
% Training in Hospital Outpatient Clinics	17	Programs offering Multiple Start Dates	1
		Programs allowing Moonlighting	8
% Training in Non-Hospital Community Ambulatory Clinics	6	Programs offering a Hospitalist Track	3
AOA-Approved Programs	2		

For more information, contact:

- American Academy of Facial & Reconstructive Surgery, (703) 229-9291; www.aafprs.org.
- American College of Osteopathic Surgeons, (800) 888-1312; www.facos.org.
- American Society of Plastic Surgeons, (847) 228-9900; www.plasticsurgery.org.
- Association of Academic Chairmen of Plastic Surgery, (800) 526-9884; www.aacplasticsurgery.org.

Preventive Medicine, General *

Specialty Overview: Preventive Medicine requires entry through one of its three subspecialties: Public Health & General Preventive Medicine, Aerospace Medicine, and Occupational Medicine. Physicians in this field are committed to population-based approaches to disease prevention and health promotion. Training includes both clinical preventive medicine and education in epidemiology, biostatistics, informatics, environmental health, health promotion and disease prevention, and research. These physicians work in primary care settings, managed care organizations, public health, government agencies, industry, and academia.

In some cases, Family Medicine programs have made arrangements so that training in both specialties can take place concurrently. Two subspecialty certifications are available: Medical Toxicology (2 programs) and Undersea & Hyperbaric Medicine (1 program). Preventive Medicine specialists average 53 hours per week in clinical work.

Training: At least one year of clinical training and a Master of Public Health or equivalent degree are required to complete the program and to be eligible to take the specialty examination. Recently, the ACGME proposed that Preventive Medicine no longer require a Master of Public Health degree, but rather require a minimum of 24 months in the core Preventive Medicine residency program. This would, presumably, include much of the didactic material now taught in the MPH course.

Match: Few General Preventive Medicine programs participate in the NRMP Match. Most physicians begin the two-year programs after some other clinical training. Applicants can usually make arrangements with individual programs to begin at the PGY-2 level. The intern year is obtained through the NRMP PGY-1 Match.

Preventive Medicine, General

ACGME-Approved Programs	71	AOA-Approved Programs	0
1st-Yr. Spots for M.D. Students	4	Funded Entry-Level D.O. Spots	0
Adv. Spots Avail. to M.D. Students	1	% IMG Residents	214
All Entry-Level M.D. Spots	284	Avg. Res. Work Hours/Week	42
% Women Residents	46	% Training in Non-Hospital Community Ambulatory Clinics	28
Avg. Ratio of Full-Time Physician Faculty to Residents/Fellows	2.8	Programs offering Multiple Start Dates	12
% Training in Hospital Outpatient Clinics	12	Programs With Childcare	9
		Programs allowing Moonlighting	14

For more information, contact:

- American College of Preventive Medicine, (202) 466-2044; www.acpm.org.
- American Osteopathic College of Occupational & Preventive Medicine, (800) 558-8686; www.aocopm.org.

Psychiatry *

Specialty Overview: Psychiatrists diagnose and treat disorders of the mind. They deal with the entire spectrum of mental illness, from mild situational problems to severe, incapacitating psychotic illnesses. Psychiatrists practice in a variety of settings, including private offices, community mental health centers, psychiatric hospitals, prisons, and substance abuse programs. The majority are office- rather than hospital-based. While there may be night call, it is easier than it might otherwise be, since many Psychiatrists use other health care workers to screen their calls for them. The wide diversity of new potent psychotropic medications has given the Psychiatrist a powerful pharmacological armamentarium.

As of 2012, the demand for psychiatrists is rising faster than any other medical specialty, and it is the third most heavily recruited for jobs after Family

Physicians and Internists. Yet, the shortage of psychiatrists is projected to increase as the aging workforce retires. Fewer than 5% of medical students choose to specialize in Psychiatry, due in part to lower earnings despite spending the same amount of time in training as procedural-based specialties. Those who go into Psychiatry do so because of the intellectual challenge, a desire to return to a humanities/social science background, their patients' novel and unique problems, or because they want to treat the "whole person." Psychiatrists average 47 hours per week doing patient care.

Training: Training is three years following a clinical internship that is usually very similar in structure to a Transitional year. The residency consists not only of training in Psychiatry, but also a significant amount in Neurology. Subspecialty fellowships and certification are available in Addiction Psychiatry (44 programs), Forensic Psychiatry (42 programs), Geriatric Psychiatry (58 programs), and Psychosomatic Medicine (46 programs). Fifteen programs combine Psychiatry with Internal Medicine, nine combine Psychiatry with Family Medicine, and eight combine Neurology and Psychiatry.

Fellowships exist in Child & Adolescent Psychiatry (124 programs—*see* separate listing, above) for both M.D.s and D.O.s, and consist of a minimum of three years of Child & Adolescent Psychiatry in addition to at least two years (following internship) of general Psychiatry. The Child & Adolescent Psychiatry training can start any time after the internship year. There are also ten programs with five years of training that combine Pediatrics, Psychiatry, and Child Psychiatry. All subspecialty programs are listed in *FREIDA*.

Match: In recent years, almost 100% of the available PGY-1 positions filled through the NRMP Match; about 24% of the positions were filled by foreign medical graduates.

Psychiatry (C) *

ACGME-Approved Programs	189	AOA-Approved Programs	4
1st-Yr. Spots for M.D. Students	1,118	Funded Entry-Level D.O. Spots	7
Adv. Spots Avail. to M.D. Students	3	% IMG Residents	31
All Entry-Level M.D. Spots	1,121	Avg. Res. Work Hours/Week	55
% Women Residents	54	Programs with Childcare	59
Avg. Ratio of Full-Time Physician Faculty to Residents	1.0	Programs offering a "Primary Care Track"	17
% Training in Hospital Outpatient Clinics	10	Programs offering Multiple Start Dates	65
% Training in Non-Hospital Community Ambulatory Clinics	3	Programs allowing Moonlighting	112

For more information, contact:

- American College of Osteopathic Neurologists and Psychiatrists, 28595 Orchard Lake Rd., Ste. 200, Farmington Hills, MI 48334; (248) 553-0010, ext. 295.
- American Psychiatric Association, (703) 907-7300; www.psych.org.
- American Society of Addiction Medicine; www.asam.org.
- American Academy of Child & Adolescent Psychiatry, (202) 966-7300; www.aacap.org.

Public Health *

Specialty Overview: Specialists in Public Health, an area of Preventive Medicine, deal with health promotion and disease prevention. They work in governmental and private health agencies, academic institutions, and health service research organizations. They deal with the health problems of entire communities and countries, as well as with those of individual patients. Their goals are to promote health and to understand the risks of disease, injury, disability, and death. They (1) assess information about the community's health, (2) develop comprehensive public health policies, and (3) assure the provision of services necessary to achieve the public health goals. This frequently involves dealing with the administrative and political sides of medicine. This specialty usually has no night call and very low (usually government) pay. The dearth of residency programs (a number have closed due to lack of funding) has made these specialists some of the most sought-after in medicine, although still among the worst paid.

Training: Training in Public Health consists of two years following a clinical internship. One of these years is spent obtaining an advanced degree, usually a Master of Public Health. A fourth year of training, teaching, practice, and/or research is required to take the Board examination. Some programs in Family Medicine, Internal Medicine, and Pediatrics have dual training with various Preventive Medicine specialties, including Public Health.

Match: For the most part, there is no matching program in Public Health. Applications must be made to the individual programs. Students can arrange to begin a program following a clinical year, which should be obtained through the NRMP PGY-1 Match.

Public Health

ACGME-Approved Programs	17	AOA-Approved Programs	1
1st-Yr. Spots for M.D. Students	0	Funded Entry-Level D.O. Spots	3
Adv. Spots Avail. to M.D. Students	0	% IMG Residents	n/a
All Entry-Level M.D. Spots	64	Avg. Res. Work Hours/Week	n/a
% Women Residents	n/a	Programs offering Multiple Start	4
Programs with Childcare	2	Dates	
Programs offering a "Primary Care Track"	2	Programs allowing Moonlighting	4

For more information, contact:

- American Association of Public Health Physicians, (773) 632-4400; www.aaphp.org.
- American College of Preventive Medicine, (202) 466-2044; www.acpm.org.
- American Osteopathic College of Occupational and Preventive Medicine, (800) 558-8686; www.aocopm.org.

Pulmonary Disease (F) *

Specialty Overview: Pulmonologists diagnose and treat patients with diseases of the lungs, in both the in- and out-patient settings. They deal most often with patients having lung cancer, asthma, and many types of chronic lung disease. Pulmonologists, because of their background, often act as full- or part-time Critical Care physicians. The specialty combines patient care and the performance of manipulative procedures with a deep knowledge of cardiopulmonary physiology. Procedures include: bronchoscopy, endotracheal intubation, management of mechanical ventilators, and placement of pulmonary artery catheters. Night call depends upon the type of practice. Pulmonologists average 51 hours per week (Internists) and 33 hours per week (Pediatricians) doing patient care. Pulmonary Disease Critical Care physicians average 55 hours per week doing patient care.

Training: Training consists of a two- or three-year fellowship following completion of an Internal Medicine residency or three years following a Pediatric residency. Many adult three-year programs fulfill the requirements for certification in Critical Care as well as Pulmonary Disease (*see* Critical Care for details). For Osteopathic physicians, training follows internship and two years of an Internal Medicine residency.

Match: Eighty percent of Pediatric Critical Care fellowship programs use the NRMP Pediatric Specialties Fall Match, with Match results announced in December, and just over half of the Internal Medicine Pulmonary Disease programs use the NRMP Medical Specialties Matching Program. Virtually all

Internal Medicine programs and positions, and most Pediatric Critical Care positions, are in the Match. Rank order lists are due and results of the Match are released in June, one year prior to the start of the program. Applicants for Pediatric Pulmonology training go through the NRMP Pediatric Specialties Spring Match with nearly 80% of programs participating, and 76% of positions filled.

Pulmonary Disease (Internal Medicine)

ACGME-Approved Programs	21	AOA-Approved Programs	2
1st-Yr. Spots for M.D. Students	0	Funded Entry-Level D.O. Spots	3
Adv. Spots Avail. to M.D. Students	0	% IMG Residents	87
All Entry-Level M.D. Spots	117	Avg. Res. Work Hours/Week	50
% Women Residents	29	% Training in Non-Hospital Community Ambulatory Clinics	9
Avg. Ratio of Full-Time Physician Faculty to Fellows	1.9		
% Training In Hospital Outpatient Clinics	20	Programs offering a "Primary Care Track"	2
		Programs offering Multiple Start Dates	3

Pediatric Pulmonology**

ACGME-Approved Programs	48	AOA-Approved Programs	0
1st-Yr. Spots for M.D. Students	0	Funded Entry-Level D.O. Spots	0
Adv. Spots Avail. to M.D. Students	0	% IMG Residents	45
All Entry-Level M.D. Spots	60	Avg. Res. Work Hours/Week	47
% Women Residents	49	% Training in Non-Hospital Community Ambulatory Clinics	3
Avg. Ratio of Full-Time Physician Faculty to Fellows	3.2		
% Training in Hospital Outpatient Clinics	25	Programs offering Multiple Start Dates	26

For more information, contact:

- American College of Chest Physicians, (847) 498-1400; www.chestnet.org.
- Society of Critical Care Medicine, (847) 827-6869; www.sccm.org.

Radiation Oncology *****

Specialty Overview: Radiation Oncologists use radiant energy from sealed radiation sources to treat malignancies and other diseases. A flood of new information about radiation and cancer biology has made Radiation Oncology a rapidly changing field. Over the next decade, the U.S. will need ten times the number of Radiation Oncologists than are now in practice. Radiation

Oncologists have relatively little night call, and average 50 hours per week doing patient care.

Training: Training lasts four years after internship.

Match: Medical students obtain PGY-2 positions through the NRMP Match and usually must match separately with their first-year programs (internships). In recent years, about 99% of the PGY-2 positions that were available through the NRMP Match filled.

Radiation Oncology

ACGME-Approved Programs	78	AOA-Approved Programs	0
1st-Yr. Spots for M.D. Students	15	Funded Entry-Level D.O. Spots	0
Adv. Spots Avail. to M.D. Students	156	% IMG Residents	3
All Entry-Level M.D. Spots	171	Avg. Res. Work Hours/Week	50
% Women Residents	35	Programs offering a "Primary Care Track"	3
Avg. Ratio of Full-Time Physician Faculty to Residents	1.0		
% Training in Hospital Outpatient Clinics	84	Programs offering Multiple Start Dates	7
		Programs allowing Moonlighting	22
% Training in Non-Hospital Community Ambulatory Clinics	2	Programs offering a Women's Track	4
Programs with Childcare	24		

For more information, contact:

- American Osteopathic College of Radiology, (800) 258-AOCR; www.aocr.org.
- American Society for Therapeutic Radiology & Oncology, (800) 962-7876; www.astro.org.

Radiology, Diagnostic ***

Specialty Overview: Diagnostic Radiologists use x-rays, ultrasound, radionuclides, and electromagnetic radiation to make diagnoses. While they still learn to read basic radiographs, Diagnostic Radiologists must now also learn how to interpret nuclear scans, PET scans, ultrasonography images, CT scans, and MR images. Additionally, they are trained to perform diagnostic and interventional procedures, such as angiography, guided biopsies, drainage procedures, and non-coronary angioplasty. This is an enormous body of knowledge to learn during a residency.

Most practitioners are hospital-based, although Radiologists are beginning to practice out of freestanding diagnostic facilities. Because of the increased demand for emergency CT and ultrasound studies, as well as for interventional procedures, Diagnostic Radiology night call has become very busy at many hospitals, although many studies are now being read via teleradiology from home or by "nighthawks," U.S.-trained radiologists based in countries such as Australia and Israel (where their day is night in the U.S.). Radiology has also joined Obstetrics/Gynecology as one of the most frequently sued specialties.

Diagnostic Radiologists average 50 hours per week doing clinical work. The number of hours per week Radiologists work has increased about 10% in the past 15 years, although the number of weeks per year they work has decreased by 5%. Among subspecialists, Neuroradiologists average 52 hours per week, Pediatric Radiologists average 53 hours per week, and Vascular and Interventional Radiologists average 54 hours per week doing clinical work. The field has only grown 5% in the past 15 years, although this may change as interventional procedures assume a greater role in medical care.

Training: Diagnostic Radiology programs are generally four years of training following internship. Some Diagnostic Radiology programs now require completion of a clinical first year before starting the residency. This first year can be in nearly any clinical area or combination of areas. Osteopathic training is four years after internship. Some ACGME-approved residencies in Diagnostic Radiology provide special competence in Nuclear Radiology after an additional formal year of training. This should not be confused with a residency in Nuclear Medicine, which is a distinct specialty with training only in that area.

Many residents gain an employment edge by taking one-year fellowships in Abdominal Radiology (12 programs), Cardiothroacic Radiology (2 programs), Endovascular Surgical Neuroradiology (3 programs), Musculoskeletal Radiology (13 programs), Neuroradiology (86 programs), Nuclear Radiology (22 programs), Pediatric Radiology (43 programs), or Vascular/Interventional Radiology (93 programs).

Match: The clinical year required before beginning a Diagnostic Radiology residency is obtained through the NRMP PGY-1 Match. In recent years, about 99% of the available positions filled through the NRMP Match. Vascular/Interventional Radiology and Neuroradiology go through the NRMP Specialties Matching Service. Match results are announced in June, one year prior to the start date.

Radiology, Diagnostic

ACGME-Approved Programs	188	AOA-Approved Programs	14
1st-Yr. Spots for M.D. Students	135	Funded Entry-Level D.O. Spots	30
Adv. Spots Avail. to M.D. Students	976	% IMG Residents	7
All Entry-Level M.D. Spots	1,111	Avg. Res. Work Hours/Week	51
% Women Residents	28	Programs offering a "Primary Care Track"	6
Avg. Ratio of Full-Time Physician Faculty to Residents	1.0		
% Training in Hospital Outpatient Clinics	16	Programs offering Multiple Start Dates	13
		Programs allowing Moonlighting	100
% Training in Non-Hospital Community Ambulatory Clinics	2	Programs offering a Women's Track	6
Programs with Childcare	63		

Pediatric Radiology

ACGME-Approved Programs	46	AOA-Approved Programs	1
1st-Yr. Spots for M.D. Students	0	Funded Entry-Level D.O. Spots	0
Adv. Spots Avail. to M.D. Students	0	% IMG Residents	41
All Entry-Level M.D. Spots	75	Avg. Res. Work Hours/Week	46
% Women Residents	45	% Training in Hospital Outpatient Clinics	8
Avg. Ratio of Full-Time Physician Faculty to Fellows	2.1		

For more information, contact:

- American College of Radiology, (800) 227-5463; www.acr.org.
- American Osteopathic College of Radiology, (800) 258-AOCR; www.aocr.org.
- American Roentgen Ray Society, (800) 347-7746; www.arrs.org.
- Society for Pediatric Radiology, (703) 648-0680; www.pedrad.org.

Rheumatology (F) *

Specialty Overview: Rheumatologists diagnose and treat patients with a wide variety of diseases of the joints, soft tissues, and blood vessels. These include the various types of acute and chronic arthritides. The field has grown in recent years with the increased interest in the autoimmune diseases underlying many rheumatologic conditions. Rheumatology is one of the quieter subspecialties of Internal Medicine and Pediatrics. Yet Rheumatologists often care for very ill patients. There is usually little night call and small primary or consultative inpatient services for those not mixing their Rheumatology practice with

General Internal Medicine or Pediatrics. Internist Rheumatologists average 49 hours per week doing patient care.

Training: Training consists of a two-year fellowship following completion of an Internal Medicine residency or three years following a Pediatrics residency. For Osteopathic physicians, training follows internship and two years of an Internal Medicine residency.

Match: About 90% of Rheumatology programs are in the NRMP Medical Specialties Matching Program. Match results are announced in June, a year before the program begins.

Rheumatology (Internal Medicine)

ACGME-Approved Programs	108	AOA-Approved Programs	3
1st-Yr. Spots for M.D. Students	0	Funded Entry-Level D.O. Spots	4
Adv. Spots Avail. to M.D. Students	0	% IMG Residents	35
All Entry-Level M.D. Spots	198	Avg. Res. Work Hours/Week	46
% Women Residents	58	Programs offering a "Primary	2
Avg. Ratio of Full-Time Physician Faculty to Fellows	2.4	Care Track"	
		Programs offering Multiple Start Dates	21
% Training in Hospital Outpatient Clinics	54		
% Training in Non-Hospital Community Ambulatory Clinics	5		

Pediatric Rheumatology **

ACGME-Approved Programs	30	AOA-Approved Programs	0
1st-Yr. Spots for M.D. Students	0	Funded Entry-Level D.O. Spots	0
Adv. Spots Avail. to M.D. Students	0	% IMG Residents	22
All Entry-Level M.D. Spots	24	Avg. Res. Work Hours/Week	45
% Women Residents	77	% Training in Non-Hospital Community Ambulatory Clinics	26
Avg. Ratio of Full-Time Physician Faculty to Fellows	2.2		
		Programs offering Multiple Start Dates	7
% Training in Hospital Outpatient Clinics	66		

For more information, contact:

- American College of Rheumatology, (404) 633-3777; www.rheumatology.org.
- American Osteopathic College of Rheumatology, Inc., 193 Monroe Ave., Edison, NJ 08820-3755; (732) 494-6688.

Sleep Medicine *

Specialty Overview: Specialists in Sleep Medicine assess, monitor, treat and prevent sleep disorders using a variety of techniques and medication in both outpatient and inpatient settings. Physicians use an interdisciplinary approach to treat insomnias, sleep-related breathing disorders, parasomnias, and sleep-related movement disorders.

    Training: Training consists of a one-year fellowship following completion of an ACGME-accredited residency program in Family Medicine, Internal Medicine, Pulmonology, Psychiatry, Pediatrics, Neurology, or Otolaryngology.

    Match: Fellowship programs must be contacted individually.

Sleep Medicine

ACGME-Approved Programs	72	AOA-Approved Programs	1
1st-Yr. Spots for M.D. Students	0	Funded Entry-Level D.O. Spots	2
Adv. Spots Avail. to M.D. Students	0	% Women Residents	n/a
All Entry-Level M.D. Spots	175		

For more information, contact:

- American Academy of Sleep Medicine, (708) 492-0930; www.aasmnet.org.

Sports Medicine (F) (Primary Care) *; (Orthopedic Surgery) ***

Specialty Overview: Sports Medicine fellowships are available under the auspices of Emergency Medicine (5 programs), Family Medicine (102 programs), Internal Medicine (0 programs), and Pediatrics (9 programs). This specialty is sometimes called (by the NRMP and others) "Primary Care Sports Medicine" to distinguish it from Orthopedic Surgery's Sports Medicine subspecialty. Specialists in this area diagnose and treat non-operative sports-related injuries. They also emphasize prevention and rehabilitation. Some perform epidemiological studies to determine the best preventive methods. Many practitioners incorporate Sports Medicine into their existing practices by offering fitness evaluations, acting as team physicians, or working with recreational athletes. Primary Care Sports Medicine physicians average 41 hours per week doing patient care.

    Orthopedic Sports Medicine is a subspecialty of Orthopedic Surgery. These practitioners perform many of the same preventive and therapeutic measures as other Sports Medicine physicians; in addition, they treat injuries surgically when necessary. Orthopedic Sports Medicine physicians average 55 hours per week doing patient care.

Training: Primary Care Sports Medicine training (nearly all under the auspices of Family Medicine) is one year after the initial residency. Orthopedic Sports Medicine is a one-year fellowship following the completion of an Orthopedic Surgery residency. There are three combined Osteopathic Family Medicine-Sports Medicine programs with seven positions.

Match: Applicants to Orthopedic Sports Medicine fellowships go through the San Francisco Matching Program. About 91% of applicants matched and 89% of programs are filled. Most Primary Care Sports Medicine programs are in the NRMP Medical Specialties Match. In recent years, 73% of applicants matched and 95% of available positions filled. Results are available in the January before the start date.

Orthopedic Sports Medicine ***

ACGME-Approved Programs	93	AOA-Approved Programs	0
1st-Yr. Spots for M.D. Students	0	Funded Entry-Level D.O. Spots	0
Adv. Spots Avail. to M.D. Students	0	% IMG Residents	2
All Entry-Level M.D. Spots	221	Avg. Res. Work Hours/Week	43
% Women Residents	5	% Training in Non-Hospital Community Ambulatory Clinics	41
Avg. Ratio of Full-Time Physician Faculty to Fellows	3.0		
% Training in Hospital Outpatient Clinics	45	Programs offering Multiple Start Dates	4

Primary Care Sports Medicine *

ACGME-Approved Programs	98	AOA-Approved Programs	10
1st-Yr. Spots for M.D. Students	0	Funded Entry-Level D.O. Spots	20
Adv. Spots Avail. to M.D. Students	0	% IMG Residents	5
All Entry-Level M.D. Spots	146	Avg. Res. Work Hours/Week	n/a
% Women Residents	37	% Training in Non-Hospital Community Ambulatory Clinics	48
Avg. Ratio of Full-Time Physician Faculty to Fellows	4.0		
% Training in Hospital Outpatient Clinics	37	Programs offering Multiple Start Dates	3

For more information, contact:

- American College of Sports Medicine, (317) 637-9200; www.acsm.org.
- American Orthopaedic Society for Sports Medicine, (847) 292-4900; www.sportsmed.org.
- American Osteopathic Academy of Sports Medicine, (608) 443-2477; www.aoasm.org.

Surgery, General (C) ****; (P) *

Specialty Overview: General Surgeons primarily diagnose and treat diseases and injuries of the abdominal organs and of the soft tissues and vasculature of the neck and trunk. They are also usually called in to manage, often in concert with other surgical specialists, patients suffering injuries to more than one body area. In rural settings, the General Surgeon may still be "General," doing Orthopedic, Urologic, and, occasionally, Thoracic or Neurosurgical procedures. But for the most part, today's General Surgeon primarily works in the abdomen, on the breast, on the peripheral vasculature, on the skin, and, in some cases, on the neck. Increasingly, endoscopic and other minimally invasive surgical techniques are being used.

During their 60-hour average work week in private practice, Surgeons spend about half their time on office visits, a third in surgery, and the rest on hospital rounds and other patient care activities. Nearly all surgical specialties are oversupplied with practitioners based on the population's needs. Yet there are still many areas of the country that are under-served by surgeons. General Surgeons have one of the highest incidences of malpractice claims. Growth in General Surgery has been flat over recent years, although the number of women in practice increased by 23% and female trainees increased by 21%. A recent study found that nearly 30% of surgical residents surveyed felt that general surgery was "becoming an obsolete career path," while 55% felt specialization was key to career success.

Training: Training in General Surgery is usually five years after medical school for both M.D. and Osteopathic physicians. "Categorical" General Surgery residency positions, designed for those interested in completing an entire General Surgery residency, have become relatively difficult to obtain. More than half of the available Surgery PGY-1 positions are "Preliminary" spots that only guarantee training for one or two years. They are designed for those wishing to enter other fields, particularly other surgical specialties.

Subspecialty fellowships and certification are available in Hospice and Palliative Medicine, Surgery of the Hand, Pediatric Surgery, Surgical Critical Care, and Vascular Surgery. Other fellowships are available in Minimally Invasive & Gastrointestinal Surgery (96 programs), and Abdominal Transplant Surgery (56 programs). Some educators now feel that the lack of continuity of care has harmed surgical training programs in markets dominated by managed care. Residents rarely see the same patients in the clinic, in the hospital, and during follow-up visits.

Match: In recent years, 99% of the available Categorical PGY-1 positions in General Surgery filled through the NRMP Match. Of the available Preliminary General Surgery positions, about 60% filled through the NRMP Match. Most surgical fellowship programs except Trauma (*see* Trauma Surgery/Acute Care Surgery) are available through the NRMP Specialties Match.

Surgery, General (C), (P)

ACGME-Approved Programs	291	AOA-Approved Programs	37
1st-Yr. Spots for M.D. Students (C)	1,146	Funded Entry-Level D.O. Spots	98
1st-Yr. Spots for M.D. Students (P)	1,221	% IMG Residents	19
Adv. Spots Avail. to M.D. Students	0	Avg. Res. Work Hours/Week	76
All Entry-Level M.D. Spots	2,376	Programs with Childcare	97
% Women Residents	31	Programs offering a "Primary Care Track"	10
Avg. Ratio of Full-Time Physician Faculty to Residents	1.1		
% Training in Hospital Outpatient Clinics	19	Programs offering Multiple Start Dates	28
		Programs allowing Moonlighting	35
% Training in Non-Hospital Community Ambulatory Clinics	5	Programs offering a Women's Health Track	13

For more information, contact:

- American College of Surgeons, (312) 202-5000; www.facs.org.
- American College of Osteopathic Surgeons, (800) 888-1312; www.facos.org.

Thoracic Surgery (I) *****; (F) **

Specialty Overview: Thoracic, or Cardiothoracic Surgeons operatively treat diseases and injuries of the heart, lungs, mediastinum, esophagus, chest wall, diaphragm, and great vessels. The most common surgery that these specialists perform is coronary artery bypass grafting. They also commonly perform cardiac surgery for acquired valvular disease or congenital cardiac defects, pulmonary surgery for malignancies, and surgery for trauma to intrathoracic organs. Some also perform heart and lung transplants. Postoperative care for all these patients is usually the responsibility of the Thoracic Surgeon, although they may share the duties with Critical Care physicians and Cardiologists. As might be expected from the nature of the diseases treated, very long and erratic hours are often necessary. This results in Thoracic Surgery being one of the most time-consuming and stressful of all the specialties. Those in the field, though, generally feel that the rewards are worth the price. Thoracic Surgeons average 67 hours per week doing patient care.

    Training: Thoracic Surgery is a subspecialty of General Surgery, and three mechanisms exist to qualify to take the Board examination. The first is to complete a full residency in General Surgery, including a 4/3 General Surgery/ Thoracic Surgery Joint Training Program. The second is to complete a six-year integrated Thoracic Surgery residency. The third is to complete a Vascular Surgery residency followed by a Thoracic Surgery residency. In 2008, 40% fewer physicians applied for Thoracic Surgery fellowships than in 2004, with only 67% of positions filled, down from 97%. It was the only specialty with fewer total applicants than positions offered in 2010. Osteopathic programs in Thoracic–Cardiovascular Surgery are two years in length after completing three years of General Surgery and one year of internship.

Match: Thoracic Surgery applicants go through NRMP's Thoracic Surgery Match and Thoracic Fellowship Match. Rank order lists are due and results are announced in June, one year prior to the July start date. In recent years, 90% of applicants matched and 72% of the available positions filled.

Thoracic Surgery

ACGME-Approved Programs	85	AOA-Approved Programs	2
1st-Yr. Spots for M.D. Students	20	Funded Entry-Level D.O. Spots	3
Adv. Spots Avail. to M.D. Students	116	% IMG Residents	34
All Entry-Level M.D. Spots	136	Avg. Res. Work Hours/Week	74
% Women Residents	16	Programs with Childcare	24
Avg. Ratio of Full-Time Physician Faculty to Fellows	3.9	Programs offering a "Primary Care Track"	5
% Training in Hospital Outpatient Clinics	14	Programs offering Multiple Start Dates	6
% Training in Non-Hospital Community Ambulatory Clinics	8	Programs allowing Moonlighting	2

For more information, contact:

- American College of Osteopathic Surgeons, (800) 888-1312; www.facos.org.
- Society of Thoracic Surgeons, (312) 202-5800; www.sts.org.

Trauma Surgery/Acute Care Surgery (F) **

Specialty Overview: With the wide institution of trauma centers, there is an increasing need for Surgeons with training in the treatment of patients with multiple injuries. Trauma Surgeons are generally the operating surgeon for patients with major injuries. In addition, they oversee and coordinate the large team responsible for these patients' initial and postoperative care. In-hospital call is usually required on a frequent basis. As with firefighters, there is often the need to immediately go to full speed from a dead stop. Long hours are required, and family life can be difficult. Most Trauma Surgeons are in medium- to large-sized cities. The new non-ACGME fellowship of Acute Care Surgery was developed to address the growing need for emergency and critical care surgery. It also addresses the growing shortage of on-call surgeons and surgical intensivists, while maintaining the viability of Trauma Surgery as a career.

Training: Training consists of a two-year fellowship following a General Surgery residency. At present, twelve months must be spent in continuous surgical critical care training, 2 months of which may be elective rotations. This training primarily consists of trauma surgery, surgical critical care, and emergency general surgery. A list of fellowship programs that comply with the American Association for the Surgery of Trauma (AAST) guidelines can be found at www.aast.org/Library/AcuteCareSurgery/.

Match: Applicants should register for NRMP's Surgical Critical Care match. Match results are announced in October.

For more information, contact:

- American Association for the Surgery of Trauma, www.aast.org/.

Urology *****

Specialty Overview: Urologists diagnose and treat diseases of and injuries to the kidney, ureters, bladder, and urethra. In males, they also treat disorders of the prostate and genitals. Often they work in concert with Nephrologists (Internists and Pediatricians) and have both a surgical and non-surgical practice. Renal transplantation, investigations into fertility and male sexuality, and the use of non-invasive techniques (such as lithotripsy) are all expanding areas within the field. Urologists have a moderate amount of night call and often have small inpatient services, since much of Urologic Surgery is now done in an ambulatory setting. Urologists average 56 hours per week doing patient care. The number of practicing Urologists has declined slightly (-1%) in recent years as has the number of trainees (-3%). The number of women, however, increased significantly between 2006 and 2012, both in practice (+41%) and in training (+29%).

Training: Urology training generally consists of two years of General Surgery followed by at least three years of Urology. The preliminary (first two) surgical years are at the same institution as the Urology training in about half of the programs. Eighteen programs offer Pediatric Urology fellowships. Osteopathic residents who take a "specialty-track" internship in Urology can shorten their training by one year.

Match: Urology has a separate Match run through The American Urological Association Residency Matching Program, www.auanet.org. There is a $75 application fee, and rank-order lists are submitted by early January. The results of the Match are released in late January, before participants must submit their NRMP Rank-Order Lists. The Urology Matching Program also has a list of current vacancies on its website. In recent years, 97% of positions filled, and 77% of applicants obtained positions.

Applicants generally must participate in the NRMP PGY-1 Match to obtain their preliminary surgical positions. Most of the Urology positions listed as being available to medical students through the NRMP PGY-1 Match are for individuals who have already matched at that institution in Urology through the specialty's Match, since most programs require the "pre-Urology" training to be completed at their institution. These are usually Preliminary Surgery positions.

Urology

ACGME-Approved Programs	120	AOA-Approved Programs	5
1st-Yr. Spots for M.D. Students	9	Funded Entry-Level D.O. Spots	32
Adv. Spots Avail. to M.D. Students	268	% IMG Residents	4
All Entry-Level M.D. Spots	277	Avg. Res. Work Hours/Week	66
% Women Residents	14	Programs offering a "Primary Care Track"	5
Avg. Ratio of Full-Time Physician Faculty to Residents	1.4		
% Training in Hospital Outpatient Clinics	33	Programs offering Multiple Start Dates	5
		Programs allowing Moonlighting	29
% Training in Non-Hospital Community Ambulatory Clinics	13	Programs offering a Women's Health Track	6
Programs with Childcare	41	Programs offering Hospitalist Track	3

For more information, contact:

- American College of Osteopathic Surgeons, (800) 888-1312; www.facos.org.
- American Urological Association, (866) 746-4282; www.auanet.org.

Vascular Surgery *****

Specialty Overview: As subspecialists of General Surgery, Vascular Surgeons diagnose and treat diseases of the arterial, venous, and lymphatic systems. Unless they are associated with a very large medical center, specialists in this field often have to perform General Surgery to make a living. This is partly because so many General Surgeons perform Vascular Surgery as a routine part of their practice. Vascular Surgeons average 62 hours per week doing patient care.

Training: Training for M.D.s is one or two years following completion of a General Surgery residency or a 5-year integrated curriculum containing at least 2 years in General Surgery and 3 years concentrating on Vascular Surgery.

The last year must be as Chief Resident in Vascular Surgery. There currently are 7 Osteopathic Vascular Surgery programs.

Match: The NRMP conducts the Vascular Surgery Specialty Match for residents already in a General Surgery residency, and the Vascular Surgery Fellowship Match. Fourth-year General Surgery residents generally apply for these positions. Nearly all the available positions are in this Match. In recent years, 91% of applicants successfully matched and 84% of the available positions filled in the Match. Results of the Match are announced in May, one year prior to the start date.

<table>
<tr><th colspan="4">Vascular Surgery</th></tr>
<tr><td>ACGME-Approved Programs</td><td>101</td><td>AOA-Approved Programs</td><td>7</td></tr>
<tr><td>1st-Yr. Spots for M.D. Students</td><td>41</td><td>Funded Entry-Level D.O. Spots</td><td>11</td></tr>
<tr><td>Adv. Spots Avail. to M.D. Students</td><td>121</td><td>% IMG Residents</td><td>6</td></tr>
<tr><td>All Entry-Level M.D. Spots</td><td>163</td><td>Avg. Res. Work Hours/Week</td><td>58</td></tr>
<tr><td>% Women Residents</td><td>22</td><td>% Training in Non-Hospital
Community Ambulatory Clinics</td><td>5</td></tr>
<tr><td>Avg. Ratio of Full-Time Physician
Faculty to Fellows</td><td>5.3</td><td></td><td></td></tr>
<tr><td>% Training in Hospital Outpatient
Clinics</td><td>14</td><td></td><td></td></tr>
</table>

For more information, contact:

- American College of Osteopathic Surgeons, (800) 888-1312; www.facos.org.
- Society for Vascular Surgery, (800) 258-7188; www.vascularweb.org.

Women's Health *

Specialty Overview: Every medical specialty treats women. This new area's goal, according to some advocates, is "to produce physicians with an expertise in clinical, teaching, and research aspects of women's health, and to produce physicians capable of leadership roles in the expanding field of women's health." Another program says it exists to help physicians "provide optimal care for all patients. We were clearly deficient in caring for a major sector of the population, necessitating the establishment of specific women's health activities." Hopefully, Women's Health programs will raise primary care physicians' awareness of those women's healthcare issues that are not directly related to Obstetrics/Gynecology.

Training: Training in Women's Health is available either combined with an Internal Medicine or a Family Medicine residency (3 years total), or as a two-year fellowship after the completion of residency training in Family Medicine, Internal Medicine, Neurology, Obstetrics/Gynecology, Psychiatry, or Surgery.

Virtually all residencies are currently given through Internal Medicine. Various groups sponsor these fellowships, and each program's content depends on their specialty orientation.

While more than 250 primary care programs list themselves as having a "Women's Health Track" (see *FREIDA's* "Optional Criteria"), it is unclear what this actually means in most cases. Programs that have residencies in Interdisciplinary Women's Health and fellowships in Women's Health are listed in the *Directory of Residency and Fellowship Programs in Interdisciplinary Women's Health*, published by the Association of Academic Women's Health Programs (AAWHP). A list of programs is intermittently available from the U.S. Department of Health & Human Services, Office on Women's Health: www.womenshealth.gov. There is no subspecialty certification in Women's Health.

Match: All Primary Care residencies go through the NRMP Match. There is no match for Women's Health fellowships, so applicants should contact programs directly.

Interdisciplinary Women's Health

ACGME-Approved Programs	11	AOA-Approved Programs	0
1st-Yr. Spots for M.D. Students	38	Funded Entry-Level D.O. Spots	0
Adv. Spots Avail. to M.D. Students	0		
All Entry-Level M.D. Spots	33		

Women's Health (F)

ACGME-Approved Programs	25	AOA-Approved Programs	0
1st-Yr. Spots for M.D. Students	0	Funded Entry-Level D.O. Spots	0
Adv. Spots Avail. to M.D. Students	0		
All Entry-Level M.D. Spots	37		

For more information, contact:

- American Medical Women's Association, (215) 320-3716; www.amwa-doc.org.
- AMA Women Physicians Congress, (312) 464-5622; www.ama-assn.org/go/wpc.
- Office on Women's Health, U.S. Dept. of Health & Human Services, (202) 205-2631; www.womenshealth.gov.

Figure 3.1: Length of Postgraduate Training for M.D. Physicians

* Many programs offer broad-based PGY-1 and PGY-2 training as part of their residencies.

** Emergency Medicine programs may include GY-1 through GY-3, GY-1 through GY-4, or GY-2 through GY-4.

*** One broad adult medicine year may be substituted for one year of Pediatrics.

Dotted lines indicate a variable number of training years.

Figure 3.2: Length of Postgraduate Training for Osteopathic (D.O.) Physicians

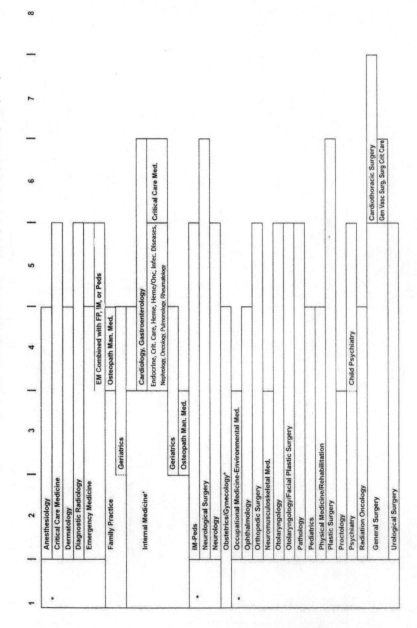

* AOA-approved 1st-year training, often in specialty.

Figure 3.3: Is This Specialty for You?

Physicians' Satisfaction with their Specialty (listed in order from Most- to Least-Satisfied)	Hours per Week Doing Patient Care
Pediatric Emergency Medicine	n/a
Geriatric Medicine (IM)	49.3
Other Pediatric Subspecialties	n/a
Neonatal–Perinatal Medicine	52.6
Internal Medicine–Pediatrics	50.7
Pediatrics	44.0
Dermatology	39.6
Child & Adolescent Psychiatry	41.8
Allergy & Immunology	41.3
Cardiovascular Diseases	58.0
Hospitalist	45.0
Critical Care (IM)	65.8
Psychiatry	40.1
Physical Medicine & Rehabilitation	47.9
Medical Oncology	n/a
Ophthalmology	43.4
Occupational Medicine	n/a
Endocrinology, Diabetes, & Metabolism	44.8
Urology	55.8
Pulmonary Diseases	51.2
Infectious Diseases (IM)	42.7
Other medical subspecialty	n/a
Otolaryngology	51.9
General Practice	n/a
Family Medicine	45.5
Gastroenterology	51.7
Internal Medicine	49.3
Other surgical subspecialty	n/a
General Surgery	59.9
Neurology	48.4
Plastic Surgery	55.7
Rheumatology	48.6
Orthopedic Surgery	60.5
Emergency Medicine	38.7

Figure 3.3: (continued)

Thoracic Surgery	66.6
Hematology-Oncology	46.6
Vascular Surgery	61.9
Obstetrics & Gynecology	48.7
Nephrology (IM)	55.2
Pulmonology-Critical Care	63.6
Neurological Surgery	61.7

n/a No information available, varies with subspecialty.

Adapted from: *AMA Statistics*, 2002; Leigh JP, Tancredi DJ, Kravitz, RL: Physician career satisfaction within specialties. *BMC Health Services Research.* 2009;9:166.

4

Choosing A Specialty

"Cheshire puss," she [Alice] began...,
"would you please tell me which way I ought to go from here?"
"That depends on where you want to get to," said the cat.
Lewis Carroll, *Alice's Adventures in Wonderland*

Your Personal Aptitudes—Assess Them Honestly

THERE ARE SEVERAL METHODS you can use to assess your interests when deciding which specialty is best for you. The first one is the "try it and like it" method. Using this option, you do a clinical rotation, like the limited experience, and decide to make that specialty your life's work. This can be very misleading.

A single exposure to a specialty can be particularly stimulating because of the attending, resident team, and patients you see—or unrealistically dismal for the same reasons. In either case, the experience may have very little to do with how well you are suited to the specialty or what the specialty is really like outside the halls of academia. Yet this is the traditional procedure that most medical students have used to make their career choices.

This method has, until recently, worked to the advantage of the entire medical system. Most students entered the specialties to which they were exposed during their third-year required rotations. At most schools, these are Internal Medicine, Surgery, Pediatrics, Psychiatry, Neurology, Obstetrics/Gynecology, and Family Medicine. When these were the specialties that needed the most practitioners, this process worked well. However, while the medical profession will continue to grow (Figure 5.5), some of these specialties currently are, or shortly will be, oversubscribed. The available first-year positions in the various specialties (Figure 4.1), though, do not necessarily reflect the number of practitioners each specialty will need.

Approximately 8% to 10% of first-year slots go unfilled each year. Specialties with more "first-year positions" than "PGY-1 positions" generally require other training, such as an internship, before entering the residency. Osteopathic programs require completion of a first year of training before entry into any residency other than a "specialty-specific" program. In 2012, there were almost 25,000 positions at the PGY-1 level in M.D. and D.O programs (not counting newly accredited programs) and about 950 one-year Transitional PGY-1 positions.

Many of the specialties listed in Figure 4.1 have positions beginning in the PGY-2 or subsequent years that are available to medical students through the NRMP or other matching programs. The training for these positions begins after a PGY-1 year. You may also want to look at Figure 23.2 to see the total number of positions available to medical students (PGY-1 and Advanced Matches), and the total number of entry-level positions that are available to both medical students and those with additional training.

Specialty Interest Tests

The second, and more scientific, method (remember, physicians are supposed to be applied scientists) is to test yourself for your interest profile. This can be done either by taking a formal, standardized test or by self-testing.

The standardized test, the Strong Vocational Interest Inventory: Gough Medical Subspecialty Scales (a Meyers-Briggs-type preference test), is available through many Dean of Students' offices. This test compares your interests with those of current practitioners in approximately seven major specialties. It has been tested and validated on large numbers of individuals practicing in the various specialties and administered to many medical students, most of whom have found it very useful. Some schools use other Meyers-Briggs-type tests. You can access some of these (for additional fees) through the AAMC's *Careers in Medicine* (*see* below). One warning: If you take any Meyers-Briggs-type test in your first or second year of medical school, it has only a fair predictive value. The farther along you are in your training, the more valid the results.

A quicker but less-accurate way of assessing your interests is to test yourself by using one of three sources. The first is *How to Choose a Medical Specialty*, by Anita Taylor (most medical libraries have a copy). This book contains short descriptions of all the approved specialties and many subspecialties, with a self-assessment quiz for each one. If you do the assessment quiz for all the specialties in the book, you will be able to rank your interests. You can then compare your interests with those of practitioners in the specialty. The second, and better, way to assess your specialty interest is to take the on-line Pathway Evaluation Program for Medical Professionals (*see* below). There is also the AAMC's *Careers in Medicine* web site, which, although at times a bit pedantic, is an excellent, complete, and mostly free (except for the Myers-Briggs-type and similar testing) source to help you evaluate what specialty you may want to enter.

Finally, while not as elegant, you can use the Personal Trait Analysis found later in this chapter.

Figure 4.1
Number of PGY-1 & First-Year Specialty Positions Offered
in 2012, and Predicted Specialty Growth

	Positions Available at PGY-1 Level	All Entry-Level Positions	% Increase Expected by 2020[#]
Radiology	135	1,033	51%
Pathology	521	521	44
Anesthesiology	919	1,412	43
Cardiovascular Diseases	0	1,165	41
General Internal Medicine	7,138*	7,138	38
IM Subspecialties (except Cardiology)	0	3,278	34
Ophthalmology	0	458	29
Family Medicine	2,740	2.740	27
Other Medical Specialties	806	1,563	26
Urology	9	277	26
General Surgery	2,376**	2,376	21
Psychiatry	1,118	1,121	21
Orthopedic Surgery	682	733	19
Other Surgical Specialties	91	753	18
Emergency Medicine	1,668	1,668	15
Pediatrics	2,475	2,475	13
Otolaryngology	285	285	10
Obstetrics/Gynecology	1,240	1,240	6

[#] These estimates were based on a relatively stable model for medical delivery systems.

*1,863 of these positions were for Preliminary Internal Medicine.

**1,165 of these positions were for Preliminary Surgery.

Adapted from: Bureau of Health Professions, Health Resources and Services Administration. *Changing Demographics: Implications for Physicians, Nurses and Other Health Workers* at http://bhpr.hrsa.gov/healthworkforce/reports/changedemo/ (accessed June 29, 2010) and other sources.

Pathway Evaluation Program for Medical Professionals

The Pathway Evaluation Program for Medical Professionals, once a live course offered by most medical schools, is now available online at http://medweb. usc.edu/pathways/intro.htm. This career-planning program provides medical students with an opportunity to determine what specialties might be the most compatible with their values and interests, helping them make informed specialty decisions. Duke University School of Medicine now administers this program in conjunction with GlaxoSmithKline.

The most interesting part of the site is the short real-time evaluation of your likes and dislikes in clinical medicine. This leads to a comparison with the results from physicians practicing in the 42 most common specialties and subspecialties. These results are based on a survey of more than 2,400 practicing physicians with a spectrum of ages and from a variety of practice settings. It also gives users a personal profile of their long-range values and interests that can be compared with practicing physicians' profiles on the site.

The physicians' profiles include their likes and dislikes about the specialty and how they rated each career evaluation factor. You can print these profiles for later perusal. You can also review each individual factor to see how the different specialties compare with each other. Take a look at "Income satisfaction." You probably won't be too surprised to learn which specialists are most pleased with their incomes.

Some schools have follow-up counseling programs for career assessment. Check with your Dean of Students to see if one is available at your school.

Careers in Medicine Website

The AAMC's *Careers in Medicine (CiM)* can be accessed after a simple registration process at http://services.aamc.org/careersinmedicine/. It is a four-phase course that helps medical students go through the process of choosing a specialty. *CiM* offers a structured, step-by-step way of thinking about this process. It uses a four-stage career-development model that includes: (1) self-assessment, (2) career exploration, (3) decision making, and (4) implementation. *CiM* also contains a variety of other resources, such as detailed information about 128 specialty and subspecialty areas, links to specialty organizations, online career planning resources (some of which you must pay for), a revised version of their Medical Specialty Preference Inventory (MSPI-R), a Physician Values in Practice Scale (PVIPS), and a bibliography. As with the Pathway Program, some medical schools use this in conjunction with formal career counseling. If you take any of the evaluation tests, your Dean of Students is probably prepared to discuss the results with you.

The resources above will broaden your field of vision beyond that which you have already experienced. Your whole professional life is at stake. Take the time to carefully think through your choice.

Personal Trait Analysis (Figure 4.2)

Neither as slick nor as rapid as the websites but available for free since you already have this book, the Personal Trait Analysis, Figure 4.2, can also help assess some medical specialty areas that interest you. As you can see in the example (Figure 4.3) completed by a sample medical student, you should put a "+" next to each "Characteristic" that you "Like" or feel is one of your "Strengths." If you neither "Like" the "Characteristic" nor consider it one of your "Strengths," put a "0" in the appropriate place. Note that you may "Like" some of the Characteristics, but not feel that they are "Strengths." Others you may feel are personal "Strengths," but you do not particularly "Like" them. In these cases, just mark the form accordingly. The statements are purposely broad, so do not be alarmed by their general nature.

Once you have completed your Personal Trait Analysis in Figure 4.2, use the Personal Trait Synthesis form (Figure 4.5) to rearrange the "Characteristics" (as our sample student has done in Figure 4.4) under the following four categories:

High Priority–Characteristics you marked (+)"Like," (+)"Strength"

Priority– Characteristics you marked (+)"Like," (0)"Strength"

Acceptable–Characteristics you marked (0)"Like," (+)"Strength"

Reject– Characteristics you marked (0)"Like," (0)"Strength"

Next, look at Figure 4.6, which summarizes the characteristics that practitioners in some major specialties feel relate to their area. Then go to Figures 4.7 and 4.8, "Selecting a Specialty for You."

Figure 4.2: Personal Trait Analysis

Characteristic	Like	Strength
1. Deal with Many Major Diseases		
2. Treat Infectious Diseases		
3. Treat Incurable & Disabling Diseases		
4. Evaluate Neurological Functions		
5. Evaluate Reproductive Functions		
6. Deal with Complex Problems		
7. Life-Threatening Problems		
8. Treat Psychosomatic Problems		
9. Deal with Intimate Personal Problems		
10. Deal with Emotional Reactions To Illness		
11. Older Age Patients		
12. Child & Adolescent Patients		
13. Dying Patients		
14. Many Patients Daily		
15. Give Comprehensive Care		
16. Home Health Care		
17. Do Preventive Care		
18. Do Genetic Counseling		
19. Marital & Sexual Counseling		
20. Family Planning Counseling		
21. Discuss Personal Relations		
22. Patient Participation in Care		
23. See Beneficial Treatment Results		
24. Use Knowledge of Musculoskeletal System		
25. Use Knowledge of Circ., Resp., Digest., & Excretory Systems		
26. Use Knowledge of Anatomy & Physiology		
27. Do Extensive, Precise Workups		
28. Use Lab Tests		
29. Use Proctoscopies & Arteriograms		
30. Use Complex Equipment		
31. Use Your Hands		
32. Do Repetitive Standard Procedures		
33. Do High-Risk Procedures		
34. Do Outpatient Operative Procedures		
35. Get & Use Family Information		
36. Use Socioeconomic Information		
37. Use Rehabilitation Services		
38. Use Social Services		
39. Give Psychological Services		
40. Get Referrals & Give Consultations		

Figure 4.3: Personal Trait Analysis, An Example

Characteristic	Like	Strength
1. Deal with Many Major Diseases	+	+
2. Treat Infectious Diseases	0	+
3. Treat Incurable & Disabling Diseases	0	0
4. Evaluate Neurological Functions	0	0
5. Evaluate Reproductive Functions	0	0
6. Deal with Complex Problems	+	+
7. Life-Threatening Problems	+	+
8. Treat Psychosomatic Problems	+	0
9. Deal with Intimate Personal Problems	0	0
10. Deal with Emotional Reactions To Illness	0	0
11. Older Age Patients	+	+
12. Child & Adolescent Patients	0	+
13. Dying Patients	0	+
14. Many Patients Daily	+	0
15. Give Comprehensive Care	+	+
16. Home Health Care	0	0
17. Do Preventive Care	0	0
18. Do Genetic Counseling	0	0
19. Marital & Sexual Counseling	0	0
20. Family Planning Counseling	0	0
21. Discuss Personal Relations	+	0
22. Patient Participation in Care	+	+
23. See Beneficial Treatment Results	+	+
24. Use Knowledge of Musculoskeletal System	+	+
25. Use Knowledge of Circ., Resp., Digest., & Excretory Systems	+	0
26. Use Knowledge of Anatomy & Physiology	+	+
27. Do Extensive, Precise Workups	0	+
28. Use Lab Tests	+	+
29. Use Proctoscopies & Arteriograms	0	0
30. Use Complex Equipment	+	0
31. Use Your Hands	+	+
32. Do Repetitive Standard Procedures	0	0
33. Do High-Risk Procedures	0	0
34. Do Outpatient Operative Procedures	+	+
35. Get & Use Family Information	0	+
36. Use Socioeconomic Information	+	0
37. Use Rehabilitation Services	0	0
38. Use Social Services	0	+
39. Give Psychological Services	+	+
40. Get Referrals & Give Consultations	+	0

Figure 4.4: Personal Trait Synthesis, An Example

Our sample student has taken his results from Figure 4.3 and grouped them according to their priority for him.

Characteristic	Like	Strength
High Priority (4)		
1. Deal with Many Major Diseases	+	+
6. Deal with Complex Problems	+	+
7. Life-Threatening Problems	+	+
11. Older Age Patients	+	+
15. Give Comprehensive Care	+	+
22. Patient Participation in Care	+	+
23. See Beneficial Treatment Results	+	+
24. Use Knowledge of Musculoskeletal System	+	+
26. Use Knowledge of Anatomy & Physiology	+	+
28. Use Lab Tests	+	+
31. Use Your Hands	+	+
34. Do Outpatient Operative Procedures	+	+
39. Give Psychological Services	+	+
Priority (3)		
8. Treat Psychosomatic Problems	+	0
14. Many Patients Daily	+	0
21. Discuss Personal Relations	+	0
25. Use Knowledge of Circulatory, Respiratory, Digestive, & Excretory Systems	+	0
30. Use Complex Equipment	+	0
36. Use Socioeconomic Information	+	0
40. Get Referrals & Give Consults	+	0
Acceptable (2)		
2. Treat Infectious Diseases	0	+
12. Child & Adolescent Patients	0	+
13. Dying Patients	0	+
27. Do Extensive, Precise Workups	0	+
35. Get & Use Family Information	0	+
38. Use Social Services	0	+
Reject (1)		
3. Treat Incurable & Disabling Diseases	0	0
4. Evaluate Neurological Functions	0	0
5. Evaluate Reproductive Functions	0	0
9. Deal with Intimate Personal Problems	0	0
10. Deal with Emotional Reactions to Illness	0	0
16. Home Health Care	0	0
17. Do Preventive Care	0	0
18. Do Genetic Counseling	0	0
19. Marital & Sexual Counseling	0	0
20. Family Planning Counseling	0	0
29. Use Proctoscopies & Arteriograms	0	0
32. Do Repetitive Standard Procedures	0	0
33. Do High-Risk Procedures	0	0
37. Use Rehabilitation Services	0	0

Figure 4.5: Personal Trait Synthesis

Now list your likes/strengths from Figure 4.2 according to their priority.

High Priority (4)

_____   _____

_____   _____

_____   _____

_____   _____

Priority (3)

_____   _____

_____   _____

_____   _____

_____   _____

Acceptable (2)

_____   _____

_____   _____

_____   _____

_____   _____

Reject (1)

_____   _____

_____   _____

_____   _____

_____   _____

Figure 4.6
Characteristics Strongly Associated with the Practice of Some Major Specialties

The following seven charts summarize the "Characteristics" practitioners feel relate to their specialties in Pediatrics, Surgery, Family Medicine, Internal Medicine, Obstetrics and Gynecology, Psychiatry, and Emergency Medicine. While there are *many more specialty fields than are listed here*, these charts should give you a starting point from which to look into similar, related specialty areas.

When you finish looking these over, turn to Figures 4.7 and 4.8, "Selecting a Specialty for You," to determine how your own rating of the Characteristics compares to those of specialists practicing in these fields.

Emergency Medicine

Very Common
- Life-Threatening Problems
- Many Patients Daily
- Use Your Hands

Common
- Use Lab Tests
- Child and Adolescent Patients
- Use Knowledge of Musculoskeletal System
- Use Knowledge of Circ., Resp., Digest., & Excretory Systems
- Use Knowledge of Anatomy & Physiology
- Many Major Diseases
- Beneficial Treatment Results
- Outpatient Operative Procedures

Rare
- Deal with Emotional Reactions to Illness
- Preventive Care
- Use Proctoscopies & Arteriograms
- Incurable & Disabling Diseases
- Discuss Personal Relations
- Use Rehabilitation Services
- Family Planning Counseling
- Use Psychological Services
- Evaluate Reproductive Functions
- Home Health Care

Very Rare
- Marital & Sexual Counseling
- Genetic Counseling

Family Medicine

Very Common
- Comprehensive Care
- Use Lab Tests
- Outpatient Operative Procedures
- Child & Adolescent Patients
- Older Age Patients
- Many Patients Daily
- Intimate Personal Problems
- Use Family Information
- Treat Infectious Diseases

Common
- Many Major Diseases
- Deal with Life-Threatening Problems
- Psychosomatic Problems
- Dying Patients
- Home Health Care
- Preventive Care
- Marital & Sexual Counseling
- Family Planning Counseling
- Discuss Personal Relations
- Patient Participation in Care
- Beneficial Treatment Results
- Repetitive Standard Procedures
- Use Socioeconomic Information
- Use Rehabilitation Services
- Use Social Services

Rare
- Genetic Counseling
- Use Complex Equipment
- Do High-Risk Procedures
- Get Referrals & Give Consults

Figure 4.6 (continued)

Internal Medicine	Obstetrics And Gynecology

Internal Medicine

Very Common
- Complex Problems
- Use Lab Tests
- Get Referrals & Give Consults

Common
- Many Major Diseases
- Treat Infectious Diseases
- Incurable and Disabling Diseases
- Life-Threatening Problems
- Psychosomatic Problems
- Intimate Personal Problems
- Older Age Population
- Dying Patients
- Comprehensive Care
- Patient Participation in Care
- Knowledge of Circ., Resp., Digest., & Excretory Systems
- Extensive, Precise Workups
- Proctoscopies & Arteriograms
- Use Family Information

Rare
- Child & Adolescent Patients
- Genetic Counseling
- Family Planning Counseling
- Psychological Services
- Use Knowledge of Musculoskeletal System
- Evaluate Reproductive Functions

Very Rare
- Outpatient Operative Procedures

Obstetrics And Gynecology

Very Common
- Marital & Sexual Counseling
- Use Your Hands
- Family Planning Counseling
- Intimate Personal Problems
- Evaluate Reproductive Functions

Common
- Many Patients Daily
- Preventive Care
- Beneficial Treatment Results
- Use Lab Tests
- Repetitive Standard Procedures
- Get Referrals & Give Consults

Rare
- Incurable & Disabling Diseases
- Older Age Patients
- Dying Patients
- Home Health Care
- Use Knowledge of Musculoskeletal System
- Use Complex Equipment
- Do High-Risk Procedures
- Use Socioeconomic Information
- Give Psychological Services

Very Rare
- Use Rehabilitation Services
- Use Proctoscopies & Arteriograms
- Evaluate Neurological Functions

Figure 4.6 (continued)

Pediatrics	Psychiatry

Pediatrics

Very Common
- Preventive Care
- Comprehensive Care
- Many Patients Daily
- Child & Adolescent Patients
- Treat Infectious Diseases

Common
- Beneficial Treatment Results
- Use Lab Tests
- Repetitive Standard Procedures
- Use Family Information

Rare
- Incurable & Disabling Diseases
- Family Planning Counseling
- Deal with Emotional Reactions to Illness
- Use Knowledge of Musculoskeletal System

Very Rare
- Older Age Patients
- Marital & Sexual Counseling
- Use Complex Equipment
- Do High-Risk Procedures
- Dying Patients
- Evaluate Reproductive Functions
- Use Proctoscopies & Arteriograms

Psychiatry

Very Common
- Psychosomatic Problems
- Intimate Personal Problems
- Emotional Reactions to Illness
- Discuss Personal Relationships
- Patient Participation in Care

Common
- Get Referrals & Give Consults
- Give Psychological Services
- Use Social Services
- Use Socioeconomic Information
- Use Family Information
- Marital & Sexual Counseling
- Complex Problems

Rare
- Use Lab Tests
- Extensive, Precise Workups
- Genetic Counseling
- Home Health Care
- Life-Threatening Problems
- Evaluate Reproductive Functions
- Use Knowledge of Anatomy & Physiology
- Use Rehabilitation Services

Very Rare
- Use Your Hands
- Do High-Risk Procedures
- Outpatient Operative Procedures
- Many Patients Daily
- Use Complex Equipment
- Use Proctoscopies & Arteriograms
- Treat Infectious Diseases
- Use Knowledge of Musculoskeletal System
- Use Knowledge of Circ., Resp., Digest., & Excretory Systems

Figure 4.6 (continued)

Surgery

Very Common
- Life-Threatening Problems
- Beneficial Treatment Results
- Get Referrals & Give Consults
- Use Your Hands
- Outpatient Operative Procedures
- Use of Knowledge of Anatomy & Physiology
- Use Proctoscopies & Arteriograms

Common
- Many Major Diseases
- Complex Problems
- Dying Patients
- Extensive Precise Workups
- Use Lab Tests
- Use Knowledge of Musculoskeletal System
- Use Knowledge of Circ., Resp., Digest., & Excretory Systems

Rare
- Comprehensive Care
- Preventive Care
- Deal with Emotional Reactions to Illness
- Intimate Personal Problems
- Evaluate Neurological Functions
- Psychosomatic Problems
- Evaluate Reproductive Functions
- Use Socioeconomic Information

Very Rare
- Genetic Counseling
- Marital-Sexual Counseling
- Family Planning Counseling
- Psychological Services

Adapted from: Zimny GH: *Manual for the Medical Specialty Preference Inventory* (revised draft). St. Louis, MO, 1977; and Zimny GH, Iserson KV, Shepherd C: A characterization of emergency medicine. *JACEP.* 1979;8(4):147-49.

Figure 4.7: Selecting a Specialty for You, An Example

This form summarizes the prior pages (Figure 4.6) and briefly describes those characteristics favored by current practitioners in seven common specialties. Our sample student, whose Personal Trait Synthesis can be found in Figure 4.4, would fill out the blank Figure 4.8 as seen below.

Every characteristic that the student rated as a *"High Priority"* [Like (+), Strength (+)] gets *4 points;* each one rated as *"Priority"* [Like (+), Strength (0)] gets *3 points;* each one rated as *"Acceptable"* [Like (0), Strength (+)] gets *2 points;* and each one rated *"Reject"* [Like (0), Strength (0)] gets *1 point.* That student would then fill in the numerical values for each of the characteristics [rated as Very Common (VC), Common (C), Rare (R), or Very Rare (VR)] in each of these specialties.

Once the individual numbers are filled in, a score can be calculated based upon the correlation of personal traits with the specialty characteristics.

Characteristic	IM	SUR	FM	PED	OB	PSY	EM
1. Deal with Many Major Diseases	C 4	C 4	C 4	-	-	-	C 4
2. Treat Infectious Diseases	C 2	-	VC 2	VC 2	-	VR 2	-
3. Treat Incurable & Disabling Diseases	C 1	-	-	R 1	R 1	-	R 1
4. Evaluate Neurological Functions	-	R 1	-	-	VR 1	-	-
5. Evaluate Reproductive Functions	R 1	R 1	-	VR 1	VC 1	R 1	R 1
6. Deal with Complex Problems	VC 4	C 4	-	-	-	C 4	-
7. Life-Threatening Problems	C 4	VC 4	C 4	-	-	R 4	VC 4
8. Treat Psychosomatic Problems	C 3	R 3	C 3	-	-	VC 3	-
9. Deal with Intimate Personal Problems	C 1	R 1	VC 1	-	VC 1	VC 1	-
10. Deal with Emotional Reactions To Illness	-	R 1	-	R 1	-	VC 1	R 1
11. Older Age Patients	C 4	-	VC 4	VR 4	R 4	-	-
12. Child & Adolescent Patients	R 2	-	VC 2	VC 2	-	-	C 2
13. Dying Patients	C 2	C 2	C 2	VR 2	R 2	-	-
14. Many Patients Daily	-	-	VC 3	VC 3	C 3	VR 3	VC 3

Figure 4.7 (continued)

Characteristic	IM	SUR	FM	PED	OB	PSY	EM
15. Give Comprehensive Care	C 4	R 4	VC 4	VC 4	-	-	C 4
16. Home Health Care	-	-	C 1	-	R 1	R 1	R 1
17. Do Preventive Care	-	R 1	C 1	VC 1	C 1	-	R 1
18. Do Genetic Counseling	R 1	VR 1	R 1	-	-	R 1	VR 1
19. Marital & Sex Counseling	-	VR 1	C 1	VR 1	VC 1	C 1	VR 1
20. Family Planning Counseling	R 1	VR 1	C 1	R 1	VC 1	-	R 1
21. Discuss Personal Relationships	-	-	C 3	-	-	VC 3	R 3
22. Patient Participation in Care	C 4	-	C 4	-	-	VC 4	-
23. See Beneficial Treatment Result	-	VC 4	C 4	C 4	C 4	-	C 4
24. Use Knowledge of Musculo-skeletal System	R 4	C 4	-	R 4	R 4	VR 4	C 4
25. Use Knowledge of Circ., Resp., Digest., & Excretory Systems	C 3	C 3	-	-	-	VR 3	C 3
26. Use Knowledge of Anatomy & Physiology	-	VC 4	-	-	-	R 4	C 4
27. Do Extensive, Precise Workups	C 2	C 2	-	-	-	R 2	-
28. Use Lab Tests	VC 4	C 4	VC 4	C 4	C 4	R 4	C 4
29. Use Proctoscopies & Arteriograms	C 1	VC 1	-	VR 1	VR 1	VR 1	R 1
30. Use Complex Equipment	-	-	R 3	VR 3	R 3	VR 3	-
31. Use Your Hands	-	VC 4	-	-	VC 4	VR 4	VC 4
32. Do Repetitive Standard Procedures	-	-	C 1	C 1	C 1	-	-
33. Do High-Risk Procedures	-	-	R 1	VR 1	R 1	VR 1	-
34. Do Outpatient Operative Procedures	VR 4	VC 4	VC 4	-	-	VR 4	C 4

Figure 4.7 (continued)

Characteristic	IM	SUR	FM	PED	OB	PSY	EM
35. Get & Use Family Information	C 2	-	VC 2	C 2	-	C 2	-
36. Use Socioeconomic Information	-	R 3	C 3	-	R 3	C 3	-
37. Use Rehabilitation Services	-	-	C 1	-	VR 1	R 1	R 1
38. Use Social Services	-	-	C 2	-	-	C 2	-
39. Give Psych Services	R 4	VR 4	-	-	R 4	C 4	R 4
40. Get Referrals; Give Consultations	VC 3	VC 3	R 3	-	C 3	C 3	-

Figure 4.8: Selecting a Specialty for You

Your rating number, *taken from Figure 4.5,* for each "Characteristic" is inserted below the associated strength of the characteristic ("VC"= Very Common; "C"= Common; "R"= Rare; "VR"= Very Rare) for each specialty. *Note that your rating number for each characteristic will be the same under each specialty. (See Figure 4.7 for the numbers to use.)* Once the individual numbers are filled in, a score can be calculated based upon the correlation of personal traits with the specialty characteristics.

Characteristic	IM	SUR	FM	PED	OB	PSY	EM
1. Deal with Many Major Diseases	C	C	C	-	-	-	C
2. Treat Infectious Diseases	C	-	VC	VC	-	VR	-
3. Treat Incurable & Disabling Diseases	C	-	-	R	R	-	R
4. Evaluate Neurological Functions	-	R	-	-	VR	-	-
5. Evaluate Reproductive Functions	R	R	-	VR	VC	R	R
6. Deal with Complex Problems	VC	C	-	-	-	C	-
7. Life-Threatening Problems	C	VC	C	-	-	R	VC
8. Treat Psychosomatic Problems	C	R	C	-	-	VC	-

Figure 4.8 (continued)

Characteristic	IM	SUR	FM	PED	OB	PSY	EM
9. Deal with Intimate Personal Problems	C	R	VC	-	VC	VC	-
10. Deal with Emotional Reactions to Illness	-	R	-	R	-	VC	R
11. Older Age Patients	C	-	VC	VR	R	-	-
12. Child & Adolescent Patients	R	-	VC	VC	-	-	C
13. Dying Patients	C	C	C	VR	R	-	-
14. Many Patients Daily	-	-	VC	VC	C	VR	VC
15. Give Comprehensive Care	C	R	VC	VC	-	-	C
16. Home Health Care	-	-	C	-	R	R	R
17. Do Preventive Care	-	R	C	VC	C	-	R
18. Do Genetic Counseling	R	VR	R	-	-	R	VR
19. Marital & Sex Counseling	-	VR	C	VR	VC	C	VR
20. Family Planning Counseling	R	VR	C	R	VC	-	R
21. Discuss Personal Relationships	-	-	C	-	-	VC	R
22. Patient Participation	C	-	C	-	-	VC	-
23. See Beneficial Treatment Result	-	VC	C	C	C	-	C
24. Use Knowledge of Musculo-skeletal System	R	C	-	R	R	VR	C
25. Use Knowledge of Circ., Resp. Digest., & Excretory Systems	C	C	-	-	-	VR	C
26. Use Knowledge of Anatomy & Physiology	-	VC	-	-	-	R	C
27. Do Extensive, Precise Workups	C	C	-	-	-	R	-

Figure 4.8 (continued)

Characteristic	IM	SUR	FM	PED	OB	PSY	EM
28. Use Lab Tests	VC	C	VC	C	C	R	C
29. Use Proctoscopies & Arteriograms	C	VC	-	VR	VR	VR	R
30. Use Complex Equipment	-	-	R	VR	R	VR	-
31. Use Your Hands	-	VC	-	-	VC	VR	VC
32. Do Repetitive Standard Procedures	-	-	C	C	C	-	-
33. Do High-Risk Procedures	-	-	R	VR	R	VR	-
34. Do Outpatient Operative Procedures	VR	VC	VC	-	-	VR	C
35. Get & Use Family Information	C	-	VC	C	-	C	-
36. Use Socioeconomic Information	-	R	C	-	R	C	-
37. Use Rehabilitation Services	-	-	C	-	VR	R	R
38. Use Social Services	-	-	C	-	-	C	-
39. Give Psych Services	R	VR	-	-	R	C	R
40. Get Referrals; Give Consultations	VC	VC	R	-	C	C	-

Figure 4.9
Correlation of Personal Traits and Specialty Characteristics

It is now time to see how your own traits, likes, and strengths match with the seven specialties analyzed. Using Figure 4.8, add the numbers associated with a particular rating for each specialty and put the result in the appropriate box in the chart below. For example, our sample student (Figure 4.7), in the Internal Medicine column, put two "4" and one "3" rating for traits listed as Very Common (VC). This equals "11." So our sample student would put the number "11" in the top left box in the chart, labeled "Very Common, IM." (See Figure 4.10 for an example.)

Complete the remainder of your chart in a similar manner. Then, to get the scores you will need, divide by the number specified in the box. This will give you an average score for the traits in that category.

As you can see, the higher the scores in the "Very Common" and "Common" boxes, and the lower the scores in the "Rare" and "Very Rare" boxes, the better your personal traits, strengths, and likes correlate with the practice in a particular specialty.

For an example of this form filled out by our sample student, turn to Figure 4.10.

	IM	SUR	FM	PED	OB	PSY	EM
Very Common Total:							
Divided by:	3	7	9	5	5	5	3
Score =							
Common Total:							
Divided by:	14	7	15	4	6	7	9
Score =							
Rare Total:							
Divided by:	6	8	4	4	9	8	10
Score =							
Very Rare Total:							
Divided by:	1	4	-	7	3	9	2
Score =							

Figure 4.10
Correlation of Personal Traits and Specialty
Characteristics, An Example

	IM	SUR	FM	PED	OB	PSY	EM
Very Common Total:	11	24	26	12	8	12	11
Divided by:	3	7	9	5	5	5	3
Score =	3.67	3.43	2.89	2.40	1.60	2.40	3.67
Common Total:	37	23	35	11	16	19	33
Divided by:	14	7	15	4	6	7	9
Score =	2.64	3.29	2.33	2.75	2.67	2.71	3.67
Rare Total:	13	15	8	7	23	18	15
Divided by:	6	8	4	4	9	8	10
Score =	2.17	1.88	2.00	1.75	2.56	2.25	1.50
Very Rare Total:	4	7	-	13	3	25	2
Divided by:	1	4	-	7	3	9	2
Score =	4.00	1.75	-	1.86	1.00	2.78	1.00

This example demonstrates a pattern, which should point our sample student toward a specialty choice. Surgery and Emergency Medicine have characteristics closest to the student's likes and strengths. These two specialties also rarely deal with many of the aspects of medicine the student feels are neither personal "Likes" nor "Strengths."

In general, you should look for the highest scores in the "Very Common" and "Common" characteristic areas, and the lowest scores in the "Rare" and "Very Rare" areas. A specialty that shows a reversal of this trend will be a poor match for you. The presence of very similar numbers in all four categories indicates that you may not be able to generate much enthusiasm for the specialty.

However, there is one major caveat to using this scoring sheet: *the subspecialty areas are not really considered in this schema.* For example, while Internists very rarely do outpatient operative procedures, the subspecialty of Cardiology, especially those Cardiologists who do heart catheterizations, considers this a "Very Common" aspect of their practice. So, use these charts to get an estimate of areas that you would like to explore further. *Do not use them rigidly or without thinking beyond the results.*

5
Important Factors When Choosing A Specialty

The more alternatives, the more difficult the choice.
Abbé D'Allainval, *L'embarras des richesses,* 1726

MANY FACTORS COME INTO PLAY when you are trying to choose a specialty. The elements you find important may not be the same ones that your classmates value. Yet it might be instructive to look at what recent graduates felt were important factors in their choice of specialty.

Figure 5.1 shows a variety of factors that can influence specialty choice. The most important factors that students believe influenced their specialty choice relate to how they will interact with patients. Interest in helping people, the opportunity to make a difference in people's lives, and the type of patient problems encountered in the specialty were the major influences for most students. This suggests that most students' altruistic reasons for entering medicine still influence them after the four-year grind of medical school. Very reasonably, other persuasive factors cited are whether their own personality fits with the specialty and whether they possess the required skills or abilities.

Some medical students seem to make bad specialty choices—either being attracted to or rejecting specialties—based on the nature of the people with whom they have worked, especially during their third-year rotations. There are, however, inherent personalities in different specialties. Associating with specialists both at the academic center and in the community, for example at the regional society meeting, may help you decide whether your personality fits that specialty.

Unlike previous generations of medical students, recent graduates have wisely relied much less on a particular physician or a specific medical school course when choosing their specialty. However, they do still rely a bit too heavily on their experience during subspecialty clerkships. Brief and isolated experiences such as these can be misleading—both positively and negatively—so beware.

Other common factors considered when making a specialty choice are the *intellectual content* of the specialty and whether the specialty has *challenging*

Figure 5.1
Factors Influencing Medical Students' Specialty Choice

Factor	No Influence	Strong Influence
Fit with personality, interests & skills	1%	83%
Specialty content	1	80
Role model's influence	11	44
Work/life balance	8	38
Advisor/Mentor	26	34
Future family plans	18	26
In-house extramural electives	20	25
Fellowship training options	22	24
Specialty interest groups/sponsored panels & presentations	7	23
School-sponsored career planning workshops & courses	3	13
Careers in Medicine Website	2	12
Family expectations	44	11
Expected income	27	10
Length of residency training	30	8
Specialty's competitiveness	40	6
Personal educational debt	55	6

Adapted from: Association of American Medical Colleges: *GQ Medical School Graduation Questionnaire, All Schools Summary Report (Final)*. AAMC, 2009:35-7.

diagnostic problems. Basically, students prefer not to be bored by the career path they take. Significantly, these are the same factors cited by physicians in practice who still enjoy their specialty 20 and 30 years after completing their residency.

Most students claim that how a specialty's practice *fits with what they enjoy doing in medicine* has the most influence. Good for them! This may make them much happier than prior generations of physicians. Other factors also influence career choices, but few people readily acknowledge being swayed by them. These include income, length of training, work hours, availability of jobs in the future, and the difficulty of getting a residency position.

Monetary Rewards

One aspect of selecting a specialty, which is rarely, if ever, spoken about except in a humorous fashion, is the financial remuneration you can expect. While it may be both noble and consistent with the values that brought you into the medical field to try to ignore financial considerations completely, it is unrealistic. No physician is likely to be poor, but most medical students accrue enormous debts to finance their education.

Specialty Income

Medical students generally believe that their educational investment will pay off handsomely. More than one-third of graduating medical students expect to be earning more than $200,000 annually within ten years of completing their postgraduate training.

Procedure-oriented specialties are the most lucrative for physicians. And the difference between the income for physicians in these specialties and that of their non-procedurally oriented colleagues can be truly amazing. This is because, at present, the insurance payment schemes reward *doing* (procedures) at a much higher level than *thinking* (cognition). One study found that while Pediatricians have a median annual income of about $203,000, Cardiothoracic Surgeons earn nearly two and a half times as much (Figure 5.2). Another study showed similar discrepancies between specialties when comparing salaries on an hourly basis (see Figure 5.3). This list accounts for the variability in the hours worked; Neurosurgeons may earn more than two and a half times as much as Pediatricians, yet they work only one more hour a week on average. Neither study takes into account the huge malpractice premiums paid by some specialists.

Due to physician shortages, median salaries are increasing, creating a more competitive marketplace. In some specialties, graduating fellows are being offered starting salaries close to those of more experienced colleagues, most notably in Infectious Diseases and Hematology/Oncology. Non-primary care physicians receive starting salaries that are 25% to 50% higher than those received by physicians in primary care. Unlike other physicians, in their first three years following residency, physicians in General Internal Medicine, Family Medicine, and Pediatrics have expenses exceeding after-tax income.

For decades, some policy makers have predicted changes in this system as mechanisms for physician payment are rearranged at the federal, state, and private levels through "health-care reform." So far, it hasn't happened. Across the United States, the highest physician incomes continue to be in the central Southeast states (AL, KY, MS, TN) and the central Southwestern states (AR, LA, OK, TX), while the lowest are in the Mountain (AZ, CO, ID, MT, NM, NV, UT, WY) and Pacific states (AK, CA, HI, OR, WA). Real physician income (adjusted for inflation) has remained relatively unchanged for the past decade.

Figure 5.2
Median Physician Annual Income

Specialty	Income*
Neurological Surgery	$605,000
Cardiothoracic Surgery	507,000
Orthopedic Surgery	476,000
Diagnostic Radiology	438,000
Vascular Surgery	403,000
Cardiology	400,000
Gastroenterology	390,000
Urology	390,000
Plastic Surgery	389,000
Colon & Rectal Surgery	367,000
Otolaryngology	365,000
Dermatology	350,000
Pathology	344,000
General Surgery	340,000
Ophthalmology	325,000
All Physicians	**$ 316,000**
Hematology/Oncology	$315,000
Anesthesiology	312,000
Obstetrician/Gynecology	294,000
Allergy & Immunology	241,000
Physical Medicine & Rehab	237,000
Neurology	230,000
Infectious Disease	222,000
Rheumatology	219,000
Emergency Medicine	215,000
Occupational Medicine	214,000
Endocrinology	212,000
Hospitalist	212,000
Geriatrics	211,000
Psychiatry	208,000
General Internal Med	205,000
Pediatrics	203,000
Family Medicine	198,000

*Reports of specialty salaries vary widely. These numbers are only an approximation.

Adapted from the *2009 Physician Compensation Survey* by the American Medical Group Association (AMGA).

Figure 5.3
Physician Median Hourly Income & Hours Worked Per Week

Specialty*	Hourly Unadjusted Income**	Hours Worked/Week (Mean)***
>$100/hour		
Neurological Surgery	$132	58
Radiation Oncology	126	53
Medical Oncology	114	60
Plastic Surgery	114	54
Allergy & Immunology	112	49
Cardiothoracic Surgery	110	65
Orthopedic Surgery	108	61
Ophthalmology	104	52
Dermatology	103	45
Hematology/Oncology	100	55
Other Surgical Specialties	100	62
$80 to $99/hour		
Cardiology	94	60
Gastroenterology	93	57
Otolaryngology	93	55
Neurology	93	52
Physical Medicine & Rehab	92	46
Emergency Medicine	87	47
Nephrology	87	58
General Surgery	86	61
Urology	86	58
Occupational Medicine	85	44
Obstetrics/Gynecology	83	57
Vascular Surgery	80	68
$60 to $79/hour		
Rheumatology	78	53
Pulmonary-Critical Care	76	62
Neonatal-Perinatal Medicine	76	65
Psychiatry	72	45
Hospitalist	72	60
Endocrinology	72	48

(continued)

Figure 5.3 (continued)

Specialty*	Hourly Unadjusted Income**	Hours Worked/Week (Mean)***
Pediatrics	69	45
Critical Care-Internal Medicine	69	68
Child & Adolescent Psychiatry	67	46
Infectious Disease	66	52
Pediatric Emergency Medicine	66	41
<$60/hour		
Family Medicine	58	52
General Internal Medicine	58	54
General Practice	58	48
Other Pediatric Subspecialites	53	56
Internal Medicine-Pediatrics	50	57

*Specialties not included are Anesthesiology, Diagnostic Radiology (high salaries); Colon/Rectal Surgery, Pathology (intermediate salaries); and Geriatrics (low salary).
**Unadjusted hourly income rounded to nearest dollar. Salaries vary widely; consider these only as an approximation.
***Rounded to nearest whole number.
Adapted from: Leigh JP, Tancredi D, Jerant A, et al.: Physician wages across specialties: informing the physician reimbursement debate. *Arch Intern Med.* 2010;170:1728-34.

If the past is any indicator, the disparity in salary between doers and thinkers will persist. In fact, it has been shown that primary care physicians have a substantially lower return on their investment in professional education than do medical or surgical subspecialists, attorneys, dentists, and individuals in business. Based on the costs of a medical education, the "hours-adjusted net present value" of the money invested in education is $12.61 for attorneys, $12.22 for procedure-based physicians, $10.45 for dentists, $9.72 for businessmen, and $7.01 for primary care physicians. After their mid-20s, lawyers, businessmen, and dentists also work fewer hours than do physicians. Yet no matter which specialty a physician chooses to enter, he or she is in no danger of going on the dole.

In 2012, almost half of new physicians were hired to work in hospital-owned practices, perhaps in part because the starting salaries for both primary care and specialty care physicians in these practices are now generally higher than for non-hospital-owned practices. Another reason for moving to hospital-based practices is that these provide a sustained income and practitioners are shielded from the uncertainty associated with third-party reimbursements in a rapidly changing environment. However, eventually the need for, and the income of, many specialists will decrease. This is because managed healthcare systems generally make money by keeping their patients away from medical specialists. So far, they have been only partially successful at doing this.

Then there is the malpractice insurance dilemma, which has cycled from a crisis level to merely being uncomfortable and will continue to affect some specialties until broad tort reform is enacted. More than 60% of physicians aged 55 years or older have been sued, including half the Obstetricians over 40 years old and 90% of General Surgeons 55 years or older. In some locales, Obstetricians still find it difficult to deliver babies at a cost that new families can afford, while paying ever-increasing malpractice insurance premiums.

In many cases, Family Practitioners have completely abandoned the portion of their practices that previously included Obstetrics, outpatient Orthopedics, and Surgery. Radiologists have joined the unlucky group of the most-frequently-sued specialties, mainly due to inaccurately reading mammograms. General Surgeons, Neurosurgeons, Plastic Surgeons, and many other specialists now face similar stiff increases in the already astronomical cost of malpractice insurance. While the highest-income specialties are still lucrative even after subtracting the cost of their malpractice premiums, the net remuneration is not quite as attractive as it would first appear. Note, however, that less than 30% of Pediatricians and Psychiatrists are sued.

Overall, physicians earning the highest net income live in metropolitan areas with fewer than one million people, are not in solo practice, are not linked to a managed care group, and are between 46 and 55 years old.

Debt & Specialty Choice

While no study has shown that medical students make career choices based solely on the level of their debt, some studies suggest a trend in that direction, and one-third of graduating medical students admit that their educational debt influenced their specialty choice. Although a May 2009 report by the U.S. Government Accountability Office found that most physicians make career choices based on their intellectual interests and lifestyle preferences rather than indebtedness, other surveys have shown that as medical students' debt rises, it has more impact on their specialty choice. Of students with a debt less than $50,000, only 18% say it influences their choice. However, their debt influences more than half of those with debts above $150,000, although how it influences them is uncertain. For example, an AAMC survey of graduating medical students showed that medical students choosing Radiology (very high income) had less debt, on average, than those going into Pediatrics (relatively low income). Not measured, though, was whether the difficulty of obtaining a position in the highest-paying specialties or the longer period of residency training also influenced their specialty selection.

Few medical students escape amassing huge amounts of debt from educational loans. The 85% of 2011 medical school graduates who borrowed money to pay for their education owed an average of $156,000, and 25% had debt exceeding $200,000. This debt level has increased 300% since 1985! For perspective, the average graduating student's debt in 1971 was only $8,435 ($45,440 in 2010 dollars).

This debt level will continue to rise, given that in 2010, the mean annual tuition plus fees was almost $27,000 at public medical schools, and was more than $45,000 at private medical schools. Many public medical schools' costs exceed $50,000 and at one, Southern Illinois University, the cost is about $75,000 for non-residents. Even so, if present trends continue, the average medical student debt at public and private medical schools is expected to stay at the same level in constant dollars (meaning adjusted for inflation) until 2033. But, the ability to repay the loan will change. Rates of indebtedness are growing by about 6% a year, which is far more than the estimated 3% growth in physician salaries. In addition, nearly 16% of medical school graduates' spouses have their own debts exceeding $50,000. To make matters worse, nearly 15% of medical students take more than four years to graduate, thus increasing their debt.

Because of the accrued interest, many medical students eventually pay back up to three dollars for every dollar they borrow. Therefore, those who select a poorly remunerated specialty without understanding the ramifications may have a rude awakening at the end of residency training.

An excellent, comprehensive source of information about how to handle medical student debt—conveniently staged for each level of training—can be found on the AAMC's web page "Financing Your Medical Education" (www. aamc.org/students/financing/start.htm). Periodically updated to reflect changes in lending practices and related laws, it contains nearly all the information you will need to manage your medical school debt. One useful section is a searchable database, Loan Repayment/Forgiveness and Scholarship Programs, which lists state and federal programs open to medical students and other health professionals.

Most residents now use the Income Based Repayment (IBR) plan to repay their loans. Payments are based on the difference between your adjusted gross income and 150% of the current federal poverty level (www.cms. gov/MedicaidEligibility/Downloads/POV10Combo.pdf). It provides partial deferment (i.e., reduced payments) for those who can demonstrate some financial hardship. Most residents qualify for some reduction in their loan repayments. The AMA has an excellent information sheet (www.ama-assn. org/ama1/pub/upload/mm/15/ibr-issue-brief.pdf) with details on IBR and web addresses where you can calculate various repayment options.

Importance of Income

A final note is in order about the importance of income to physicians at various stages of their career. For the entry-level physician, income is extremely important. This makes sense, since most new physicians have enormous debts, no money, and increasing financial responsibilities. At mid-career, however, income is of only medium importance—with job security being the most important factor keeping the physician in practice. At this stage of physicians' careers, job satisfaction is equally as important as income. Job satisfaction becomes of overwhelming importance for physicians in the last third of their career. Those who have high job satisfaction presumably keep working longer than those who do not, and have more fun while they are working.

Length Of Training

The majority of medical students do not make specialty choices based on the length of required training. The pleasure they get out of practicing a specialty that interests them generally pays them back for the time they spend as residents and fellows.

Studies show that the length of training does influence some medical students' specialty choice, particularly those selecting generalist or support specialties. The amount of this influence increases as the student's debt rises, becoming particularly strong at debt levels above the mean debt level (about $150,000 in 2011). While this may be understandable, it is sad to think that after expending so much effort, an individual might make a life-long career decision on such a flimsy basis.

One point worth noting, however, is that longer training does not always equate to additional income. In the medical subspecialties, for example, Gastroenterologists, who frequently perform high-reimbursement procedures, have large incomes while Rheumatologists, who do few procedures, make scarcely more than a General Internist. This doesn't mean that those who have a calling in Rheumatology should not pursue this specialty, only that extra education does not always equal an increased income.

Work Hours/Lifestyle

While income is one factor to consider, work hours and lifestyle become much more important once you complete residency. Having a controllable lifestyle has become increasingly important to medical school graduates. Over the past 20 years, the proportion of women choosing "controllable lifestyle" specialties (such as Anesthesiology, Dermatology, Emergency Medicine, Ophthalmology, Otolaryngology, Pathology, Psychiatry, and Diagnostic Radiology) rose from 18% to 36%. During that same period, the proportion of men choosing controllable lifestyle specialties rose from 28% to 45%. These changes persisted even after controlling for income.

An important element of lifestyle is the hours worked. During residency, the hours worked by PGY-2 and higher-level residents, even under the new work-hour rules, often parallel practitioners' work hours in that specialty. Figure 3.3 shows the hours different specialists work in patient care; Figure 5.4 shows the number of patient-care hours in relation to the total time some specialists devote to professional activities. A comparison with Figures 5.2 and 5.3 shows that the hours worked do not correlate with income.

The hours a physician puts into work will markedly influence his family life and extracurricular activities. If you expect to have any life outside of medicine, consider this carefully. Also, note that Surgeons and Obstetricians have lots of "down time" while waiting for an available operating room or for a woman in labor. Much of this time may be in the middle of the night, on weekends, and on holidays. On average, Diagnostic Radiologists work the least time each year (44 weeks), closely followed by Anesthesiologists (45 weeks/year) and by Urologists, Dermatologists and Neurologists (about 46 weeks/year). Most other specialists work between 47 and 48 weeks/year.

Many specialists now join group practices to decrease their work hours and on-call time. Depending on the nature of the group, some physicians have found this quite helpful. The result is a large variation in work hours not only among specialties, but also within each individual specialty. Therefore, a specialty's work hours should not be your only issue when choosing a specialty—but it is a factor that you should seriously consider.

The Potential Future

Anticipating future physician and specialty supply and demand is an inexact science. Physician oversupply and mal-distribution has been an issue in the

Figure 5.4
Average Weekly Work Hours & Workload of Various Specialists

Specialty	Patient Care	All Professional Activities*	Patient Visits*	% Time in Primary Care Activities
Cardiovascular Diseases	61	64	98	6%
Anesthesiology	59	61	n/a	<1
Radiology	59	58	n/a	2
Gastroenterology	58	64	80	8
General Surgery	58	63	81	4
Urology	57	63	98	<1
Gen Internal Medicine	56	62	104	62
Obstetrics/Gynecology	56	61	101	24
Neurology	54	61	78	1
Orthopedic Surgery	54	60	112	4
Otolaryngology	52	58	91	3
Family Medicine	51	56	127	86
Emergency Medicine	50	56	118	30
Pediatrics	49	55	111	73
Ophthalmology	44	49	121	6
Psychiatry	44	47	n/a	1
Dermatology	42	47	152	<1
Pathology	42	46	n/a	<1

* Average hours per week.

Adapted from American Medical Association. *Physician Socioeconomic Statistics,* Chicago, IL: AMA, 2003; and other sources.

United States since at least 1895, when a *Journal of the American Medical Association* discussion of the topic concluded, "our 'excess of doctors' would disappear at once" if the physician population was equitably distributed. At present, more than 6,000 U.S. communities have been designated Primary Care Health Professional Shortage Areas (HPSAs).

Analysts currently predict there will be a shortage of 100,000 physicians in the United States by 2020, with a shortage of primary care physicians reaching 21,000 by 2015. The following factors support this prediction:

- A rapidly aging patient population.
- An increasing supply of women in medicine (with 20% fewer hours worked over their professional lives).

- Faster-than-expected population growth.
- An aging physician population.
- Shorter work hours for all physicians because of the increase in alternative health plans, legislative requirements, and changing lifestyles.

In recent years, physician retirement rates have increased significantly; this is partly due to physicians retiring earlier. The probability of a physician retiring between the ages of 55 and 74 has increased by 60% in the past decade. Above the age of 60, employed physicians consistently retire earlier than those in solo or group practices. According to AMA estimates, increasing retirement rates may absorb as much as one-third of the projected growth in physician supply by the year 2020.

Figure 5.5 shows estimates of the numbers of physicians in the major specialties over the next ten and next twenty years. While they are based somewhat on projected future needs, these numbers are highly speculative. For example, a decreasing birth rate may suggest a need for fewer Pediatricians, but health care reforms allowing children greater access may increase the need. Despite numerous studies, no one knows whether advances in the treatment of coronary artery disease will favor a need for more Invasive Cardiologists (those who pass catheters under x-ray guidance) rather than for more Cardiothoracic Surgeons. Changes in both the treatment of chronic renal disease and the government's and public's attitudes toward chronic renal dialysis programs will profoundly affect the need for Nephrologists. Finding an organic basis for more major psychoses may reduce the need for Psychiatrists, while new medical and invasive treatments for neurological diseases may alter the need for practitioners who deal with those problems (e.g., Neurologists, Neurosurgeons, and Physical Medicine/Rehabilitation physicians).

And, if history is any guide, AIDS and annual worldwide influenza pandemics will be only two of many widespread infections requiring more Family Physicians, Internists, and Infectious Diseases specialists. The number of primary care physicians will most likely increase. Whether that will result in too many primary care physicians is uncertain.

Basically, medicine is not static. Rather, it is an ocean of care with many storms and currents. The storms are the major new medical discoveries, new diseases, and changes in the population's demographics. The currents are the changes in attitudes, by both the medical community and the public concerning the popularity of various medical practices. (Yes, unfortunately, medicine is guided by more than pure science.) Your ship will sail this ocean. Care, foresight, and a willingness to occasionally alter course slightly will keep you afloat.

Figure 5.5
Change in Number & Percentage of M.D. Physician Specialists,
2005, 2010, and 2020

Specialty	Number of Physicians			% Change, 2005 to 2020
	2005	2010	2020	
TOTAL M.D.s & D.O.s	**811,800**	**860,000**	**926,600**	**14**
PRIMARY CARE	**267,000**	**313,200**	**344,700**	**29**
Gen. Family Medicine	107,600	121,400	134,700	25
Gen. Internal Medicine	107,500	131,400	143,900	34
Pediatrics	51,900	60,400	66,100	27
MEDICAL SPECIALTIES	**86,400**	**96,100**	**101,300**	**17**
Cadiovascular Diseases	20,600	22,200	22,900	11
Other Internal Medicine	65,900	73,900	78,500	19
SURGERY	**159,400**	**167,800**	**169,800**	**7**
General Surgery	33,000	31,400	30,800	-6
Obstetrics/Gynecology	41,500	48,000	51,600	24
Otolaryngology	9,800	10,300	10,300	5
Orthopedic Surgery	24,100	25,500	25,500	6
Urology	10,400	10,100	9,600	-7
Ophthalmology	18,400	19,200	19,100	4
OTHER PATIENT CARE	**200,900**	**230,900**	**250,600**	**25**
Psychiatry	38,300	41,000	43,100	13
Anesthesiology	37,800	45,400	50,000	32
Emergency Medicine	26,300	32,200	36,300	38
Radiology	30,900	34,700	36,500	18
Pathology	17,200	18,000	18,200	6
Other Specialties	50,400	59,700	66,400	32
NON-PATIENT CARE	**42,200**	**52,700**	**60,200**	**43**
U.S. POPULATION (000)	**294,100**	**310,333**	**341,387**	**16**

Adapted in part from: Bureau of Health Professions, Health Resources and Services Administration. *Physician Supply and Demand: Projections to 2020.* Washington, DC: U.S. Dept. of Health and Human Services, September 2006:22; and other sources.

Difficulty Of Getting A Residency Position

The difficulty you have in getting an individual residency position will vary with the amount of preparation you do, including correctly matching your aptitudes and accomplishments with a program's needs. However, you can "guesstimate" how difficult it will be to match with each specialty using the tables in the annual National Resident Matching Program's *Results and Data*, posted online at www.nrmp.org.

For example, in 2012, the average specialty offering PGY-1 positions through the NRMP PGY-1 Match filled 95.6% of the available spots. (Additional spots were filled outside of or after the Match.) Those filling higher percentages, and thus being more difficult to match in, were General Surgery-Categorical (1,146; 99.7%), Orthopedic Surgery (682; 100%), Emergency Medicine (1,668; 100%), Internal Medicine-Pediatrics (362; 95%), and Pediatrics-Primary (67; 95.5%).

Of note, however, is that U.S. senior M.D. students filled a relatively small number of positions in some specialties, including Family Medicine (48%), Internal Medicine (56%), Preventive Medicine (25%), Primary Care Internal Medicine (60%), Pathology (55%), Psychiatry (55%), Physical Medicine & Rehabilitation (59%), and Neurology (59%). This means that U.S. seniors should have little difficulty matching into a program in these specialties.

The numbers in the NRMP's charts do not include all the positions available to you. A more accurate picture can be seen by comparing some of these numbers with those in *FREIDA* or in Figure 23.2. Several specialties, including Child Neurology, Ophthalmology, and Urology, hold separate matches for some or most of their positions (see Figure 23.10). These matches occur both through the NRMP and outside of it. Direct application is required for many programs in Preventive Medicine (Aerospace, Occupational, Public Health, and General Preventive Medicine), Nuclear Medicine, many Internal Medicine specialties, and many Osteopathic residencies.

Usually, programs that accept students for an advanced-level position require applicants to match separately in a Preliminary or Transitional internship program for their first year. The students themselves must usually arrange for this training, which means going through the NRMP Match to get a first-year slot. On occasion, the specialty program will arrange the first-year position. Find out how it usually works in the specialty of your choice by writing the specialty's board or society. However, you also need to check with the individual programs, as first-year arrangements may vary from program to program, even within the same specialty. To make things even more complex, the rules for some specialties change frequently.

6

Starting the Process

There are three types of people: those who make things happen,
those who watch things happen, and those who wonder what happened.

Anonymous

Choosing An Adviser/Mentor

SELECTING A MENTOR is *one of the most important career decisions you will ever make*. Most students, however, don't have mentors—they only have "advisers." These faculty members, usually chosen by the Dean, often have multiple advisees and little time for any of them. They may not even have any interest in actually helping students advance their careers in the right direction. You need a mentor!

Selecting a mentor is serious business. When you were born, you could not choose your parents. You now, however, have a choice of mentor. And make no mistake about it, you are choosing a surrogate parent. At best, your mentor can simplify the whole process of selecting your specialty, choosing a desirable residency program, and getting into that program. At worst, a mentor can obstruct your decision-making process by putting the roadblocks of guilt and favors in the way of a correct personal choice.

Your mentor is the individual who will help you make the most of your medical school education. He or she will get you over the rough spots, show you opportunities that you otherwise might miss, guide your career, and generally think of your interests above those of other medical students. Your mentor is your guide, your teacher, your role model. But finding one is up to you. It will take effort, initiative, and assertiveness on your part to locate the right individual. The choice is yours—you can either find a mentor or resign yourself to struggling through on your own.

Choose Early

You should select your mentor early to have the widest possible selection and to fully use his or her expertise. "I'm only in my second semester," you say. "I'll wait until I have had some clinical experience." Baloney! The longer you wait, the less likely it is that your mentor will be:

- your first choice
- a mentor, rather than a standard "adviser"
- able to actually help you very much

A young man showed up in my office one day. Asking if he could have a few moments to talk to me, he explained that he had just been accepted into medical school. He would be starting classes in about six months and wanted to know if I would be his adviser. (His approach was correct. Using the word "mentor" often frightens faculty members.) He explained that he was not sure what field of medicine he wanted to enter, but thought that he had an interest in Emergency Medicine. I agreed to "advise" this student. As his mentor, I was able to introduce him to early clinical experiences, guide him to research opportunities, and help him over some rough spots in his life. Even though he had an interest in my specialty, I repeatedly challenged him on this decision—especially asking him to "tell me the worst parts about the specialty." As with any specialty, if he couldn't answer that question, he didn't know enough about the field.

During his clinical years, I showed him alternative paths to enable him to get the most out of his clinical experiences, prepared him for the entire residency matching process (in General Surgery, which he finally decided upon), and used personal contacts to get him interviews that he desired. He got into his first choice of residency programs. That, in part, was because he was savvy enough about both medical school and the residency selection process to have a mentor help him get the most out of those experiences. But, in fact, getting a supportive mentor is no different in medicine than it is in any field of endeavor. The trick is, start early!

What Type of Person?

When Odysseus went on his travels, Mentor was the person he entrusted with caring for his house and son. He looked for a wise and faithful counselor. That is also what you seek.

The individual you want as your mentor has five characteristics: clinical experience, approachability, the understanding and willingness to work through your insecurities, the character to act as your personal and professional role model, and a vested interest in helping you become successful, regardless of the specialty you ultimately choose.

How do you find a mentor? This will take some effort on your part. Start by making contacts with upper-level (third- and fourth-year) students. They should be doing clinical rotations, and so can be found at the hospital in the evening and at night. Two good places to make contact are in the hospital cafeteria and in the library. Introduce yourself as a fellow medical student and tell them that you need some advice. Unless they are in a rush to get somewhere (the life of a medical student is a harried one) they will be honored by your interest. The question you need to ask is, "Who are the best clinical teachers at the school?" Ask several students for their opinions. This will get you started.

Usually Clinical

Some students select their advisers by picking faculty members who are professors or department chairs. A few students may be lucky enough, using this method, to get counselors who are both interested in them and still knowledgeable about what they will need to do as medical students to get into a residency. But the primary requirement for becoming a full professor is research. Teaching really plays very little, if any, part in their promotion. So choose a mentor from the faculty members who are still involved in teaching, rather than from those who have "retired" to their offices and laboratories. *Your mentor must be reasonably accessible.*

Why choose a clinician rather than a basic scientist? There are three reasons. First, your career will probably be in clinical medicine. You need someone who knows the clinical ropes—not just those in the lecture hall and the lab. Second, the most difficult decisions you will face as a student will revolve around your clinical rotations. In what order should you take the required rotations? What should you do in your senior year? Clinicians are the most qualified people to answer such questions. Finally, your role model should live in the same world that you plan to enter—clinical medicine.

Pick a Known Teacher

Now you have a list of clinical teachers that other students consider excellent. Why did they choose these people? Being an excellent teacher takes effort. This effort stems from an interest in helping students to learn. It is also based on a deep and abiding interest in student welfare. Doesn't this sound like the type of person you want for a mentor? Of course, given the recognition of their excellence by other students, some of these individuals may already have many students whom they are counseling. If they cannot add another student, ask if they can recommend an individual whom they feel would be an excellent adviser. These people can usually spot the gems among their faculty, so take their suggestions seriously. If one of them feels that they can add you to his or her group, go for it. You already stand out by showing initiative so early. You can now do several other things to enhance that positive image.

Be visible. This means showing up with some regularity at your adviser's doorstep. The best and most productive way to accomplish this is to spend clinical time with him or her. This could mean doing afternoon or Saturday morning ward rounds, scrubbing in on a Saturday morning operation or procedure, or tagging along during an evening clinic or an emergency department shift. Since you have chosen a great teacher, it probably will be no time at all until you are actively participating (at your level of expertise) in patient care. If you do this, be sure to wear appropriate attire. This is the time to start looking professional. And bring along a stethoscope. Here is where you will begin to learn to use it.

Develop an image in your mentor's mind of a likable, courteous, and considerate individual. It is always pleasant to have a cheerful person around. But fawning and flattery generally have a negative effect. Mentors can quickly see through this facade.

Be respectful of your mentor's time. Once a clinician has agreed to be your adviser/mentor, make an appointment to see that individual whenever necessary. This is the professional thing to do and your mentor will appreciate your consideration of his or her valuable time.

Be clear about what you desire from your mentor (advice) and what your mentor can expect from you (hard work and dedication). Don't push for anything else. If you demonstrate the hard work and dedication, all else will follow.

Notice that nothing has been said yet about your mentor's specialty. Having examined your options, you probably have a general idea of what you are aiming for in the future. But, at best, it will be a very rough guess at this point. Try to select a mentor who is in a field compatible with your interests. For example, if you are contemplating Thoracic Surgery, a Dermatologist should probably not be your first choice as a mentor. If you do get a mentor who is in the specialty you finally choose, so much the better. However, *your choice of the appropriate person as your mentor actually depends more upon the individual than on his or her specialty.*

Steer Clear of Those with Blinders

Selecting someone who cannot see beyond his own chosen field of specialization is a real danger. You quickly may discover this attitude from such comments as, "The only real doctors are Surgeons," or "The only satisfaction in medicine comes from delivering babies." The key here is the word "only." At this point in your career, there is no "only," merely a lot of "maybes."

Too many medical school advisors and other faculty say "That's a bad career move" as they denigrate other specialties that students are considering. This statement is often accompanied by incorrect information about the other specialty. Instead, they should be supporting their students who are searching for the best fit of a specialty with their personality, needs, and abilities.

If you find that your selection for mentor wears specialty blinders, bail out—fast. This is the right time to get another adviser—one with a broader outlook about medical practice.

Supplement Later, If Necessary

Congratulations! You have gone through the process of getting a mentor early. This should help you through many of the rough spots in the road ahead. But now, after your exposure to Pediatrics, you are certain that you are destined to be a Pediatrician. Your mentor is an Anesthesiologist. What should you do?

First, make an appointment with your mentor. Explain that you have given the question of specialty choice a great deal of thought, and have decided on Pediatrics. If you have chosen your mentor correctly, he or she will understand and support your decision. He or she may also ask you why you made that decision and if you have thought about some important points related to your specialty decision. Being able to answer those questions may serve to deepen your resolve and help assure you that you have made the correct (initial) decision.

Next, ask if your adviser knows any Pediatricians, either from within the faculty or in the community, who could assist you in gathering more specific information about the specialty. Could he or she arrange an introduction or telephone ahead to say that you will be calling for an appointment? Then, visit these referrals and get all the information and special help from them that you can.

But don't forget your mentor! He or she is still the physician who has your interests most at heart. Keep in close contact, and continue to run your major decisions by him or her for an honest appraisal. Your mentor can be a close contact and source of advice for the rest of your career—don't abandon that individual now.

No Available Specialty Advisor?

While most students will have at least one local physician in their specialty of interest to act as a mentor, no medical center has specialists in every field. Therefore, some students will find that no one practices that specialty (or trained in the field) at their medical school. What should you do if this happens to you?

First, get an advisor who is sympathetic to your plight rather than someone who wants to steer you toward his or her specialty. Talk with the Dean of Students about this to get an appropriate person.

Next, contact the geographically closest physician practicing that specialty. If you have difficulty locating such a person, contact the national specialty organization for assistance. (See the contact information in each specialty's description in Chapter 3.) You can also check the "Doctor Finder" section of the American Medical Association's website (https://extapps.ama-assn.org/doctorfinder/home.jsp). Use the "Patient" option to indicate your location and the specialty that interests you. This list includes both AMA members and non-members. Contact an individual on the list and see if they are willing both to give you long distance advice (e-mail, phone, mail) and to allow you to visit their practice when you have time (weekends, holidays). Another option is to use the Administrator in Medicine website (www.docboard.org/aim/). Choose the heading "DocFinder," and search for the locale and the specialty that interest you to find the physicians' work addresses and phone numbers. While not all states participate in this database, those that do list both M.D. and D.O. physicians.

Testing Your Specialty Choice

Once you think you know which specialty you might like, why don't you give it a try? Would you buy a car without taking it for a test drive? Of course not! Then why consider investing time, effort, and money to train in a specialty when you really don't know if you have found the correct one?

At graduation, only 20% of medical students are still interested in entering the same specialty that they wanted when they entered medical school. That is certainly understandable. More troubling is that nearly 25% of all physicians change their specialties after graduation, either during their training or shortly thereafter. In many cases this is due to poor planning. Be smart. Test your specialty choice before you invest too much of yourself in it.

Volunteer Time

One of the best ways to learn about a specialty is to spend some of your free time on that clinical service. This is especially true if that specialty rotation is not available early in your third year of medical school. If your mentor is in this field, you should have no problem arranging this. Otherwise, he or she might help you contact a physician in that specialty with whom you can work.

No matter where you are in your training now, you are probably saying, "What free time?" The answer is that you have time to do anything that is important to you. *This is important.* Certainly you can arrange to have a half-hour or forty-five minutes to participate in a portion of morning rounds before class. How about Saturday or Sunday mornings?

What information are you seeking as you do this? First, look at the specialists you're with. Do they seem happy doing what they do? Would you enjoy doing what they do? Do you want to have the same type of clinical practice as they have? Will it provide enough intellectual stimulation for you? What don't you like about it? Could you put up with it for your entire career? These are just a few of the questions that you should ask yourself during your volunteer stint. Some of the questions you will ask yourself, and the clinical experiences that you will have, will differ depending upon your level of training and prior clinical experience. The farther along you are in your training, and the more in-depth your clinical experiences have been, the more subtle the questions you will be able to ask yourself about the specialty.

But this doesn't mean you should delay volunteering for clinical experiences to explore your choices. Rather, it means you should start early. The more of this type of volunteer time that you spend, the faster you will gain experience and be able to probe your specialty choice in depth. *Also, spend some of your time in a community hospital or office setting.* This will give you a broader view of how the specialty is practiced away from the academic medical center.

Pre-med

This is an excellent time to volunteer in a specialty. You have time to spare. And you can find out something even more important than what specialty you want to enter: *You can determine if you really want to become a physician.* This must be *your* choice, not your parents', teachers', or friends' choice for you. And in volunteering, you will be able to see the amount of dedication, hard work, and commitment to continued learning that the profession requires. If a medical career is really what you want, this experience will renew your motivation. If not, it may save you a lot of frustration and help you to redirect your energies.

How do you volunteer at this stage of your training? Undoubtedly, it will be more difficult to get a volunteer position in a specific specialty now than it will be after you enter medical school. You may have fewer contacts in the medical field and less knowledge upon which to base a specialty decision.

Your best bet is to first approach your family's doctor. Tell him or her of your interest in the medical profession and of your desire to experience medicine firsthand by "tagging along and helping out." Usually the clinician will be flattered that you asked, and will let you participate in at least a limited fashion. After a few months of this (stick it out, you are learning vital information on which to base lifelong decisions), it may become obvious that you have progressed beyond the level of knowledge that this practitioner can offer. If the practitioner does not spontaneously suggest it, you should inquire as to whether there is a more in-depth (read "active") medical experience available to you. If you know this physician really well, you might even address the possibility in your first meeting. In many cases, of course, working with a practitioner of this sort will be interesting and intriguing. If that is true for you, stick with it.

Okay, you don't have a family physician and neither of your parents are physicians. (Physician–parents should generally be able to help you to arrange these experiences.) What do you do now? If you are not quite gutsy enough to walk in on a physician unannounced, try to get some leads from the staff at your college's student health center. If this does not prove useful, go to a major hospital in your area and volunteer to work in a clinical area.

The hospital you choose depends upon your interests. To start, you may want to pick the hospital that gets most of the accident victims (Level I Trauma Center). Ask to work in the emergency department. There you will see both a wide variety of illnesses and injuries and some of the activities of practitioners in many different specialties. You may even make some contacts that you can use in the future. If you have the opportunity and the time, it might even be useful for you to work as an emergency department aide. These positions are often available to individuals with little or no experience. Then you will really be part of the team and be able to interact with patients in an even closer manner. You will also get paid.

Preclinical Years

If you are reading this between studying for Physiology or Pharmacology, you may question where you will find time to volunteer clinically. You can use nights, weekends, and holidays for this clinical activity, after the demands of studying (and the absolute imperative to find some time for yourself) have been satisfied.

Volunteering to work clinically during the preclinical years is an essential part of your career preparation—not only to help you choose a specialty, but also to remind you of why you struggled so hard to get into medical school. You have more clinical opportunities available than does an undergraduate student. Remember, you are a *medical student*. You will soon be a physician, and the entire profession stands ready to help you.

Basically, you will find yourself in one of two situations, depending upon the nature of your medical school. The first results from the traditional medical school structure, in which the major teaching hospital is adjacent to the school. There you will bump into "white coats" every day. And you will have little difficulty finding the time between classes to approach clinicians about working with them. The hospital and the physicians working there are oriented toward education and will, in general, be ready to accommodate you.

The second type of medical school is less consolidated than the first type. This makes it somewhat more difficult to get a meaningful clinical experience early in your training. Either the basic science and clinical campuses are geographically separated or there is no specific or adjacent teaching-oriented hospital. (These latter are the "community-based" medical schools.) A mentor, if you have one, can be invaluable in assisting you here. If you don't have a mentor, you will have to approach local hospitals and practitioners on your own. Success depends upon your persistence; keep trying if you are initially turned down.

With community-based medical schools, there are several options for locating volunteer opportunities. As when choosing a mentor, get leads from upper-level medical students. If your school offers Physical Diagnosis courses in the first and second years, use your instructor as a resource. He or she might actually be an individual with whom you can work in a real clinical setting. You can also approach physicians at the largest of the affiliated community teaching hospitals. They are more attuned to education than other practitioners. And even if the first physician you contact can't help you, that clinician can probably give you some excellent leads. If nothing else proves fruitful, try the county or state medical societies. Some branches have programs designed to pair students with practitioners.

The most important reason to obtain clinical experience in your preclinical years is to learn the relationship of the basic sciences to the practice of medicine. "But why will this be important to me as a physician?" asked a first-year medical student after a rather mystifying biochemistry lecture. The lecturer, a Ph.D. who proudly proclaimed whenever he had the chance that he had never been in a hospital as an adult, could not answer the student's question. He did not even understand it.

You are in medical school to become a physician. In almost every case, physicians interact with the ill and injured on a daily basis. If you wonder why the basic sciences are important, you may find the answers in the real and immediate classroom of clinical experience. The basic sciences are not just "important": They are vital to understanding clinical practice and the changes that will occur in medicine during your career. Spend some time in clinical activities. It's worth it.

Clinical Years

If you are already in your clinical years, mere additional clinical exposure is not what you need. You must spend time testing your tentative specialty choices.

"But when do I have the time?" you ask. The answer is, during "slow" rotations, on weekends, and in the evenings. If you find spending time with specialists in the field you plan to enter to be too much work, rather than a joy, perhaps you have discovered the answer to whether you are really interested in that specialty. If you don't enjoy the work now, how will you feel about it in 20 years? Or 20 years after that?

By your fourth year, if you have put in some effort, you should have made a reasonably definite and educated decision regarding a specialty choice. Some students wait until their elective time to test their specialty choices. That is too late. Unless there is an elective opportunity in the third year, you cannot afford to wait that long to make a decision. You should use the prime elective time early in your fourth year for two vital electives: First, take a rotation that will allow you to make decisions and take responsibility for them, such as an Internal Medicine or a General Surgery subinternship. These experiences will help you to be a "star" when you take your second vital elective in your chosen specialty. Use this elective to "show your stuff" to the specialists who will be writing your letters of recommendation.

At many schools, students are now allowed to postpone some required clerkships, such as Psychiatry, Neurology, and Family Practice, until their fourth year. This allows them time earlier in their training to experience other fields, such as Anesthesiology and Radiology, which have traditionally been reserved for fourth-year elective time. If it is not overdone, this may be a good chance to get a more in-depth look at an area you have strongly considered as a career.

Reading (See Annotated Bibliography)

There are several sources for material dealing with every specialty and subspecialty. The first (often easiest-to-access) is the Internet, although finding the right URL may be difficult. The current URLs are listed under each specialty description in Chapter 3; most provide you with additional "links." The bibliography contains more URLs, and others are listed in appropriate sections throughout this book. They were up-to-date at the time of publication but, as you know, the Web constantly changes, so if the supplied URLs don't work, use a search engine and look for the organization's name. If you use Google, go to the "Advanced Search" mode (www.google.com/advanced_search) and put the name in the "exact phrase" box. Rarely, some specialty organizations dissolve, change names, or merge. If you still can't find it, look at the links on related websites.

Your medical school's library is another great source of information. If you are interested in any of the more popular specialties, there should not only be factual material on the specialty, but also biographies of individuals in the field. Also, look for articles highlighting the specialty in *The New Physician*, which regularly prints such reviews. Specialty journals, especially the "throwaways," may also give you an idea of the discipline's breadth. This is particularly true for some of the smaller specialties, which do not get significant coverage in journal articles. The reference librarians can also help you locate online information that you haven't been able to find.

Two other excellent sources of information are the American Medical Association Medical Student Section's Specialty Information web site (go to www.ama-assn.org/go/mss and scroll down to "Resources You Can Use"—"Residency Resources") and the Pathway Evaluation Program's "Specialty Profiles" (http://medweb.usc.edu/pathways/intro.htm). In addition, the AAMC offers a brief review of many specialties on its *Careers in Medicine* web site (www.aamc.org/students/cim/specialties.htm). Generally, these sources review the history, economics, and practice of most of the medical specialties.

For information about the smaller or newer specialties, you may have to turn to other sources. One, discussed in more detail in Chapter 10, is the

Directory of Graduate Education Programs. The section "Essentials of Accredited Residencies in Graduate Medical Education" provides a wealth of information about each officially recognized specialty and subspecialty.

Ask your mentor or adviser for material about the specialty that you are considering. This individual may have information from a variety of sources, or may have produced some herself. Finally, you may want to borrow a standard text for the field, assuming that you are considering a lesser-known specialty that is not well-represented in the library. This should also give you a broad idea of the discipline's scope.

Talk to Many Specialists in the Field

Specialty choices are often based on a student's interaction with one physician in a given field. Often this specialist is a parent or the family's doctor. Other times it is an assigned adviser or a respected faculty member. But no matter who the role model is, basing your entire career on only one individual's experiences can lead to disaster.

It is essential that you get input from a wide variety of practitioners as you try to decide on your medical specialty. If your interest is Dermatology, this does not mean talking only with the faculty at your school. You should also visit Dermatologists in private practice, group practice settings, and health maintenance organizations in your community. If there is a county or state society meeting for the specialty, try to attend it as a student observer. Normally, these specialty societies will welcome you. You will then have a chance to talk with a variety of specialists practicing in that field, and will also hear about the problems they face in their practices and about their general attitude toward their own specialty choice.

Many physicians practicing today would not choose the same specialty if they had it to do over again. While some of this may be due to "the grass is always greener" syndrome, in large part, it is because they made career decisions without adequate information and with inappropriate expectations. Get as much information as you can directly "from the horses' mouths." The grief you save will be your own.

Match Your Choice to Your Needs

It is vital that you consider your personal desires when choosing the direction your career will take.

Abraham Maslow, in his famous book, *Motivation and Personality* (Harper & Row, New York, 1954), sought to explain why people are driven by particular needs at particular times. He felt that all human needs are arranged in a hierarchy, from the most pressing to the least pressing (Figure 6.1). As each level of need is satisfied, it is no longer a driving force for that individual. For nearly all medical students, the basic physiological needs, such as hunger and thirst, have been satisfied. The safety needs of security and protection will be satisfied if you believe you will complete medical school, get into a residency program, and earn a living. The factors on this level, plus those on the next most important level, the esteem needs of recognition, self-esteem, and status, are very often the driving forces behind a medical student's specialty choice. (Most medical students can see that the social needs of love and belonging will be fulfilled in the future, if not now.)

What you must do, however, is look beyond these levels and try to visualize what you will need to reach the highest level—*Self-Actualization.* Basically, you must try to determine *what will be fulfilling to you for the rest of your life.* Will you be happy in your specialty choice at age forty? Will you be able to meet your life goals? (You are about to be a doctor, so you have essentially achieved that goal.) Assessing your future self is something that, though easily stated, is very hard to do. Yet if you give it some serious thought—reflecting on it and talking it over with those close to you, you may very well make a much better decision than you otherwise might have made.

Figure 6.1
Maslow's Hierarchy of Needs

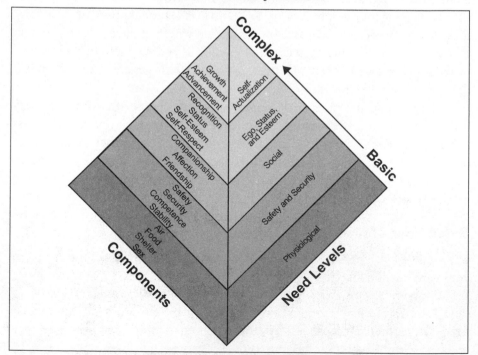

7
Grades, Research, Summers, Clinical Clerkships, & Awards

*Choose a job you love and
you will never have to work a day in your life.*

Confucius (551-479 BC)

Putting Your Effort Where It Counts, Part 1

SUCCEEDING IN MEDICAL SCHOOL takes a lot of work. But since there are many areas in which to work hard and only a finite amount of time and energy available to put into them, it is important to determine where you should put your greatest effort—and how to make it pay off.

Residency programs will use your grades, test scores, and, occasionally, "audition electives" to evaluate your medical school performance. Institutions, and specific residency programs at those institutions, vary widely in how they assess the individual components of any candidate's application. Thus, how a particular program will evaluate the various criteria is almost impossible to ascertain. The best you can do is to put as much effort as possible into each of the areas listed in this chapter, which discusses grades, research, clinical rotations, awards, and summer work, and in Chapter 8, which discusses tests. Your personal strengths will help determine the areas in which you excel.

Honor Grades

Grades reflect your abilities over a wide range of activities. Therefore, they are one of the major factors used to differentiate you from other applicants. In the basic sciences, grades reflect your ability to gather, memorize, regurgitate, and, occasionally (especially in schools with problem-based learning), synthesize information. Grades from clinical services reflect your ability to perform basic patient care, to memorize information, and to work well with patients, staff, and physicians. This is measured by how well you regurgitate the information for exams and synthesize it on the wards. Grades from clinical rotations also reflect your social and interactive skills.

Getting "Honors" (equivalent to an "A" or a "4.0" on a four-point scale; also equivalent to "High Honors," "Outstanding," or "Superior" at some schools) sets you apart from your classmates—and, more important, other applicants. But it will be the rare individual, indeed, who will be able to get all, or even a majority of, "Honors" grades. So, it may benefit you to set your sights on particular courses and clerkships in which to make an all-out effort for "Honors," and to settle for lower (but passing) grades in the remaining classes.

If your school happens to be on a strict pass-fail system, you will have a slightly lower chance of getting into the most competitive residencies. You cannot change the grading system your school uses—at least not by yourself. So you will have to concentrate on other demonstrable honors, awards, and letters of recommendation.

Order of Importance

Okay, so you have decided to put extra effort into certain courses to get "Honors" grades in them. How do you decide which ones? Actually, it is not that difficult.

Third-Year Required Clerkships

Your most important grades (and letters of recommendation) for getting a residency are those from required third-year clerkships. While the level of difficulty and the types of experiences a student has during the preclinical years can vary widely among medical schools, junior-year clinical experiences are, for the most part, very similar. Therefore, even though the grading for them varies from school to school, residency programs still find third-year clinical grades the easiest way to compare applicants. *Residency directors know that high-honors grades in core clerkships are excellent predictors of outstanding clinical performance—and consider them one of the most important factors in resident selection.* Also, unless you are going into Pathology, patient care is the job for which you will be applying. Therefore, residency programs must know whether you are competent in this area. Since you will apply to the programs very early in your fourth year, most of the clinical grades that the evaluators see when selecting candidates for interviews will be those from the third year.

If you are entering a specialty that is required in the third-year curriculum, such as Internal Medicine, General Surgery, Pediatrics, Psychiatry, Obstetrics and Gynecology, and often Neurology or Family Medicine, it will obviously be to your advantage to do well in that area. Otherwise, the two clerkships that normally carry the most weight in residency selection are Internal Medicine and Surgery. Make an extra effort to do well on these rotations.

Now for a note about your third year in general: You will probably find your junior year of medical school to be both the most exciting and the most confusing period of your professional career. As you rotate through the various specialties, you will be barraged by their differing attitudes, rules of behavior, and personalities. Even if you have a good idea about which discipline you want for a career, don't close your mind to the experiences that you encounter. You might find a field that interests you more than your original choice. But don't rely on a single experience at a single institution with a single group of physicians to make your career decision. It may be very misleading.

In what order should you take your junior clerkships? Basically, it boils down to deciding whether to take Medicine and Surgery early in the year or later, after you have been "seasoned" by completing the "lesser" clerkships. The answer depends upon two things:

1. **The amount of clinical experience you had before medical school or obtained during your preclinical years.** If you have had significant clinical experience, it matters little when you take any particular clerkship.

2. **Do you want to go into a specialty that is offered in the third year?** If you think that you do but you are not sure, take that clerkship early to find out if you like it. On the other hand, if you are sure, take it at a time when you can be certain of doing well on the rotation. Again, if you already have a great deal of clinical experience, take it when it is convenient. If you are a clinical novice, then wait until later in your third year to "show your stuff." Going through other clinical areas first will improve your performance—and your grade.

Specialty Clerkship

Next in importance to your third-year clerkships, and often of equal or greater importance in some specialties (such as Ophthalmology and Orthopedic Surgery), is your performance in your chosen specialty's senior clerkship. Where and with whom you take this clerkship is critical. If you plan on going into Radiology, taking a Radiology clerkship at the local suburban hospital won't work, no matter what the quality of teaching or your experiences. Use that site for extra volunteer time.

For a senior specialty elective "Honors" grade that residency programs view favorably, and to obtain a beneficial recommendation letter, take this rotation *at a major teaching hospital with an attending physician who is well-known to residency directors in the field.* Since you have ample leeway in setting up your senior schedule, there is no reason why you cannot find a suitable clerkship.

Remember that the smaller specialties (e.g., Neurological Surgery, Otolaryngology) and the smaller programs in most other specialties prefer to take applicants they know. Use this to your advantage.

Preclinical

Third on the list of priorities for getting "Honors" grades are the preclinical courses. This, of course, does not include those of you who are interested in going either into Pathology or into a research-oriented career. In both of these cases, "Honors" grades in the preclinical years are very important. For a Pathology residency, preclinical "Honors" grades will often be the most important selection factor.

If you are interested in a clinical career, you should pick and choose carefully where to focus your main effort during the first two years. For those entering the Surgical specialties, "Honors" in Anatomy and Pathology are very helpful. Those contemplating any of the Neurosciences (including Psychiatry) should strive for excellence in their Neuroscience course. And for almost everyone else, the key courses are Pharmacology and Physiology. This is not meant to imply that you shouldn't try to make a clean sweep by getting more "Honors" grades. But in reality, this is just not possible for most mortals. So, direct your efforts where they will count the most.

A strategy that some students find successful is to pick one major course each semester (or quarter) in which to try to achieve an "Honors" grade. Then, when you have a little extra time to study, concentrate on that course. While this strategy does not always work, many individuals have found that it gives them motivation to study just a bit harder.

Senior Electives

The grades from senior electives are the least significant to most programs when choosing residents. *This does not include electives in your chosen specialty.* Other senior grades are considered very minimally—except in extraordinary cases, such as getting all "Honors" or, at the other extreme, failing or getting "Incomplete" in a course. All experienced residency directors know that "grade inflation," that is, a higher percentage of excellent scores than is warranted, is rampant on senior electives. This is especially true for electives taken outside the main teaching hospitals. So don't expect to correct a dismal record with a lot of "Honors" grades from fourth-year electives. Everyone will see through that ploy.

One problem for some individuals is that the grades for senior specialty electives will not be recorded in time to affect their selection for an interview. If you have done very well on a rotation in your chosen specialty, have your

Dean's office send an updated transcript to the programs to which you are applying and get a letter from the elective director to give to the residency directors during your interview. Of course, if you didn't do well in some senior electives (too much time at the beach?), not having the grades on the transcript sent to residency programs will be to your advantage.

Clinical Honors = Effort + Effort + Effort

Since so much emphasis is placed on doing well during clinical rotations, understand that you do not have to be either a genius or a saint to get "Honors" grades. All it takes is a realization that you will have to expend *effort, effort, and more effort*. This includes *in-depth reading* about the patients that you have seen, are taking care of, or will see (such as those in the operating room). If you have time, also read about the other patients on the ward. If you are scheduled to do a procedure, read about it in advance. And don't just scan the *Cliff's Notes* version; get a book that will give you detailed information. If you can, also learn a few pieces of arcane trivia about the disease or procedure. These are always fun to introduce into discussions when making rounds.

Know the ropes. New rotations initially confuse all students and residents. Each service has its own culture, its own rules, its own body of basic knowledge, and its own stumbling blocks for the unwary. One way to ease your transition into a new rotation is to discover exactly what the service expects of you. (See Figure 7.1 for a list of questions to ask.) If you don't receive this information at least a week before the rotation begins, call or visit the rotation director's office to ask your questions. Often, the secretary will have a pre-printed list of information that is normally handed out the first day; get it in advance.

Round early and stay late. If you show up before the rest of your team to find out what happened on the ward overnight, you will be able to help the housestaff immeasurably. This often translates into glowing recommendations about you to the attendings. Stay late to complete any work that was left undone. If you are still there (doing something useful, not just hanging around) when the other students are gone, you will stand out as the hard worker you are.

Volunteer for extra or onerous work. Of course no one wants to put an IV into Mrs. Smith for the twentieth time or to push Mr. Jones down to radiology, but volunteer to do it with a *smile*. Not only will you make points, but you also may get priority in doing things that you want to do, such as the next thoracentesis or hernia repair.

Figure 7.1
Questions about Clerkship Expectations

- What are the goals and objectives for the rotation?
- What clinical responsibilities do students have?
- Where and when should I report the first day?
- At which facilities will I work?
- What is the call schedule? Is there in-house call for students?
- Is there a conference and lecture schedule?
- Do students carry pagers?
- Are there non-clinical responsibilities (such as a presentation)?
- Who is the attending? How often will I meet with him or her?
- Who will be the senior resident on the service?
- Which other students will be on the rotation?
- Is there a list of required or suggested readings?
- Are there printed descriptions of special clinical procedures?
- Are there study questions?
- Will there be written or oral exams? How many and when?
- Who evaluates students? On what basis?
- Can I see a copy of the student-performance evaluation form?
- Is housing available for out-of-town students?
- Can I interview for a residency position during the rotation?

Show enthusiasm in everything that you do on the clinical services. Be pleasant. Smile, even if it is after your bedtime—or maybe you haven't been to sleep and it's 6 A.M. Everyone gets tired, but if you use the energy you still have to bolster everyone's spirits, you will earn big points—and will have a better time doing it than if you are sullen.

Clinical services are increasingly using problem- and case-based small-group instruction during clerkships. The hints below have helped other students perform well in these groups.

Small Group Participation
- Show up for all sessions.
- Read required material in advance.
- Listen actively (i.e., focus on the speaker).
- Participate an appropriate amount of the time.
- Ask questions that improve discussion and understanding.
- Show respect for other group members' opinions.
- Relate positively and constructively to other group members.
- Encourage other group members to participate.
- Help to keep the discussion on track.

Problem-Based Learning Hints
(Also useful for presenting cases on the wards.)

- Show up for all sessions.
- Read and research the Problem Case(s) and Learning Issues in advance.
- Prepare using MEDLINE, textbooks, journal articles, and expert faculty.
- Critically interpret information and information sources.
- Identify case issues that may lead to Learning Issues.
- Share information appropriately.
- Identify pertinent facts in the case.
- Present information in an organized manner.
- Formulate hypotheses.
- Identify the information needed to progress further with the case.
- Apply previously learned and new information to the case problems.

Finally, if there are written or oral exams at the end of the rotation—*study.* Find out early if there will be such a test (there usually is) and try to ascertain what will be on it. Then use your extra time (believe it or not there will usually be a lot of "down time" on the wards) to study. If you know what you have to study at the beginning of the rotation, the reading that you do about your patients will complement, enhance, and, often, shorten your study time.

The key to success on clinical rotations, as one student wrote in her personal statement, is to "Work like a duck: appear smooth on the surface, but paddle like crazy underneath."

Summer Work

The Beach Boys sang "you'll have fun, fun, fun 'til your daddy takes the T-Bird away." Even if you don't have any idea what a T-Bird is (a car) or who the Beach Boys are (a '60s California singing group), you certainly know about summer fun. Unfortunately, now that you are in medical school, the sun and fun will have to be put in proper perspective. Summer, especially the summer between your first and second years of school, is your only free time to explore the tentative selections you have made concerning a specialty choice. But it also will probably be the last "free" summer that you will have for many years. The question for you is, "What is most important?"

There is no question that there's a great pull to escape after a year of bookwork and laboratories. That is only natural. But escape into the world of clinical medicine. This should be an exciting and interesting experience on several counts.

First, it will be completely different from the classroom you have labored in for the past nine-plus months. Second, it will allow you to do what you got into medical school to do—practice medicine. This might rejuvenate you for your second year of studies. Third, it will enable you to see in more detail just what aspects of medicine you enjoy and what parts you dislike. Finally, you might even make some money.

The two places to start when exploring options for summer work are your mentor and the Student Affairs office. The latter will probably have lists of those clinical (and research) fellowships that are offered to medical students. While some fellowships are available through national programs (though not necessarily to first-year students), others are generally specific to a particular institution.

What you are looking for is *clinical experience*. In some cases, this will be obvious, e.g., it is labeled as a student clinical fellowship. Other times the clinical experience may come disguised as research, as in a Pediatric project where you will have to do specific parts of a physical examination on children to collect the necessary data. The point in summer work is to try, if at all possible, to be around clinicians, learning and doing some of what they do.

The second source to use for finding a summer clinical experience is your mentor. This individual may not only be aware of opportunities at your institution of which the Dean's Office is uninformed, but also may know of opportunities in the community or at other institutions. Your mentor may also invite you to work with him or her during the summer. This could be an outstanding experience. But you may not receive any money for it.

If you are in serious need of money to continue living through the next year, you may have to balance the time you spend in an unpaid clinical experience with time spent in a paying job. However, do not neglect this unique opportunity to get your feet wet and your hands dirty in the clinical sphere. It will help crystallize your idea of what specialty you want to enter when you finish medical school, as well as improve your attitude and ability to learn in your second year.

Research

Common wisdom nowadays, meaning the scuttlebutt among the rest of your class, is that it is vital to do research if you are going to get into a good residency program—especially if it is in one of the competitive specialties like Orthopedics, Neurological Surgery, or Otolaryngology. As with all rumors, there is a kernel of truth imbedded in the lie. It isn't mandatory to do research. If you have no desire to do research at this time, if you have no knack for it, or if you have no access to research opportunities, forgo it for now. Put your energy into other areas in which you do have an interest and that, therefore, will pay off more handsomely for the amount of energy that you expend.

If you do have an interest in research, it is important to make any such endeavor a meaningful experience. First of all, try to do a project that is clinically related to the field to which you will be applying. Too many applications list research projects dealing with such obscurities as the genetic makeup of the hummingbird. This is not the kind of research that will endear you to most clinicians. Though that type of research can be important and the students who do it probably learn many fine laboratory techniques, they are misdirecting a lot of energy if their goal is to get into a clinical residency program. So, how do you go about getting the most out of your research effort?

Begin by choosing the correct preceptor. Hopefully, your mentor either will be willing to act as your research preceptor or can direct you to someone else who is suitable. Make certain the individual you choose has previously worked on student and resident research projects. Many students suffer under the tutelage of either experienced researchers who see medical students only as "gofers" or individuals without adequate research experience (the blind leading the blind).

Doable Project

Next, select the project. It can be your idea or, more likely, it will be your preceptor's idea. The key to choosing the correct project is to select one that interests you. You should also be able to do the project with relatively little assistance. This usually rules out the use of a linear accelerator or other complicated instruments unless you have prior experience, or the time and interest to learn how to use such equipment. It must be a project that you can do in the time that you will have available to you. If you will only be working on it at night and during weekends, it is foolish to take on a project that requires your intervention six times a day for a month. If you have a period of time, say a month or six weeks, that you want to block out to do the research, make sure that you plan to do the work in less time than that. Research *always* takes much more time and energy than is initially allotted.

Finally, make sure that your research is at least somewhat related to your specialty choice. If you are not certain yet of what that is, aim for something with broad clinical applicability—something that affects all aspects of medicine. Projects dealing with an aspect of hypertension, diabetes, wound healing, or sepsis are some examples.

Make It Count

Other than the factors listed above, there are several key parts of the project that will provide you with extra benefits. There are *two things that must be decided before any work is performed*. The first is to make sure that a *publication* will come out of the research, and that the work won't just be either relegated to the circular file or used as a footnote in a larger piece of work. While nearly half of all medical students are involved in research projects, only one-third of this group gets listed as authors on publications. The issue of *authorship* is very important. Even if you do 90% of the work, you may only get fifth billing on any publications, meaning that you will be listed after four other individuals. You would like to be listed first, or at least second, on the paper that comes out of the research. Of course, make sure that you do enough work on the project to warrant this.

You should also be aware that clinical research seems to be much easier to publish than basic science research. It also often seems to require less time to actually perform the research—particularly if you retrospectively study already available data, such as in a chart review. (Institutional Review Board approval for projects with student participation, however, may take much longer than for other projects. So start that part of the process ahead of time.) And, if you do not wish to or do not have the time to do actual research, a case report with a literature review is a reasonable alternative. All these are excellent learning experiences. Okay, so you won't get a Nobel Prize for it, but that publication will help you get the residency you want. If you broach this subject at the start of discussions about your research project, you may find that you will have a much easier time getting both a publication and appropriate authorship.

The other item to arrange in advance is the question of presentation at a scientific meeting. A scientific article may take a long time to get published, often a year or more after submission. And the words "submitted for publication" next to an article on a résumé or application are not as impressive as "published" or "presented." The quickest way to upgrade the firepower of your paper and the research behind it is to present the findings at a national scientific meeting. If the research is of decent quality, you should have no problem doing this. If it is to be presented, an abstract of your paper is normally published ahead of time in a scientific journal; you will still be able to submit the entire paper later for publication. But if you are considering this, be sure to think, early in the planning stages, about both the project's content and the deadlines for the meeting. That way you will be able to finish the project in time to meet the meeting's deadline. Plan ahead.

Sources of Funding for Student Research

Aside from programs associated with your school, several national sources provide funding for students with identifiable research projects. These include:
- Alpha Omega Alpha (AOA) Student Research Fellowships, www.alphaomegaalpha.org/student_research.html
- American College of Rheumatology, www.rheumatology.org/ref/awards/index.asp?aud=stu
- American Federation for Aging Research (AFAR), www.afar.org/grants.html
- American Urological Association/AUA Foundation Research Scholars Program, www.urologyhealth.org/researchpage
- American Gastroenterological Association/Foundation for Digestive Health and Nutrition, www.fdhn.org/html/awards/awards.html
- American Heart Association Student Scholarships in Cardiovascular Disease & Stroke, www.americanheart.org
- American Society for Clinical Nutrition/National Clinical Nutrition Internships, www.nutrition.org/education-and-professional-development/graduate-and-professional-development/nutrition-internships-for-medical-students/
- American Society of Hematology, www.hematology.org/awards
- Society for Academic Emergency Medicine/Emergency Medicine Foundation, www.saem.org/saemdnn/GrantsAwards/grants.htm/tabid/68/Default.aspx
- U.S. Dept of Health and Human Services, Substance Abuse and Mental Health Services Administration, Minority Fellowship Program, http://mentalhealth.samhsa.gov/publications/allpubs/NMH02-0143/default.asp

Organizations that provide funding for students who will devote a year or more to specific research projects:
- Howard Hughes Medical Institute, www.hhmi.org/resources/students.html
- National Institutes of Health Clinical Research Training Program, www.training.nih.gov
- Stanley J. Sarnoff Fellowships, www.sarnoffendowment.org
- American Academy of Orthopaedic Surgeons, Washington Health Policy Fellowship Program, http://www.aaos.org/news/bulletin/nov07/reimbursement5.asp

For those with no clue about a project, but who would like some research experience over a one- to two-month period, these may be of interest:

- American Academy of Child and Adolescent Psychiatry Minority Fellowship, www.aacap.org/research/spurlck2.htm
- American Pediatric Society/Society for Pediatric Research, www.aps-spr.org/Programs/programs.htm
- Memorial Sloan-Kettering Cancer Center Summer Student Fellowship Program, www.mskcc.org/mskcc/html/2637.cfm
- National Institutes of Health Summer Research Fellowship Program, www.training.nih.gov/student/index.asp

Arranging Your Senior Schedule

One of the major questions that medical students ask their advisers is "How do I arrange my senior schedule?" Although there is a movement away from the previous laissez faire attitude toward the senior year at many medical schools, most, if not all, of the senior year is still wide open for anything that the student wants to take. But, by now you understand that you will need to arrange your schedule so that you maximize the results of your hard work and have the best chance of getting into a residency. So your choices, or at least your timing, become somewhat more limited. How do you arrange your schedule?

Let's start with the second half of your senior year. Mid-February until June of your fourth year is when you should take the balance of your allotted vacation, any exotic international electives for which you have a yearning, and electives in areas in which you feel that you need more training. The average senior medical student takes more than seven weeks of electives outside his or her medical school; the average school allows students to take 24 weeks of electives.

Many senior students bolster their training in Radiology, Anesthesiology, Emergency Medicine, Pediatrics, Orthopedics, Cardiology, and Critical Care with senior electives. This is definitely not the time to take more electives in your chosen specialty. It is, instead, an opportunity to fill in some of the gaps in your training. However, when planning these exciting electives, remember that there is a cost for travel, housing, and maybe even tuition for electives away from your school. Look into it before you sign onto an away experience.

Working backward, you need to block out the next period for interviews. Remembering that you want to interview as late as possible, this means January and early February for those matching through the NRMP, and December for those in one of the early Matches. You will either have to use up some of your vacation or be on a very flexible rotation during this period.

Now we need to consider those critical months *at the beginning of your fourth year. First, do not take any vacation between your third and fourth years.* Immediately following the end of your third-year clerkships, start your subinternship (described below). You will need both the intense experience of this rotation and an excellent reference letter from the clinicians with whom you work for your application. Next, take a rotation in the specialty that you have chosen. If you think it will be useful to you, opt for more than one. But remember, your time is limited to those months between the end of your subinternship (often up to eight weeks long) and the beginning of your interviews.

Once these rules for arranging your senior year have been laid out, it doesn't seem so difficult, does it? If you remember that your twin goals are to use the first half of your senior year preparing to get into a residency and the second half obtaining training in your areas of clinical deficiency, you won't go wrong. And as you can see, such rotations will give you the type of solid clinical experience that no adviser can fault.

Subinternship

As a subintern, medical students are given more responsibility and authority than they have previously experienced. This is the rotation, if done correctly, in which the student assumes all or part of the intern's role on a clinical service. This is where learning how to practice medicine actually takes place. Advisers often disparage the subinternship (a.k.a., junior internship, advanced clerkship). They say, "Why do your internship early?" Your answer is that you need to learn how to practice medicine, and that *you learn best when you take responsibility for patient care.*

The most effective subinternships for senior students to take, therefore, are the ones that offer the most responsibility for patient care. These are often located at the municipal or Veteran's Administration hospitals. While these rotations are never as "cushy" as others that are available, they do provide the experiences that teach you the independence of thought and action, which a good clinician, and a "standout" senior student, must learn.

Most frequently, the rotation, no matter what career specialty you have selected, will be on an Internal Medicine service. Because of these services' large patient loads, and the difficulty of doing any major damage before being stopped, students often can be given enough responsibility to become effective clinicians. In some cases, this will also be true of other services, but it is less likely. For the most part, because so much of the decision-making on Surgery services is irreversible, the staff will be less likely to offer this kind of responsibility to students. But this varies from institution to institution.

Try to get information from the class ahead of you and from your Dean of Students about the nature of the various subinternships available. If possible, get a prestigious individual as an attending so he or she can write a letter about your performance. You can do this primarily by investigating who will attend at the institutions that are available to you during the appropriate time period. But don't pick a stellar attending over a stellar experience. The latter is much more important.

A second option available to some of you may also give you the same responsibility. This is working at a medical mission in a remote, usually foreign, area. While this is often an exciting and broadening learning experience, there are some drawbacks. This experience may not be universally available or affordable. In addition, it may teach you some thought processes and methods that are frowned upon in the United States, at a time in your training when it may be hard to distinguish these adequately. And, most important of all, many faculty may look upon it as mere senior student flightiness.

Senior-Year Specialty Rotations

Questions constantly arise about whether, when, and how many rotations you should take in your chosen specialty field. You have by now heard at least some snatches from the debate on this subject. From the halls of academia, the pronouncement often goes something like, "Don't use your senior electives to train in the specialty for which you are applying. You will get enough of this training in your residency. Use your senior year to broaden your medical education." This, of course, is advice from academicians who are firmly ensconced in tenured posts. But is this the advice that they followed as medical students? Is it advice that they would give to their children? Probably not. Nearly 95% of medical students take electives in their first-choice specialty, and more than a third take three or more such electives.

What should you do? This depends first upon your perceived competitiveness for the specialty. As a candidate for a particular specialty, you fall into one of three categories: a star, middle-of-the-pack, or a struggler. How should students in each of these categories approach the idea of a senior-year specialty rotation? Assuming that you have done adequate preparation and now are reasonably certain that you do want to enter a particular area of medicine, your use of the senior specialty rotation should be directed toward maximizing your chance of getting the residency you want.

Advantages and Disadvantages

For the few of you who qualify as stars, you can use the rotation to demonstrate to residency programs that you are as good as your file says. Physicians, being generally conservative in nature, tend to prefer working with people whom they know, in lieu of those whom they have not met or have met only briefly in interviews. Some residency directors require that candidates do student rotations at their program if they wish to be considered. More than 35% of programs suggest to applicants that they are more likely to be seriously considered for selection if they take an elective at that program. If you truly are a "star" academically, personally, and clinically, show them your stuff!

If you fall into the struggler category, where it is obvious that your paperwork will not even get you an interview, much less the residency slot of your choice, you will need to do more than one specialty rotation. Put your greatest effort forward; you need to demonstrate to the faculty at the residency programs not only that you are capable of doing a solid job as a resident, but also that you will fit in well with their department. Demonstrate to them that you are a pleasure to have around and that you will acquit yourself well now that you have found the area of medicine for which you have been searching. Many students, after doing poorly in medical school, have used this strategy to land excellent residency positions. The key to succeeding with this strategy, however, is to work very hard—both clinically and at fitting in with the team.

Most of you are in the middle-of-the-pack group. While you should do at least one senior specialty elective, both to confirm your interest in the specialty and to get an additional reference letter, you run a great risk if you do more than that. There are only two types of performance for senior students doing electives in their chosen specialties. They are either "standouts" or "shutouts." There are relatively few individuals who shine both clinically and personally. If you can achieve that status, you are as good as in the residency. But even the "stars," and these are the best of the best, cannot always achieve that ranking in the minds of the specialty faculty during a rotation.

If you do not become a "standout," you are a "shutout." As Dr. Alan Langlieb wrote after he went through the interviewing process, "One experience shared by me and other students I have met on interviews was the 'so-this-is-what-we're-getting' or the 'we-can-do-better' phenomenon. Faculty are honored that someone took the trouble and had the interest to spend from four to six weeks at their institution, but often do not know the best place to put you. They don't want to work you too hard. Anyway, you spend half your time getting accustomed to a new hospital . . . The program may see too much of the student and feel as though they could do better. . . . My advice is to spend a night or weekend on call. This lets the program know of your interest and makes you stand out from other applicants, but you are not around long enough to become a part of the wallpaper."

The student who looks really good on paper, but who has not rotated through the department, will be seen as a potentially much stronger candidate than one who has rotated through and done anything less than a stellar job. Simply getting "Honors," while essential, does not necessarily mean that you were perceived as a "standout." It may only be a reflection of easy grading or it may have been based upon your clinical performance alone. The faculty may have thought that you would be impossible to work with for the duration of a training program. And there is no way to really know this. So, you take a big risk by doing a rotation at a residency where you would like to go.

But if programs require that all applicants do a rotation at their facility, you are stuck. More than one-third of students report that programs to which they applied at least suggested that they were more likely to be considered if they did a rotation with them. If you really want to go into such a program, you will need to do the rotation. These are normally rather small programs in selected specialties. In most cases, Orthopedics, Ophthalmology, and Neurological Surgery only rank students who have done an "audition clerkship" at their program. However, this requirement severely limits their applicant pool and, therefore, you may stand a better chance than you would otherwise expect. There are, of course, ways to improve your clinical performance on the specialty rotation. This takes a little preparation.

Preparation

How do you prepare for an elective rotation in the specialty that you have chosen? First, of course, you should have been preparing over the past several years by reading about the specialty, talking with many practitioners in the field, and spending volunteer time with physicians in the specialty.

But now you are getting ready to "show your stuff" to a residency faculty and you want to be a "standout." Clinically, a residency faculty is looking for an individual who

1. Knows enough of the specialty's factual material to have a solid basis for future training.
2. Is able to use these facts in an intelligent manner to deliver good patient care.
3. Delivers patient care in a manner consistent with the specialty's personality.

This almost sounds as idealistic as "motherhood and apple pie." But it is what you have to achieve.

The first requirement, **knowing the basic facts**, can be satisfied through exposure to specialists in the field, reviewing your notes from the relevant basic science courses, and reading specialty textbooks. Make sure to read at least one cover-to-cover prior to taking the rotation. If you are pressed for time, it can be the shorter "Essentials of . . ." version.

The second requirement, **using those facts in an intelligent manner to deliver good patient care**, is more difficult to achieve. This means having the skill to integrate the facts that you have learned and then apply them in clinical situations. It also means, in almost all cases, demonstrating a certain degree of independence by devising and carrying out diagnostic and treatment plans without guidance, though not without supervision. How, as a fourth-year student, will you possibly be able to do this? You will be able to do this as a result of the training and experience you gained while doing a subinternship.

The third attribute specialty faculties look for is whether you **deliver care in a manner consistent with that field's personality**. What does this mean? One of best examples of this is expressed in a story about a new General Surgery intern at a prestigious institution. As he was walking across the hospital's cafeteria one day, he was pointed out to the surgical chief residents by the chairman of the department with the comment, "He's just not aggressive enough to be a real surgeon. He'll have to go." Perhaps this quiet, studious physician was too stubborn to be kicked out (also maybe too good), but he didn't go. And, as is true in all such stories, he went on to succeed—in fact, he became a world-famous Pediatric Cardiovascular Surgeon. But the fact remains that a particular type of person tends to be drawn to each specialty, and the medical care in that field is generally given with a certain overlay of that personality.

While there are many exceptions (you probably know of some), a certain aggressiveness is expected in applicants for Surgery, most Surgical subspecialties, and Emergency Medicine. Warmth and understanding is looked for in applicants to programs in Psychiatry, Pediatrics, Family Practice, and Physiatry. Calmness and a low-key nature are often sought in applicants for Internal Medicine, Radiology, Anesthesiology, Pathology, and Neurology residencies. It is not clear whether current practitioners' personalities guide the specialty's personality, or whether the nature of each specialty attracts and molds particular individuals. But the important point to remember is: if you stand out as a significantly different personality type than individuals already in the specialty, it will be more difficult for you to get a training position in that specialty.

Home or Away?

Many factors involved in taking a specialty rotation at home or away have already been discussed. However, there are still three points worth noting.

First: *There can be significant expenses* involved in the travel, meals, and lodging associated with taking an away rotation. While you may assume that there is housing available for rotating medical students, and some of you might even expect free meals, much of the time you would be mistaken. Find out about these costs before arranging the rotation.

Second: *The expense might be worth it.* If you rotate at the site of your first-choice residency only to find out that it really does not meet your needs, you have spent the money wisely. In such a case, the one-month rotation may possibly save you several years of unhappiness. Remember, specialty rotations work both ways—they look you over and you look them over.

Third: *Apply for externships early!* Very popular clerkships, either at your own school or away, are often filled a year or more in advance. Even if you make your specialty choice at a late date, you may still have a good chance of obtaining a rotation in the specialty at your own school. This is not true of away rotations. If you are strongly considering doing an away elective in your chosen specialty, get information and sign up for the externship as early as possible. If you change your mind later, you can always cancel.

The Association of American Medical Colleges (AAMC) has a website with information about medical student electives (www.aamc.org/students/medstudents/electives/start.htm). Unfortunately, it is not organized by specialty, but only by medical school, state/province, and geographic region. The University of Kansas School of Medicine has a wonderful website (www.kumc.edu/som/medsos/opp.html) listing many types of "Unique Electives" and summer "Fellowships" with their URLs.

The AMA's Medical Student Section also has a great site with International elective opportunities. (Go to www.ama-assn.org/go/mss and scroll down to "*Resources You Can Use*"—"*International Opportunities.*") Another source for finding year-long international medical student fellowships is via the AAMC's "Resources for Medical Students" page (www.aamc.org/students/medstudents/). Many specialty societies also have lists of electives in their specialty.

Timing

When should you do your specialty rotation? If you are applying to one of the specialties that does not match early, you have some leeway. But if you will be in an early Match, you may be pressed for time. In either case, you should do a strong subinternship immediately following your junior year, usually on an Internal Medicine service. That's right—no vacation for now; you will have to wait until much later in the year.

A subinternship is usually a six- or eight-week block, so you should finish near the end of August. Then you should take a specialty rotation. If you take it at a program to which you are applying, you will probably be able to interview near the end of the rotation—especially if you notify them of your desire to do this in advance and reconfirm your intent upon arrival. If you have the time, and you feel that you will be exceptionally weak clinically for a fourth-year student in your selected specialty, you may want to first do a specialty rotation at a program that you do not rank highly. Then, if you think that doing another rotation will help your individual chances, you can do it at one of your top choices. Consider, though, that many students have found that the programs that they thought would be lowest on their rank-order list ended up at or near the top.

As you did with your third-year clinical rotations, try to arrange your schedule so you can work with an attending who is well-known by residency directors in the specialty. Ask that individual at the start of the rotation if, contingent upon your performance, he or she would be willing to write you a letter of recommendation. Attendings are normally very amenable to this. Then make sure that you supply the necessary names and addresses so that the letters can be sent. There won't be much time. These letters will have to go out fast.

You will have now used up all the time that you have available for rotations that will be of any help (or hindrance) in getting into a residency. You can finally spend some time broadening your medical horizons and, certainly, taking a well-deserved vacation.

Awards

Not everyone receives awards during medical school. But getting them may help you obtain a residency position, and make you feel good in the process. Who doesn't like getting an award? The acknowledgments you received as an undergraduate are passé. Not that you shouldn't list Phi Beta Kappa or other undergraduate achievement awards on your résumé, but remember that everyone else has similar achievements. That is why you were accepted into medical school. And anyway, you received those awards a long time ago. Residencies want to know what you have done recently. Awards, in part, answer that question. They are also an important factor in making you and your application stand out as being unique among the crop of applicants to the programs.

AOA

Alpha Omega Alpha (AOA) is the national M.D. medical school honorary society. (Note that this is not the American Osteopathic Association [AOA].

Residency directors know the difference.) Students are elected to AOA based primarily on their grades. In most schools, students can be elected to AOA either at the end of their third year or during their fourth year. Because it is found in most schools, AOA is the best-recognized medical school award. Students elected to the honorary are generally assured of serious consideration by residency programs. This means that many will get most of the interviews they desire. After that it will, of course, be up to them to do well in those interviews.

Some schools do not have AOA chapters. Generally, this is due to the school's philosophy that they should attempt to reduce competition among students. Other schools do not elect anyone to AOA until late in the senior year. Their assumption is that this gives those students at the bottom of the class a better chance of competing against their classmates for residency slots. It is, however, not just your classmates but rather, all medical students who are the competition.

If your school has an AOA chapter, find out from the Dean of Students what the requirements are to be elected. If you think that you can satisfy these requirements, then go for it. Getting into AOA can somewhat ease the burden and anxiety of getting a residency position.

If you are elected to AOA after you submit your residency applications, or even after you have been interviewed, send the programs an official notification from the registrar. Most schools will ask you for the necessary addresses since they know this is very important.

But AOA is not the only award that you can get.

Just For Women

The American Medical Women's Association gives several awards to its members. These include a merit-based scholarship, an essay award, a certificate to top medical school graduates, and a research award. They also occasionally have month-long, special-project "internships." For further information, contact AMWA, (215) 320-3716; www.amwa-doc.org (go to "Member Services").

Special Awards

Many other awards are given out both nationally and locally. However, they may have to be sought out. Your Dean of Students should have a list of the awards given at your school, and probably knows a good bit about other national prizes. The University of Kansas School of Medicine website also has a fine list of nationally available scholarships and awards (www.kumc.edu/som/medsos/opp.html).

The most obvious awards are those that you probably investigated as soon as you were accepted into medical school. These are *scholarships*. Since these are awards, they should be noted as such on program applications. If your scholarships have been renewed because of your good performance in medical school, so much the better. Note, however, that bartering service for money, such as signing up for the Health Professions Scholarship Program, doesn't count.

Another type of award given in most schools is for *excellence in particular courses or clerkships*. For example, the outstanding student in Anatomy or in Family Practice may get an award (often with money as well as a plaque). If you have been selected for such recognition, it is a big deal! Note it prominently on your applications. If the specialty for which you are applying has an award, find out the requirements for it and see if you can be the one to receive it. Your interest in the specialty alone should go a long way toward getting you this honor.

Unfortunately, many schools do not announce award recipients until graduation. This is long past the time when it will help you to get a residency position. While speaking to your Dean of Students about awards in general, find out if this is your school's policy. If it is, can it be changed? If it can't, and you know that you have been designated for such an award, try to at least have it mentioned in your Dean's Letter or in a separate letter that you can include with your applications.

One way you can get recognition and also buff up another area of your application is to receive a *research grant*. Very often either medical schools or individual departments, or both, have monies specifically set aside for medical student research. If you plan to do research anyway, it wouldn't be a bad idea to apply for some of this research money. Not only is it a significant accolade, but it will also make your foray into research much easier.

There are also awards, usually given by major drug companies, for *medical writing*, *biomedical illustration*, and other specialized endeavors. If you have talent in any area where such a prize is given, go after it. You will often be able to find out about these awards from your Dean of Students, notices on your class's bulletin board, or advertisements in *The New Physician*.

8

Examinations

Whether you think you can or think you can't, you're right.

Henry Ford

Putting Your Effort Where It Counts, Part 2

THE UNITED STATES MEDICAL LICENSING EXAMINATION (USMLE) is now the standard licensing examination for M.D.s who wish to practice in the United States or Canada, no matter where they were educated. Osteopathic physicians may take either the USMLE or their own licensing examination, the COMLEX. These tests assess examinees' understanding and application of biomedical and clinical sciences and medical knowledge to the practice of clinical medicine. They are generally taken over a period of years during medical school and early clinical training.

Licensing examinations, however, are not used solely to obtain medical licenses; residency programs use them to screen applicants, many medical schools require students to pass them to advance or graduate, and some states require that physicians pass specific USMLE Steps before beginning or continuing residency training. Repeated studies in many specialties have shown that residents' performance during training and on their specialty Board examinations directly correlates to how well they do on the USMLE. Residency directors know that and select residents accordingly.

Many schools use USMLE Steps 1 and 2 as a part of their student evaluation system: 124 (of 126 total) U.S. M.D. medical schools require students to take Step 1, 124 schools require Step 2 Clinical Knowledge (CK), and 123 require Step 2 Clinical Skills (CS). For advancement or graduation, 100 U.S. M.D. schools require a passing score on Step 1, 93 schools require passing Step 2CK, and 75 schools require passing Step 2CS. Only 17 schools do not require students to pass any USMLE Steps to advance or graduate. Residency directors are hesitant to "rank" applicants who have not completed their school's graduation requirements.

The Federation of State Medical Boards recommends that all medical students pass USMLE Steps 1, 2CS, and 2CK prior to entering residency programs. This means that applicants may have to prove that they have passed these exams before the date that residency directors submit their rank-order lists to the NRMP (or sooner for the "early" Matches). More than 67% of residency programs require applicants to pass Step 1, 43% require passing Step 2 CK, and 41% require passing Steps 1, 2CK, and 2CS. Applicants who have taken both Step 1 and the two components of Step 2 before applying to residencies may have a better chance of matching with the programs they rank highly—if they have done well on the exams. As a result of the rapid scoring possible after a computer-based exam (generally sent within six weeks) and the automatic transmission (if requested by the applicant) of scores to residency programs, more applicants are reporting their Step 2 scores.

The Educational Commission for Foreign Medical Graduates (ECFMG) also administers Steps 1, 2CK, and 2CS. These three exams fulfill the medical science examination requirement for ECFMG Certification. All international medical graduates (IMGs), including U.S. citizens, should apply directly to the ECFMG to take the USMLE. When you initially apply to the ECFMG, download their Medical Education Credentials Submission Form (Form 344) at www.ecfmg.org/forms/form344.pdf. Use this form as a checklist to remind you to send all the correct documents to them.

United States Medical Licensing Examination (USMLE)

Overview

The USMLE (which some students paradoxically call "You Smile") replaced the old "National Board" exams in 1992. The computerized versions were introduced sequentially from May 1999 to June 2004. The advantages of using computerized exams are:
- Enhanced security (questions are drawn from a pool of content-parallel questions in a very large question bank).
- Increased flexibility for examinees when scheduling their exam (all Steps are offered throughout the year).
- Shorter testing times for Steps 1 and 2.
- Wider access to the exam.
- Faster score reporting.
- The ability to add new assessment methods to the exams.

The computerized Step 1 is a one-day (eight-hour) examination consisting of seven 60-minute blocks of approximately 50 multiple-choice "one-best answer" questions each.

Step 2 has two parts: Step 2 Clinical Knowledge (CK) and Step 2 Clinical Skills (CS). Step 2CK is a one-day (nine-hour) examination consisting of eight 60-minute blocks of a maximum of 45 multiple-choice questions each. Step 2CS is a one-day (eight-hour) examination broken into 25-minute segments, during which students interact with 12 "standardized patients." While Step 2 was designed to be taken near the end of the final year of medical school, many U.S. medical students take it at the end of their first clinical year (year 3 in most schools). Basic science and clinical science topics are becoming more integrated throughout all the Steps, and the content is constantly monitored by the governing bodies. This will lead to the restructuring of Steps 1 and 2CK.

Step 3 is a two-day (eight hours each day) exam, with a day and a half to take 480 multiple-choice questions and a half day to complete 12 computer-based Case Simulations (CCS). However, the NBME and FSMB have announced their intention to divide Step 3 into two distinct exams, each one day in length. This change will not occur before 2014.

All three Steps have many tables and graphs to interpret. While the exact questions each examinee gets will vary, everyone is tested on equivalent content. The difficulty of the questions may vary, but the results are statistically adjusted so that all examinees are treated fairly. How well an examinee does on the initial blocks of questions may determine which subsequent blocks he or she gets. Within the time period allowed for a block, examinees may answer questions in any order, go back to review responses, and change their answers. However, once the time is up, the questions and responses in that block cannot be accessed.

Examinees may take Steps 1, 2CS, and 2CK in any sequence; the components are scored and the results are reported separately. You must pass Steps 1 and 2 (both CK and CS) before taking Step 3.

How to Apply

All applicants should obtain the *USMLE Bulletin of Information* from www. usmle.org. A separate booklet on the Step 2CS exam can also be downloaded.

Students in and graduates of accredited U.S. and Canadian M.D. and D.O schools, including foreign nationals or "Green Card" holders attending these schools, apply to the National Board of Medical Examiners (NBME) to take Steps 1, 2CK, and 2CS; they apply to their state's medical board for Step 3. Application materials are available on the NBME's website at www. nbme.org. For additional questions, contact NBME's Department of Licensing Examination Services, 3750 Market St., Philadelphia, PA 19104; (215) 590-9700; e-mail: webmail@nbme.org.

Students and graduates, including U.S. citizens and "Green Card" holders, from medical schools outside the United States or Canada (IMGs) should get information about the requirements to take the examination, and apply for it, through the ECFMG website (www.ecfmg.org) or by contacting them at 3624 Market St., Philadelphia, PA 19104-2685; (215) 386-5900. Fifth Pathway students will already have taken part of the USMLE through the ECFMG. As with other candidates, IMGs apply to the state medical board for Step 3.

Follow the instructions on the appropriate website to apply for the USMLE. Usually you can complete the application on-line, but you can also mail it to them. Submit your application at least three months before you expect to take the test.

When you apply, you must select a three-month "eligibility period" during which you prefer to take the exam. Be sure that the three-month time period begins at least six weeks from the date you submit (or mail) your application, to allow time for your application to be processed. If you need to, you can ask later for a three-month extension to your eligibility period (in *writing*; the form is on the website). USMLE officials may grant an extension—*but only once, and for an additional fee*. If you do not take the test during the original or extended eligibility period, you will need to submit a new application and pay the full fee again.

After you application has been processed, you will receive your "Scheduling Permit," which will detail the Step for which you registered, your eligibility period, your testing region, your Scheduling Number (SN), and your Candidate Identification Number (CIN), which is a private code that you will need to take the exam. Information and instructions necessary to schedule your exam with a Prometric® Center are also included. If you do not receive this material, or if you lose it, call the NBME, Monday to Friday between 8 A.M. and 5 P.M. Eastern Time.

Eligibility (See Figure 8.1)

Steps 1, 2CK, and 2CS
Medical students should be officially enrolled in or a graduate of: (1) a U.S. or Canadian medical school accredited by the Liaison Committee on Medical Education (LCME) or the American Osteopathic Association (AOA); or (2) a medical school recognized by the ECFMG (year of graduation and the medical school must be listed in the *International Medical Education Directory* [*IMED*] of the Foundation for Advancement of International Medical Education and Research [FAIMER®]).

Figure 8.1
USMLE Eligibility Requirements and Contacts

Type of Applicant	USMLE Step	Contact to Take Examination	Contact to Have USMLE Transcript Sent
Students officially enrolled in or graduates of medical schools in the U. S. and Canada accredited by the Liaison Committee on Medical Education (LCME) or the American Osteopathic Association.	Step 1 or Step 2 (CK and CS)	NBME Dept. of Licensing Examination Services 3750 Market St. Philadelphia, PA 19104-3190 (215) 590-9700 e-mail: webmail@nbme.org www.nbme.org	NBME If registered through the NBME, (most U.S. and Canadian medical students) and going to recipients (e.g. residency programs) other than licensing bodies (e.g., state medical boards). Results can also be sent through ERAS.
Students officially enrolled in or graduated from Foreign Medical Schools. A "foreign" medical school is one that is located outside the U.S., Canada, and Puerto Rico that, at the time of application to take the USMLE (student) or at graduation, is listed in the FAIMER International Medical Education Directory.	Step 1 or Step 2 (CK and CS)	ECFMG 3624 Market St. Philadelphia, PA 19104-2685 (215) 386-5900 e-mail: info@ecfmg.org www.ecfmg.org	ECFMG If registered through the ECFMG (most international medical graduates) and going to recipients (e.g. residency programs) other than licensing bodies (e.g., state medical boards). Results can also be sent through ERAS.
All medical graduates who have: (1) Passed Steps 1, 2CK, and 2CS (2) Met their licensing authority's requirements (varies in different locales) (3) If an IMG, obtained an ECFMG Certificate or successfully completed a Fifth Pathway program.	Step 3	Medical Licensing Authority (State Medical Board) - or - FSMB Dept. of Examination Services P.O. Box 619850 Dallas, TX 75261-9850 (817) 868-4041 email: usmle@fsmb.org www.fsmb.org	FSMB For any transcript going to a medical licensing body (e.g., state medical board).

Step 3

Applicants must: (1) have an M.D. (or equivalent) or D.O. degree; (2) have passed USMLE Steps 1, 2CK, and 2CS (if a recent graduate) or, if an IMG, hold an ECFMG Certificate or have completed a "Fifth Pathway" program [**Note:** USMLE will no longer accept Fifth Pathway certificates to meet eligibility after January 1, 2017]; and (3) meet any other requirements set by the Medical Board through which they are applying (see Figure 8.9). Initial applicants for a medical license who do not meet the standard eligibility criteria but who otherwise meet all other requirements of the licensing board may be allowed to take the examination if the licensing board makes a request to the USMLE's Secretariat.

Special Testing Arrangements

Test accommodations, such as a separate room or increased examination time limits for students with disabilities, can be arranged. If you have special needs due to a documented physical or learning disability that is covered under the Americans with Disabilities Act (ADA), contact the group that administers the Step (NBME, ECFMG, or state medical board) as early as possible. They will supply you with additional information and a supplementary application for special accommodations. Much of this information is also on the USMLE, NBME, ECFMG, and FSMB (www.fsmb.org) websites.

Any request for special accommodations must be submitted, with the supporting documentation, at the time you apply to take the Step. Although you should submit these forms at the same time as your application, *send the application separately*. Special accommodations that the USMLE may provide include assistance with keyboard tasks, audio renditions of the material, extended testing time, extra breaks, large-print versions, and other adaptations. Any special accommodations used during the testing are noted on the USMLE score reports and transcripts.

Scheduling the USMLE

Test scheduling is on a "first-come, first served" basis. Therefore, contact the ProMetric scheduling representative immediately after receiving your permit to schedule your exam. (The phone number will be on the permit.) You can also schedule it online at www.prometric.com and receive confirmation via e-mail, although this may be slower than speaking to the representative.

Before calling ProMetric, select several alternative dates and testing locations. Find ProMetric test centers near you by using their website. To schedule your exam, you will need to have your Scheduling Number (SN).

To unlock your test at the Center, you will need your Candidate Identification Number (CIN). *Keep these numbers confidential.* The representative will give you information about available dates at the centers near you, including, if necessary, alternative centers with open dates. Note that May, June, July, November, and December are the most popular months to take the exams in the United States and Canada. The test centers are closed on major U.S. holidays and for the first two weeks of January.

Note: To avoid problems, re-confirm your testing appointment a week prior to your scheduled testing date!

If you want to reschedule your test date within your eligibility period, you do it at least 14 calendar days before your scheduled date or you will have to pay an extra fee (see below). If you do not get your first choice of test centers or dates, it is worthwhile checking back, since openings occur when other examinees change their test dates.

Cost

The fee (in 2012) to take Step 1 or Step 2CK is $535 and for Step 2CS is $1,140. Note that if you take Step 1 or Step 2CK outside the United States, U.S. territories, or Canada, the fee increases. If you will be doing this, call the NBME Department of Licensing Examinations at (215) 590-9700 or e-mail USMLEreg@nbme.org before submitting your application to determine the correct fee.

If you cancel or reschedule your test appointment later than noon (Eastern time) 14 calendar days before the scheduled exam date, there is an additional charge ($150 in 2012); this increases substantially ($400) if you miss your appointment without rescheduling. These fees are due when the exam is rescheduled. No rescheduling can occur after 12:00 AM (Eastern time) on the day of the exam. For applicants who need to extend their designated eligibility period (3 months for Step 1 and Step 2 CK; 12 months for Step 2 CS), there is a $65 fee.

Since individual state licensing boards administer Step 3, the fees and rules vary. In 2012, Step 3 cost $745 in all states except Iowa ($795), Vermont ($780), and South Dakota ($895). The number of times candidates can take Step 3 varies from once (Alaska) to no limit (in 11 states). Candidates generally have up to seven or ten years to complete all USMLE Steps, although Michigan and Minnesota give candidates five years and five states (ID, LA, MI, NY, NC) have no time limit.

The total cost (2012) for Step 3 plus a medical license ranges from $945 in North Dakota, South Dakota, and Utah to $2,745 in Vermont. Osteopathic physicians' total costs range from a low of $260 in Pennsylvania to a high of over $1,200.

Preparing for the USMLE

Free orientation materials for all Steps are on the USMLE website at www. usmle.org. (Click on "Orientation and Practice Materials" and then on the link to the year in which you want to take the test.) The downloadable software contains more than 100 practice test items for each Step, two videos describing Step 2CS, and five sample case simulations for Step 3. The practice test items can be taken in either a timed or an untimed mode. Be certain to remove any prior copies of these programs before downloading the new versions. This material can also be obtained on a CD-ROM from the entity (NBME, ECFMG, FSMB) through which you are registering for the exam. The NBME also sells downloadable assessment tests (www.nbme.org).

It may be worthwhile for you to purchase a scheduling permit for a 3½-hour practice session at a ProMetric test center. Although the practice test contains the same materials as are on the USMLE website, it gives you a chance to experience it in the setting you will be in when you take the actual test. (Practice sessions prices ranged from $60 in the United States and Canada to over $220 in Japan in 2012.) Private tutoring companies also run preparation courses.

Taking the Test

On test day, get to the test center at least 30 minutes before the exam time listed on your confirmation notice. If you are more than 30 minutes late, you will not be admitted and must pay a rescheduling fee within your assigned eligibility period. For Step 2CS, if you arrive after the on-site orientation, you cannot take the test; if you arrive during the orientation you can continue, but must sign a Late Admission Form.

Wear comfortable clothes. For Step 2CS, wear comfortable professional clothes and bring a stethoscope and a white lab/clinic coat. (They may be able to supply a white coat and stethoscope if you forget them.)

On arrival, you will sign in, be photographed, and show your Scheduling Permit and a photo ID with your signature, such as a driver's license, a passport, a national identity card or other form of unexpired government-issued identification, or an ECFMG-issued identification card. The name on the photo ID must *exactly match* the name on your Scheduling Permit. You will also be fingerprinted as part of ProMetric's Biometric Identity Management System (BIMS). An electronic copy of your fingerprint, along with your name, address, date of birth or age, identification document number, and a scanned copy of your identification document (which may include your digitized photograph) will be collected and stored for up to 48 hours after the test; then it is deleted.

Once you have completed the sign-in process, you are required to place all personal items (including food, beverages, hats, watches, coats, wallets, book bags, handbags, backpacks, books, notes or study materials, and any mechanical or electronic devices) in a small locker. If you need to keep a personal item (such as food for a diabetic) with you, you will need to apply in advance for a Personal Item Exception. For Step 2CS, only a coat rack and open cubbyholes are available for personal storage; do not bring anything of value other than a white coat and a stethoscope, which you will keep with you. For all exams, there is no place to store luggage and no place for non-examinees to wait.

For Steps 1, 2CK, and 3, a proctor will offer you an erasable writing board, marker, and tissues to use as erasers. They will then escort you to a testing room and show you how to adjust the mouse and monitor. Entering your Candidate Identification Number (CIN) will initiate a 15-minute tutorial that explains how the test works. If you wish, you can immediately exit this tutorial and begin the test. For Step 2CS, there will be an on-site orientation, after which staff members will direct you how to proceed.

One of the keys to doing well on the USMLE is time management. Each day there are at least 45 minutes of "break time" (including the lunch period) that you can take as you wish. For Steps 1, 2CK, and 3, doing the tutorial in advance will give you 15 more minutes for lunch and breaks. By limiting the number of breaks you take, you save time signing in and out each time (and you have longer breaks). Completing sections early also gives you additional time for breaks or lunch. Those who have taken the USMLE recommend that you pre-plan when and for how long you will take your breaks so that, under stress, you do not shortchange yourself on the allotted time for the test sections. Be careful not to use up all the break time early in the testing day.

For Step 2CS, the entire day is spent in the testing area. Once you check in and enter the secure testing area, you cannot leave until the exam is over. There are two breaks. The first is 30 minutes long, during which they serve a light meal (you can bring your own) and make vending machines available. Later, there is a 15-minute break.

Upon completing the test, give your Permit to the proctor, sign out of the Center, and get a Test Completion Notice.

You must complete the entire examination to receive a score, although you may not have time to answer all the questions. If you leave Step 1 or Step 2CK early without at least beginning each block, "incomplete examination" will appear on your USMLE transcript. If you leave Step 2CS early, your score will be based on the cases you completed and "Pass," "Fail," or "Incomplete Examination" will be reported. If computer or technical problems develop, notify a proctor and he will make the necessary adjustments. If you wish to file a complaint, you must do so at the testing center that day or within three days (in writing) to NBME Test Administration.

Scores

Scores for Step 1, Step 2CK, and Step 3 are usually available four weeks after the exam, although the report may take as long as eight weeks to arrive. For Step 2CS, look for their Schedule for Reporting Results on the USMLE website. Unless you send a written request to the USMLE, the scores will automatically be reported to all accredited M.D. and Osteopathic schools in the United States and Canada. No scores are ever reported by telephone, e-mail, or fax.

The pass/fail standards for all Steps are set before the exam begins. There is no set percentage of examinees that must pass or fail. This standard is statistically maintained at the same level across test administrations. Generally, examinees must correctly answer 60% to 70% of the questions on each Step or Component to pass. Although the USMLE program recommends a minimum passing score for each Step, each medical licensing authority (i.e., state medical board) may establish the passing scores for their own jurisdiction. The mean three-digit scores range from 215 to 235 with a standard deviation of 20 points. In 2012, the minimum passing score for Step 1 was 188; for Step 2CK, 196; and for Step 3, 187. Changes to these scores can be found on the USMLE website. Scores are also converted to a two-digit score, since most state medical boards require a "75" to pass. This generally equates to at least one standard deviation below the mean three-digit score.

How do you interpret the scores? Your score report will list the minimum three-digit score needed to pass that Step; the minimum passing two-digit score is always 75. The percentile score once used to rate examinees against a standard group is no longer being reported, resulting in a more-or-less "Pass-Fail" system. This makes it more difficult for residency directors and licensing boards to determine how well examinees who passed the exam actually did on the USMLE (although many residency directors try to interpret the relative scores that individuals get).

The unintended consequences of these "Pass-Fail" scores include bland recommendation letters and the granting of more applicant interviews for each residency position, thus increasing the costs for applicants and programs. Figure 8.2 shows the recent performance on the test by various groups. Although it may not be clear from the chart, the NBME says that about 1% of graduates of U.S.- and Canadian-accredited schools never pass the USMLE, while as many as 25% of IMGs are unable to pass the exam.

Figure 8.2
Recent USMLE Pass Rates

Examinee	Pass Rate	
	First-time taker	**Repeater**
Step 1		
U.S./Canadian M.D. Students	94%	70%
D.O. Students	89%	65%
ECFMG-registered Students	73%	36%
Step 2CK		
U.S./Canadian M.D. Students	97%	68%
D.O. Students	93%	57%
ECFMG-registered Students	82%	50%
Step 2CS		
U.S./Canadian M.D. Students	98%	91%
D.O. Students	88%	N/A
ECFMG-registered Students	79%	67%
STEP 3		
U.S./Canadian M.D. Graduates	97%	74%
D.O. Graduates	94%	N/A
ECFMG-registered Graduates	84%	60%

Adapted from USMLE materials, June 2012.

For Step 2CS, the standardized patients assess examinees' data-gathering and communication skills, including spoken English. Physician raters assess examinees' ability to complete an appropriate patient note. Performance on Step 2CS is reported as "Pass" or "Fail," with no numerical score. Examinees who fail will receive a performance profile, which reflects the relative strengths and weaknesses of their performance on the subcomponents of the exam.

In Step 3, the computer-based case simulations (CCS) are scored against answers given by practicing clinicians and experts in the field. The closer you come to matching what these practitioners deem to be "ideal management," the higher your score. Potentially dangerous and unnecessary actions significantly lower your score. Scores are mailed approximately two weeks after the examination. Most state licensing boards have the results sent simultaneously to them and to the examinee. Some state boards have the scores reported to them first, and then they send results to the examinee.

Retaking the USMLE

If you fail a Step or a Component (CK/CS), you must resubmit the same application as you did the first time and pay the fee again. You cannot take a USMLE Step or Component more than six times. Also, you *cannot take a failed or incomplete Step more than three times in a 12-month period.*

The USMLE recommends that state licensing boards require examinees to pass all components within a seven-year period. They also recommend that they allow candidates a maximum of six attempts to pass any Step or Component (CS or CK) without demonstrating additional educational experience. Just when this seven-year "clock" begins differs among states: This can pose difficulties for M.D./Ph.D. students, who often take from seven to nine years to complete their programs. Most states will make exceptions for them.

If you *pass* a Step or a Component (CK/CS), you may not retake it unless the licensing authority requires you to do so (usually because of the seven-year rule) or you are still enrolled as a medical student six or more years after you first passed Steps 1 or 2. In either case, if you previously passed the Step but fail when you take it the second time, you must retake and pass that Step to complete the USMLE requirements.

Sending your USMLE Results (Transcript)

Unless an examinee writes to request that test scores not be sent, they will automatically be sent to all accredited M.D. and Osteopathic schools in the United States and Canada. Requests that scores be sent to other agencies or institutions depend on which Step(s) you have taken and where you want to send them. Most residency applicants have their results sent electronically via the Electronic Residency Application Service (ERAS). Other requests must be made in writing to the appropriate body (see Figure 8.1).

Upon receiving your request, either in writing or online, plus a small fee, the NBME (ECFMG for IMGs) will send copies of your USMLE transcript to residency programs. The form to use and the current cost can be obtained from the NBME, ECFMG, or your Dean of Students. This USMLE transcript includes results of all your attempts to pass USMLE Steps, as well as your results from any NBME Parts or FLEX examinations (old licensing tests). It also includes notes about any examinations for which no scores were reported (incomplete examinations or indeterminate scores), any special accommodations that were provided, any incidents of irregular behavior (e.g., cheating), and any actions that credentialing or licensing authorities have taken against you. After physicians take the USMLE Step 3, the Federation of State Licensing Boards, rather than the ECFMG or NBME, sends out the transcripts.

Irregular Testing Behavior

A USMLE examinee's "irregular behavior" is serious and, if confirmed, becomes a part of the USMLE record that is sent to medical licensing authorities and residency programs. The examinee may also be barred from taking future USMLE exams (if they haven't completed the series), meaning that they cannot be licensed in the United States if they are an M.D., or that they may be required to take the remaining USMLE Steps under special conditions. "Irregular behavior" includes:

- Seeking or obtaining access to examination materials prior to the exam.
- Falsifying information on the application or registration forms.
- Taking the exam without being eligible for it.
- Impersonating an examinee or hiring a proxy to take the exam.
- Copying answers from another examinee or looking at another examinee's computer screen.
- Allowing your answers to be copied.
- Making notes of any kind during the exam except on the non-removable, erasable writing surface provided for examinees.
- Failure to adhere to test center staff's instructions.
- Disruptive behavior at the test center.
- Possessing photographic, communication, or recording devices, including electronic pagers and cellular telephones.
- Altering or misrepresenting examination scores.
- Theft of or other unauthorized possession of examination materials.
- Any unauthorized reproduction (including memorization and distribution) of examination materials.

USMLE Step 1

Step 1 is a one-day (eight hours), 322-item multiple-choice examination that assesses examinees' understanding of and ability to apply key basic biomedical science concepts. All questions in Step 1 require "one best answer." The exam emphasizes the principles and mechanisms of health, disease, and therapeutic modalities. Most test items present basic science principles in the context of clinical vignettes. Step 1 covers anatomy, behavioral sciences, biochemistry, microbiology, pathology, pharmacology, and physiology, as well as interdisciplinary topics such as nutrition, genetics, and aging (Figure 8.3). The questions are not grouped by subject area (e.g., anatomy), but appear randomly.

The test is given in seven 60-minute blocks; each block has from 25 to 50 questions that cover all the subjects. The test items include pictures and tables, and require the identification of normal and pathologic gross and microscopic specimens and the integration of basic science with clinical problems. Recently, the number of factual-recall questions has decreased, while more questions requiring examinees to answer based on integrating information from various subject areas have been added.

Of the 22,021 U.S. and Canadian medical students who took the exam in 2011, about 92% passed; this is expected to rise to 99% after accounting for repeat attempts. Non-U.S./Canadian first-time takers numbered 14,855.

Most U.S. medical students take this Step after completing their second preclinical year. The NBME's Comprehensive Basic Science Subject Examination (CBSE)—given at most U.S. medical schools—seems to predict whether students will pass the USMLE Step 1. Like the USMLE, these are computer-based tests.

USMLE Step 2

Step 2 consists of two examinations: Step 2 Clinical Knowledge (CK), a multiple-choice component, and Step 2 Clinical Skills (CS), a simulated-patient encounter to assess clinical and communication skills.

Step 2 Clinical Knowledge (CK)
Step 2CK is a one-day (nine hours), 346-item multiple-choice examination divided into eight 60-minute blocks. It assesses whether examinees have sufficient knowledge and understanding of the clinical sciences to provide safe and competent patient care under supervision. It emphasizes health promotion, disease prevention, and clinical situations commonly seen during a primary care internship (Figure 8.4). There are two types of questions: (a) the single-best answer, as in Step 1, and (b) "extended matching", where there is one list of up to 20 answers available for a series of questions.

The test includes material from Internal Medicine, Obstetrics and Gynecology, Pediatrics, Preventive Medicine and Public Health, Psychiatry, and Surgery. Nearly all questions are clinical scenarios where the examinee must provide a diagnosis, a prognosis, an indication of the underlying disease mechanism, or the next step in medical care, including preventive measures. Examinees must interpret tables, laboratory data, imaging studies, photographs of gross and microscopic pathology specimens, and the results from other diagnostic studies.

Figure 8.3
USMLE Step 1 Content*

1. Systems

General Principles	25%-35%
Normal & abnormal processes not limited to specific organ systems	
Organ Systems	65%-75%
(Normal and abnormal processes that are system specific.)	

- Cardiovascular
- Endocrine
- Gastrointestinal
- Hematopoietic/Lymphoreticular
- Immune
- Musculoskeletal
- Nervous/Special Senses
- Respiratory
- Renal/Urinary
- Reproductive
- Skin/Connective Tissue

2. Process

• Normal structures and functions	20%-30%
• Abnormal processes	40%-50%
• Principles of therapeutics	15%-25%
• Psychosocial, cultural, occupational and environmental considerations	10%-20%

*All percentages are subject to change.
Adapted from the *USMLE 2012 Bulletin of Information*.

Of the 19,295 U.S. and Canadian medical students who took the exam in 2011, about 95% passed; this is expected to rise to 99% after accounting for repeat attempts. Non-U.S./Canadian first-time takers numbered 11,594.

Step 2 Clinical Skills (CS)

Step 2CS was added to provide a minimum national standard for interpersonal and clinical skills, which a large body of literature has shown to be strongly correlated with the incidence of malpractice suits and patients' treatment compliance and satisfaction. For IMGs, Step 2CS replaces the Clinical Skills Assessment (CSA) that was administered by the ECFMG. The Medical Council of Canada has also adopted Step 2CS as part of their medical licensing exam.

The exam takes one-day (eight hours) and is broken into 25-minute segments, during which examinees interact with 12 "standardized patients."

Figure 8.4
USMLE Step 2CK Content

1. Normal Conditions and Disease Categories

Normal growth and development and general principles of care
Individual organ systems or disorders:
- Blood and Blood-forming Organs
- Cardiovascular Disorders
- Endocrine and Metabolic Disorders
- Gynecologic Disorders
- Immunologic Disorders
- Mental Disorders
- Musculoskeletal System and Connective Tissue
- Nervous System and Special Senses
- Nutritional and Digestive Disorders
- Pregnancy, Childbirth, and the Puerperium Disorders
- Renal, Urinary, and Male Reproductive Systems
- Respiratory System
- Skin and Subcutaneous Tissue

2. Physician Task*

• Applying principles of management	15%-25%
• Establishing a diagnosis	25%-40%
• Promoting preventive medicine & health maintenance	15%-20%
• Understanding mechanisms of disease	20%-35%

*These percentages may change.
Adapted from the *USMLE 2012 Bulletin of Information*.

It closely parallels many elements of the Objective Structured Clinical Examination (OSCE; described later in this chapter) given at most medical schools. The secure test area is a series of exam rooms equipped with standard exam tables, blood pressure cuffs, otoscopes, ophthalmoscopes, non-latex gloves, sinks, and paper towels. Outside each exam room is a cubicle with a computer where the patient note can be written or typed. Bring a stethoscope and white coat; they provide you with a clipboard, blank paper, and a pen.

The test is meant to present examinees with a broad spectrum of cases from a physician's typical workday in U.S. medical practice. The cases are the kinds of medical problems that would commonly be encountered in a clinic, doctor's office, emergency department, or hospital. The "standardized patients" are people that have been trained to act like patients from a broad range of age, racial, and ethnic backgrounds. Presentation categories include cardiovascular, constitutional, gastrointestinal, genitourinary, musculoskeletal, neurological, psychiatric, respiratory, and women's health. A few of these cases may, in fact, be tests of possible new cases; these will not be scored. You should treat the SP as a "real" patient, and assume that you are responsible for their immediate and follow-up care.

While the specific cases used vary from day to day, each examinee will get a combination of cases with an equal degree of difficulty. Each group of cases will reflect common and important symptoms and diagnoses. In any case, the simulated patients will respond to similar questions in the same way.

Examinees can spend up to 15 minutes in the exam room with each patient. Use this time to establish a rapport, elicit pertinent information, and perform a physical examination. Then you have 10 minutes to record a patient note, including pertinent history, and initial diagnostic studies to be ordered. As of June 17, 2012, you are also expected to present a focused Differential Diagnosis (maximum of 3 diagnoses) listed in order of likelihood. For each diagnosis, you must indicate the finding from the history and physical exam that supports or refutes it. Also include diagnostic impressions and plans for possible further evaluation. The cases must be taken in the order that they are presented and be completed in the time allowed.

Before entering an exam room and once an announcement tells you to begin, you will read an instruction sheet about the patient's case, including the chief complaint and the patient's vital signs. (Consider these vital signs to be accurate.) If laboratory results are included, it means that the patient is returning for a follow-up appointment. Make notes of the relevant information. After entering the room, take a *focused* history based on the chief complaint and do a *focused* physical exam, if indicated. Wash your hands before and after you do the exam. Listen *empathetically* to the patient; be careful not to interrupt patients, a common mistake when taking a history.

Do a *gentle exam*. (If you don't normally do a gentle exam, have someone teach you how; all your patients will appreciate it.) If you would normally do an exam that is not part of the test (genitourinary, pelvic, female breast, and corneal reflexes), note that on your proposed "diagnostic workup" when you write up the case. In some cases, you may be asked to perform the exam on a mannequin or a simulator.

Scoring for the Communications Skills portion of the patient encounter will focus on how well you

- Foster the doctor-patient relationship.
- Gather information.

- Provide relevant information to the patient, including explaining the possible diagnosis and any tests you are ordering.
- Make basic decisions.
- Support the "emotions" of the patient by addressing their concerns and answering questions.

Immediately after the patient encounter, you will have ten minutes to write or type (on a computer) a patient note. If you finish the patient encounter early, you can use that extra time for your note. If you choose to write your note by hand, *write or print it legibly!* If the scorers cannot read it, it will count against you. You may use the abbreviations on the sheet posted at every station and other common medical abbreviations. However, if in doubt that your abbreviation will be understood, write it out. Be sure to clearly document your analysis of possible diagnoses. You can write your note in full sentences, in the short phrases more typical of physicians' notes (e.g., "Abd: non-distended, NL BS"), or a combination of both.

In some instances, the case may require that you make a telephone call. Follow the instructions and, once connected, do not press any button on the phone until you are done. As with the patient encounter, you only get one chance. Once you leave the room or hang up the phone, you cannot go back. An announcement will tell you when you have five minutes left with the patient. Although no children will act as simulated patients, you may need to discuss a child's case with their caregiver.

You must pass all three components of the CS examination during a single administration: (1) an Integrated Clinical Encounter (ICE), which assesses your data collection skills and your recorded patient note; (2) an assessment of your Communication/Interpersonal Skills (CIS); and (3) an assessment of your Spoken English Proficiency (SEP). (See Figure 8.5.)

For Step 2CS, if you do not begin every case, your performance will be assessed only on those cases you completed. If this assessment would result in a "Pass" no matter how poorly you might have done on the skipped case(s), you will get a "Pass" score. The reverse is also true: if you failed the completed cases, you will get a failing score. Otherwise, your attempt will be noted as an "incomplete examination."

Of the 29,818 students who took the exam between July 2010 and June 2011, about sixty percent were U.S. or Canadian medical students, with a 97% pass rate; IMGs, who made up the rest of the students, passed 79% of the time.

Fifth Pathway students must have taken either the prior CSA exam or Step 2CS to be eligible to take Step 3.

Figure 8.5: USMLE Step 2CS Content

Components

1. Integrated Clinical Encounter (ICE)
- Data gathering: Take a patient history and perform a physical examination. (The standardized patient scores only the physical exam by using a checklist.)
- Documentation: Complete a Patient Note summarizing the findings of patient encounter, diagnostic impression, and initial patient work-up.

2. Communication and Interpersonal Skills (CIS)
  (The standardized patient scores all CIS components using a checklist.)
- Questioning skills: includes the ability to tailor open-ended questions to the patient's specific needs and respond accordingly, without interrupting the patient.
- Information-sharing skills: such as avoiding jargon, responding to patient questions/concerns, and providing counseling when appropriate.
- Professional manner and rapport: such as showing concern for patient's comfort/modesty, the examinee's personal hygiene (wash hands before and after physical exam), and expressing interest in the impact of the illness on the patient.

3. Spoken English Proficiency (SEP)
- Clarity of spoken English communication within the context of the doctor-patient encounter, including pronunciation, word choice, and minimizing the need to repeat questions or statements.

Patient Note

The written form and computer form are essentially identical. Remember to focus on the patient's chief complaint.

History: Include significant positives and negatives from the patient's history of present illness; past medical, social and family history; and a review of system(s).

Physical Examination: Indicate only pertinent positive and negative findings related to patient's chief complaint. If no physical exam was required or possible (e.g., you spoke on the phone with a patient or caregiver), leave this section blank.

Differential Diagnosis: In order of likelihood (with #1 being the most likely), list up to 3 potential or possible diagnoses for this patient's presentation. Document why you include each diagnosis in your analysis.

Diagnostic Workup: List immediate plans (up to 5) for further diagnostic workup. If a part of the physical exam (i.e., a pelvic exam), is indicated, list it here. Do not include treatment, consultations, or referrals.

Adapted from: *USMLE 2012 Bulletin of Information.*

USMLE Step 3

Step 3 is a two-day *examination (eight hours each day), with 480* multiple-choice items divided into blocks of about 50 items and 12 computer-based Case Simulations (CCS). Unlike Steps 1 and 2CK, all the multiple-choice questions in each block relate to the same clinical setting. You will have from 45 to 60 minutes to complete each multiple-choice block and either 20 or 10 minutes to complete each CCS. Note that the USMLE has announced that this Step will be restructured in 2014 at the earliest.

Step 3 is administered after graduation, usually during the PGY-1 year. It assesses whether examinees have sufficient knowledge and understanding of biomedical and clinical science to practice medicine without supervision. The knowledge base is what would be expected of a generalist physician, including non-emergency and emergency encounters with regular and new patients in various settings, such as clinics, offices, nursing homes, hospitals, emergency departments, and via telephone. The exam now also includes question sets requiring you to critically evaluate drug advertising and journal abstracts. It is heavily weighted toward clinically oriented knowledge and situations (Figure 8.6).

Candidates can take this exam only after they have: (a) passed Steps 1, 2CK, and 2CS; (b) received an M.D. or D.O. degree from a school accredited by the LCME or the AOA; and (c) completed their state medical Board's required amount of graduate medical education (GME). (See Figure 8.9.) Graduates of foreign medical schools must have an ECFMG Certificate or have completed a "Fifth Pathway" program. (**Note:** USMLE will no longer accept Fifth Pathway certificates to meet eligibility requirements after January 1, 2017. See Chapter 14, International Medical Graduates.)

Of the 26,334 physicians who took the exam for the first time in 2011, about two-thirds were graduates of U.S. or Canadian medical schools. They had a 96% pass rate; this is expected to rise to 99% after accounting for repeat attempts.

Registered applicants should write to their state's board for the additional information contained in *USMLE Step 3 General Instructions, Content Outline, and Sample Items.* The address, telephone numbers, and website of individual state licensing boards are listed in the *USMLE Bulletin of Information*, and on the Federation of State Medical Boards of the United States, Inc., website (www. fsmb.org). Depending on state requirements, this Step can be taken during or after the PGY-1 year.

Note that the application material for Step 3 is sent to your residency program director. If you change training programs after the Match or you

---

Figure 8.6
USMLE Step 3 Content*

1. **Physician Tasks**
   - Obtaining history and performing physical examination   8%-12%
   - Using laboratory and diagnostic studies   8%-12%
   - Applying scientific concepts and mechanisms of disease   8%-12%
   - Formulating most likely diagnosis   8%-12%
   - Evaluating severity of patient's problems   8%-12%
   - Managing the patient: 45%-55%
     Health maintenance
     Clinical intervention
     Clinical therapeutics
     Legal and ethical issues

2. **Clinical Encounters**
   - Continued care   50%-60%
   - Emergency care   15%-25%
   - Initial Care   20%-30%

*These percentages may change.
Adapted from: *USMLE 2012 Bulletin of Information*.

---

do not receive an application, contact your state licensing board or the Test Administration Office, Step 3, National Board of Medical Examiners, 3750 Market St., Philadelphia, PA 19104-3190. Include your full name as it appeared on Steps 1 and 2, your NBME Identification Number that is on your Step 1 and 2 results, your medical school, the year of graduation, and your current address.

Step 3: Computer-based Case Simulation (CCS)

In the CCS, the examinee provides care to approximately nine simulated patients. Using the information received in the clinical problem, examinees must decide what treatment to give and when to initiate it. They must also monitor each patient's responses to their interventions (or non-interventions). The cases must be completed in the order presented.

During the CCS, examinees type their requests on the "order sheet"; including information from the history and physical, orders for laboratory studies and procedures, requests for consults, and instructions to begin medications and other therapies. These are drawn from thousands of possible entries. As the case progresses, you can advance the time clock and re-evaluate the patient, check on test results, and learn the results of any interventions. By looking at the patient's chart, you can review vital signs, progress notes, nurses' notes, and test results—all under different tabs. Time is suspended (neat idea) as you consider what steps to take next. You cannot go back in "time," but you may change orders as the situation changes and as you move the patient between the office, home, emergency department, intensive care unit, and ward.

The computer monitors each action you take: the highest score is given for thoroughness, efficiency, avoiding risks, timeliness, and avoiding unnecessary or potentially dangerous actions.

To do well, you must become familiar with the CCS software and understand how the simulated cases work before taking the exam. Review all the orientation materials and do all the practice cases sent with your application packet, plus those available at the USMLE website (www.usmle.org) or at LCME- and AOA-accredited medical schools. The NBME recommends that all Step 3 applicants review the Primum® CCS tutorial and the practice cases well in advance of the testing day to have a thorough understanding of how Primum CCS works.

USMLE Sample Questions

Three types of questions (described below) make up the multiple-choice part of the exam: single-item, matching sets, and case clusters (multiple item sets). The questions concentrate on therapy and management. They are based upon audio and graphic presentations of data (radiographs, EKGs, pictures of patients, photomicrographs, patient charts, etc.) and patient-management problems designed to simulate actual patient encounters.

One-Best-Answer Questions: Steps 1, 2CK, and 3

Single-item questions are typical multiple-choice questions in which you must select the one best answer. The question can be phrased in the positive, such as "What is the next appropriate laboratory test?", or in the negative, such as "What organism is NOT likely to cause the patient's problem?". For both types of questions, first read the case and the question carefully and eliminate the answers you know are wrong. Then, from those remaining, select the answer you think is the most correct. (This strategy does not work for extended-matching questions, where there are up to 20 choices.) A typical single-item question is:

1. A 32-year-old man comes to your office with severe flank pain radiating into his right groin. The pain began suddenly about one hour before his arrival. On physical examination, you find normal bowel sounds, no abdominal wall guarding, rigidity or mass, no costovertebral angle tenderness, and no evidence of a hernia. His chest and rectal examinations are normal. The most appropriate next step is to:

(A) do an non-contrast CT scan.
(B) get a surgical consultation.
(C) obtain abdominal radiographs.
(D) obtain blood for a complete blood count and electrolytes.
(E) test his urine for blood.

(Answer: E)

Matching Sets: Step 2CK

Matching sets questions also require one best answer, but with a twist: You are given a series of questions on a common topic with a list of between 4 and 26 possible answers. The questions are not linked, and each answer may be used more than once or not at all. An example of a matching set question is:

> The response options for the next two items are the same. You will be required to select one answer for each item in the set.
>
> For each patient with a cough, select the most likely diagnosis:
> A. Asthma   D. Pneumonia
> B. Cancer   E. Pulmonary embolus
> C. Congestive heart failure   F. Tuberculosis
>
> 1. A 62-year-old, previously healthy man has had several days of right-sided pleuritic chest pain, a cough productive of yellow-green sputum, fever, sweats, and increased difficulty breathing. He has never used tobacco. His chest radiograph shows consolidation of a portion of the right lower lobe.

(Answer: D)

> 2. A 62-year-old, previously healthy man has had progressively increasing right-sided pleuritic chest pain, recent hemoptysis, increased difficulty breathing, and weight loss. He has never used tobacco and has had no fever. His chest radiograph shows mediastinal fullness on the right with obstructive atelectasis and a right-sided pleural effusion.

(Answer: B)   **END OF CASE**

Case Clusters: Steps 2CK and 3

Case clusters are single-patient vignettes followed by from two to six questions. These questions may each test a different point, or may be linked sequentially, where one provides information needed to answer the next question. Therefore, it is extremely important to answer these questions in the order presented. Generally, once you proceed to the next item in the set, you cannot change a previous answer. An example of this format is:

> A 5-year-old girl's parents bring her to the emergency department because of difficulty breathing. She has previously been in good health and began complaining of pain in her throat about three hours ago. She now is wheezing, sitting forward, and drooling.

1. When auscultating her lungs, you most likely hear:
   (A) diminished breath sounds   (D) rales in both bases
   (B) expiratory wheezes   (E) unilateral inspiratory wheezes
   (C) inspiratory wheezes

   (Answer: B)

2. The patient's oxygen saturation on room air is 87%. She does not want an oxygen facemask and pushes it away. Your next step should be:
   (A) admit her to the intensive care unit
   (B) do an arterial blood gas analysis
   (C) examine her throat for a foreign body
   (D) have her parent hold the oxygen near her mouth
   (E) perform a thoracostomy

   (Answer: D)

3. Soft-tissue radiographs of the neck demonstrate [a swollen epiglottis. *On the test you would interpret the radiograph.*] The most likely etiologic agent is:
   (A) Bacteroides melaninogenicus
   (B) Haemophilus influenzae, type B
   (C) Mycoplasma pneumoniae
   (D) Parainfluenza virus, type 1
   (E) Staphylococcus aureus

   (Answer: B)

4. If you saw a similar patient who presented with a barky cough and whose chest radiograph showed "steepling" of the tracheal shadow, immediate treatment might include:
   (A) endotracheal intubation
   (B) immediate tracheostomy
   (C) inhaled albuterol
   (D) inhaled racemic epinephrine
   (E) topical cocaine

   (Answer: D)   **END OF CASE**

Comprehensive Osteopathic Medical Licensing Examination-USA (COMLEX-USA)

The National Board of Osteopathic Medical Examiners, Inc. (NBOME™), first established in 1934, administers this licensing examination for Osteopathic physicians in the United States. All 50 states accept the COMLEX-USA for licensure (in this book, referred to as "COMLEX"). It is designed to assess whether the Osteopathic physician has the requisite knowledge to practice medicine without supervision.

This examination parallels the USMLE in content and format. COMLEX consists of three computerized tests (Levels 1, 2 Cognitive Evaluation [CE], and 3) and a clinical skills test (Level 2 Performance Evaluation [PE]). The computer-administered versions of the exams were introduced between February 1995 and June 1998. Level 2PE is similar to the OSCE exams and USMLE Step 2CS, and was first given in September 2004. COMLEX Levels 1, 2, and 3 must be taken in sequence, but the two parts of Level 2—CE and PE—can be taken in any order. COMLEX will probably be restructured beginning in 2014; check the NBOME website for details.

The primary difference between the COMLEX and the USMLE is that COMLEX has elements of Osteopathic Principles and Practice in all Levels. Osteopathic medical students and graduates may take the COMLEX, the USMLE, or both exams.

Eligibility

For Level 1, individuals may apply for the exam only after having satisfactorily completed the first year at (or graduated from) a medical school accredited by the AOA's Commission on Osteopathic College Accreditation (COCA). For Levels 2CE and 2PE, applicants must have passed COMLEX Level 1 and satisfactorily completed the second year in a COCA-accredited medical school. The Dean's office at each Osteopathic school submits a list of students eligible for Levels 1, 2CE, and 2PE to the NBOME.

Applicants for COMLEX Level 3 must have a D.O. degree from a COCA-accredited medical school and have passed Levels 1, 2CE, and 2PE. (D.O.s who graduated prior to January 1, 2005 don't have to take Level 2PE if, before June 30, 2005, they had passed Level 2CE.) Requirements for post-graduate training vary among states. Generally, all candidates for Level 3 must submit verification that they are in or have successfully completed the requisite training program.

Registration/Scheduling

To register for COMLEX Levels 1, 2CE, and 2PE, the applicant's name must be on the list from their Dean. If the candidate has already graduated, a notarized copy of his medical school diploma will be accepted.

You *must* use the online access system at the NBOME website (www.nbome. org) to register and pay for, schedule, cancel, withdraw from, or reschedule an examination. Once the NBOME has proof of your eligibility, they will send you and e-mail with a unique link you must use to initially access the system and establish an account. You will then choose a username and password and enter and verify personal information. Follow the instructions; you must complete all the steps in sequence to be able to schedule the exam. After a short delay, you may then schedule your exam and pay by credit card.

Levels 1, 2CE, and 3 are given at more than 300 testing centers in the United States. The exact location of the test centers and the availability of the site for the scheduled test dates are listed on the NBOME's Examination Scheduling web page. Level 2PE is administered at NBOME's National Center for Clinical Skills Testing in Conshohocken, Pennsylvania (about 15 miles from Philadelphia International Airport).

Eligible candidates may register for and schedule an examination as early as six months in advance of a scheduled test date for COMLEX Levels 1, 2CE, or 3. For Level 2PE, once you are eligible, you may register for and schedule it as early as a year before the exam. For the best choice of dates and locations, you should schedule it at least 90 days before your desired test date. To schedule the exam, you must have your NBOME six-digit identification number. After scheduling, you will receive a confirmation number from the NBOME and an e-mail confirmation notice.

Warning: You must schedule any computer-delivered exam at least 120 hours before your selected date and time. If you fail to do so, you will be denied access to the examination and will be charged a non-refundable fee (in addition to the regular fee) when you schedule a new test date.

For more complete instructions about how to register, see "Registration Information" in the current NBOME *COMLEX-USA Bulletin of Information* or the CBT Tutorial at www.nbome.org. The NBOME website has the most current information about policies and procedures applicable to testing, as well as other items of interest to candidates.

Canceling/Rescheduling

For COMLEX Levels 1, 2CE, and 3, you may cancel any time before 30 days prior to the scheduled test date with no penalty. If you cancel between 30 full days and 120 hours before the exam, you will be charged an additional fee ($85, in 2012) when the test is rescheduled. If you cancel less than 120 hours and up to 24 hours before the start of an exam, the additional fee is $190: if you simply don't appear for the exam or withdraw on the test date, the fee is $225.

For COMLEX Level 2PE, applicants who cancel or reschedule their exam from 90 days to 30 days before their original test date are charged an additional $50 when they re-register. Cancellations made from 30 days to 48 hours before the test cost $150, and if within 48 hours, $400. *Warning:* if you don't show up for a Level 2PE exam and haven't notified the NBOME prior to the start of the exam, you will be charged $650. (All fees are as of 2012.)

In the event of severe inclement weather, contact your scheduled test center to determine whether the test will still be administered. For Level 2PE, contact the NBOME National Center for Clinical Skills Testing (610-825-6551; or the power-independent emergency line, 610-825-4240). In the unlikely event that a test center is closed or is forced to close during testing, candidates will be rescheduled by the NBOME (Level 2PE) or the Thomson ProMetric Help Desk (Levels 1, 2CE, 3) on the next available test date.

Special Testing Accommodations

If a candidate has a disability as defined under the Americans with Disabilities Act (ADA) and requires special accommodations to take the test, the individual must submit a written request using the form provided on www.nbome.org (search for "Test Accommodations") to NBOME, 8765 W. Higgins Rd., Suite 200, Chicago, IL 60631-4101; (773) 714-0622; fax: (773) 714-0631. ADA candidates should submit the required ADA-accommodation application 90 days in advance of the test for Levels 1, 2CE, and 3, and 180 days prior to Level 2PE; a review of an application will take a minimum of 45 days. The NBOME strongly recommends that all requests for accommodation and the supporting documentation be sent to the NBOME by a traceable means of delivery (e.g., UPS, FedEx, Certified Mail). Keep copies of everything you send.

Candidates will be notified in writing of their accommodation status prior to the examination. If approved, contact the appropriate NBOME office in Chicago for registration instructions. If the request is rejected, schedule the exam on-line without accommodation. **NOTE** that the NBOME will not provide additional time to complete the patient encounter portion of Level 2PE.

Retaking COMLEX

If you fail a Level or a Part (CE/PE), you may apply to retake the test on the next available date after you receive your Score Report. You must still meet the eligibility criteria and re-apply as if you are taking the examination for the first time. Candidates may not take the same level more than three times in any 12-month period. Examinees who have passed a Level or Part may not retake that exam to improve their score.

Applicants requesting special accommodations who must retake a Level or a Part (2CE or 2PE) must contact the NBOME office and re-apply for the appropriate accommodation. A candidate may not reschedule an accommodation exam without notifying the NBOME office.

At this time (July 2012), the NBOME does not limit the number of times a candidate who fails a Level may retake it; however, they recommend that medical licensing authorities consider that the candidate [should] successfully complete Levels 1, 2CE, 2PE, and 3 within a seven-year period, beginning when the candidate passes COMLEX Level 1; and not allow more than three attempts to pass each Level without demonstration of additional educational experience acceptable to the medical licensing authority. Since this is not a mandate, the time period within which all Levels must be completed, the allowed number of attempts to pass a Level without additional education, and the required passing scores vary among the state medical licensing authorities. Each state's licensing board website (accessed through www.fsmb.org) has more specific information. However, effective July 1, 2016, candidates will be limited to a total of six attempts for each examination.

Cost

The standard fees (2012) for COMLEX are: Level 1, $535; Level 2CE, $535; Level 2PE, $1,185; and Level 3, $715. Additional fees may be assessed for cancellations within 30 days of the exam or for not showing up (see above).

Taking the Test

Levels 1, 2CE, and 3

Dress comfortably, since testing may take the full day. If you will need to use hearing aids or earplugs during the test, contact the NBOME prior to your test date. Bring one piece of identification, such as a current driver's license or passport. You will be required to have a digital photograph and biometric ID (fingerprint) taken when you check in. Candidates are not permitted to bring any food or drink into the testing area. If you will require food or drink during the testing period, you may request an unscheduled break that will be charged against your allocated time for the test session during which the break is taken.

Be sure to arrive early for the test; candidates who arrive at the test center 30 minutes after the scheduled start time can take the test, but are given no additional time. If you arrive 30 minutes or more after the test has started, you can take it only at the discretion of the proctor. Otherwise you will be considered a "no show."

There are three optional breaks: one 10-minute break during the morning after completion of Section 2 and another 10-minute break in the afternoon after Section 6. The actual time spent on breaks is deducted from the total time allocated to complete the exam. There is also an optional 40-minute lunch break following the morning session that does *not* count against the total exam time.

Level 2PE

Dress professionally for Level 2PE, and bring a white lab coat and a stethoscope. You should arrive 30 minutes before the scheduled starting time for the exam. Be sure to allow extra time: travel delays are common in the greater Philadelphia area. If you need to cancel due to a travel delay, immediately contact NBOME's National Center for Clinical Skills Testing. You will be given a boxed lunch at the first of the two scheduled breaks; you may bring your own food (not requiring refrigeration) and beverages for use during the breaks, if desired. During the 7-hour test session, candidates will not be allowed to have contact with anyone outside the test center. This includes the use of cellular phones. The testing sequence details are in the *[annual] Orientation Guide for COMLEX Level 2PE*, available on the NBOME website.

Scores

Scoring for COMLEX is essentially the same as for the USMLE; the number of items answered correctly (the raw score) is converted to 3-digit and 2-digit standard scores. The passing score for all COMLEX Levels is based solely on a candidate's performance, and the percentage of examinees that pass or fail is not predetermined.

The mean standard score for each of Levels 1, 2CE, and 3, regardless of when the exams were given, is 500. A minimum standard score of 400 (75 using 2-digit scores) on Level 1 or Level 2CE is required to pass the exam. A standard score of at least 350 (75 using 2-digit scores) on Level 3 is required to pass the exam.

Levels 1 and 2CE results are available online about 4 to 6 weeks after the test. Score reports are mailed to both examinees and their Dean approximately 8 to 10 weeks after the test. Examinees and Deans' offices may access COMLEX scores online using a secure system. (Examinees establish a secured NBOME web account during the registration process.) Level 3 score reports also may be released to the Director of Medical Education at the candidate's internship hospital. No scores will be reported by telephone, e-mail, or fax.

Level 2PE scores are reported only as "Pass" or "Fail." To achieve a "Pass," you must pass both the Humanistic Domain, which is a measure of physician-patient communication, interpersonal skills, and professionalism, and the Biomedical/Biomechanical Domain, which includes history-taking, physical examination, Osteopathic principles and Osteopathic manipulative treatment, written communication (synthesis of clinical findings in a SOAP Note format), integrated differential diagnosis, and clinical problem-solving. Examinees who "Fail" receive additional feedback to help them identify their areas of strength and weakness.

Sending Your COMLEX Results (Transcript)

To have an NBOME transcript with COMLEX scores sent to a third party, such as ERAS, a residency program, or a licensing Board, send a written or electronic (via the online registration system) request and the appropriate fee to the NBOME. Instructions and the form are on NBOME's website. Requests are processed within two weeks; additional fees can speed the process.

NBOME transcripts include: a complete history of all exams taken, including scores if reported; information documenting "indeterminate" results for any exams; information concerning any irregular behavior during testing; and notification of any actions taken against the candidate by a medical licensing authority or other credentialing entity that were reported to the NBOME.

The NBOME transcript will only reflect a Pass/Fail grade for Level 2PE. The candidate's certified transcript is the only verification sent by the NBOME to state boards for licensure applications. Processing of a certified transcript for candidates who have passed Level 3 begins no earlier than two weeks after the original release of scores. Additional certified transcripts will be sent only upon receipt of a written request from the candidate, and the normal processing time applies.

Preparing for COMLEX

The COMLEX Levels are not "computer-adaptive," therefore, the questions are determined before the test is administered. Usually, the questions will be identical regardless of when and where the test is administered. (For testing hints, see "Tips for taking USMLE-type Tests," below.)

Materials for COMLEX preparation, including the *NBOME Bulletin of Information,* are available at www.nbome.org. For additional questions, contact the National Board of Osteopathic Medical Examiners (NBOME), Inc., 8765 W. Higgins Rd, Suite 200, Chicago, IL 60631-4174; (773) 714-0622.

The NBOME provides a wealth of information on their website for those traveling to the Philadelphia area to take Level 2PE. This includes maps and written directions for those coming by train, shuttle, and car. In addition, they have arranged airline discounts. For additional information about Level 2PE, contact the National Center for Clinical Skills Testing, 101 W. Elm Street, Conshohocken, PA 19428; (610) 825-6551. Inquiries about any part of COMLEX can also be sent via e-mail to admin@nbome.org or testing@nbome.org.

COMLEX Content

The computer-based Levels 1, 2CE, and 3 each have 400 multiple-choice questions, grouped into 50-question blocks. You can review and change answers only on the questions in the current section. You cannot return to a prior section to change your answers. A clock on the screen assists with time management, and you will be warned about the amount of time remaining.

The majority of the test items are "one-best-answer" questions, although a few will be matching questions. Most of the one-best-answer questions are single, stand-alone items; the rest consist of a case history with two or more related, one-best-answer questions. Some have "exhibits" or "lab values" that can be accessed by pressing the appropriate buttons.

COMLEX is designed to assess the Osteopathic medical knowledge and clinical skills considered essential for Osteopathic generalist physicians to practice medicine without supervision. It is constructed in the context of medical problem-solving, which involves clinical presentations and physician tasks. Candidates are expected to utilize the philosophy and principles of Osteopathic medicine to solve medical problems.

All Levels follow the same two-dimensional "Examination Blueprint," although the emphasis changes to reflect examinees' educational level (see Figure 8.7). This blueprint has two main components: "Dimension I," or Clinical Presentation, identifies high-frequency and/or high-impact health issues that Osteopathic generalist physicians encounter in practice. "Dimension II," or Physician Task, specifies the major steps Osteopathic physicians generally undertake to solve medical problems. Details of the topics covered by each category are in the CBT Tutorial, available on the NBOME website.

Level 1

Level 1 is usually taken in June of the sophomore year, is a one-day exam comparable to USMLE Step 1. It covers the basic medical sciences of anatomy, behavioral science, biochemistry, microbiology, Osteopathic principles, pathology, pharmacology, and physiology. Examinees must demonstrate that they understand the mechanisms of health, medical problems and disease processes.

Figure 8.7
COMLEX-USA Examination Blueprint
Dimension I: Patient Presentation

Levels 1, 2CE, 3

Asymptomatic/General Symptoms	8%–16%
Symptoms/Disorders of Digestion & Metabolism	4%–10%
Symptoms/Disorders of Sensory & CNS Systems	28%–38%
Symptoms/Disorders of Musculoskeletal & Motor Systems	6%–12%
Symptoms/Disorders Related to Human Sexuality & Genitourinary System	3%–8%
Symptoms/Disorders of Respiration & Circulation	8%–16%
Symptoms/Disorders of Thermoregulation	2%–6%
Symptoms/Disorders of the Tissues and Trauma	8%–16%
Symptoms/Disorders of Pregnancy & Human Development	3%–8%

Dimension II: Physician Tasks

	Level 1	Level 2CE	Level 3
Health Promotion/Disease Prevention	1%–5%	15%–20%	15%–20%
History & Physical	5%–15%	30%–40%	10%–20%
Diagnostic Technologies	1%–5%	10%–20%	15%–25%
Management	2%–7%	10%–20%	25%–40%
Scientific Understanding of Mechanisms	70%–85%	5%–15%	5%–10%
Health Care Delivery	1%–3%	5%–10%	5%–10%

Adapted from the NBOME website (www.nbome.org), May 2012.

Level 2CE

This Level, usually taken in August of the senior year, is a one-day exam comparable to USMLE Step 2CK. It integrates the clinical disciplines of Emergency Medicine, Family Practice, Internal Medicine, Obstetrics and Gynecology, Osteopathic Principles, Pediatrics, Psychiatry, Surgery, and other areas necessary to solve medical problems. Examinees must demonstrate the clinical concepts and principles necessary to make appropriate medical diagnoses through patient history and physical examination findings.

Level 2PE

Level 2PE is a one-day (7 hours) exam comparable to USMLE Step 2CS. It uses 12 standardized patients in simulated ambulatory medical settings with problems and symptoms that are acute, chronic, or provide opportunities for health promotion and disease prevention. It is designed to test the following clinical skills: doctor-patient communication, interpersonal interactions, professionalism, medical history-taking, physical examination, Osteopathic principles, Osteopathic manipulative treatment, and written communication— including synthesis of clinical findings, integrated differential diagnosis and formulation of a diagnostic and treatment plan. The NBOME website has the *(Annual) Orientation Guide for Level 2PE*, as well as a video. The video is also available at all Osteopathic medical schools' Dean's offices.

Level 3

Level 3, usually taken in December of the first postgraduate year, is comparable to USMLE Step 3. It is a one-day problem- and symptom-based assessment integrating the clinical disciplines of Emergency Medicine, Family Practice, Internal Medicine, Obstetrics and Gynecology, Osteopathic Principles, Pediatrics, Psychiatry, and Surgery. Examinees must demonstrate that they can make the appropriate patient management decisions and solve medical problems at the level of an independently practicing Osteopathic generalist physician.

Irregular Testing Behavior

Examinee behaviors that are not tolerated are essentially the same as those for the USMLE (see above). The penalties are also similar.

Comparing COMLEX and USMLE Scores

With increasing numbers of D.O. students applying to M.D. residencies, the question naturally arises, how do the COMLEX and USMLE scores compare? While the tests themselves cannot fairly be compared, COMLEX scores can be converted into their USMLE equivalent. The formulas were developed by Philip Slocum, D.O. and Janet Louder from the Kirksville College of Osteopathic Medicine, and published in the *Journal of the American Osteopathic Association* (September 2006). For COMLEX Levels 1 and 2 three-digit scores, the formulas are:

USMLE Step 1 score = 67.97 + (0.24 x COMLEX Level 1 score)
USMLE Step 2 score = 102.2 + (0.18 x COMLEX Level 2 score)

You can provide these comparisons to program directors if they are interested. **Warning**: these are only approximations, since the numbers they are based on vary slightly each year. It might be better to give them the "COMLEX-USA at a glance" sheet, found on the NBOME web site.

Licensure

Passing all three parts of the USMLE or COMLEX (for D.O.s only) and completing the required amount of ACGME- or AOA-approved graduate medical training are both necessary to gain an initial medical license (Figures 8.8 and 8.9).

In most states, since the licensing bodies are the same for both M.D.s and D.O.s, physicians can use either examination for licensure. However, Arizona, California, Florida, Maine, Michigan, Nevada, New Mexico, Oklahoma, Pennsylvania, Tennessee, Utah, Vermont, Washington, and West Virginia have separate Osteopathic licensing boards. These states, as well as some others, have distinct requirements for D.O. licensure. For further information about licensure, see *State Medical Licensure Requirements and Statistics*, published annually by the American Medical Association.

One important note: NBME policy states that individuals who demonstrate "irregular behavior" and/or those who "subvert the NBME assessment or certification process" (i.e., cheat) will be permanently barred from certification by the Board. In addition, reports will be sent both to the individual's medical school and to the Federation of State Medical Boards. NBOME has similar policies in place. Don't say that you weren't warned.

Figure 8.8
Examination Pathways for U.S. Licensure

U.S. Graduate Pathway

M.D. Student   D.O. Student
USMLE Step 1*   USMLE Step 1*
USMLE Step 2CK* & 2CS*   USMLE Step 2CK* & 2CS*
USMLE Step 3   USMLE Step 3
                                        -or-
                                COMLEX Levels 1-3

IMG Pathway
ECFMG Certification:
    USMLE Step 1*
    USMLE Steps 2CK* & 2CS*
    USMLE Step 3

*May be taken in any order.

Figure 8.9: Graduate Education Requirements for Licensure

Number of years of accredited U.S. or Canadian graduate medical education (residency) required for a medical license.

One Year

Alabama[1]	Idaho[1]	Missouri[1]	South Carolina[1]
Arizona[1]	Indiana[1]	Nebraska[1]	Tennessee[1]
Arkansas[1]	Iowa[1]	New Mexico[3]	Texas[1]
California[1,10]	Kansas[1]	New York[1]	Vermont[1]
Colorado[1]	Louisiana[1,9]	North Carolina[1]	Virginia[1]
Delaware[1]	Maine[3]	North Dakota[1]	Washington[3]
District of Columbia[1]	Maryland[1,4]	Ohio[1]	West Virginia[1]
Florida[1]	Massachusetts[1]	Oklahoma[1]	Wisconsin
Georgia[1]	Michigan[3]	Oregon[1]	Wyoming
Guam[1,6]	Minnesota[1]	Pennsylvania[3]	
Hawaii[1]	Mississippi[1]	Puerto Rico	

Two Years

Alaska[1]	Indiana[2]	Minnesota[2]	Oklahoma[2,8]
California[2,10]	Iowa[2]	Montana[1]	Pennsylvania[8]
Connecticut	Kentucky	New Hampshire	Rhode Island[1]
Florida[2]	Maryland[2,4]	New Jersey[7]	Utah
Hawaii[2]	Massachusetts[2]	New Mexico[2,8]	Virginia[2]
Illinois	Michigan[2,8]	Ohio[2]	Washington[2,0]

Three Years

Alabama[2]	Guam[2,6]	Nebraska[2]	Rhode Island[2]
Alaska[2]	Idaho[2]	Nevada	South Carolina[2]
Arizona[2]	Kansas[2]	New York[2]	South Dakota[5]
Arkansas[2]	Louisiana[2,9]	North Carolina[2]	Tennessee[2]
Colorado[2]	Maine[2,8]	North Dakota[2]	Texas[2]
Delaware[2]	Mississippi[2]	Oregon[2]	Vermont[2]
District of Columbia[2]	Missouri[2]	Pennsylvania[2]	West Virginia[2]
Georgia[2]	Montana[2]		

[1] Graduates of U.S. or Canadian M.D. or D.O. medical schools only.
[2] International medical graduates only.
[3] D.O.s only.
[4] Additional year of residency required if applicant failed any Step of licensing exam three or more times.
[5] Must complete a residency program.
[6] Canadian training not accepted.
[7] 2 years GME with a contract to do a third year.
[8] M.D.s only.
[9] Only ACMGE-approved (M.D.) training accepted.
[10] Must include at least 4 months of General Medicine.
Adapted from: *State Medical Licensure Requirements & Statistics: 2010.* Chicago, IL: AMA, 2010:Tables 7 & 9; and *State-Specific Requirements for Initial Medical Licensure*, FSMB, 2012.

Are the Examinations Fair?

Some subgroups have consistently different results when taking both the USMLE and the COMLEX. This has raised some doubts about these exams' fairness. Although neither the NBME nor COMLEX releases this information any longer, it may be instructive to look at the information they previously released.

At least in the past, both gender and race seemed to influence students' USMLE scores on Steps 1 and 2. (These findings were actually drawn from the very similar NBME Parts I and II.) White men had the highest pass rate, followed in order by Asian/Pacific Islander men, white women, Asian/Pacific Islander women, and Hispanic men. Trailing badly in order, were, Hispanic women, black men, and black women. Many of the differences in test results could be predicted from the MCAT scores on reading or science problems.

On the COMLEX precursor, the NBEOPS exam, men consistently scored higher on Part I, and women scored higher on Part III. Men and women performed equally well on Part II. These findings remained consistent for all Osteopathic schools. Some researchers suggest that these findings result from a difference in men's and women's academic growth rates.

The debate continues as to whether the variance in scores on the USMLE and COMLEX reflects real differences in individuals' clinical competence.

Special Purpose Examination (SPEX®)

State licensing authorities use this one-day, computerized examination (containing 420 multiple-choice questions) to test the knowledge of physicians who have held a valid, unrestricted medical license in a U.S. or Canadian jurisdiction and are seeking licensure in a new state, or re-licensure in the same state, *at least five years after graduation from medical school.*

More state medical boards are requiring physicians who were previously licensed in another state to pass the SPEX to obtain a license in the state. Medical boards also require passing SPEX before they will reinstate the license of physicians who have been inactive for a period of time. In recent years, the pass-rate has been about 68%. This test is *not* available as a licensing mechanism for graduating medical students. As with the USMLE, ProMetric administers the exam.

Importance of Passing the Tests

Do not underestimate the importance of these tests! If you do not eventually pass the USMLE (or the COMLEX for Osteopaths), you will never practice medicine in the United States. That alone should give you a good reason to take them seriously. Another is that you may need to pass the tests to get a residency position.

How Important Are the Scores in the Resident-Selection Process?

Residency directors prefer to rank only those applicants who have fulfilled their school's requirements for graduation: If a matched candidate fails to graduate, the residency program ends up with an unfilled position in July. That is why even moderately competitive residencies may require you to submit evidence that you have passed all examinations required by your medical school for graduation. Therefore, students whose schools require passing Step 2 to graduate may need to take this Step early in their senior year to assure residency directors that they have passed the test and, presumably, will graduate on time.

Although the tests are not designed for this purpose, many, if not most, residency programs use applicants' USMLE or COMLEX scores as a *primary screening device*. Because of the unavailability of other information about candidates, the scores on licensing examinations, especially Steps 1 and 2 of the USMLE, have become outrageously important. This is not the fault of program directors. They would like nothing better than a useful transcript (not all "Pass" grades) and a specific Dean's Letter (not saying that everyone "will be a fine clinician"), as well as for school honors (such as AOA election) to be given out before they have to make Match decisions. However, the licensing examination scores are often the only objective way to evaluate the large pool of candidates from multiple schools with varying amounts of background and supporting material.

Residency directors also want their residents to be able to pass the specialty's Board examination, because both residency applicants and the individuals who approve residency programs look at how many of a residency's graduates pass their Board examination. (This information is in *FREIDA.*) As one residency director said, "Our residency program is judged, in part, on how well our graduates do on their Board examinations. Doing well on the USMLE says that they are at least good test takers—and that's important." Good USMLE scores do correlate with passing specialty board examinations. In general, they also correlate with residents' clinical performance in at least their PGY-1 year.

Although this practice has been officially condemned, the NBME has sent residency directors information on how to interpret the USMLE scores to screen applicants. At the most competitive programs and in the most competitive specialties, you must obtain minimum scores on the exams for them to consider you, despite any other credentials. The specific minimum scores vary directly with the specialty's and the program's competitiveness. Scores may not be considered at all in non-competitive programs, while some highly competitive specialties and programs reportedly grant interviews only to applicants with USMLE scores greater than 210 (the mean score ranges from 200 to 220; standard deviation is 20 points). This alone suggests that the scores may be very important to you and that you should take the test very seriously.

How Much Effort Should You Expend?

Since the USMLE is so important to your career, it is worth the extra effort to do well. Educators refer to these tests as "high-stakes evaluations," because they may determine whether you graduate from medical school, the type and quality of the residency program you enter, and whether you are ever licensed to practice medicine. Take heed.

Most medical schools use USMLE-type questions for many of their examinations, so you will already be familiar with the format. (Some courses, however, have not changed their examinations in years, so they still use the format that the USMLE has abandoned; i.e., single questions with multiple true-false options.) You have probably also learned some of the tricks about how to take these kinds of tests. A few basic tips are listed in the next section.

Each of you knows how you learn best. For some, it is by reviewing their own notes and textbooks. For others, it may be by going over any one of the available specialized review texts. Nearly all students use the special USMLE review texts, rather than their textbooks or the study materials that the NBME supplies. Many students recommend using the books from the National Medical Series for Independent Study (John Wiley & Sons) and the "Blueprints Series" (Blackwell Science). Regardless of the source, remember to focus on "high-yield" information (start with the "high-yield" section of *First Aid for the USMLE Step 1* or *2*). Don't get mired in unimportant details!

For *Step 1*, begin by reviewing your notes and books from your two basic-science years. Focus on the basic science principles related to common life-threatening and debilitating conditions, to normal development, and to prevention.

For *Step 2*, be able to diagnose and initially manage common life-threatening and debilitating conditions, and review normal development across the lifespan (including pregnancy) and anything pertaining to prevention. Definitely study for Step 2—no matter what your buddies say. The test has become harder in recent years, with Steps 2 and 3 requiring you to integrate material from several sources. Also, it will help you stay sane if you pass Step 2 before starting residency; once you graduate, you will have much less time to study for the exam.

For each Step, review previously studied material. The key is to *review* material rather than trying to learn it for the first time. This builds on your strengths and minimizes your weaknesses. Take practice tests to identify content areas that you need to study further. Start with the free tests on the USMLE website.

The well-publicized national review courses are primarily for those students whose academic performance has been marginal, for those who have failed the test once, or for IMGs who are not native American-English speakers. These courses can be expensive. If this list doesn't include you, use your money to have dinner with a spouse/friend once a week as a reward for studying or to have a nice vacation after the test. Take the test and, until you get your score, assume that you have passed. Over 90% of test takers do!

Whatever the method or methods you use, it is important for you to *take this test seriously and to do the best that you possibly can.*

If you passed the test but did not do as well as you thought you should—or could—have, *you do not have the option of repeating it.* You can retake the exam only if you fail. If you retake and pass a Step, the passing score becomes the official National Board record, although transcripts that are sent out will list all your attempts to pass the USMLE. Even if you successfully complete several subsections of a Step on the initial attempt, the entire Step must be retaken. Steps 1 and 2 may be taken as many times as are needed to pass.

Many of the students who fail Step 1 do so because of reading problems or learning disabilities. Most medical schools are not prepared to deal with these issues. If you fail Step 1 and feel that a learning disability is the reason, you might want to contact either your school's education department or one of the following medical school-based programs:

- **Rosalind Franklin University of Medicine and Science**. Their Step 1 review course lasts 15 weeks between January and May (five days/wk with an occasional practice exam on weekends). Contact Dr. Gordon Pullen, Ph.D. at (847) 578-8603; e-mail: gordon.pullen@rosalindfranklin.edu; http://66.99.255.20/cms/educationalaffairs/.

- **University of Missouri–Kansas City, Institute for Professional Preparation.** Their programs, held since 1981, are available to enrollees in or graduates of U.S. medical schools. They provide programs of varying length (up to 17 weeks) for those with problems at any stage of the licensing exam process. Specific information and applications can be found at www.umkc.edu/ipp/.
- **The Medical H.E.L.P. Program at Marshall University in West Virginia.** This 5-week program is designed for those with learning disabilities and dyslexia. Call (304) 696-6315 or (800) 642-3463; e-mail Ryan Orwig at orwigl@marshall.edu; www.marshall.edu/medicalhelp.

If an applicant fails Step 3, the licensing board may require evidence of the completion of additional training before allowing him to retake the exam. For licensure, most states require that all Steps be completed within a seven-year period. The time limit begins when an applicant first passes a USMLE Step.

Tips for Taking USMLE-Type Examinations

Listed below are several things you can do to maximize your scores on licensing examinations. The first, of course, is to know the material as well as you can. If you don't know the material, there are few tips that can help, especially on tests that have been written and field-tested by experts.

1. Know the material.
2. Get enough sleep the night before.
3. Follow a normal routine the day of the exam.
4. Wear comfortable clothing.
5. Arrive early enough to sign in and get your entire allotted time for the exam.
6. Check the test information to be certain that you bring all needed materials, e.g., admission card or identification with picture.
7. Be familiar with the test format so that you don't waste time taking the tutorial or floundering with the computerized test. (Do this by taking a computerized practice test and the tutorial on the CD supplied with the registration materials.)
8. Be familiar with the types of questions (single answer) that will be used.
9. Know how the test will be scored.
10. Use your time efficiently.

Mental preparation is the next key. Most people are familiar with pretest anxiety. Butterflies in the stomach, sweaty palms, rapid heartbeat and respiratory rate, and fear of failure do not necessarily mean you have lost the war of nerves. You merely have to steady yourself. It is said that *Tonight Show* host Johnny Carson (during whose show you were probably conceived) had a heart rate approaching 160 just before he went out to do his monologue. And he did this for twenty-five years! The trick for you is to do everything as normally as possible. Get enough sleep the night before the exam and follow your normal routine the day of the test. Dress in comfortable clothes. Large testing sites are often too warm, too cold, or alternate between these extremes. Wear clothing that can be removed or loosened to cool off and bring something extra to wear in case it gets too cold. Arrive at the testing site early to avoid hassles. Do not be caught short by failing to bring your picture ID or the admission card.

Read over testing materials well in advance of the exam date. For the USMLE, if you become familiar with the testing method by taking a practice session, you can skip the tutorial and gain 15 minutes of time. COMLEX candidates can review a CD-ROM with a practice test at their school's Deans office.

The testing materials you receive in advance will also tell you how the test will be scored and explain the types of questions used on the exam. The USMLE is scored by crediting the correct answers; there is no numeric penalty for getting a question wrong, although it will affect the subsequent questions you get for that block. (COMLEX does not alter the questions during the exam based on the examinee's responses.) If you don't know the answer, it pays to guess. Therefore, you need to know how to guess effectively.

Guessing effectively means knowing how to best answer the types of questions on the test. As medical students, most of you will be very familiar with the standard A-Type (single-answer, multiple-choice) questions used on the exams. These are essentially variations of simple true-false questions. To answer them correctly, use the following hints:

- Even if "A" seems to be the correct answer, look over the other answers to be certain that a more correct answer does not exist. This is especially important on USMLE Steps 2 and 3.
- If you cannot spot which answer is "true," read each alternative and mark the ones you believe are "false." If you can mark three answers (out of five) as "false," you have increased your chance of correctly answering the item from 20% to 50%.
- Use the information you get from other parts of the test to help answer questions you otherwise would not know. A great deal of

information is given in the stems (first part) of the exam's questions. Use this to your advantage.

- Try not to change your answers. Change an answer only if you are *certain* that your initial answer was incorrect.
- Look for long introductory clauses (foils) or the qualifying word "may" in true answers. Look for the limiting words "never" or "always" to spot false answers.

When faced with questions concerning a clinical case, first review the questions. These will often suggest the parts of the case that are most important and the key points to look for when reading the clinical description.

When taking computerized tests, two-thirds to three-fourths of examinees who go back and change their answer for a prior question go from a wrong to a right answer. This is true if they change the answer because they (1) reread and better understand the test item, (2) use clues or cues from subsequent items, or (3) are correcting a clerical error. Examinees are less likely to select a correct answer if they are replacing one wild guess with another or if they just have a "gut feeling" that the new answer is better.

Finally, use your time effectively. This is possibly the most important strategy for successful test-taking. Do not spend too much time on any one question. If you don't pace yourself and then have to randomly guess the answers to too many questions, you will fail the exam. On the USMLE, you have only about one minute per question. During each USMLE and COMLEX timed computer module, you may answer the questions in any order, review your responses, and change your answers. Since each question counts the same, if a question is too difficult to be answered in a reasonable amount of time, make an educated guess at the answer immediately and make a note to go back to it after you have finished the rest of the items in that module. (For the USMLE, mark questions to review with the available check mark [√]. These marks will appear on the navigation bar on the left side of the screen.) After you exit the module, or when time expires, you can no longer access those test items.

Simulated Patient cases (Step 2CS and Level 2PE) and Step 3 case simulations must be answered in the order presented. After you exit the case or session, or when time expires, you no longer have access to those test items or cases and their answers.

If you run out of time in a module, but are still working on a question, you are allowed to finish that question. The time, however, is deducted from your total time allotment. Even so, it is generally worthwhile to try to answer that last question.

Note that the NBME suggests that examinees answer each question as it appears. Since you have taken examinations of this sort in medical school, you should know which method works best for you.

If You Don't Have To Take the USMLE

Take Steps/Levels 1 and 2 while you are in medical school. A number of schools do not require their students to take Steps 1 and 2 of the USMLE. Some only require that the student pass Step 2. But unless you are an Osteopathic student, there is only one route to getting a medical license in the United States—the USMLE. You must pass all three USMLE Steps. In general, you will never be as prepared to take the basic-science-oriented Step 1 as you are during medical school. Take the test: Remember your priorities. While a low score on Step 1 might put you out of the running for some residency positions, you will have passed the first hurdle to practicing medicine.

"But I took Subject Exams (also called "Shelf Exams") in my preclinical courses," you say. Residency directors place little stock in these test results, with good reasons. Performance on these tests (the questions are taken from prior Board examinations) is not directly comparable to performance on the USMLE Step 1. That is because rather than having to study for, and know, all the basic sciences at once, you take the Subject Exams immediately after you have intensively studied each subject, usually as a final examination for the course. These exams do not contain the newer type of test questions or the integrated-subjects questions now found on the USMLE. This is similarly true for Subject Exams given in the clinical years. For example, students with marginal passing scores on the Subject Exams for Biochemistry, Physiology, Pathology, Pharmacology, and Microbiology had a 25% or greater chance of failing the same section when they took their licensing examination.

Objective Structured Clinical Examination (OSCE)

The Objective Structured Clinical Examination (OSCE) tests a student's clinical abilities. The OSCE uses "standardized patients"—either patients with stable physical findings (e.g., arthritis, heart murmurs) simulating disease symptoms or staff members trained to simulate such symptoms. These tests evaluate how well students deal with real patients' problems, not just how well they score on tests, in class, or on the licensing examinations. Ideally, the OSCE tests whether a student can

- perform a focused history and physical examination.
- recognize pathological processes.
- interpret laboratory data.
- establish a relevant differential diagnosis.
- develop a management plan.
- clearly document clinical findings and plans.

OSCE examinations normally take about 6 hours (including breaks): each station requires from 5 to 40 minutes to complete. Some stations may be coupled, so that the second station relies on clinical information from the first station. Time and the number of stations are the two variations that do not seem to affect the test's validity. Students are scored at each station using a standardized checklist of tasks.

More than 58 U.S. and all Canadian medical schools now use the OSCE for clinical evaluations. Many require their students to pass it before graduation. The results will also appear in Deans' letters, most probably showing the student's results in comparison to his or her classmates. Since all specialties value clinical abilities in their residents, these test results may carry enormous weight with residency directors.

OSCE-type "simulated patient" encounters became part of USMLE Step 2 in June 2004. They also are part of the Medical Council of Canada's licensing exam.

9

Putting Off A Decision

Even if you are on the right track,
you will get run over if you just sit there.
Will Rogers, American Humorist (1879-1935)

NOT MAKING A DECISION about a specialty choice is, as the saying goes, equivalent to deciding not to enter a specialty—at least for the present. Fifty years ago, medical students routinely put off choosing a specialty until they were well into their internship year. This is the tradition of Ben Casey and Marcus Welby (maybe you saw them in reruns on TV) and of *Arrowsmith* (perhaps you read it in high school). This tradition stemmed from a time, now happily past, when many, if not most, physicians went into practice with little more than an internship as their postgraduate training.

Today, it is dangerous—if not insane—to go into practice so unprepared. Advanced training is now necessary to understand medicine's increasing complexity. Without advanced training, today's medical school graduates will often neither qualify for malpractice insurance nor be granted hospital privileges. They also may not be able to get a medical license.

Sadly, we still routinely allow physicians with only an internship to practice in both our Public Health Service (treating Native Americans and poor people) and the military. If you plan to follow these career paths, you can do so with only PGY-1 training, although you will probably not progress very far.

Admittedly, making a specialty choice is difficult. It is yet another step in the maturation process, and it will make you more uncomfortable than you have felt for a number of years—ever since you received your acceptance into medical school.

Now, instead of seeing yourself as "a doctor," you must generate another image of yourself. Looking in the mirror, you now must see a Pediatrician, a Pathologist, a Family Physician, a Surgeon, or another specialist. This much narrower focus may be an uncomfortable fit if you have envisioned yourself as the omniscient healer. But it is a fit to which you are going to have to adjust. The only question is, when should you make the decision?

More medical students make their initial specialty decision during their third year of medical school (46%) than at any other time. Another 24% select a specialty during their fourth year, while 23% make a decision before beginning their clinical years of medical school.

The Fine Art of Procrastination

Despite the common wisdom, making a life-changing decision is not easy and may not completely succumb to rational analysis. A decision about which specialty to enter is just such a decision. Writing a list of pros and cons will just not hack it. Such a decision must take into account many intangible factors, such as your past experiences, willingness to take risks, and unspoken dreams.

Everyone has procrastinated about making a major decision. The question to ask is why are you procrastinating? Usually it is because you fear making a "wrong" decision, especially if that decision seems irrevocable. Any major decision involves risk—personal, financial, or both. Some decisions don't work out the way you planned. That's okay. Obviously, choosing a specialty to enter is a gigantic step. It is not, however, permanent: approximately 20% of physicians change their career direction at least once.

Several techniques may help you make a decision, especially if you have already gathered the basic information about the specialties you are considering, including spending time with both academic and community physicians practicing those specialties.

Discuss your options with close friends and family. Allow yourself to express your emotions, not just "the facts." Your career choice is emotional, so "let it all hang out."

Weigh what is most important in your own life: personal satisfaction, family, money, prestige, or time off. Actually give each one a weight (like in the "Must-Want" Analysis in Chapter 11) and see how each specialty you are considering will fulfill them.

When you are alone, *imagine yourself in each of the specialties* you are considering. Are you enjoying yourself or stressing out? Do you feel satisfied or frustrated? Maybe most important, do you want to go to work tomorrow?

The key is to not hem and haw while you are in the middle of the road about which way to go. It will only make you middle-of-the-road kill—not a pretty picture.

Taking Time Off

There are several reasons to take time off during or immediately after medical school. Residency directors are used to seeing this type of hiatus in medical training, so this should not hurt an applicant's chances of getting into a program.

If you have a choice, when should you take time off? One student suggested that if she took time off between her first and second years, she could go straight into third year without losing any clinical skills or knowledge. Some students take time off between their second and third years, others between the third and fourth years. Few take time off immediately after graduation.

Taking leave for medical, personal, and family reasons, especially to have a baby, is now fairly common. If you do that, be sure your reason for taking time off is clearly stated in your personal statement. With the increasing debt many medical students carry, some schools allow students to take a year off to work. In the long run, this is probably not a wise financial decision, but it should not penalize residency applicants. If you include something in your personal statement, however, it is fair game to ask about during the interview. For example, if you mention your chronic illness, they may ask if it is under control or how often you have exacerbations requiring time off.

If the time off was to acquire another degree, do extended research, or have an unusual medical experience (such as doing volunteer work in a disaster area), describing what you learned and why you did it should probably be the focus of your personal statement. This may also be the focus of most of your interviews. In many cases, this type of extra experience and knowledge may make you an even *more desirable* candidate.

Others who take time off may have less-clear motivations. Often, the individuals were not sure whether they really wanted to pursue a medical career, or they had so much academic difficulty that they were asked to temporarily drop out. These types of breaks during training may seriously hurt applicants' chances of getting a desirable residency position, especially if they cannot demonstrate that they have used the time to make certain that medicine is the career they want or to correct their academic deficiencies.

Win-Win Decisions

Fear of making decisions often keeps people from moving ahead with their lives and their careers. The motto for most medical students—those who have traveled the normal route to medical school—is often "Be careful! You might make the wrong decision." They believe that, at any juncture, an incorrect career choice could deprive them of those things that the "correct" decision is supposed to bring: money, love, respect, and security. They may also, by making the "wrong" decision, find that they are neither perfect nor in complete control of their lives. But, like the donkey that couldn't choose between two bales of hay, it is possible for them to waiver in their decision just long enough to starve to death.

To feel better about making a career decision, you must readjust your view of the possible outcomes. First, realize that this is not a life or death decision. The decision need not be permanent. It can be reassessed at a later time when you have more information. Second, instead of thinking of your career decision in terms of the "right" path (you win) versus the "wrong" path (you lose), consider that any of the paths you have reasonably investigated can offer you exciting, although not necessarily equivalent, opportunities.

By thinking of your career decision as a Win-Lose situation (Figure 9.1), you will doom yourself to forever thinking "What if I had taken the other route?" every time something in your career, or your life, is not perfect. This results in a life of misery and depression. By following a Win-Win model (Figure 9.2), you allow yourself to feel good and gain the rewards you desire from whichever path you take.

Figure 9.1
Win-Lose Decision-Making Model

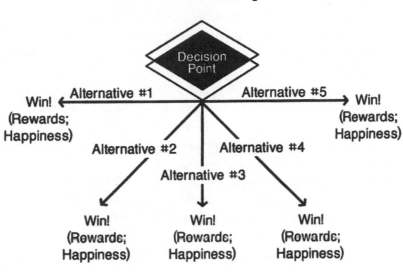

Figure 9.2
Win-Win Decision-Making Model

Advantages & Disadvantages of a Transitional Year

Taking a transitional internship without having obtained a commitment for PGY-2-level training has both advantages and disadvantages.

The Transitional internship is similar to the "Rotating" internships of old. It exposes physicians to Internal or Family Medicine, Surgery, Emergency Medicine, Obstetrics and Gynecology, Pediatrics, and, perhaps, Psychiatry. Very similar in many ways to a repeat of your third year of medical school, albeit with upgraded responsibility, it provides another general overview of medical practice. The additional knowledge and abilities you acquire may be useful throughout your career. This is especially true if you are thinking of using this as your first year of training prior to beginning a program that starts in the second year, such as Anesthesiology, Radiology, or Ophthalmology. But if you are merely postponing a decision about which specialty to enter, and assume you will use the Transitional year to decide, you may be in for a rude awakening.

First, look at the time schedule for the NRMP application process (Figure 23.5). You will see that going into a Transitional year allows you to put off making a decision, at best, only until the end of your senior year of medical school. Matching in the advanced Matches (PGY-2 and above) and with programs not participating in the Match usually occurs even earlier. If you plan to start specialty training the year after your internship, you will have to have made a decision before the end of your senior year. So, what price do you pay for procrastinating?

Internship is tough on both body and soul. You will work long hours and get little sleep. That is the nature of the beast, even with ACGME-regulated duty hours. So, now you have moved the very grueling process of applying for a training position to what will probably be the most difficult time in your entire life—the first half of your internship. Not a pretty prospect. It is so difficult to deal with the added stress that many interns give up and take the easiest route to a decision. That is, they agree to take virtually any open position, even if it is not in the specialty they want. They promise themselves that they will look for a better position later. They rarely do.

Another problem relates directly to the Transitional year. Many specialties, including most Surgical areas, Internal Medicine, Pediatrics, and Family Medicine, will not accept a Transitional year as counting toward completion of a residency (Figure 23.1). Therefore, you may have to either avoid going into these specialties or repeat your internship—a dismal thought and nearly always an unhappy experience. No matter how much you think you won't mind repeating the intern year—you will hate it. I have seen many individuals, all of whom truly believed they would not mind going through internship again, be absolutely miserable when having to repeat the experience. Most people emerge from their internship with a wealth of new clinical knowledge and the ability to make clinical decisions and work in a clinical setting. Repeating this experience will not substantially increase these abilities. Instead, it often causes frustration, since your supervising residents may not be as knowledgeable as you.

An alternative, if you can at least decide between Surgery and Medicine, is to take a "Preliminary" Surgery or Medicine internship. These are not broadly based, as are the Transitional programs. They are essentially the same training that the Categorical Medicine or Surgery interns go through. (For more explanation of the types of internships, see Chapter 23.) The benefit is that you will have more options following such training. Surgery and its associated areas will accept a Preliminary Surgery internship; Medicine will accept a Preliminary Medicine internship. Some Preliminary spots may be relatively easy to obtain: only 60% of Preliminary Surgery spots filled in the 2012 Match, although 93% of Preliminary Internal Medicine positions filled. Specialties that accept Transitional programs will also accept either of these. So perhaps part of a decision is better than none.

You may still decide to do a Transitional year, as did nearly 5% of 2012 M.D. graduates, either because you cannot make up your mind about a specialty or because your specialty requires a preliminary clinical year before beginning specialty training, such as in Anesthesiology, Radiology, and Ophthalmology. About 80% of residents in a Transitional year plan to follow that year with a residency. Another 12% intend to follow the year with required federal service, and a small number plan to go into research. With more confidence than common sense, 1% plan to go into practice after just this one year of training!

Quick Decisions & Forty Years of Sadness

More than half of all medical school graduates believe that deciding on a specialty before beginning their third year gives them an advantage in obtaining their choice of residency program. While this may have some validity, there are dangers in making a specialty decision too quickly. Many physicians whom I have met or have counseled over the years are disappointed, if not frankly frustrated and bored, by their specialty. This is not as surprising as it may seem. When asked how they had made a specialty decision in the first place, many said that they were influenced by an exciting third-year rotation, a dynamic teacher in medical school, a childhood physician, or a physician-parent.

During training, some got a hint that the specialty was not for them. They may have lacked a feeling of excitement when they were about to go to the operating room. Or they became depressed taking care of patients with chronic illnesses on the wards. But they did not listen to their feelings and continued their training. By the time they finished their residencies, they felt that they had committed too much time to the specialty to change.

Others liked their training immensely. The diagnostic challenges and therapeutic dilemmas seen in the tertiary-care teaching facility stimulated them. But once they got into practice, they found that they rarely used most of their skills. Rather, they dealt with a parade of patients with the same mundane problems. And this was not what they had anticipated.

Physicians also change specialties because of the process of self-discovery that accompanies most educational endeavors. It is not uncommon for medical students (maybe not you, but certainly most of your friends) to be service-oriented, obsessive-compulsive individuals. They receive much of their stimulus to achieve from a self-sacrificing posture designed to win approval from superiors, relatives, and acquaintances. Yet, while training in clinical medicine, some individuals find that their route to personal satisfaction is not through their chosen specialty; some find that the route does not include medical practice at all.

In the past, I have gotten calls not only from physicians in practice, but also from their spouses. Our discussions were always variations on the same theme. The physicians had been in practice from eight to ten years and were very unhappy, even though they were often in what most people consider to be very desirable specialties. The physicians repeatedly stated that life would be much better if only they could change their specialty. The caller now wanted advice about how to make that change. What could not be ascertained, however, was whether the initial specialty choice, or something much more profound, was the problem.

I am saddened when I see a 45-year-old physician who is unhappy that he or she ever entered the field of medicine. It is less sad, but still somewhat unnerving, to see the same physician reenter a training program to change specialties at such an advanced stage in his or her career. So there definitely can be reasons to wait to make a specialty decision. Investigating your options early will help to prevent you from making a foolish or uninformed choice. But just procrastinating in making that decision will not make the final selection either easier or better.

Some residency programs may now hesitate to take physicians who have completed too much prior residency training. The federal government, through the Medicare program, reimburses hospitals for much of the cost of resident education. The most support is given during the time necessary to meet the requirements for initial Board certification—with a maximum of five years. They calculate this time period beginning with the first year of Categorical residency (not counting a Transitional or Osteopathic internship year). Although the amount of money is relatively small, the impact makes some programs wary of accepting residents who have already done training in another specialty or who are in a Transitional year but want to go into another PGY-1 position. This also applies to those who entered one field, even decades ago, and now want to retrain in another specialty.

In reality, the Medicare payments hospitals receive for these residents are not decreased as much as one might believe. They continue to get substantial "indirect" reimbursement; only the "direct" payment is partially decreased. While programs and hospitals may consider this factor, generally it does not prevent residents from changing their residency program. *This relatively minor reduction in hospital reimbursement should never cause residents to work without pay, as some have suggested.*

Switching Careers

Medicine, more than any other profession, tenaciously hangs onto its practitioners. Physicians are expected to remain committed to the field until death or voluntary retirement, either through a sense of altruism, because of the benefits they gain, or simply because they believe that their focused education precludes other forms of employment. Each year, however, about 3% of U.S. medical school graduates leave medicine to pursue other careers.

Numerous physicians have successfully either combined other careers with medicine or switched completely. Most of these individuals' names are well known to you, although you may not know that they were physicians. These include:

- *Philosophers:* John Locke and Oliver Wendell Holmes, Sr.

- *Astronomers:* Nicholas Copernicus (physician to the Heilsberg Bishopric)

- *Scientists:* Luigi Galvani (Italian physiologist), Carol Linnaeus (Swedish taxonomist), and Thomas Huxley (English biologist)

- *Politicians:* Jean Marat (French Revolution), Georges Clemenceau (World War I French Premier), Sun Yat Sen (first president of the Chinese Republic), and Che Guevara (modern communist revolutionary)

- *Writers:* Arthur Conan Doyle, Tobias Smollett, A.J. Cronin, Thomas Campion, Anton Chekhov, Johann Schiller, John Keats, William Somerset Maugham, and Michael Crichton

- *Others:* Galileo, Charles Darwin, and Gertrude Stein went on to fame after dropping out during medical school. (In Ms. Stein's case, it was during her 4th-year OB/Gyn clerkship at Johns Hopkins.)

So there is life outside medicine. One of the most common alternative careers that physicians now consider is the law. The AMA estimates that there are as many as 6,000 physician-lawyers in the United States. Each year, many physicians enter law school for uncertain reasons, but drop out because they find it tedious or boring. If you consider changing from a medical career, don't just run away—go toward a positive goal.

Dangers of Indecision

Some students think that because they have been unable to make a specialty decision, they will let the luck of the Match—not at all like the luck of the Irish—decide for them. They interview in two or more specialties. And, although they may give preference in their rank-order list to one field or another, it is clear that they are not committed to a particular specialty. (This is not to say that you should not list some appropriate internships at the bottom of your rank-order list—that is just being careful. See Chapter 23.)

In such cases of indecision, the question must be raised, "Is the indecision based upon a lack of knowledge about the specialties, or about one's self?" Unfortunately, it is common for students to apply to multiple types of specialties. If you are contemplating such a move, it is time to get some serious counseling. And one of the items that needs to be discussed is *whether you really want a career in medicine*. Of course you have already spent a lot of time in school, but consider that residency will be another three to seven years. Nevertheless, if you still think you really do want to work as a physician and you intend, for some reason, to apply to multiple specialties, consider the two biggest problems involved.

The first, and most obvious, problem with applying to multiple specialties is the time and cost involved. If you plan to research the specialties, and perhaps take senior electives in them, you will use up your available time very quickly. Expenses also mount up rapidly if you are applying to multiple specialties.

The second problem is that you will have broken a basic tenet of the residency application process. You will have shown that you are not committed to a specialty. And if the reason you are applying to multiple specialties in this fashion is to stay within a defined geographic area, be assured that most of the programs will know or soon discover this. If the programs are anything more than "bottom-rung" and you are anything less than a "star," they probably will not consider you seriously. Consequently, you may very well end up in a poor, nondescript program, which probably will, either then or later, make you very unhappy. It is better to make an informed choice about a single specialty and then go after the position with maximum effort.

10

Gathering Information

Just to look costs nothing.

Folk saying

NOW THAT YOUR SPECIALTY DECISION IS MADE, it is time to collect information on individual training programs. You need to discover the differences among programs, where they are located, how difficult it is to get a position at each, and what variables and options exist for completing your training.

You probably have limited time and money to invest in searching for the best programs. Therefore, it is essential that you do some priority shopping—spending your resources in a manner that gives you the highest probability of finding what you want. To do this, you must get enough information about each program that you seriously consider to allow you to complete your own "Must/Want" Analysis (Figure 11.1). If you know where to look, much of this information is readily available.

First, get organized! You need to be able to easily sift through the mountain of information about programs that you will accumulate. One method that many students find useful is to set up a paper or computer file for each program they consider. If you do this, then you can put the material in the file as you collect it. Put a copy of your "Must/Want" Analysis in each computer folder or paste it on the *inside* cover of each paper file folder. When you go to an interview or "audition" elective, take this file with you so you can fill in your "Must/Want" Analysis immediately. (Also include a copy of Figure 18.2, "Interview Notes".) If you use paper file folders, you may find it useful to purchase a sturdy cardboard file box (sometimes called a "bankers box") to hold them. Of course, many applicants will simply put the information in a file in their computer or PDA. One warning: be sure to back up these files frequently!

Now that you have a method for organizing program information, let's consider some information sources in detail. (For more sources and how to get them, see the *Annotated Bibliography*. Also see *Contact Information* for addresses.)

Graduate Medical Education Directory ("Green Book")

The American Medical Association (AMA) issues this substantial book annually. Usually referred to as the "Green Book," it lists all "approved" M.D.-run training programs, i.e., those accredited by the Accreditation Council for Graduate Medical Education (ACGME). Most of the information in this book has been supplanted by the AMA's *FREIDA* system (see below). However, there are a few areas that are particularly useful to residency applicants, including Section I, which lists key resources for students and residents, and Appendix B, which lists the requirements for Board certification in each medical specialty. This information is also available on the AMA's annual *Graduate Medical Education Library* CD-ROM. Both the "Green Book" and the CD-ROM should be in the Reference section of your medical school's library.

Section I: Graduate Medical Education Information

Extensively revised in 2010, the four subsections contain a wealth of resources for students and residents about graduate medical education (GME).

- Residency Application and Career Planning Resources provides information about *FREIDA* Online, the *GME Library* (CD-ROM), ERAS, and other useful resources.

- Information on Matching Programs gives information on the NRMP and other Matches.

- GME Information for IMGs contains extensive information on how to obtain residency positions in the United States, visa options, and ECFMG certification.

- AMA Medical Education Products, Services and Activities contains information about many of the AMA's resources, including the *GME e-Letter*, available free via e-mail (www.ama-assn.org/go/gmenews), and the *Medical Education Bulletin*.

Section II: Specialty/Subspecialty Information and Programs

This section constitutes the bulk of the book. It contains a list and description of all specialties and subspecialties accredited by the ACGME, as well as each accredited residency program (listed by the sponsoring institution's state and city). Each specialty's, and some subspecialties', listing includes the number of programs and residents, work schedules, benefits, and employment policies, most of which is also listed in *FREIDA*. Each program's listing includes the director's name, basic contact information, the length, and the number of approved residency positions. **Note**: Check *FREIDA Online* for the most accurate and up-to-date information, especially for a program's length.

Section III: New and Withdrawn Programs

Here you will find a list, by specialty, of new programs, as well as of withdrawn programs. This section may be useful, especially if you cannot find the program you are looking for; it may no longer exist.

Section IV: Graduate Medical Education Teaching Institutions

A list, by state and city, of the "sponsoring" hospitals/organizations for GME programs. This information is also in *FREIDA* under "Medical School Affiliations Search," with additional facts about each program.

Appendices

Several of the appendices are useful. The most important for all applicants is *Appendix B*, which contains the requirements for Certification by each of the 24 recognized American Specialty (M.D.) Boards, including examination fees, deadlines, and policies about taking a leave of absence during training. Figure 10.1 lists specific information you should obtain about your chosen specialty's Board requirements. Now would be a good time to look at these requirements, especially if you are not going directly from medical school into residency training, or if you are anticipating something out of the ordinary while you are in training. It is better to learn the rules now than to suffer later.

Appendix A lists details about the combined-specialty training programs; use *FREIDA* to search for individual programs. *Appendix E* lists some non-ACGME-approved subspecialty and fellowship programs. Check out *Appendix F* for extensive information, by state, about medical licensure for M.D.'s, D.O.'s, and IMGs. There is also a glossary of frequently used terms.

AMA *Graduate Medical Education Library* (CD-ROM)

This resource is expensive, so use the copy in your medical library or in the Dean's office. The CD-ROM has an easy-to-use Web browser interface with a standard HTML version to accommodate all users, as well as an advanced XML version (for Microsoft® Windows® users only) with sophisticated search options and other useful features. In addition, the CD-ROM contains archived copies of all editions of the *Graduate Medical Education Directory* since 1996.

The CD-ROM features several broad categories. Under "Specialties," users select a specialty from the drop-down menu and then choose: (a) General Information, which contains information similar to that in the "Green Book", and has links to the professional organizations; (b) Program Requirements, which details the requirements to sit for the specialty's Board exam; or (c) Certification Requirements, which lists the fees, dates, and requirements for certification, and has a link to that specialty's certification board.

Figure 10.1
Questions to Ask About Requirements for Specialty Certification

1. Is this residency program accredited? If not, will I still be qualified to take the Boards if I take my training here?
2. Can I take the specialty Boards if I do my residency outside the United States?
3. Will I be penalized (i.e., additional required time in training) if I switch programs within this specialty, or if I switch into this specialty from another specialty?
4. What are the Board's rules about taking sick leave, family leave, and other breaks during my training? Is there a maximum time period allowed for absences or for completing training?
5. When can I take the Board exam? Are there requirements in addition to residency training (e.g., time in practice, advanced degree) that I will need? When should I apply for the exam(s)?
6. Are there different ways to become certified in this specialty?
7. Do I need an unrestricted U.S. medical license to take the Boards?
8. How many times can I take the exam? What are the pass-fail rates?
9. What are the rules regarding recertification?

Under "Programs," users can select a specialty from the drop-down menu to find links to individual programs organized by state and city. Each program listing has many details, including work schedules, curriculum, employment policies/benefits, resident evaluation, and links to the medical school and to the program director's e-mail. At the bottom of each listing, there is a link to *FREIDA Online*, where you can find additional and updated information. "Institutions" allows users to search by state to find teaching institutions, arranged alphabetically by city.

The "Certification" category gives basic information about Board certification, as well as links to certification requirements for each approved specialty and subspecialty. These requirements detail each specialty's training philosophy, programs' expected general characteristics, the required scope of training (including special exceptions, acceptable prerequisite training, and alternative routes to accomplish training, if they exist), programs' expected content, the nature of the teaching staff and facilities, and any other requirements unique to the specialty.

The CD-ROM also contains information about *FREIDA*, ERAS, the National Resident Matching Program (NRMP), and other matching programs, including the Military Match. Finally, "Licensure" provides basic information on licensure, with links to state licensing boards. In addition, there are links to many states' lists of approved and disapproved international medical schools.

Fellowship and Residency Electronic Interactive Database Access (FREIDA)

The AMA's *Fellowship and Residency Electronic Interactive Database Online®* (commonly called *FREIDA*) will be your major source of information about training programs. This system provides so much information that the unprepared can be overwhelmed. *FREIDA* now lists about 8,800 ACGME-approved residency and fellowship programs and almost 200 combined-specialty residency programs. It also offers specialty-specific workforce information and an overview of each specialty's residency programs.

Before using this database, the prudent move would be to review the sections of this book on the "Must/Want" Analysis to determine which residency program characteristics are important to you.

FREIDA can be accessed online through the American Medical Association's website. There is NO CHARGE to access *FREIDA*, simply go to either www.ama-assn.org/go/freida to get to the main page or www.ama-assn.org/vapp/freida/srch/ to begin a search.

To search in the specialties, click "Residency Fellowship Training Program Search" on the *FREIDA* homepage for a list of all ACGME-approved specialties, combined specialties (such as Internal Medicine–Pediatrics), and subspecialties. Select the specialties that interest you and press "Continue" at the bottom of the page, or "Clear" to start over. At that point, *you can get a brief overview of up to 250 programs in the specialty by selecting "Search Plus."* This is a side-by-side comparison of the programs using basic information such as first-year salary, duty hours, and number of positions. This function can be used again to compare programs selected with the criteria listed below. (If the specialty you choose has more than 250 programs, you must narrow your search, as described below, before the information can be displayed.)

You now have the option of narrowing your selection criteria. By clicking "Choose Location," you can limit your search to specific states or regions. Use "Optional Criteria" to search for programs meeting any or all of the criteria chosen from the various information items below. For example, you can search for programs that participate in the NRMP, require prior residency training, offer preliminary or shared-schedule/part-time positions, and offer starting dates other than in June or July.

Each program with a complete *FREIDA* listing has more than 100 information items available in the database. *FREIDA* divides the data into several categories.

1. **Basic Information**: This information includes the program name, FREIDA identifier (useful for returning to this entry), e-mail, snail-mail address, and telephone/fax numbers for the program director and the contact person (if different); their website's URL (if any); program length; whether they are accepting applications for the current and following years; program start date(s); whether they participate in ERAS; whether they are affiliated with the U.S. government; and which institutions are sponsors and participants. You can link to information about each listed institution from this location.

2. **General Information**: Extra information is in a "Comments" section. Examples are the number of positions in each post-graduate year (PGY); primary teaching site and type of hospital (such as university, military, or community); whether prior residency training is required; availability of "preliminary" positions; if applicants must pass USMLE Step 2CS before beginning residency; participation in, and the code number for, the NRMP or other Matching programs; the number of interviews granted in the past year; the number of required reference letters; the deadline for applications; and the interview period.

3. **Program Faculty**: The number of physician and non-physician full- and part-time faculty; percentage of full-time female physician faculty; and the ratio of residents to full-time-equivalent paid faculty.

4. **Work Schedule**: Average hours on duty per week, excluding beeper call; maximum consecutive hours on duty during first year, excluding beeper call; number of 24-hour off-duty periods per week during the first year; whether moonlighting is allowed within the institution; whether there is a "night float" system; whether the program offers help with resident fatigue; and the "most taxing" schedule and the beeper or home-call schedules for each year of the program.

5. **Educational Environment:** Frequency of educational conferences; hospital/non-hospital ambulatory experience; formal mentoring program; educational benefits/features (such as debt management/ financial counseling, international experiences, resident/fellow retreats, off-campus electives, hospice/home-care experiences, cultural-competence curricula, instruction in medical Spanish or other languages, alternative medicine curricula, MPH/MBA/Ph.D. training, research rotations); and evaluation methods (annual in-service exams required, patient surveys); and methods for evaluating program quality (completion rate for program, in-training exam scores, board-certification rates).

6. **Employment Policies/Benefits:** Availability of part-time/shared-schedule positions; on-site or subsidized childcare; stipends for professional expenses, housing, or moving; educational leave and reimbursement; on-call meal allowance; PDAs; job placement assistance; salary and vacation/medical or maternity/paternity/family leave policies for each year in the program; whether written policies exist on substance abuse, mental health impairment, and physical disability; and who pays for residents' and their dependents' medical, dental, mental health, and disability insurance.

7. **Institutional Information** (for each clinical site in the program): Size of hospital and the medical staff; number of annual admissions and emergency/non-emergency department outpatient visits; type of specialized inpatient units; and other GME programs sponsored by or affiliated with that institution.

If you like what you see in a program's description, add it to your personal folder by clicking the icon labeled "Add to Folder." However, to create a permanent folder so you can use the information later, you must be an AMA member; join at www.ama-assn.org/ama/pub/membership.shtml. The saved programs (up to 100 in a 12-month period) can then be downloaded to a spreadsheet program. Members can also print address labels from their folder. **Note:** *FREIDA* will send updates with changes to the program information you've downloaded if you supply them with your email address.

FREIDA contains an enormous amount of information, but the necessity of molding the database to all specialties has resulted in a poor fit for some. For example, applicants often want to know the number of procedures performed for some specialties (especially Surgery, Radiology, Anesthesiology, and Pathology), but this information is not available. Even so, the *FREIDA* system represents a vast improvement over the "Green Book."

Three caveats: First, residency directors supply their own program information and no one verifies its accuracy. When using *FREIDA,* be careful how you interpret the information, and double-check it if it seems questionable. Verify all information before and during your interview. Programs may not have updated their information recently: The date listed under "Basic Information" is the last time the information was updated. Second, *FREIDA* may not list very new programs and programs (e.g., Trauma Surgery, Alternative-Integrative Medicine) which are not ACGME-approved or for which program requirements are not yet approved. Contact these programs directly for their information.

Finally, the AMA asks every GME program to provide data for its listing. So, while all ACGME-approved programs are listed, the listings may be incomplete for some fellowships and residencies with few positions, showing only their name, contact information, and the number of positions offered. This suggests that you should double-check the "Green Book" to be certain that you locate all the programs which may interest you.

Program Codes. Each program's NRMP Code (listed in *FREIDA*, on the NRMP website, and in the "Green Book") specifies *the specialty and the institution*, as well as whether the program is Categorical, Preliminary, or Advanced. *FREIDA* allows searches using these categories. For example, the program code *110-03-12-056* means that the program is in specialty #110 (Emergency Medicine) and is at institution #03-056 (University Medical Center, Tucson, AZ).

Other Information. *FREIDA's* main page offers additional information. On the left side of the page, you can access "Graduate Career Plan Statistics" or "Training Statistics," which provide more information about each specialty.

Mailing Labels. *FREIDA* allows AMA members to print mailing labels at no charge. Labels are generated for all programs saved to your folder. (It is a good deal to join the AMA for this service, plus you receive the *Journal of the American Medical Association* (*JAMA*) and other benefits.) Another option is to print the program information and then cut out the address.

FREIDA is remarkably easy to use, even for the computer illiterate. Just turn on the machine or connect to the website and follow the instructions. Have fun with it.

AOA Website

The American Osteopathic Association maintains a list of AOA-approved intern and residency programs and parallels the AMA's *FRIEDA* system. Go to www. osteopathic.org/inside_aoa/education/ and click on "Interns and Residents." The database, called "Opportunities," can be found under "Additional Resources."

ACGME Website

The ACGME (Accreditation Council for Graduate Medical Education) controls M.D. residency and fellowship programs. Their website, at www.acgme.org, contains several items of interest to residency applicants.

The most important are the information concerning residents' duty hours (they make the rules; select "Duty Hours" from the menu), and the listings under "Special Requirements" for each specialty and subspecialty. Each program in the specialty must adhere to these requirements if they want to remain accredited. Knowing these requirements and finding out how closely they adhere to them can help you decide on a program's quality (select "Review Committees" from the menu).

One caveat: Remember that these Program Requirements are what the specialty's leaders would like their ideal residency program to encompass. Few, if any, training programs ever meet all these requirements. To be accredited, they are expected to have met most of them and, where possible, to work on meeting the others. The pertinent questions for you to ask will be: (1) Does the program meet enough requirements so that it will most likely remain accredited throughout my period of training? and (2) Are the factors that I consider important present at that program?

National Residency Matching Program (NRMP) Online Directory

The *NRMP Directory* is no longer supplied in printed form. Instead, a list with up-to-date, but basic, information for registered residency programs is posted at the National Resident Matching Program's website (www.nrmp.org/). Only the programs registered for the current year are listed. Although programs can post their information in the Directory earlier in the year, many can't get their act together to submit their information before November or December. Both M.D. medical students and Independent Applicants (IMGs, Osteopathic students, and non-medical-school-sponsored physicians) use the same website, which can be accessed only after you register for the NRMP Match.

You can searach the *Directory* for "All Programs" in one or more specialties, up to a limit of 250 programs. You can also search for "Advanced Programs (A)," "Categorical (C)," "Preliminary (P)," "Physician Only," or "Primary Care" (labeled "M"). Primary care programs can be searched only for Pediatric and Internal Medicine programs. Once you are in the *NRMP Online Directory*, click on "Details" for additional information about a program.

More detailed information about residency programs, including whether they plan to participate in the NRMP Match and their NRMP Program Code, can be found in *FREIDA*.

NRMP Data and Reports—Listing of Filled & Unfilled Programs

This information, released on the NRMP website two days before Match Day each year, shows, by specialty, the positions offered *through the current NRMP Match* and what percentage filled, as well as similar data from previous years. The website also shows the percentage of couples that matched. This is vital information for you to read, especially if you think that you might have difficulty getting a position, as it shows you which programs might be a bit easier to enter in the coming year. In July, the NRMP publishes this information as *NRMP Results and Data: [Year] Main Residency Match Book* in "hard copy" and online.

Individual Programs

Once you have used the information from the sources described above to narrow your program choices at least a little, send an e-mail directly to the programs for additional information. You can obtain the address from *FREIDA*. Be certain that you put "Residency Information Request" on the subject line. In the body of the e-mail, ask for information on residency programs beginning in a specific year. If you want to know about student elective rotations, include that request as a separate line or in a separate e-mail so that it has less chance of being overlooked. Also, include your full name, a good mailing address, and a phone number in case they need to contact you. Be sure to proofread your e-mail, including the address and subject lines, before pressing that pesky "send" button.

One caveat about e-mail: If you have a "cute" name as part of your e-mail address, for example "sexyguy@xyzmail.com" or "most-wanted-gal@xyzmail.com," change it to your name, your initials, or the anonymous moniker that large systems automatically provide to clients. You're a professional and your e-mail address should reflect that. Also, change those too-cute messages that callers hear on your cell phone, answering machine, or similar device. "Thanks for calling. I'll get back to you as soon as possible" is the type of bland message that you should use.

If you cannot use e-mail, send a letter, postcard, or fax. While the rumors about programs keeping this first request letter on file are not true—they start a file when they actually receive application materials—it doesn't hurt to make these requests legible. Also, include a *legible return address*. Each year our program receives about ten requests without legible, or even any, return addresses. It also helps to print or type your name. Many information requests have only signatures. And true to form, fewer than half of these can be deciphered.

If you write or call early—that is, before the interviewing process is over for the prior year—be prepared to get material applicable to trainees a year ahead of you. Usually this will not be much different from the material that is finally ready for your year, but be sure to compare the information you received with more current information for those programs with which you interview. In some cases, there may be substantial changes from year to year. Also, if you request your information during the early part of the year (February to April), be prepared for some delay while new material is being prepared. It is best to get preliminary information that may change a bit, and then update the materials for the "short list" of programs to which you intend to apply.

Information from residency programs varies widely. It ranges from websites with all the bells and whistles or glossy brochures with lots of pictures but very little solid information to detailed descriptions of the program, institutions, faculty, resident responsibilities, and benefits. You will probably not be able to tell the good programs from the marginal ones based only on the material you view on the Web or receive in the mail. Essentially, that is because there are no set guidelines for this material. Also, some residency programs are good at marketing; others are not. Nevertheless, the information that you receive directly from the programs may assist you in working out your own "Must/Want" Analysis (Figure 11.1) and in winnowing the programs down to a reasonable number for further consideration.

The *FREIDA* system supplies information in a more consistent format than that from the individual programs and institutions. Yet the programs' materials may supply you with more recent, as well as additional, information, so requesting it is worthwhile.

Other Internet Sites

Nearly every specialty has a website with extensive information, and many individual residencies also have websites. Check the specialty listings in Chapter 3 and at the end of this book for some of these Web addresses.

One good website for those who are undecided about their specialty choice is the *Careers in Medicine* site, described in Chapter 4. When considering an away rotation, visit www.scutwork.com. This student-run website has detailed reviews of individual programs from those who have done rotations there and provides some enlightening information. The American Medical Student Association (AMSA) website also has a similar section, under "Career Development Program," where medical students can both fill out their own assessments and read other students' comments about residency programs. To find the programs, search either by state or for individual programs. Unfortunately, only a limited number of program reviews are featured.

Many specialties have online discussion groups that you may be able to join. These may provide you with valuable information. You can find them through the specialties' national organizations. To participate, you may be required join their medical student/resident organization (usually very inexpensive). If you are seriously considering the specialty, it is worth the minimal cost to join their Society.

Specialty Society Directories

Many specialties maintain online directories of residency programs. Nine of these are:

- Emergency Medicine,
  http://saem.org/saemdnm/ResidencyCatalog/tabid/680/Default/aspx

- Family Medicine, www.aafp.org/residencies and
  www.acofp.org/ResidencyDirectory/

- Internal Medicine, www.acponline.org/residency and www.sgim.org

- Obstetrics & Gynecology, www.apgo.org/residencies

- Pathology, www.pathologytraining.org

- Physical Medicine & Rehabilitation,
  www.physiatry.org/education/index.html

- Preventive Medicine, www.acpm.org/education/residency/ataglance.htm

- Psychiatry, http://archive.psych.org/career_corner/careers_psych/
  clearinghouse/CHsearch.cfm

- Urology, www.urologymatch.com/urology_program_directory_links

Each directory contains significantly more information than can be obtained by writing to the residency programs. And, though their information is updated only sporadically, they provide an excellent picture both of the scope of residencies in the specialty and of the individual programs. Each directory is described in the *Annotated Bibliography*.

Specialty Faculty

Your mentor or specialty adviser is another source of information about programs. This individual may have enough knowledge about the programs in the specialty to assist you in your search. Usually, he or she will be familiar with programs in one or more specific geographic areas. If the individual has been in the field for some time, he may have visited other training programs in the course of professional activities. This will provide a wider knowledge base from which to counsel you. But an adviser's input must still be considered in light of both your personal needs and the other information you collect.

Remember, no matter what your specialty adviser or mentor thinks is the best program, *you* are the one who will be going through the training. However, do not discount his inside information about, and personal contacts at, specific programs. You will not find this in any book. And your adviser's influence may get you an interview at your most desired program.

Journals

If you are looking for programs with a strong academic or research bent, scan the major specialty journals to see which programs are most heavily represented. In addition, you can discern which programs are most heavily represented at national scientific meetings, either from journals or from mailings your specialty adviser receives. Obviously, this is only supplemental knowledge. But it may be useful when selecting programs; and that knowledge can also give you an inside track during interviews.

If you seek a program that will be relatively easy to match with, look at the advertisements in *The New Physician*. Programs normally advertise here if they have difficulty filling their slots. Many such programs are at well-known institutions, and some are even in hard-to-match-with specialties. Similar advertisements also appear, although not in as great a quantity or with as much information, in *JAMA* and the *New England Journal of Medicine*.

A program's or an institution's national reputation is not usually of major importance unless you are shooting for a high-profile research or academic career. In that case, your training institution's reputation may play a role in helping you obtain a desired position. Information about some institutions and their reputations for treating certain disease processes can be found in the annual "Best of" issue of *U.S. News & World Report*. This issue normally comes out in late July. Note that this listing says nothing about the quality of their training programs.

Dean of Students

Another source of information about specific residencies is your Dean of Students. You should already have had numerous opportunities to contact him or her while you were searching out a mentor, trying to decide upon how your interests match with different specialties, and arranging your schedule to best meet your needs. While this person may not know very much about specific programs in the specialties, he or she is usually very conversant about the difficulty or ease of getting into various fields. Often, the Dean can be invaluable if you perceive that you will have difficulty getting a position in your chosen specialty. The Dean of Students often knows, or can find out, where extra positions will open up, and about Preliminary or Transitional programs and other first-year slots that you might be able to fill.

Some Student Affairs' offices have a "contact book" that lists the links various faculty members have with programs around the country. So, especially if you think you are in trouble, go see your Dean of Students—the sooner the better.

Residency Fairs

Many medical schools and some hospitals have residency fairs where students have an opportunity to hear residency directors talk about their specialties. Students can often talk with physicians involved in several specialties' training programs. Some schools combine these fairs with the distribution of NRMP Match materials. Often, residency programs from within the institution (and elsewhere) have booths with glossy materials and people to answer questions. These fairs may give you some leads, as well as some additional program and specialty information.

Information about Unfilled Residency Positions

The AMA's Resident and Fellow Section publishes a list of "Residency and Fellowship Vacancies" provided by program directors. You may also want ask the appropriate specialty society about unfilled positions. Also check on the AAMC's FindAResident website (www.aamc.org/students/findaresident/). And finally, there is ResidentSwap (www.residentswap.org/how_it_works. php), which lists vacant residency positions as posted by programs, as well as spots that are currently filled by residents who would like to swap locations or specialties with another resident.

11
Finding Programs That Meet Your Needs

If the doors of perception were closed, everything would appear as it is—infinite.
William Blake, *A Vision of the Last Judgment*

The First Cut

NOW THAT YOU HAVE SOME initial information about residency programs, it is time to start weeding. But like any good gardener, be cautious. Don't be so anxious to get rid of the "bad choices" that you inadvertently discard the daffodils with the dandelions. Be prudent when eliminating potential programs from your list. Only reject them after you have carefully reviewed their information. Don't eliminate programs simply because you suspect you are not a strong enough candidate—at least wait until after they tell you they do not want to interview you.

You will probably want to consider about thirty programs seriously enough to get all their information. Out of this group, apply to from fifteen to twenty programs (more if you are stretching to get into some very competitive programs or have a poor scholastic record) and interview at ten or twelve. These numbers will vary depending upon your personal needs and the difficulty of getting a residency slot in that specialty. Nearly 40% of medical students have interviews at ten or fewer programs, and nearly two-thirds interview at fifteen or fewer (see Figure 12.2).

There are good reasons to be liberal in your selection criteria and leery of discarding programs from consideration too soon. The main reason is that residencies that may appear superficially unacceptable often turn out to be the ones that best fit your personal needs. Program websites and their written material vary with the marketing sophistication of the residency and their hospitals. You do not want to miss a great opportunity just because a program does not know how to present itself; you also don't want to pursue only those programs with excellent marketing departments.

What Do You Want in a Program?

What do *you* want in a residency program? You can't get to the right place until you figure out what the "right place" looks like. Your situation is similar to that of a pilot who says to his passengers over the intercom, "I have good news, and I have bad news . . . We are making good time, but I have no clue where we are going." Take the time to figure out where you want to go.

Both your residency and your subsequent career will differ markedly from medical school. In deciding about the best residencies for you, you will consider a large number of factors that you may never have had to think about previously. Most of these factors apply to everyone. But how much weight you put on each factor will be a function of your personal needs. Although it may be somewhat onerous to find some of the information you need to make the decision, the sources listed in the previous chapter, especially *FREIDA,* make it much easier than it was in the past.

Weighing the Factors—The "Must/Want" Analysis

How do you weigh the many factors involved in deciding to which residencies you should apply (and then how do you rank them in the Match)? The simplest method is to use a "Must/Want" analysis.

As shown in Figure 11.1, you make a list of all the possible factors that could influence your decision about the type of program that you would like. (Do not complete your own "Must/Want" Analysis or fill in Figure 11.1 now; wait until after you have read all the following descriptions of the factors to consider.) Some of the items may be absolute necessities for you, such as paid family health care. *If an item is an absolute, a "MUST," you have decided that the factor is so important that it must be present or else you will eliminate the program from consideration regardless of the program's other qualities.*

Other items will be relatively more or less important to you. For example, you may have compelling personal reasons for living in a certain part of the country or in a certain city. In that case, you would rate "geography" higher than other factors. However, if where you live is less important than other factors, you would give "geography" a low rating, or you might even eliminate it from your list.

Assigning "Weights" to each factor rates their relative importance to you. Refer to Figure 11.2 to see how a sample student assigned "Weights" to the factors important to her. After you have read the descriptions, use Figure 11.1 as a master form from which to build your own list.

Deciding What You Want—The Most Difficult Task

Completing the "Must/Want" Analysis has consistently been each student's most arduous task in the residency selection process. It is not because the concept is difficult, but because it requires you to assess what you really are searching for in a training program. It helps you answer three questions:

1. What "MUST" I have to go to a program?

2. What do I "Want" in a program?

3. How important is each of the various factors to me?

I require my advisees to complete their own list of important factors and assign "Weights" to each before discussing which programs they might want to consider. (Our medical students get this book free from the Arizona Medical Association Foundation.) This process often precipitates constructive discussions between students and their families, significant others, and mentors, especially about where they feel they would like to (or must) live during residency training.

Once students have puzzled through what is important to them, they find that they are much better prepared to discuss why they might want to apply to certain programs. The focus of the discussion changes from what the adviser thinks are the "best" programs to which programs best meet the needs described by a student's "Must/Want" Analysis.

I have talked with numerous students who followed much of the advice contained in this book, got the residency they wanted, and then found that it did not meet their needs or expectations. As the saying goes, "Be careful what you wish for—you might get it." In nearly every case, they neglected to complete their "Must/Want" Analysis, and found out later that their "wish" was not what they really wanted. In many cases, the program's reputation or location overwhelmed every other consideration, to the individual's subsequent regret. Avoid years of dissatisfaction: Take the time to complete your own "Must/Want" Analysis. And once you complete it, be sure to use it!

Now, skim Figure 11.1 and read the descriptions of the various factors you may want to consider. Then I will explain in detail how to complete your own "Must/Want" Analysis using Figure 11.1 as a base.

Figure 11.1
"Must/Want" Analysis—The Instructions

Read the following instructions before filling out this form. Once you have adapted this form to reflect your needs and wants, you should make several copies. One copy of this form will be used for each residency program you consider.

1. Add any personal factors that are not already listed.

2. Select any factors that absolutely MUST be present for you to consider the program. Put the word "MUST" in the "Weight" column instead of assigning it a number value. This means the factor is so important to you that if it is not present, you will not go to that program.

3. Next, select those factors that are not at all important to you and, therefore, that you will not consider in making your decision. Put a "0" next to these in the "Weight" column. Delete these factors from your final list.

4. Finally, determine how important each of the remaining factors is to you in selecting a residency position. Put a number next to each factor in the "Weight" column, so the total of all the "Weights" equals 100. To do this easily, first rate factors of minimal importance with a "1," and rate those of slightly more importance "2." Continue in this fashion until the total for all assigned "Weights" equals "100." You will probably need to make multiple changes until you are happy with the result.

Congratulations! You have now completed the most difficult part of the process. Make multiple copies of your "Must/Want" Analysis Form with the "Weight" column completed. You will use one of these for each residency program you consider. Figure 11.2 shows how one hypothetical student completed this first step.

Later, as you get information about each program, you will assign a "Score" (on a 1-10 scale; 10 is "perfect") that is your estimate of how well that residency program fulfills your initial expectations in the category. Then you multiply the "Weight" by the "Score" to give the factor "Total" for that program. All factor "Totals" are added to give your "Program Evaluation Score." Examples of this are shown in Figures 11.7, 11.8, and 11.9. These "Program Evaluation Scores" will be what you use to make your Rank-Order List (ROL) for the Match. (Don't worry; I'll explain this in more detail as we get to it.)

Figure 11.1
"Must/Want" Analysis—The Form

PROGRAM _____

	WEIGHT	x SCORE	= TOTAL
Clinical Experience			
On-Call Schedule			
Patient Population			
Responsibility			
Setting			
Volume			
Geographic Location			
Inner City, Suburb, Rural			
Part of Country			
Specific City			
Spouse/Mate/Dependent Needs			
Reputation			
Institution's Reputation			
Program's Reputation			
Program Age and Stability			
Faculty			
Availability			
Interest			
Stability			
Curriculum			
Curriculum Structure			
Interaction with Other Specialties			
Number of Conferences			
Special Training			
Types of Conferences			
Esprit De Corps			
Research Opportunities/Training			
Knowledge			
Materials			
Time			
Local Job Prospects After Training			
Facilities			
Clinical Laboratory Support			
Computerized Records/Lab Results			
Hospitals' Ages, Atmosphere			

Figure 11.1 (continued)

	WEIGHT	x SCORE	= TOTAL
Library/On-Line Journal Access			
Parking			
Resident Call Room Ambiance			
Safety/Security			
No Restrictive Covenant			
Health Benefits			
Dental			
Drug Prescriptions			
Employee Health Services			
Health Insurance			
Health Promotion			
Hospitalization			
Optical			
Psychiatric Counseling			
Sick Leave			
Non-Health Benefits			
Association Dues			
Childcare			
Disability Insurance			
Educational Leave:			
Funding Available			
Time Off			
Family Educational Benefits			
Housing (Allowance)			
Laundry/Uniforms			
Liability Insurance			
Life Insurance			
Parental Leave			
Meals			
Photocopying			
Vacation			
Organized Housestaff/Union			
Moonlighting			
Shared/Part-Time Positions			

TOTAL OF ALL WEIGHTS = ___100___

PROGRAM EVALUATION SCORE =

Figure 11.2
"Must/Want" Analysis, An Example

	WEIGHT	x SCORE =	TOTAL
Clinical Experience			
On-Call Schedule	5		
Patient Population	2		
Responsibility	14		
Setting	7		
Volume	10		
Geographic Location			
Part of Country	1		
Specific City	1		
Reputation			
Program Age and Stability	2		
Faculty			
Availability	5		
Interest	7		
Stability	3		
Curriculum			
Number of Conferences	1		
Special Training	6		
Types of Conferences	2		
Esprit De Corps	8		
Research Opportunities/Training			
Knowledge	5		
Materials	2		
Time	7		
Facilities			
Clinical Laboratory Support	1		
Library/On-Line Journal Access	2		
Safety/Security	3		
No Restrictive Covenant	MUST		
Health Benefits			
Health Insurance	MUST		
Hospitalization	MUST		
Non-Health Benefits			
Childcare	MUST		

Figure 11.2 (continued)

	WEIGHT	x SCORE =	TOTAL
Disability Insurance	MUST		
Educational Leave:			
Funding Available	1		
Time Off	2		
Liability Insurance	MUST		
Vacation	1		
Moonlighting	2		

TOTAL OF ALL WEIGHTS = ___100___

Note that this individual, who is a single mother, feels that disability, liability, and health insurance, as well as childcare, are absolute necessities for any position she might take. She also gives rather a high priority to research and subspecialty training, because she plans to have an academic career. However other educational benefits, local job prospects after training, and the availability of a shared-schedule position are of no interest at all, and her interest in the geographic location of the program is minimal. This allowed her to shorten her "Must/Want" Analysis form to include only the items she considered important. How this individual will score specific programs will be discussed in the text accompanying Figures 11.7, 11.8, and 11.9.

Factors To Consider

The following is a discussion of the most common factors encountered when choosing a residency program. The importance of some factors, which may not seem obvious at first, is explained. Read the discussion carefully. Next, complete your own "Must/Want" Analysis form (Figure 11.1) by adding any factors that are applicable to your situation and deleting those factors that are not. Then assign either "MUST" or a "Weight" to each factor on your list.

Fellow students, residents, and faculty often advise medical students: "If you can get into that [big name] program, go for it!" This advice is worth just what you have paid for it: Nothing! No residency program, no matter what its reputation, is right for everyone. You are an individual. Start treating yourself like one. Look at your own needs, both for now and those you can foresee for the future. Examine your personal desires and your dreams. The program you choose, the contacts you make during training, and the type of training you receive will determine the course of your future professional and, possibly, your personal life.

A resident I knew at a very prestigious, high-powered, research-oriented institution spent most days moping through the halls. She was halfway through her second year of training and completely miserable. She confided that she had come to this program because of its great reputation, but was now completely disheartened because she was not receiving the "nuts and bolts" primary care experience she knew she would need when she went into rural practice. Rather than deciding for herself what needs she wanted filled by a residency program, she had let others make her choice for her. After some soul-searching and counseling, she switched to a program that emphasized rural primary care—where she was much happier. Choose carefully. Choose for yourself. It's your life, not your peers', friends', mentor's, or family's.

Clinical Experience

Clinical experience is the basis of any residency program. This is true whether you go into a field that acts as a primary provider, such as Family Medicine or Internal Medicine, or one that acts as a consultant, such as Radiology or Pathology. It is important to your training that the entire clinical experience, from the volume and types of patients treated to the setting of the program and the amount of responsibility that you are asked to assume, is as close to optimal as possible for your needs. *If the clinical experience isn't right for you, it is unlikely that any other factor or combination of factors can make up for it.*

On-Call Schedule

The frequency of night and weekend call varies depending upon the specialty, type of institution, specific service, and year of training. In the wake of threatened federal legislation and continued concerns about patient safety and physician fatigue, the ACGME revised its mandatory work-hour regulations for all specialties. These new regulations went into effect in July 2011.

The new rules state that the total hours worked cannot exceed 80 hours/week, averaged over four weeks. Moonlighting (within and outside of the training institution) and the time spent taking call from home or returning to the hospital for an emergency are included in the 80 hours. PGY-1 residents (interns) may not have duty periods longer than 16 hours, while upper-level residents may work a maximum of 24 hours continuously, with some leeway allowed for continuity and caring for a critical patient. PGY-1 residents must also have 10 hours off and 8 hours free of any duty between each scheduled duty period. All residents must have 24 hours off per 7-day period (averaged over 4 weeks) during which they may not take call from home.

However, even under the new rules, some specialties may be granted an 8-hour/week increase in permitted work hours: Neurological, Orthopedic,

General, and Thoracic Surgery make up the majority of the 68 programs allowed to use this higher 88 hours/week limit. The guidelines for each specialty are listed in Section II of the "Green Book" (the AMA's *Graduate Medical Education Directory*).

In 2008, a survey conducted by the ACGME found that the majority of residency programs appeared to be complying with the weaker 2003 regulations: 80% of the responding residents said they "always" or "frequently" worked no more than 80 hours/week. The survey also found that fewer programs had received citations for non-compliance with duty-hour limits. During the 2004-2005 academic year, the ACGME received 16 resident complaints for such violations, compared with 53 complaints the previous year.

Programs use a variety of approaches to deal with the decrease in available resident work hours. Some hire more residents, while others designate a person as a "night float" to handle excess new admissions for the on-call resident. Depending upon how it is structured, this may relieve much of the stress of being on-call at busy institutions—until you get tapped to be the night floater. Inner-city hospitals have been affected the most, since they rely heavily on housestaff for service needs.

Carefully investigate the call schedules at the programs that interest you. Basic work duty hours and call schedule information are included under "Work Schedule" for each program in *FREIDA* and in the *GME Library*. Be certain that you will be able to survive with the sometimes paltry amount of rest that these schedules imply. In general, Surgery programs, particularly in the PGY-1 and Chief Resident years, have more brutal call schedules than other specialties. (We'll have to see how that changes for PGY-1s with the new rules.) But this is certainly not always the case. And remember to ask about the amount of call "from home." No matter how benign this sounds, it will also deprive you of sleep. The key is to investigate the call schedule thoroughly—by asking the residents.

Patient Population

The types of patients and their prevalent problems vary greatly among institutions and in different parts of the country. Consider whether the institution offers the diversity of patients and diseases necessary for your training. Knowing only the number of patients seen tells you nothing about this important element.

Will you see a general cross section of patients that are normally encountered by practitioners in your specialty? Or will you see a population restricted to the narrow subspecialty or tertiary care interests of a particular program or institution? Will you see only middle-class neurotics at a Psychiatry program in a well-to-do suburb? Or will you see the full range of psychiatric diseases?

Will you see only tertiary referrals for complicated procedures at the world-famous mecca of surgery? Or will you get to see patients with "hot" appendices and gallbladders as well? Are virtually all the admissions scheduled and the major procedures done electively? Or is there a large population with unexpected, urgent, or traumatic disease? In large part, these answers can be ascertained from the type of institution in which a program resides.

Responsibility

As the traditional expression says, a physician "sees one, does one and then teaches one." This is how you will learn to practice medicine. Yet it is not only learning to do procedures, but also deciding *whether* to do procedures (or to admit patients or how aggressively to pursue "work-ups") that constitutes the essence of clinical maturity. Performing procedures is relatively easy; making the hard decisions about when, and if, they should be done is difficult. To learn this, trainees must (with adequate backup, of course) assume responsibility for all aspects of patient care for many patients. What does this mean?

First, this means having primary clinical responsibility. The pertinent questions for you to ask are:

- Will you be the one to make the moment-by-moment decisions necessary for acute patient care? Or will every decision have to be approved in advance?

- Will you really be responsible for managing a group of patients? Or will you only be the "scut puppy" for attendings and the more senior residents?

- Will you be doing the critical care procedures, or are these relegated to the subspecialty fellows?

- Will you be responsible for your patients when they enter the intensive care unit? Or will they be turned over to another specialty team?

You learn by taking responsibility. When investigating programs, find out if you will have actual responsibility for patient care.

Second, if you choose a specialty in which procedures are a large part of the practice, make certain that you will do those procedures. Procedures are essential in all Surgical specialties, including Obstetrics and Gynecology. But procedures are also a vital part of Anesthesiology, Emergency Medicine, Radiology, Cardiology, Internal Medicine, Family Medicine, Gastroenterology, and Pathology.

Not only do you need to perform an adequate number, but you also need to do the types of procedures that you expect to be doing when you go into practice. It does you little good as an Ophthalmology resident to become an expert at drilling burr holes, or as a Family Medicine resident to refine your laminectomy skills. You certainly will not be performing these operations when you go into practice. You need to gain proficiency in at least those skills that all Board-Certified specialists in your field are expected to know. A list of these procedures can, in most cases, be obtained from the specialty's Board, or, for ACGME-accredited residencies, from the list of "Special Requirements" for that specialty in the "Green Book" or at the Residency Review Committee's page on the ACGME website (www.acgme.org/acWebsite/navPages/nav_comRRC.asp). Concentrate on learning whether the procedures you will need are offered in sufficient quantities to hone these skills during your training.

If you are going into a Surgical specialty, you may want to know not only how many and what type of procedures you will perform as a resident, but also how soon you will get to operate. In many programs the first-year residents, though working harder than they may have thought possible, get little or no actual operating experience. They certainly go to the operating room, but often only to watch and hold retractors. At some programs, this can last well into the second or third year. Remember, unless you are a very unusual individual, you not only will become very frustrated by this, but you also will not learn very much. For Surgeons, the question "When do I actually operate?" is vital. However, be smooth about when and of whom you ask this question, since it can raise the hackles of many faculty members. If you cannot ascertain this from the program's literature, find out from the residents when you make your visit. It will save you a lot of frustration in the future.

One caveat: Personnel other than resident physicians should be available to do minor procedures (scut work), such as blood draws and the placement of peripheral intravenous lines or routine catheters, once these have been mastered. While it is necessary for most clinicians to learn to do these procedures, constant repetition serves little purpose and may become an impediment to a resident's education. It is worthwhile to find out how this is handled at each institution.

Setting

The institution(s) at which a residency program is located often determine the volume of patients that you will personally see, the responsibility that you will have for these patients, and the procedures that you will perform. Hospitals in large urban areas tend to offer more patients and more responsibility to the resident physician. They are often understaffed with attendings and have an overabundance of patients. At the other end of the spectrum are those community hospital programs with an abundance of attendings and a dearth of patients.

Neither situation is ideal. What you should look for is something in-between—enough patients to satisfy your personal training needs, and sufficient attendings to give you adequate guidance without taking away your responsibility for most decisions and procedures.

Sometimes major deficiencies, such as the lack of major trauma in a Surgery program, are corrected by using "away" rotations. These short rotations, taken at institutions particularly known for their expertise in specific areas, serve to fill gaps in the home institution's training program. How well these "away" rotations work varies widely. It depends upon the residents, the other institution, the deficient areas, and the amount of time spent away. To evaluate this type of rotation with any accuracy, you will need to speak to the residents in the program who have already "been there and done that."

Adequate training in ambulatory, rather than inpatient, settings is becoming more desirable due to changes in the practice of medicine. Training programs in all specialties should provide you with significant exposure to the systems for, the problems found, and the patients treated in outpatient settings. The type of outpatient setting is also important. If you are planning a primary care practice, it may be helpful, for example, to have some experience working at a managed care facility. (Less than 20% of all teaching hospitals have residents spend time in health maintenance organizations.) Find out how high the acuity is in the program's outpatient clinics. This can be measured by the ratio of number of patients admitted to number of patients seen. Emergency departments usually admit from 15% to 18% of the total patients they see. Judge clinics using that number.

Volume

The actual volume of patients to which you will be exposed, either as the primary provider or as a consultant, is of paramount importance to the quality of your training. However, information about numbers of patients can be very misleading—and often is deliberately skewed in order to attract medical students to an institution's training programs.

The size of a particular institution, the number of patients seen at the facility or by a particular service, and the number of procedures done give you, a prospective trainee, only a snapshot of the information you need. You also need to know the ratio of house officers to patients. If you are going into General Surgery, and the hospitals used by a training program do a total of 4,000 resident-performed operations per year, it sounds like an adequate number. But if there are fifty General Surgery residents, each resident does only eighty cases—with probably only about forty of these being major cases. This means that at the PGY-1 and PGY-2 levels you will rarely, if ever, hold a scalpel.

In other specialties, where ward and outpatient activities comprise most of the training, there is another danger: too few residents. *While it is important to guarantee that there will be enough patients, it is also necessary to find out if there are enough residents.* Both extremes can be harmful to your training. If the ratio of residents to patients is too high (too few patients), you may not be exposed to enough medical activity to get the training you desire. But if the ratio of residents to patients is too low (too few residents), you will be robbed of valuable reading, thinking, and discussion time. You will use this time attempting to care for an ever-multiplying patient load.

Over the past decade, the ratio of postgraduate trainees to inpatient beds has been highest at training programs in the western United States, programs at university-operated institutions, and those at state-owned institutions. Programs in the southern United States, programs with limited university affiliation, and those that are church-owned have had the lowest ratio.

Numbers can also deceive in another way. While a residency program may note that there are over 1,500 babies delivered per year at the hospital, it may not tell you that private practitioners deliver more than half of these with no resident involvement. This affects the amount of responsibility that you can assume as a resident in that program. But it also influences the volume of patients that you personally will encounter. Your individual patient load should be at the forefront of your mind when assessing any residency program.

Geography

Geography often plays a more important role in the selection of a residency program than it rightfully should. But, geography probably will be the most personal factor for you. Those most likely to do a residency in a particular state have also lived in that state prior to medical school. Remember, though, that geographical ignorance and prejudices should not be allowed to limit your choice of programs.

If you, like many of your cohorts, have not had time to visit most of our country, then spend some time getting an accurate picture of both the geography and the medicine in different parts of the nation from people who have actually been there. No, it's not true that everything east of the Mississippi River is concrete. Likewise, it's not true that physicians practice "cowboy medicine" out West. Wherever you are now, I have no doubt that you have heard horror stories about other areas of the country. Find out about these areas from faculty who have lived and worked there. Don't assume anything. You may be surprised by what you discover.

There may be a special reason to carefully consider the location of residency programs. About half of all physicians set up practice in the state where they did their residency or fellowship; more than two-thirds stay if they completed both medical school and residency in the state. Those most likely to stay are those who do their residency in the same state where they went to medical school, are generalist physicians, or are women.

Note that the number of residency programs varies greatly by region (Figure 11.3). If you concentrate on a region with a small number of residency positions, your chance of matching may decrease.

The following factors will help you determine how important it is for you to obtain a training position in a specific part of the country, a specific state, or a specific city.

Figure 11.3
Percent of Residency Programs, Residents,
and Fellowships by Geographic Region

Regions	Programs*	Residents**	Fellowships*
Mid-Atlantic (NJ, NY, PA)	22%	24%	22%
East-North Central (IL, IN, MI, OH, WI)	17	17	16
South Atlantic (DE, DC, FL, GA, MD, NC, SC, VA, WV)	17	15	17
Pacific (AK, CA, HI, OR, WA)	11	11	12
West-South Central (AR, LA, OK, TX)	9	9	9
New England (CT, ME, MA, NH, RI, VT)	8	8	9
West-North Central (IA, KS, MN, MO, NE, ND, SD)	7	6	7
East-South Central (AL, KY, MS, TN)	5	5	5
Mountain (AZ, CO, ID, MT, NV, NM, UT, WY)	4	4	4
Territories (PR)	<1	<1	1

* ACGME-accredited residency programs only.

** Includes both M.D.s and D.O.s. The location of AOA-accredited programs generally correlates with these numbers.

Sums may not equal 100% due to rounding.

Adapted from Appendix II, Table 4, *JAMA.* 2009 Sept;302(12):1364-65; and *FREIDA*, accessed June 2012.

Family Needs

Many students have family obligations which limit where they can go for training. These may include having a spouse or "significant other" in a job that he or she cannot leave or transfer, a spouse or child at a critical point in school, ill parents, and family members who need specialized medical care. In dual-profession relationships, the ability of the other partner to meet professional requirements in another locale (often for the second time) carries great weight. Dentists, lawyers, accountants, architects, and others may find obtaining a new license difficult, if not impossible, in another state. For some people, being near their extended family or religious group may also be an important consideration.

One of these constraints may make a particular geographic location a "MUST" for you. Since this is so personal, I can't give you much advice other than to tell you to talk this factor over with the individual involved before you assume that you need to limit your search for that person's benefit. You may be amazed at the amount of flexibility you actually have.

Personal Needs

Other needs may influence how much weight you will give to geography. Besides a desire to "see the mountains (or ocean, or trees) every day," the most common personal geographic need is compatibility with leisure-time activities. Although you probably won't have much spare time, especially during your first year of training, the desire to make the most of the free time that you do have is very reasonable. But even this may not restrict you as much as you think.

Of course, if you are a mountain climber, you need mountains (or at least some good climbing walls). And if you are a surfer, you will need surf. But if you are involved in running, swimming, hiking, or the more cerebral activities of music, art, and theater, you can find many locations that will meet your needs. By the way, if you are a skier, remember that the snow only lasts a little while—and anyway, you can always fly to the slopes.

Range

Although several comments have already been made about expanding your geographic horizons when choosing programs, a word needs to be said specifically about hesitancy to leave the "nest." The "nest" is your medical school, where you know the rules, know the faculty, and generally feel at home. It would be very comfortable to stay. And, unless you are a top student from a highly respected medical school, you may feel that you are not prepared to go out into the world and work, as I have heard many students say, "with students who really know something."

My advice is, *leave if you possibly can.* You are just as capable as the medical students from other or "big name" schools. In fact, you may have much more clinical experience. And, if you stay at your medical school's hospital for residency training, you will probably be working under a handicap that will not afflict your fellow residents. That is the "Once a medical student, always a medical student" syndrome.

The faculty and staff know you as a medical student. Of course, they will know, deep down, that you are now a resident, but you may have some frustrating attitudes directed your way. You certainly will have to work harder for their respect. By the way, this factor has an exponential effect upon residents joining the faculty where they completed their residencies. They spend an inordinate amount of time making the switch, in their colleague's minds, from resident to staff physician. So, if you have aspirations of joining the faculty at a specific institution, especially your medical school, go elsewhere for residency training.

Salary
In general, resident salaries have remained stable (in constant dollars) since the late 1960s. This means that although the total amount on the paycheck has increased, when it is adjusted for inflation, its purchasing power has remained unchanged.

Although it may seem that salary should be discussed under benefits, there is an element of salary that is geography-dependent. The cost of living varies significantly across the country. In general, costs will be lower in the Deep South and in the Midwest. The farther northeast or west you go, the higher the average cost of living will be. Normally this will not be a significant factor, since residents' salaries usually reflect the local cost of living. If, however, you need to repay a monster-sized school loan, this difference may be important.

Reputation

The institution's and program's reputations naturally influence applicants. Few reputations derive from excellent education. Rather, other achievements bring recognition to the institution and faculty. Nearly all residency applicants do best if they look beyond a reputation to the factors that are important to their own professional development.

Institution's Reputation
Some venerable institutions, such as Harvard, Johns Hopkins, Stanford, and the University of Chicago, have built their reputations largely on research over decades or centuries. The prestige envelops all their programs, whether

deserved or not. How should this institutional reputation affect an applicant's decision about whether to go there? If the institution has a residency program that is competitive in all aspects with similar programs elsewhere, some applicants may want to consider another factor: prestige. Those physicians aspiring to careers in academia or to clinical practices in posh locales may benefit from "gold-plated" credentials. Problems arise when an applicant sacrifices an excellent education for this prestige, as sometimes happens. In general, it is best to choose programs that provide an optimal educational experience, regardless of the institution's perceived status.

Program's Reputation

Some programs in every specialty have a reputation for excellence. Many of these provide superior education. But some programs' reputations linger long after the glow has faded. Other programs have not yet acquired a reputation for excellence, either because they are new or because information about program alterations has not permeated the specialty's intelligence network. Changes in the residency director, affiliated institutions, the patient population, and institutional funding may all affect a program. Applicants cannot simply rely on a program's reputation for past excellence; they must analyze each program as it currently exists, based on their personal needs.

Nevertheless, more than one-fourth of all applicants use a program's reputation as their primary factor in deciding among programs. Many later regret this.

Program's Age and Stability

No one wants to enter a residency program only to learn partway through training that the program will merge with another institution or close, that crucial faculty members are leaving, or that the program has lost accreditation. In these times of financial upheaval within the health care industry, no guarantees exist. Large teaching hospitals and individual residency programs are closing; faculty members leave for better personal opportunities.

Increasing numbers of teaching hospitals are now merging for economic reasons. This provides them with economies of scale, may reduce operational expenses by eliminating redundant services, and makes them more attractive for managed care contracts. These mergers, though, may disrupt resident education. Teaching faculty, especially in subspecialty areas, may be diminished, as may indigent or resident clinics and ancillary services that ease resident workloads. Remaining faculty may be pressured to decrease teaching and increase patient care while shifting many of their duties to physician assistants, nurse practitioners and other allied health personnel. While these changes are ongoing in many institutions, the rate may be accelerated during and just after large mergers. It would be wise to check to see whether such a merger is in the works at programs to which you are applying.

A reasonable method for testing a program's stability is to look at its history. How long has it existed? Has it ever had difficulty with accreditation? Has the program's faculty been stable? The answers to these questions cut two ways. They may indicate a stable program, but they also may point to programs and faculty that are rigid and unable to change with the times. And none of this information provides a guarantee. For example, the Mount Sinai Medical Center in Cleveland and the Manhattan Eye, Ear and Throat Hospital in New York suddenly closed their facilities (and thus their residencies) in June 1999, just as 150 new residents were arriving. On July 31, 2000, St. Elizabeth Medical Center in Dayton, Ohio, closed its doors, eliminating the positions for its 32 Family Practice residents. And, in 2001, Des Moines' Metropolitan Medical Center closed their residency program, making 28 residents jobless just a week into the new training year. In 2005, Hurricane Katrina forced the abrupt closure of the renowned Charity Hospital's many residency programs. And, in 2008, Chicago's venerable Michael Reese Hospital closed its last residency and shuttered its doors.

Strong Faculty

A large part of what makes any residency program unique is the faculty. Their interests, strengths, and involvement in the institution, national specialty activities, and the local community are all important factors in making any residency solid. Without a dynamic faculty, it does not matter what else is present—the residency will be weak.

Current residents can best answer your questions about the faculty. They interact (or don't) with the faculty every day, and will either highly praise them or barely give them a lukewarm endorsement. There is rarely a middle ground.

Availability

Even if the faculty is intensely interested in teaching, there might be either too few of them or too much extra work, such as administrative duties, added clinical responsibilities, student teaching, research, or writing, for them to be around when you need them. Specifically, you need to know whether teachers are readily available to you in three situations.

Clinical setting. Do program faculty just make rounds or take morning report, or are they there for you whenever you feel that you have gotten in over your head? Can they be relied upon to respond in the middle of the night and on weekends? Will you be left "hanging" in clinics without anyone to guide you through tough or unfamiliar territory? And do they show up promptly when you need to go to the operating room or do an emergency procedure? Sadly, the answers to these questions are not optimal at many programs. Recently, non-physician staff members have begun supervising residents at some programs. While this is not permitted under ACGME rules, find out if it occurs at the programs you are considering.

Personal counseling. The second time you need faculty to be available is for personal counseling. As with any job, no residency will be without its ups and downs—moments of personal crisis and indecision. More mundane will be the day-to-day administrative problems of scheduling your days off appropriately, getting your research started, or getting a nagging administrator off your back. Eventually, there will also be the question of a job search and the process of going out into the "real world." All of this can, and should, be eased by personal interaction with your faculty. That is one of the reasons they are there. If they are not available for this, you may have nowhere to turn.

Formal teaching. Last, and perhaps least important, is the faculty's participation in formal teaching. This includes grand rounds, journal clubs, and other formal conferences. While generally regarded as the most important of a faculty member's duties, it will actually be of less importance to you than the other activities.

The point is, for faculty to be effective, they not only have to be interested, they must also be available. Part-time faculty, those with too many other duties, and those who just don't have the concern to be available to residents are not what you are seeking. Reviewing the often-inflated faculty-to-resident ratios that many programs advertise will not help you to answer this question. Get this information during your program visits.

Interest

The key ingredient for any individual faculty member, or any faculty group, is that they have a strong interest in training residents.

This may seem to be a foregone conclusion. They are faculty members at a training institution, aren't they? But individuals choose the academic path for a variety of reasons, many of which do not include teaching. They may have a strong research interest, want to avoid night call as much as possible, or just want the easier or more distant clinical experience that teaching institutions often permit. Or, they may have had, at one time, a strong interest in teaching, but are now burned out. This is not to say that there aren't many wonderful teachers at residency programs. But the quality varies widely, and it is up to you to check it closely. Without real faculty interest, you will essentially be on your own.

Stability

Along with faculty interest and a presence, there needs to be some continuity. Look for how long faculty members have been with the program, especially the residency director. Each year, about 20% of residency directors quit their positions. If there is a high turnover, there may be significant problems. How much experience have the faculty members had in the specialty? If most of them are fresh out of residency training themselves, you will probably not get the wisdom (yes, indeed—there really is some) that comes with experience, if not age. You may be getting instruction from a group who are themselves still "wet behind the ears" in their practice of medicine. While some individuals at this level may give a program an instillation of vigor and enthusiasm, too many may lead to a less-than-satisfactory training experience.

The key, then, is to check into the interest level, availability, and stability of the faculty. They are the residency program's foundation.

Curriculum

What educational opportunities, in what settings, and with what outcomes does the residency program say it offers? Standard specialty requirements may determine some of this. Some of what they say may be exaggerated. Remember that whatever they say about the curriculum is always subject to modification based on financial changes, institutional reorganization, faculty transitions, and patient care needs.

Structure

What will you do and when? Which services will you be on, for how long, and in which training years? These elements, the most basic part of a program's curriculum, are the easiest to compare among programs. Will you do the intensive care service in the first year? Do you work in the clinic during your second and third years? If particular programs interest you because of either specific rotations or the order or length of rotations, ask about these during your interview to be certain that the program does not anticipate changing them.

Curriculum structure matters more in some specialties than in others. Child/Adolescent Psychiatry programs, for example, may mix the Psychiatry and Child Psychiatry years in different ways. Similarly, all the "hyphenated" programs, such as Pediatrics–Physical Medicine and Rehabilitation, Internal Medicine–Emergency Medicine, or Psychiatry–Neurology, have unique methods to combine time in each specialty. If this is important to your educational needs, find out how the program has structured its curriculum.

Interaction with Other Specialties

To get the most benefit from a residency program, residents should be exposed to the knowledge that other specialists provide. During the course of your training, you will most often interact with the residents (rather than attendings) from other specialties. They are an excellent, non-threatening source of information about the diseases and procedures common to their specialty. Such interactions also provide you the opportunity to learn about the thought processes used by other specialists. In addition, other specialty training programs often have organized conferences and teaching rounds that you can attend.

In some cases, the presence of another specialty's residents or fellows may interfere with your residency training. Family Medicine seems to be the most commonly affected, since other residents' involvement in cases often precludes Family Medicine residents from first-assisting in surgery, delivering babies and doing Cesarean sections, or getting adequate experience in Orthopedics. Many Family Medicine programs use rotations at alternative institutions to solve this problem. Not so obvious may be the decreased experience some residents get due to the presence of subspecialty fellows. Surgery residents may not get a full thoracic surgery experience if fellows perform or first-assist on most of the cases. Internal Medicine or Pediatric residents may lack some procedural skills if Critical Care, Hematology-Oncology, or Cardiology fellows constantly upstage them.

The presence of other specialists and subspecialists is a mixed blessing. Consider each institution's blessings in light of your own needs.

Conferences

How many conferences does the residency program offer? This number is usually a prominent part of the program's literature. Rather than the absolute number, however, look at the amount of time devoted to conferences per month. Use "conferences per month" to compare the programs, since some programs hold their conferences only once or twice a month, while others may have them daily or weekly.

Conferences do you no good unless you can attend them. So, also ask these important questions: How many of these conferences will I be able to attend? Is coverage of my clinical duties provided? Which takes precedence, conferences or patient care? Also, does the program require attendance at a minimum number of conferences? If so, do penalties exist for non-attendance? Ask the residents these questions to get a more balanced answer.

Not only is the quantity of conference time important, but so are the *types and quality of these conferences*. Some types of conferences are mandated by the specialty's Board. Others are at the whim of or reflect the educational savvy of the residency's faculty.

It is relatively easy to determine what conferences a program holds. More difficult to determine is how good an educational experience they provide. Conference quality varies with the organization, faculty participation, relevance, and ambiance. Relevance refers to the importance of the topics to your education, rather than to the faculty's research interests or a sponsoring drug company's latest wonder drug. Do the conferences regularly enhance your ability to perform patient care or expand your knowledge of the specialty? Are some conferences joint projects between your department and complementary specialties? These are the qualities that make conferences useful.

Ambiance refers to the amount of tension that faculty and senior residents produce, especially during morbidity and mortality conferences. Education need not be an ego-destructive experience, although some residency programs have yet to figure that out.

Lastly, how many of these conferences are resident-run? This is less important than the conference quality, although it points to another area of resident responsibility.

Special Training

Residency programs differ in their orientation. This is true for all specialties. This orientation depends partly on the institution's values and philosophy, partly on the residency director, and in large measure on the faculty's interests and abilities.

At present, there are recognized subspecialty areas within nearly all medical specialties (Figures 2.7 and 2.8). Some are well defined and have subspecialty boards in place. Others, such as Trauma Surgery and Hospitalist Medicine, have been defined both through need and by the medical community's acceptance. If you think you have a desire for training in a subspecialty, make sure that you will be exposed to it during your residency program. If you are not certain about your long-term goals, you should make sure that you will at least have exposure to several of these areas. You might just develop an interest in one of them.

If you are certain you want to enter a specific subspecialty training program after residency, find out if that area is particularly strong at the institution(s) in which the residency is located. Will you have an easier time getting into the subspecialty program (if one exists) at that institution if you do your residency there? Find out now. It may save you time, money, and a great deal of effort in the future. Or, even better, if you're certain of your career choice, apply to "integrated programs," which allow medical students to directly enter Thoracic Surgery, Vascular Surgery, and Plastic Surgery, as well as the combined programs that exist in many non-surgical specialties.

Esprit de Corps

An important factor for your well-being is the amount of esprit de corps (i.e., fellowship and camaraderie) found in the department. This aspect of a training program is hard to measure, and can only be assessed by your gut feeling about the program. But it is important to most residents, and affects how much they enjoy their residency experience. About one out of five applicants rates this as their main consideration in deciding among programs.

The attitude that pervades any department helps to determine the ease with which residents, faculty, and staff perform their duties. If there is a feeling of calm serenity, with people genuinely liking and trusting their coworkers, then the residents' job is much easier. But if there is a feeling of strain, anxiety, and perhaps fear, a resident's entire life becomes much more difficult.

The important attitudes are the day-to-day interpersonal interactions at all levels within the department, rather than those during episodic medical crises. Do the secretaries respond to you as if you are a welcome guest, or a miserable underling? Do the residents and faculty seem to get along with each other? Is there an underlying feeling of tension and bitterness?

The problem, of course, is how to assess this nebulous quality. The trick is to open your personal sensors and record your experiences after every interaction, including telephone calls, with each program. When you visit the program, try to discover their feelings. Pump the residents, and if possible the ancillary staff, for their attitudes toward the people in the department. While inexact, this is the best method for assessing the departmental attitudes that may be very important for your happiness during your training.

Research Opportunities/Training

If you plan to skip this section because you don't have any interest in research, please stop and reconsider. The availability of research opportunities and training at a residency program means that you will:

1. Sharpen your ability to critically read the medical literature—as you know, there is a lot of junk out there.

2. Keep abreast of the latest knowledge—at least in the areas being researched.

3. Be exposed to enough research to see whether you actually get "turned on" by it.

Quite a few residents have entered residency programs intending to never do any research after their training, only to discover that they actually liked searching for answers to pithy questions. In fact, some of them found that research added a necessary and fulfilling dimension to their professional life.

While they are still in the minority, an increasing number of new medical school graduates seem to be interested in research. More than 40% plan to include a period of research in their postgraduate training.

The presence of research activity suggests that clinical service, such as patient care, is not the only reason that the faculty and residents are at a particular institution. There is more to that department and institution than merely treating patient after patient. To have research, a spirit of learning and education must be present. This is what you are looking for in a training program. Value it highly when you find it.

Knowledge

No one learns to do research by him- or herself. You may have done some research as a medical student. However, it is unlikely that you either had the primary responsibility for the project or had to acquire the in-depth knowledge of scientific methodology, statistical analysis, writing, or any of the other elements of a successful research project. You are looking for faculty members who are experienced in doing (and publishing) research in your specialty. If you have developed an interest in one particular area, you may look for that. The important thing is to find at least one faculty member experienced in research who will be willing to work with you during your training. This individual will act as a research mentor, much like your mentor in medical school.

Of course, it is best to have a selection of experienced researchers to choose from, but this is not always possible. The things you should learn about research from any particular program are:

- How to design a research project.

- How to work with the Institutional Review Board.

- How to perform those techniques needed to complete the project.

- How to statistically analyze your research.

- How to coherently write a scientific article.

- Where and how to present and/or publish your results.

How is this information about doing research presented? Is it given as lectures, assigned readings, personal tutelage, or learned by trial and error? Usually, programs use a combination of these methods. But the most important element is exposure to a faculty experienced in all phases of research.

Materials

If you plan to do research, especially if your time will be limited, find out what materials for research are available to you. The more that are readily available, the less time and energy you will have to spend hunting down needed supplies, space, and equipment.

The first, and often the most essential, material is *money*. While it is the root of all evil, money is also the key to getting research done. Does the department or institution have funds set aside for resident research? Are there other sources that can be tapped easily? Are the amounts limited? Does their availability depend on the type of research being done?

The second material you may need is *laboratory facilities*. If you are planning on doing either bench or animal research, you need both laboratory space and equipment at your disposal. You will often be able to "squeeze into" a faculty member's lab and use "borrowed" equipment. But these first have to be available. Also find out if there are support personnel, such as veterinarians and technicians, to help you. Are there animals for research? This will vary markedly due to both state law and the amount of funding you have at your disposal. Are there individuals outside the department who are supportive enough of resident research to help with space, equipment, or expertise?

Often forgotten is the question of whether you can get *secretarial support*. Whether or not you are a "hunt-and-peck" typist, those keys can get mighty blurry when you are doing the third revision of a manuscript after making ward rounds at 8 P.M. Although not essential, secretarial support is a great asset.

Finally, how about *computers?* Is the network up-to-date with fast internet connectivity and the software you will need, such as statistical software? Is IT training and support available? If IT support is available, can you talk to a live person at 3 A.M. when the computer quits in the middle of running your program?

Even if you aren't interested in any other aspect of research, *inquire about computers*. Most medical students are sophisticated computer users. If you aren't, know that it is essential for any modern physician, no matter what their specialty, to be acquainted with at least basic computer operation—which means being computer literate. All large hospitals in the country, as well as most physicians' offices, use computers for business management and, most recently, electronic medical records. In research, computers are essential. Knowledge of databases, spreadsheets, statistical packages, and word processors is necessary for all but the simplest research being conducted today. Be sure that you are computer literate when you complete your residency training.

Time Allotted

If you anticipate doing serious research during your residency training, you will need adequate time. Programs vary widely in how they supply that time. Some assign specific blocks of time in which to do research. Often this is because of, or at least consistent with, specialty-Board requirements.

Other options are either doing research during an elective time period or working on research while attending to other clinical duties. The former may deprive you of necessary extra clinical experiences, which are often in subspecialty or complementary areas (such as neonatal ICU for an Obstetrics resident). The latter, unless the clinical load is very light, will deprive you of sleep. And during a residency, as you will find out, sleep is a commodity in very short supply. As early as possible, determine how research time is allocated in the programs that you investigate.

Local Job Prospects after Training

You may believe that you already know where you want to live and set up practice once you have finished training. If that is true, you might want to think about this when selecting a residency site. But first, consider whether jobs in your chosen specialty are even available in that geographic area. More important, with the ongoing changes in health care delivery systems, will jobs still be available by the time you complete your training? Will doing training there help you get a local job when you finish? Will you still be interested in living in that area when you finish?

Remember, your attitudes will change as you age. In some instances, residents who train in a particular area have an advantage getting local jobs, since they have been able to make contacts during their residency. In other cases, it may be a better strategy to train at a respected program and then look for jobs in the geographic region that interests you. Determine this by checking with clinicians or the medical society in the communities you are considering. Do not make a residency selection based on erroneous assumptions. Always check the facts first.

Also, career counseling should not end with deciding upon a specialty or entering a residency. With the proliferation of subspecialties and the wide variety of practice options, residents should actively seek advice on career decisions, beginning as soon as they enter their residency program. This may stimulate the faculty to provide some of this information in a standardized fashion, and even if they do not, it suggests to them that you are a top-notch resident who has his or her eyes focused on having a fulfilling and meaningful career. Is such counseling available at the residency program?

Facilities

As a resident, many factors will influence your day-to-day stress and comfort levels. The nature and organization of the facilities in which you work, however, are major contributing factors. While many residency applicants discount these elements, you would be wise to consider how important they will be to your education, your lifestyle, and your sanity.

Clinical Laboratory Support

Waiting for the results of an urgent, pre-operative, or outpatient laboratory test can cost both residents and patients their most valuable resource, time. Delays can frustrate everyone involved. Questions about the speed and comprehensiveness of clinical laboratories may be very important. How extensive are the tests an institution's clinical laboratories run? Is a stat lab available? Can you only get commonly needed tests during certain hours? Will lab technicians (or nursing staff) draw blood at all hours?

The days of running your own laboratory tests came and went and now have come again—at least to a limited extent. Performing these and similar tests are part of medicine's new age. Will you learn to perform the common "point-of-service" tests, such as Strep screens, pregnancy tests, electrolytes, CBCs, ABGs, and enzymes? Some laboratories have barred clinicians from performing tests in the clinics in the name of quality control (or is it revenues?). Yet you need this experience to be prepared for medical practice after residency.

Electronic Medical Records

The world has embraced computerization, and the government is pushing medicine to accelerate their adoption of electronic medical records (EMRs). You need to know how to use these systems, even though the ones you will use in your practice will, undoubtedly, be different. The basic principle is the same, though: you have rapid access to old records, labs results, and imaging studies. However, you must often type in, or at least dictate, medical encounter information and orders. If the training institution is not "on-board" with EMRs, it will weaken your educational experience.

Hospitals' Ages and Atmosphere

The bricks and mortar (and plastic, steel, and wood) that make up the institution(s) in which you work may look chic and modern or staid and ivy-covered on the outside, but you will work on the inside. How well is the facility maintained? Is its structure so outmoded that it makes working there difficult? Do its piecemeal additions mean that you will be walking endless miles to do the simplest tasks? Or are the new "modern" conveniences unworkable? Does the place look shabby and unkempt, or does it look neat and clean, despite its age?

You are going to spend many hours here. The hospital's or clinic's appearance and structure may not be your first consideration, but it will impact your daily existence.

Library/On-Line Journal Access

How good is the library? Even if you do not plan to do research, the library is essential for house officers to prepare talks and investigate unusual findings in their patients. Likewise, what facilities are there to do *computer searches* and to access *electronic journals?* Are reference librarians available to help you hone your searches and suggest other information sources? These services are an essential part of medical education and are available through most medical libraries. Also, do residents have wireless or at least hard-wired Internet access on the wards, in the clinics, in the emergency department, and from their on-call rooms?

Parking

Parking may not only be expensive, but it can also be a hassle—as you probably already know from your medical school experience. The amount of frustration involved in parking a vehicle can be ascertained by talking to current residents. The cost, though, is a commonly offered benefit. Seventy-two percent of teaching hospitals pay at least part of the parking costs for PGY-1 housestaff. Additional questions to ask are: How safe is the parking area? How safe is the area between where I will park and the hospital?

Resident On-Call-Room Ambiance

The on-call rooms will be your home-away-from-home. Don't expect them to resemble even the quality or size of a low-rent motel room. They should, however, be clean and quiet, have ready access to a telephone, have reasonable air flow and temperature control, and be private. The rooms should be cleaned daily and have fresh bed linens, although this is not the case at some institutions. Privacy is necessary so that your sleep will not be interrupted by telephone calls or pages to other residents sharing the sleeping quarters. The room should also have a lock so that both you and your personal items remain safe. Ideally, you should have easy access to a bathroom and shower.

These requirements do not describe five-star accommodations, but rather one step above tent camping. Yet if the on-call rooms meet them, they should suffice for your nocturnal hospital stays. Ask to see the on-call rooms during your visits.

Safety/Security

Most medical students feel that they are immortal, at least until they take Pathology. Since age brings some wisdom, most residents recognize that they must not only learn but also be safe in their clinical environments. News stories about physicians being killed only suggest the level of danger physicians face in and around hospitals. Many institutions in traditionally high-crime areas have tight security in place. Yet even there, injuries and deaths have occurred. Some institutions have not yet come to grips with their changing environment and lack adequate security. If you recognize that no place is absolutely safe, you can reasonably balance your security concerns with your educational needs.

Restrictive Covenants

Restrictive covenants, also called "non-compete clauses," are sections of employment contracts that prevent individuals from subsequently working within a specified geographic radius. For residents and fellows, this often meant not being allowed to work in the city where the residency was located or within a specified number of miles of the residency's main clinical site.

The AMA's Council on Ethical and Judicial Affairs has said, "it is unethical for a teaching institution to seek a non-competition guarantee in return for fulfilling its educational obligations. Physicians-in-training should not be asked to sign covenants-not-to-compete as a condition of their entry into any residency or fellowship program." According to ACGME rules, residencies must not require individuals to sign these types of covenants in order to become or remain a resident.

Unless there are extenuating circumstances, *do not apply* to programs that have restrictive covenants. Therefore, in your Must/Want Analysis, "No Restrictive Covenants" should be completed as a "MUST."

Benefits

The benefits a training program provides determine your real compensation level, and, in part, how endurable your life will be during residency. They suggest how much of your salary will have to be spent on some of life's necessities, or whether you can afford to do your residency at all.

At present, programs may offer any benefit package that allows them to compete for applicants. They must, however, provide professional liability (malpractice) coverage for the duration of a resident's training and for any lawsuits filed after they leave the program that arise from events that occurred as part of their educational program. The AMA, through its representation on the ACGME, is urging that residency programs be required to also provide health, life, and disability insurance for all residents. As of early 2011, the only requirement for ACGME-approved programs is to "provide access to insurance to all residents for disabilities resulting from activities that are part of the educational program."

When you are told about the benefits that programs offer, be aware of the fine print. Many programs offer certain benefits only if the resident contributes a share of the cost. Often this portion of the cost can be considerable. If you need a particular benefit, such as parking, dental care, or insurance, find out in advance how much you will need to pay to get it.

Note that you pay no tax (or very little) on most benefits offered by a program. And, since these are expenses that you otherwise would have to pay, essentially they are additional salary. But a benefit is only worthwhile to you if you need it. Obstetric care and family education fee waivers probably do you no good if you are a single male. About 62% of all institutions now offer flexible (cafeteria-style) benefit plans in which the employee selects the specific benefits that he or she wants from a menu of available options.

Salary

Salary is the bedrock of all other benefits. Unlike most individuals aspiring to a professional position, residency applicants never negotiate salary—it is fixed in advance. Generally, an institution pays the same salary to all residents in the same postgraduate year of training. Yet, these salaries can vary considerably among institutions, and from one region of the country to another.

In general, PGY-1 residents receive the highest average salary ($52,316) in the northeastern United States and the lowest ($47,134) in the South. Nationwide, PGY-1 average salaries also vary depending on who owns the hospital: medical school-owned hospitals pay the least ($47,745) and not-for-profit private hospitals pay the most ($50,449). Salaries increase about 5% per year during training. Housestaff salaries have remained fairly constant over the past 37 years, if adjusted for inflation. (A 2011 salary of $49,394, the national average PGY-1 salary, is just 22% more in "constant dollars" than the $6,200 that your older professors earned as interns in 1968.)

If there is a large variation in housestaff salaries among local institutions, think about why some have to pay higher salaries to their housestaff. Often it is because the housestaff have reasons, such as a deficient training program, to be dissatisfied.

Salary is not an absolute number. Rather, it should be compared to the cost of living in a particular locale. An apparently high salary may not go very far in Washington, DC; San Francisco; Boston; New York City; or parts of Los Angeles. (Los Angeles, by the way, has one of the lowest average first-year housestaff salaries.) However, a much lower salary may allow a rather nice lifestyle in many smaller, southern, or midwestern cities.

Health Benefits

Health benefits vary. Since you really are getting older and you probably don't plan to sit in a chair and vegetate during your time off, you need an affordable way to stay healthy and to get necessary medical treatment. This is without even considering the needs of any dependents (e.g., spouse or children) that you have or might acquire along the way.

Health benefits you might find available through your employer at a residency program include coverage for hospitalization, dental services, drug prescriptions, employee health services, psychiatric counseling, vision services (glasses), and additional health insurance. These are often grouped under various types and styles of health insurance. The bottom-line question, though, is: What services are paid for by the employer? (See Figure 11.4.)

You may never have had to purchase *health insurance*. In the past your parents or your school may have paid for your health insurance. If so, you will be shocked at the cost. Health insurance is very expensive. In addition, what you get for your money varies a great deal. The major elements to consider when looking at insurance that a residency program offers are: (1) who is covered, (2) what is covered, and (3) how much you will still have to pay. If you have dependents, it is very important to know whether they will also be covered. If you expect to need obstetric care, or if you or a member of your family needs special medical services, be certain that these will be covered by the policy. In addition, are prescriptions, glasses, and dental care covered? If they aren't, these items can take a big bite out of your salary.

Figure 11.4
Health Benefits Provided to Housestaff & Dependents*

Benefit		Resident	Family
Group Medical Insurance	Offered/Fully Paid	41%	29%
	Offered/Cost Shared	55	67
	Not Offered/Not Paid	1	3
Dental Insurance	Included in GMI	21%	
	Offered/Separate Plan	73	
	Not Offered/Not Paid	3	
Drug Prescriptions	Included in GMI	91%	
	Offered/Separate Plan	6	
	Not Offered/Not Paid	3	
Psychiatric Treatment	Included in GMI	95%	
	Offered/Separate Plan	1	
	Not Offered/Not Paid	3	
Vision Plan	Included in GMI	41%	
	Offered/Separate Plan	49	
	Not Offered/Not Paid	7	

GMI = Group Medical Insurance
* Some totals may not add up to 100% due to rounding, and "No Response."
Adapted from: Association of American Medical Colleges. *AAMC Survey of Resident/Fellow Stipends and Benefits.* Autumn 2010 Report. AAMC Division of Health Care Affairs.

Finally, if the insurance does cover your specific health needs, what is your co-payment? *A co-payment is the amount that you must pay*, and may be a flat fee or calculated as a percentage of the charges for specific health services. If the co-payment is large or the total amount of covered services is relatively small, you could be put at financial risk if you or your family members need extensive health services. More than half of all institutions charge residents co-payments for inpatient medical care, ranging from $5 to more than $1,500. For ambulatory services, about two-thirds have co-payments, ranging from $5 to $50 or more. Most programs state whether they offer, pay for, or share the cost of medical, mental health, and dental insurance under "Major Medical Benefits" in *FREIDA* (if the residency director completed it).

Group medical coverage is offered to residents and their families by nearly all teaching institutions. Most hospitals have from two to eight plans, with varying benefits, to choose from. In recent years, more hospitals in the South and the West (43% and 66%) have paid the full cost of residents' medical insurance than did those elsewhere in the country (<38%). Programs in the West also most commonly pay in full for a resident's family to be covered (48%); this is the least common in the Midwest (21%). Who owns the hospital also influences whether they are likely to pay for this coverage. HIV/AIDS coverage is included in most policies.

Dental plans for housestaff are offered by about 83% of hospitals, with about 78% offering this benefit for dependents. *Prescription drug* benefits for residents are offered by more than 97% of teaching hospitals. *Psychiatric* benefits are offered to housestaff by 96% of teaching hospitals, but only 37% fully pay for it. *Vision plans* are offered at low or no cost at about 80% of teaching hospital residency programs. Although this may appear to be a minor benefit, prescription glasses can be expensive.

Health promotion has become a cost-effective benefit for an increasing number of non-hospital employers. At least one-third of major employers have on-site exercise facilities and classes. An additional one-third provides employee discounts for health club memberships. The increasing awareness of and interest in fitness should soon make this benefit available at many teaching hospitals. Health promotion comes in two forms: *screening* and *risk-avoidance*. Residency applicants dislike pre-employment screening, such as that for drugs or HIV. They respond positively, however, to risk-avoidance measures, such as a smoke-free workplace.

Sick leave is one benefit few people look forward to using. Since you will work around ill patients and colleagues, you will probably get sick enough to stay home at some point during your residency. What provisions does the program have for this? The other side of the coin is: What requirements are there for you to act as "back-up" for other residents who take sick leave? The general requirements are often set by the specialty's residency review committee, but the amount of time and how to use it are set by the institutions and programs.

Non-Health Benefits

Non-health benefits are designed to make your life as an employee easier. They include some of the necessities that you will have to pay for if the teaching institution does not. So, if you need a particular benefit, having it paid for by your employer will make your salary go that much farther. Of course, if the benefit is of no use to you, do not consider it as a real part of your benefit package.

Non-health benefits that may be offered to housestaff or their dependents include: life insurance, disability insurance, parking, housing allowance, meals, vacation, educational time off, educational funding, liability insurance, childcare, laundry (uniforms), association dues, family educational benefits, and photocopying allowances. It is important to consider each institution's salary and benefit package to ensure that you will have the means to survive. You may find it useful to compare a program's benefits with those offered nationwide (Figures 11.5 and 11.6).

Life insurance is a necessity if you have dependents (especially if they are children). If anything should happen to you, this is what they will use for survival for the first several months after your death. Premiums are fully paid by most teaching institutions, and partially paid by nearly all others. Most teaching hospitals also have provisions for housestaff to purchase additional life insurance if they so desire. The amount of life insurance provided averages about $48,000, and ranges from $1,000 to $600,000 or more.

Disability insurance is an absolute necessity for you from now on. You have invested an enormous amount of time, effort, and money getting into and through medical school. Your potential earning power is sizable. However, if anything should happen to you that would prevent you from practicing medicine, or even practicing in your specialty once you have been trained, you will lose it all. Disability insurance will cover some of this loss. Currently, standard policies for residents pay a maximum of 60% of their annual salary each year.

Figure 11.5
Non-Health Benefits for First-Year Housestaff*

Benefit	Hospital Contribution	Percentage with Benefit
Parking	Offered/Fully Paid	55%
	Offered/Cost Shared	17
	Not Offered/Not Paid	23
Housing	Offered/Fully Paid	<1%
	Offered/Cost Shared	5
	Not Offered /Not Paid	89
Meals when on call	Offered/Fully Paid	72%
	Offered/Cost Shared	18
	Not Offered/Not Paid	6
Meals when working	Offered/Fully Paid	20%
	Offered/Cost Shared	26
	Not Offered/Not Paid	48

* Some totals may not add up to 100% due to rounding and "No Response."

Adapted from: Association of American Medical Colleges. *AAMC Survey of Resident/Fellow Stipends and Benefits*. Autumn 2010 Report; AAMC Division of Health Care Affairs.

It is worthwhile to consider purchasing additional disability insurance, especially since you, like nearly 80% of residents, may have substantial education-associated debts. Depending upon the type of coverage, you will be paid a set amount regularly for a defined period of time if you cannot work as a physician (or as a specialist once you have been trained). A special "HIV Indemnity Plan" is available through some insurance companies, including the AMA, that pays a lump sum if a resident becomes HIV-positive. Many disability policies will not pay unless the individual becomes incapacitated.

Most teaching hospitals pay some or all of the costs of disability insurance for housestaff. These policies usually may be continued (are "portable") after a resident leaves the program, if someone (usually the resident) continues to pay the premiums. Often, additional coverage can be purchased. Most programs state whether they offer, pay for, or share the cost of disability insurance under "Major Medical Benefits" in *FREIDA*.

Housing is a necessity, although you may not see much of your home as a PGY-1. Few teaching hospitals still offer to pay all or part of the cost for housing. Most programs state whether they offer a housing stipend under "Employment Policies and Benefits" in *FREIDA*.

Meals are provided at no cost for most (72%) first-year housestaff while on-call, and to many (20%) when they are working but not on call. Many other hospitals subsidize a portion of housestaff meals. Two important considerations are whether the food is edible and whether it will be available when you have time to eat, such as at 3 A.M. Most programs state whether they offer an "On-Call Meal Allowance" under "Employment Policies and Benefits" in *FREIDA*. You will need more information about this, so ask the residents and also sample the cafeteria's food when you visit the program

Vacation and **educational leave** are important to rejuvenate your mind and body. Housestaff typically get three to four weeks of vacation. Educational leave to attend conferences in excess of vacation time is granted by most teaching hospitals. While many institutions have a general vacation policy, two-thirds let individual programs determine the amount of a resident's educational leave. Most hospitals contribute about $400 toward conference registration and per-diem costs for PGY-1s and $700 for PGY-2s. Programs usually state the amount of vacation and sick days allotted each year under "Compensation and Leave" in *FREIDA*.

Lab coats are less critical than many other benefits, but their purchase and upkeep are often expensive. Will the hospital pay for your lab coats and also wash them?

Liability (malpractice) insurance is a "MUST" for all residents. The cost is astronomical if you pay for it personally, and is even higher if you should need it and not have it. This is one expense that *must* be covered by the institution. It is not too difficult to consider as a "MUST" since, for their own protection, all teaching institutions cover your malpractice insurance. There is no harm in double-checking, however.

House-officer groups have questioned whether hospitals are supplying residents with the appropriate type of malpractice insurance. The more inclusive type of coverage is the "occurrence" policy, which covers all alleged negligent acts occurring during the policy period. "Claims-made" policies are less comprehensive, and cover policyholders for all lawsuits filed during the period of coverage. (The alleged negligent act must also have occurred during the period of coverage).

In essence, an occurrence policy will cover you for any malpractice allegations that happen during your residency—no matter when the lawsuit is filed. This is the type of professional liability coverage that the General Requirements for residency accreditation strongly suggest that all programs have in place. Governing bodies also strongly suggest that occurrence-type professional liability coverage be provided.

The claims-made policy only covers you while you are still at the same institution. If lawsuits are subsequently filed, you are not covered by the insurance unless separate "tail coverage" has been purchased. So far, no former resident is known to have been forced to pay damages. But it could happen.

Although the General Requirements for all residency programs mandate that applicants must be provided with the details of the professional liability coverage, programs might forget to do so—especially if the coverage is inadequate. Ask for details, including the type of insurance and the amount of coverage the hospital provides.

Childcare, a benefit resulting from the increased number of working parents, is offered by about one-third of teaching institutions (see Figure 11.6). Approximately 49% of medical students are now women. Nearly 13% of all graduating medical students have children, and half of these have two or more.

Childcare allows parents to perform their jobs and not spend all their earnings to pay for their offspring's care. Unfortunately, most childcare services cover only "normal" working hours, meaning Monday through Friday, 8:00 A.M. to 5:00 P.M. As a resident, your hours will be neither that regular nor that short. Only 15% of existing childcare facilities are open weekends and holidays, and only 5% are open overnight (6:00 P.M. to 7:00 A.M.).

Figure 11.6
Programs in Representative Specialties with On-Site Childcare

Specialty	Percentage of Programs
Anesthesiology	40%
Dermatology	41%
Emergency Medicine	33%
Family Medicine-	30%
Internal Medicine	38%
Neurology	38%
Obstetrics/Gynecology	42%
Ophthalmology	37%
Orthopedic Surgery	36%
Otolaryngology	40%
Pathology	45%
Pediatrics	42%
Psychiatry	38%
Radiology, Diagnostic	29%
Surgery, General	42%

Data derived from: American Medical Association. *GMED Companion: An Insider's Guide to Selecting a Residency Program 2010–2011.* Chicago, IL: AMA, 2010.

Some teaching hospitals, in recognition of the need for childcare services for parents who work long and irregular hours, have on-site childcare for housestaff. Hospitals offering childcare services to their housestaff find that this not only helps attract residents, but also decreases absenteeism. Most programs state whether they offer on-site or subsidized childcare under "Employment Policies and Benefits" in *FREIDA*.

Most teaching institutions will help residents find childcare if they don't offer it. Many subsidize childcare; the average maximum subsidy is 30% of the cost. However, even if institutions offer childcare, you may not be able to use it: 78% have waiting lists for residents' children. The average wait to enroll an infant (0 to 1 year) is six months, for children two years old and above the wait is two months.

Besides the convenience, having on-site childcare as a benefit can save you a lot of money. Hospitals normally charge residents between $45 and $100/ week per child for this service. This is usually a marked financial, as well as emotional, reward over having to arrange comparable services outside the institution. The institutional services are reliable (your only sitter does not get sick), often have flexible hours matching yours, do not require transporting your child to another site, and usually provide care for sick children. Having childcare available for children when they are ill is a new movement. This allows parents to continue working with the assurance that their children are being cared for.

If you think you could use childcare, inquire. But, since children and the responsibility that they entail are sensitive issues, inquire discreetly.

Family leave covers a wide range of reasons to take time off, including paternity and maternity leave. *FREIDA* lists maximum paid and unpaid leave for family/medical reasons under "Compensation and Leave" in the "Employment Policies and Benefits" section. For more on the topic, see Pregnancy and Family Leave in Chapter 14.

Note: Regardless of a residency program's stated policy on parental leave, childcare, or other family matters, the attitude of the residency director matters most. If a resident's supervisor is supportive, then the policies work; if not, they fail. All applicants, not just women, should ask current residents about this during their site visit. This is the only way to discern a particular department's attitude on family-related matters.

Family educational benefits are offered by some programs, especially those associated with major universities. In some cases, the benefits include free or markedly reduced tuition for college classes. While this may not be useful to most residents, who may spend much of their free time sleeping, it may be very helpful to their spouse. Many spouses are interested in pursuing the remainder of either undergraduate or graduate training. If this benefit is used, the savings can be substantial.

Recruitment incentives are commonly offered in primary care specialties. While some national groups tried to halt this practice, the Justice Department's intervention assured that it will continue. Incentives range from supplying an expense account for books and educational courses to subsidizing interview expenses. Many of these incentives are now offered only by marginal programs. In the future, better programs may also begin to adopt these tactics.

Organized housestaff/unions have become much more common. Often called Independent Housestaff Organizations (IHOs), they have helped their more than 13,000 resident members in public hospitals address training conditions, salaries and benefits, ancillary support, and patient care with a collective voice. Joining a residency where such an organization exists (if it has been effective) may help lessen the frustrations you experience during residency. Most unionized residents are located in California, the District of Columbia, Florida, Massachusetts, New Jersey, and New York, and are represented by the Committee of Interns and Residents (www.cirseiu.org/), an affiliate of the Service Employees International Union.

In December 1999, the National Labor Relations Board overturned a 23-year-old precedent by granting medical residents the right to organize in private institutions, a decision it upheld in June 2010. They had previously said that interns and residents could not collectively bargain because they were considered students, not employees. The ruling regards hospital interns and residents, and other housestaff, as "statutory employees with a right to organize."

Moonlighting

Moonlighting means working for pay during time off while you are a resident or fellow. It is not the first thing that most medical students think of when they consider residency programs. Being allowed to work clinically at another site for pay and having opportunities available to do so, however, may make the difference between eating steak or peanut butter sandwiches—or, more important, between buying gasoline for your car so you can drive to work or having to walk.

Moonlighting also offers residents an opportunity to broaden their clinical experiences, to learn about communities in which they might want to practice, to let the communities learn about them, and to find out what clinical practice is like outside a tertiary-care mecca. Most important, it lets them experience, maybe for the first time, how it feels to be treated like a professional—and to take on a professional's responsibilities.

Most residency programs have rules about moonlighting. Some allow all moonlighting. Others don't allow any. Most restrict moonlighting to either specific amounts of time or situations where it will not interfere with resident activities. Most moonlighting occurs in Internal Medicine and Family Medicine programs; about 30% of Internal Medicine residents and 18% of Family Medicine residents have moonlighting jobs. If you think that you might want to moonlight, find out under what conditions it is allowed.

States also may regulate moonlighting through licensure. A number of states require two or more years of postgraduate training prior to licensure—a requirement that is more common and more stringent for IMGs (Figure 8.9). This either discourages most moonlighting in these states or limits it to those in their last years of residency. The Federation of State Medical Boards has recommended that all state licensing boards require at least three years of postgraduate training for licensure. The ACGME's new work-hour rules, effective July 2011, include any (internal and external) moonlighting time in the 80-hour average work week total, which may effectively ban moonlighting.

Even if moonlighting is permitted, the next question is whether moonlighting jobs are available. In some institutions, moonlighting opportunities exist within the institution itself or at satellite facilities. In other hospitals, groups of residents have acquired moonlighting jobs that are available to the entire group. In most cases, however, finding these jobs is an individual endeavor. Try to find out whether current residents have found such moonlighting positions. If so, have they been within a reasonable commuting distance?

Finally, what will moonlighting cost? How expensive is a medical license in the state? How long will it take to get? In some states, it may take six months or more after applying to get a license that allows you to moonlight. How much must you spend for malpractice insurance? If there are moonlighting opportunities within the institution, it may not cost you anything. In some cases, employers furnish insurance (claims-made rather than occurrence—see "Liability Insurance," above). If you are forced to get your own insurance, it can be very expensive. Talk to the current residents about moonlighting. The information will be more reliable, and the impression that you leave with the program will be much better than if you asked these questions of faculty members.

In an interesting twist, a substantial number of teaching hospitals now arrange moonlighting opportunities, and even subsidize malpractice insurance so that residents in some specialties can moonlight. They believe this encourages students to enter these fields, or at least these residencies. Sponsoring or arranging moonlighting opportunities is most common in Family Medicine, Internal Medicine, and Pediatrics. About 20% subsidize malpractice insurance for moonlighting. Whether this will continue under the new ACGME restrictions is uncertain.

Shared-Residency/Part-Time Positions

It may be important to you, for any number of personal or professional reasons, to do your residency on a part-time basis, even though it takes longer to complete. A shared-schedule position is one in which two residents, who usually pair up before interviewing and applying to programs, agree to each spend less than full-time in a single residency slot. In essence, they share one position. These arrangements are more fully described in Chapter 14.

Other Factors

While the discussion above has covered the most common factors to consider in choosing a training position, don't forget any other personal factors that you feel are important enough to guide this decision. One rather exhaustive list of possible factors can be found in "An Applicant's Evaluation of a Medical House Officership" by Martin Raff and Ira Schwartz (1974, *The New England Journal of Medicine*). Even though the article is probably older than you are, the list is as pertinent today as it was when it was written.

Narrowing The Choices

If you have read through the description of some of the factors to consider when selecting a residency position, and if you understand the process for assigning "Weights" to the factors in a "Must/Want" Analysis, then you are ready to complete your own "Must/Want" Analysis Form. Use Figure 11.1 as a master form to develop your own list. You will use one "Must/Want" Analysis Form for each program that you evaluate, *so make several copies of the form once you have adapted it for your needs*. They will be completed first by using the programs' written information alone, and then updated using any additional information you get while interviewing.

Personal "Must/Want" Analysis

To decide on the programs to to consider applying to, complete the *Must/Want Analysis Form* (See Figure 11.1). Once you have listed the factors and assigned them either "MUST" or a "Weight" in your "Must/Want" Analysis, you should be able to go through the mass of information you have collected about the residency programs in an organized and rational manner.

How does the residency that you are assessing stack up against your ideal for that particular item? For each program you evaluate, every factor is given a "Score" ranging from "1" (farthest from your ideal) to a "10" (exactly what you are looking for). You record this result in the "Score" column of the "Must/Want" Analysis.

For example, if you ideally would like to have faculty available in the hospital for consultation 24 hours/day, you would score any program in which this was true a "10" for this factor. If faculty were available only every third Thursday, you would probably feel obliged to give this factor a "Score" of "1." (The scores do not have to add up to anything! Feel free to give any applicable score to any factor.) The scoring is subjective, but then, you are the subject and what counts is how you perceive the situation.

Let's see how our hypothetical applicant (from Figure 11.2) filled out her "Must/Want" Analysis Forms for three separate programs. Remember, she has not yet gone for interviews, so some of the information is not yet available. See Figures 11.7, 11.8, and 11.9 for her evaluations of three hypothetical programs.

Figure 11.7
"Must/Want" Analysis, Example #1

Program #1: Backwater State Hospital

	WEIGHT	x	SCORE	=	TOTAL
Clinical Experience					
On-Call Schedule	5		7		
Patient Population	2		7		
Responsibility	14		9		
Setting	7		8		
Volume	10		6		
Geographic Location					
Part of Country	1		4		
Specific City	1		1		
Reputation					
Program Age and Stability	2		3		
Faculty					
Availability	5		?		
Interest	7		?		
Stability	3		10		

Figure 11.7 (continued)

	WEIGHT	x SCORE	= TOTAL
Curriculum			
Number of Conferences	1	6	
Special Training	6	7	
Types of Conferences	2	2	
Esprit De Corps	8	3	
Research Opportunities/Training			
Knowledge	5	8	
Materials	2	?	
Time	7	9	
Facilities			
Clinical Laboratory Support	1	2	
Library/On-Line Journal Access	2	3	
Safety/Security	3	9	
No Restrictive Covenant	MUST	Yes	
Health Benefits			
Health Insurance	MUST	Yes	
Hospitalization	MUST	Yes	
Non-Health Benefits			
Childcare	MUST	**NO!**	
Disability Insurance	MUST	Yes	
Educational Leave:			
Funding Available	1	Yes	
Time Off	2	3	
Liability Insurance	MUST	Yes	
Vacation	1	4	
Moonlighting	2	?	

TOTAL OF ALL WEIGHTS = ____100____

PROGRAM EVALUATION SCORE = Not Applicable

Program #1 is completely eliminated from this applicant's consideration because of the lack of childcare. It doesn't matter what the scores are for any of the other factors—even though it scored well in several major areas. Note that a number of factors are scored as question marks. This is because the information was not available from either the written material she received or her adviser.

Figure 11.8
"Must/Want" Analysis, Example #2

Program #2: Mako General Hospital

	WEIGHT	x	SCORE	=	TOTAL
Clinical Experience					
On-Call Schedule	5		5		25
Patient Population	2		3		6
Responsibility	14		9		126
Setting	7		8		56
Volume	10		8		80
Geographic Location					
Part of Country	1		2		2
Specific City	1		1		1
Reputation					
Program Age and Stability	2		5		10
Faculty					
Availability	5		?		?
Interest	7		?		?
Stability	3		3		9
Curriculum					
Number of Conferences	1		7		7
Special Training	6		9		54
Types of Conferences	2		3		6
Esprit De Corps	8		?		?
Research Opportunities/Training					
Knowledge	5		?		?
Materials	2		8		16
Time	7		8		56
Facilities					
Clinical Laboratory Support	1		4		4
Library/On-Line Journal Access	2		3		6
Safety/Security	3		5		15
No Restrictive Covenant	MUST		Yes		OK
Health Benefits					
Health Insurance	MUST		Yes		OK
Hospitalization	MUST		Yes		OK

Figure 11.8 (continued)

	WEIGHT	x SCORE	= TOTAL
Non-Health Benefits			
Childcare	MUST	Yes	OK
Disability Insurance	MUST	Yes	OK
Educational Leave:			
Funding Available	1	?	?
Time Off	2	9	18
Liability Insurance	MUST	Yes	OK
Vacation	1	7	7
Moonlighting	2	?	?

TOTAL OF ALL WEIGHTS = ____100____

PROGRAM EVALUATION SCORE = 505 (+?)

Program #2 has scored very well against our applicant's criteria. The "Program Evaluation Score" is at least 505. However, just as in the first program, some factors could not be scored. In most cases, the same or related factors for each program will not be able to be scored without a visit to the program. These include the faculty's availability and interest, the esprit de corps of the program, and the "knowledge" of available research. Other factors may only have partial information available and may need to be further elucidated in person. The scores can then be adjusted, as necessary.

If a particular factor is either a "MUST" or a very important (high "Weight") element for you, it is worthwhile to call the program and obtain any needed information before you make your decision about where to interview. Failing to do this may either result in wasted interviews or cause you to overlook some programs that might meet your needs.

Figure 11.9
"Must/Want" Analysis, Example #3

Program #3: Saguaro Community Hospital

	WEIGHT	x SCORE =	TOTAL
Clinical Experience			
On-Call Schedule	5	6	30
Patient Population	2	5	10
Responsibility	14	4	56
Setting	7	10	70
Volume	10	3	30
Geographic Location			
Part of Country	1	10	10
Specific City	1	10	10
Reputation			
Program Age and Stability	2	7	14
Faculty			
Availability	5	?	?
Interest	7	?	?
Stability	3	?	?
Curriculum			
Number of Conferences	1	4	4
Special Training	6	6	36
Types of Conferences	2	9	18
Esprit De Corps	8	?	?
Research Opportunities/Training			
Knowledge	5	?	?
Materials	2	8	16
Time	7	4	28
Facilities			
Clinical Laboratory Support	1	?	?
Library/On-Line Journal Access	2	1	2
Safety/Security	3	5	15
No Restrictive Covenant	MUST	Yes	OK
Health Benefits			
Health Insurance	MUST	Yes	OK
Hospitalization	MUST	Yes	OK

Figure 11.9 (continued)

	WEIGHT	x SCORE	= TOTAL
Non-Health Benefits			
Childcare	MUST	Yes	OK
Disability Insurance	MUST	Yes	OK
Educational Leave:			
Funding Available	1	8	8
Time Off	2	?	?
Liability Insurance	MUST	Yes	OK
Vacation	1	4	4
Moonlighting	2	?	?

TOTAL OF ALL WEIGHTS = ___100___

PROGRAM EVALUATION SCORE = 361 (+?)

Since the information that was available for Programs #2 and #3 was not the same, they cannot be directly compared (yet). But the information available does give a general ranking for the programs. One piece of information had to be obtained by telephone about Program #3, but that residency's secretary was happy to answer a potential applicant's questions. The call provided the facts that our applicant needed in order to make an informed decision.

From this group, Program #2 is the one to which our applicant will be sure to apply. Depending upon how the other programs she rates stack up, she also might decide to apply to Program #3. Program #1, of course, has been eliminated for not fulfilling one of her required "MUSTs." By the time she finishes interviewing at programs, she should have enough information to eliminate the question marks on her forms.

12
Playing the Odds:
How Many Program Applications?

There is no certainty without some doubt.
Elias Levita, *Tishbi*

Forecasting is hard, particularly of the future.
Anonymous

MEDICAL STUDENTS FREQUENTLY ASK, "To how many programs should I apply?" There is no easy answer, since *the real answer depends upon your wants and needs, including your specialty choice.* No magic number exists. No one factor will give you an answer. As with all other aspects of the competition for a residency slot, the number of programs to which you should apply must be individualized. You must consider the competitiveness of the specialty you have chosen, the geographic and academic restrictions you are placing upon a residency choice, and your own competitiveness. Then, after discussions with your mentor or your specialty adviser, apply to a generous number of programs.

How Competitive Is The Specialty You Want?

First, consider how competitive your chosen specialty is. For example, Otolaryngology, Neurological Surgery, and Orthopedics require applications to more programs to be assured of an adequate number of interviews than do Family Medicine or Medical Genetics (see Figures 4.1, 14.8, and 23.2). For many years, students have been told (with only a little exaggeration), "If your parents did not submit your Orthopedic Surgery application while you were in diapers, it is too late." While the situation for most competitive specialties is not that bad, a few remain difficult to enter. Some specialties fluctuate widely in their competitiveness from year to year. Ophthalmology, for example, has become less competitive over the past decade. Also, one of the least competitive specialties in the 1970s, Anesthesiology, became extremely competitive in the 1980s but once again is relatively easy to enter. Generally, the more competitive the specialty, the more programs to which you should apply. Figure 12.1 demonstrates the change in total PGY-1 applicants and positions over the past fifty years. See the specialty descriptions in Chapter 3 for information on each specialty's relative competitiveness.

How Competitive Are You?

How competitive are you—really? List the qualities that are viewed as plusses in your desired specialty. Do you have strengths or weaknesses in these areas? Be objective. If you cannot be objective on your own, have your mentor or specialty adviser help you. It is generally inadvisable to have a spouse or close friend help on this—too much honesty from the wrong source can be very ego-destructive.

Do not compare yourself with others in your school who are applying to the same specialty. This will not result in an accurate assessment of your competition. *The competitive pool is made up of all students from all medical schools (throughout the world) who want to enter your chosen specialty*. Your best chance of success lies in assessing your competitiveness as accurately as possible. You do this by comparing the strengths that you have identified in yourself with those that you perceive the residency programs in your desired specialty want. The ideal candidate, the one who fits all the desired qualities, is the one you are competing against (see Chapter 19). But don't worry. That individual probably doesn't exist.

What Do You Have to Lose?

Professional photographers constantly tell amateurs to go ahead and take lots of pictures. "So what if you blow a few shots? You may end up with some beautiful pictures you wouldn't have gotten if you had been more conservative. Remember," they say, "the film—or the memory card—is the least expensive part of system."

Just so with the application process. Applying to a few extra "pie-in-the-sky" or "reach" programs (those to which you really want to go but are afraid that they won't accept you) makes good sense for at least two reasons. First, you will never have to say to yourself, as so many physicians do in their later years when they meet up with a moron graduate from their most desired training program, "I could have gotten in if only I had applied." Second, you actually may get an interview (and then a position) at that program. It takes very little extra effort to apply to a few more programs. Since you are applying to some programs anyway, follow your dreams—they may come true. If you can dream it, you can do it!

As a general guideline, the average number of applications recent

Figure 12.1: Applicants and 1st-Year Positions, 1952–2010

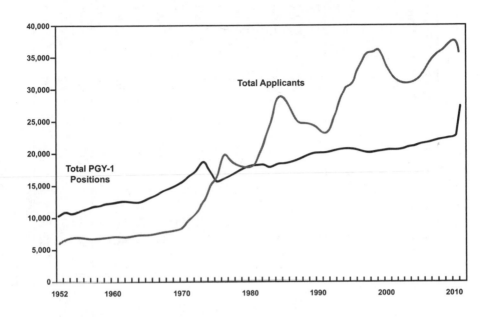

Information compiled from: Association of American Medical Colleges. *AAMC Results and Data Book.* Washington, DC: AAMC, April 2010; and from other sources.

graduates submitted through ERAS to programs in various specialties is listed in Figure 12.2. U.S. graduates who matched to the first specialty on their rank-order list submitted an average of 22 applications, while unmatched graduates submitted 35 applications. Matched Independent Applicants (prior M.D. and D.O. graduates, U.S.-citizen and non-U.S.-citizen IMGs, and Fifth Pathway graduates) submitted a median number of 42 applications; unmatched Independent Applicants submitted 50 applications.

Make your list once and then apply to those programs. Don't continue to add to the list piecemeal. The application process is hard enough and it is very difficult to keep track of the paper shuffle under normal circumstances. Adding programs as you go will only make the process harder on you, as well as on the people sending out your reference letters. Making one request for information to be sent to all your programs usually works well. Dribbling in those requests separately over time can spell disaster.

Figure 12.2

Average Number of Applications Submitted to Programs in Various Specialties (Matched/Unmatched Applicants*)

Specialty	U.S. M.D. Applicant				Independent Applicant**			
	Applications Submitted	Interviews Offered	Interviews Attended	Programs Ranked	Applications Submitted	Interviews Offered	Interviews Attended	Programs Ranked
Anesthesiology	24/32	15/5	11/5	10/4	35/49	7/3	7/3	7/3
Dermatology	66/75	11/5	9/5	9/4	10/40	2/1	2/1	2/5
Diagnostic Radiology	36/41	15/7	12/6	12/6	50/41	8/2	8/2	8/3
Emergency Medicine	26/30	17/10	11/88	10/7	30/30	10/2	8/2	7/2
Family Medicine	12/12	11/10	8/5	7/4	40/47	5/2	5/2	5/2
Internal Medicine	18/19	13/8	10/5	9/6	60/66	8/2	8/2	7/3
Internal Med/Pediatrics	16/11	13/8	10/7	8/6	25/40	8/3	6/3	5/3
Neurology	17/40	13/7	9/5	9/5	34/41	8/2	7/2	6/2
OB/GYN	25/30	16/10	11/8	10/8	35/46	9/3	8/3	7/3
Orthopedic Surgery	49/50	16/7	12/7	12/6	48/53	6/2	6/2	6/2
Otolaryngology	45/50	17/5	12/4	12/4	79/48	8/1	8/1	8/1
Pathology Anat/Clin	16/22	14/9	10/8	9/6	40/32	7/2	6/2	5/2
Pediatrics	17/18	14/13	10/8	9/7	33/41	8/2	7/2	6/2
Physical Med & Rehab	20/-	15/-	10/-	9/-	21/39	10/3	9/3	8/2
Plastic Surgery	43/42	15/6	13/6	13/5	37/36	4/6	4/3	4/3
Psychiatry	15/22	11/6	8/5	7/4	38/48	8/2	7/2	7/2
Radiation Oncology	43/48	13/6	11/5	11/5	52/64	8/4	8/4	8/4
Surgery, General	31/35	19/10	13/9	11/9	50/60	8/3	7/2	6/3
Transitional Year	10/30	10/8	8/8	7/6	32/19	1/2	1/2	1/2

* Match outcome refers to whether the applicant matched to the first specialty on their rank order list of programs.
**Includes prior M.D. and D.O. graduates, U.S.-citizen and non-U.S.-citizen IMGs, and Fifth Pathway graduates.
From: NRMP. Results of the 2009 NRMP Applicant Survey by Preferred Specialty and Applicant Type. January 2010.

13

Buffing Your File: The Paperwork

A wise man recognizes the convenience of a general statement,
but he bows to the authority of a particular fact.
Oliver Wendell Holmes, Jr.

THE KEY TO SUCCESS in preparing and gathering the information required by
residency programs is the same one that got you into medical school—being
compulsive. Four rules that will put you far ahead of the pack are:

  1. Be Thorough
  2. Look Neat
  3. Be Early
  4. Be Organized

Thoroughness means reading the application materials twice. Dot the i's
and cross those t's (figuratively, since in many cases, the computer will do
that for you). If a program requests something out of the ordinary, such as
your undergraduate transcript, then make sure that you note the requirement
and get them a copy. You can lose lots of points in this game if you don't
read each set of rules carefully. No one is prepared to go out of his or her
way to accommodate you. Some programs may not even notify you that your
application is incomplete, so it's up to you to develop a system to keep track
of your applications. Keep photocopies of all correspondence and detailed
records of your telephone calls and emails to the programs. Be thorough.

The *lack of neatness* probably destroys more potentially successful
candidates than all other factors combined. You are applying for a real job,
as well as for your lifelong career. Don't send your potential employers
anything unless it looks like it is the work of a professional. This means that
your application and résumé should never be completed in a barely legible
scrawl, in pencil, or in the middle of ward rounds. These documents are your
representatives, your entries to the goal you seek. Make them look sharp. Make
them look professional. Make them look neat. Computers and laser printers
are now accessible everywhere in the world, including rural regions in the
least-developed nations. (I know; I've worked there.) Use them.

Early birds catch the worm and *early applicants get the interviews*. More
and more students now complete their applications at the beginning of the

application "season" (August and September for programs in the NRMP PGY-1 Match). Still, many students have not even begun the application process at the time they should be making their decisions about which programs they will apply to and completing the necessary paperwork.

No matter how good the program, nor how experienced the residency director, the question that always arises at this time of year is, "Will I get enough good candidates this year?" As a result, programs have rather liberal criteria early on for granting interviews. If you walk on water and fly through the air (without assistance, of course), you can wait and file with the rest of the applicant horde. But if you don't, get your packet completed early. Even if you can do miraculous deeds, if you apply late, optimal interview dates may not be available when you're offered one. In fact, some programs may run out of interview slots, since many have only a finite number available. Get your act together early.

Get organized. You will, undoubtedly, have a mound of program information gathered from program websites. Therefore, you need to have an electronic and hardcopy filing system that allows you to quickly locate, assess, and track both the material you receive and the material you send. Develop these systems before you begin this process.

Your Name

Everyone has a name, so what's the problem? The problem is that your name may change or have several variations. In the world of medical credentialing and verification, which you entered when you took USMLE Step 1, COMLEX Part 1, or began the ECFMG process, variations aren't well tolerated. People who use their first initials and middle names, change their names when married or divorced, reverse first and last names, or hyphenate their last names may encounter difficulties. The key to avoiding problems with the various bureaucrats, who must verify that you are who you say you are, is to use the same name on all your paperwork.

For example, you used T. Michael Jones on your medical school entrance materials. (You say that you are not too keen on using Thaddeus?) Your transcript now probably reads that way—but find out from the registrar *before* you complete the USMLE Step 1 application. When you register for Step 1, use the same form of your name that is on your transcript. Do this for all subsequent official papers. That way, no one will confuse you with Tremont Michael Jones, Thomas Michael Jones, or even Theresa Michael Jones.

The same holds true for those who change their name when they get married or divorced. This has become more common with the increased number of women physicians. Those who get married after medical school usually have two names—their married name that they use in social situations, and their "professional name" that they use for work and for all official medical documents. That way, there is no bureaucratic confusion. Those who marry before or during medical school often begin using their married name for everything. Unfortunately, many of these marriages don't last, and so confusion may reign when the physician must use both her married and new (or old) names for the mounds of official paperwork throughout her career. As the number of different names increases with subsequent marriages and divorces, the confusion and resultant difficulties multiply. The best course is to have both a social name and a professional name. If possible, keep your professional name constant.

In Spanish-speaking countries (and occasionally elsewhere), a person often uses two last names—the first from their father and the second being their mother's maiden name. Therefore, a name may appear in a variety of ways on official documents, for example, Marco T. Velasco, Marco T. Velasco-Lopez, or Marco Velasco-Lopez. Others, such as those with Vietnamese names, may have their last and first names switched.

If you are in such a situation, notify all residency programs, ERAS or CAS, the ECFMG, USMLE, COMLEX, and any licensing bodies that the different names on your transcripts, Board scores, diplomas, and reference letters all belong to the same person. You do not want to be refused entrance to the USMLE because the names on your application and your ID don't match. You do not want to lose out on a possible interview because of an "incomplete file" resulting from having your materials filed under more than one name. And once you go through all this hassle, you don't want problems with the matching programs because you are not listed with the residency programs under the same name you used to apply to the Match. The best course is to *use only your full name on all official documents.*

The Application

Most M.D. residency programs now use ERAS or the Centralized Application Service (CAS), which present most information in a standard format. Some residencies and fellowships use their own applications or the Universal Application for Residency (described below). The first step is to get all the program applications you will need. Many can be downloaded from the program's website.

Application forms or the instructions specify what additional information is needed to complete the application process. Read the fine print. Make a chart of the materials each program requires. As you can see by the example in Figure 13.1, the requirements can vary widely. Nearly all will request a Medical Student Performance Evaluation (MSPE)/Dean's letter, medical school transcript, application, and reference letters. Make certain that you supply at least the minimum that they require. In most instances, you should send the maximum number (currently 4) of reference letters that ERAS allows. You are allowed to use different letters for different programs, if you wish. That is especially important when applying to two or more specialties. Whether programs ask for one or not, always send a copy of your résumé. In ERAS, this is generated automatically from the information you supply. However, you may wish to have a separate, more elegant résumé to hand to the residency director at your interview. ERAS requires that you also submit a personal statement.

Some applicants will also need to send a copy of their ECFMG Certificate, letter of waiver from the military or Public Health Service, letters and evaluations from previous residency training or work experiences, or other items. Be certain that you list all these items on your own tracking form.

Generally, the application will be the first piece of paper in your file at residency programs. The front page of the application, above all the other paperwork that you submit, must look as if the person completing it is a professional. Before you begin completing any application, it is a good idea to make copies of the form. Neatly fill out one of these copies, and then have a trusted friend review it for any spelling or grammatical errors. Such errors tend to stand out and will project a poor image of you. The reviewer, who can also evaluate your personal statement, should know you well enough to be able to suggest additional information that you were too modest to include. Then, after all your applications are ready, sit at the computer without any distractions or, in the case of non-computerized forms, give the copies along with the original blank forms to a professional typist for preparation. This process will give you the best results.

Fill in all pertinent blanks on the application form with the requested information. *Never put in the words "See résumé."* Programs ask for data that they feel is necessary to make a choice among candidates, and structure their application so they can quickly screen it for this information. Of course, you will supply a résumé to programs not using ERAS, and there will certainly be some duplicate information. Not filling in the application with the requested information, however, can be the kiss of death. It indicates that you did not think enough of the program to do the work required to fill out their application. Instead, you left them to search around your résumé for the information they desire. Is that also how you plan to act as a resident? It is the impression that

Figure 13.1
Requirements for Applications to Different Programs, Example

Hospital/ Program	Dean's Letter	Transcript	Application	Undergrad. Transcript	Personal Statement	Résumé	Reference Letters	NRMP
Saw Comm	X	X	ERAS			X	A+2	Yes
St. Marys	X	X	U	X		X	2	Yes
Amhurt Univ	X	X	ERAS		X		3	Yes
Smort Med Ctr	X	X	ERAS			X	A+3	Yes
Arden St.	X		B	X	X		2	Yes
Robin Hood	X	X	ERAS		X	X	2+P	Yes
WGMC	X	X	U		X	X	A+P	No
U of State YZ	X	X	ERAS	X	X		3	No

X--Required by program.
U--Requires use of the Universal Application.
B--Requires program's own application.
A--Requires a letter from your adviser.
#--Number of additional reference letters required.
P--At least one letter from a physician in the specialty for which you are applying.

you have delivered. That is not the impression that you want the residency program to have about you.

Finally, get your applications in early. It takes quite a bit of time to do the paperwork involved in preparing applications for submission. Since you are going to do it anyway, why not complete it early when you have a much better chance of obtaining the maximum results for your effort.

Illegal Questions

What about illegal questions? Those are the ones barred from pre-employment screening by federal and state civil rights acts. Questions dealing with race, sex, age, height, weight, national origin, military discharge status, arrest record, marital status or who lives with you, physical disability, and religion are restricted to those situations where they directly affect the job requirements or where the applicant raises them. Although they are not legal, some applications still contain these types of questions. How do you handle them?

First, remember that, in general, the programs are not being malicious in their use of these questions. Many times they are merely ignorant of the law. There is a fine line between questions that are illegal and those that are simply inept, curious, or friendly. Don't approach these questions in a hostile manner. Second, look over your Dean's letter, transcript, and other reference letters. How much new information are you supplying by answering these questions? Probably not much. What you are doing is putting the information down in a standard format for easy retrieval and comparison. So the general advice is to fill in all the blanks.

The Universal Application

The Universal Application for Residency, which was an attempt to limit the amount of medical students' application paperwork, is rarely used today. Nevertheless, you may encounter it somewhere in your application process, especially when applying to Fellowships. How should you deal with it?

ERAS and, for Ophthalmology, CAS have mostly replaced the Universal Application and individual program applications. If you find that you do need this form, you may get it from your Dean of Students or from the programs themselves (usually on their website). Print as many copies as you need. Since you generally cannot complete it on-line, you will have to either type or hand write (print neatly) your information.

Some students who use the Universal Application for multiple programs fill in one copy (but leave out the references), photocopy it, and then type in the appropriate references for each program. This looks sloppy and the program can tell that they may be receiving a different reference list than other programs. As a result, they may wonder "What is this character up to?" Don't invite this kind of curiosity. Once you have completed the application using a photocopy of your original form, give it to a professional typist with clear notes about variations for individual programs. Let the typist do the labor, so your application will look professional.

A note of caution is in order. Some programs specifically give applicants a choice between using the Universal Application or the program's own application. If you have that choice, use the program's form. It will demonstrate more commitment, better satisfy the program's information needs, and look neater (since it will probably be an original rather than a photocopied application).

Electronic Residency Application Service (ERAS)

The Electronic Residency Application Service (ERAS), run by the Association of American Medical Colleges (AAMC), transmits residency applications and other supporting documents (see below) to residency and Fellowship programs. Starting with Obstetrics & Gynecology in the 1995–96 Match cycle, ERAS participants in 2011-2012 included M.D. residencies in 43 specialties (Figure 13.2), D.O. residency programs in 26 specialties (Figure 13.3), and fellowship programs in 39 specialties (Figure 13.4). It is estimated that as of 2010, ERAS transmits more than 25 million documents each year.

In principle, programs in these specialties will no longer accept paper applications, and 95% of U.S. residencies in these specialties do participate in ERAS. The percentage may be less for some fellowships. **Note**: Just because a program participates in ERAS does not mean that it also matches through the NRMP! A list of the specialties and programs participating in ERAS is posted on the ERAS website (www.aamc.org/students/eras/start.htm). *Then, check with each individual program (usually on its website) to see if that program accepts applications through ERAS.*

You cannot apply to non-participating programs using ERAS! For programs that do not use ERAS, you need to obtain paper applications. Their contact information is available online, in *FREIDA*, or in the Green Book. *It is the applicant's responsibility to verify with each residency program to which he or she is applying that the program is participating in ERAS.* You can check this on their website or by writing or calling the program.

Ophthalmology is the sole major M.D. specialty still not using ERAS. Instead, it uses the Centralized Application Service (CAS). Many fellowships (taken after initial residency training) also require applicants to apply directly to their programs.

Figure 13.2
M.D. Specialties Using ERAS, 2013

Anesthesiology	Pathology
Child Neurology (Neurology)	Pediatrics
Dermatology	Pediatrics/Anesthesiology
Emergency Med	Pediatrics/Dermatology
Emergency Med/Family Med	Pediatrics/Emergency Med
Family Medicine	Pediatrics/Medical Genetics
Family Med/Preventive Med	Pediatrics/Physical Med & Rehab
Internal Medicine	Pediatrics/Psychiatry/Child & Adolescent Psych
Internal Med/Dermatology	Physical Med & Rehabilitation (Physiatry)
Internal Med/Emergency Med	Plastic Surgery (PGY-1 positions)
Internal Med/Family Med	Plastic Surgery (Integrated)
Internal Med/Medical Genetics	Preventive Med (Public Health, General, Occupational, & Aerospace)
Internal Med/Neurology	Psychiatry
Internal Med/Pediatrics	Psychiatry/Family Practice
Internal Med/Physical Med & Rehab	Psychiatry/Neurology
Internal Med/Preventive Med	Radiation Oncology
Internal Med/Psychiatry	Radiology, Diagnostic
Neurodevelopmental Disabilities (Neurology)	Surgery, General
Neurological Surgery	Thoracic Surgery (Integrated)
Neurology	Transitional Year
Nuclear Medicine	Urology
Obstetrics & Gynecology	Vascular Surgery (Integrated)
Orthopaedic Surgery	All Army & Navy PGY-1 positions
Otolaryngology	

Components

The ERAS is comprised of four elements: the Dean's Office Workstation (DWS), the MyERAS website (which includes the Applicant Data Tracking System [ADTS]), the ERAS PostOffice, and the Program Director's Workstation (PDWS).

The *Dean's Office Workstation (DWS)* is software that your Dean's office uses to give you your initial password, anachronistically called an "electronic token." This "electronic token" allows you to enter the MyERAS website. The DWS is also used when your recommendation letters, photograph, MSPE/Dean's

Figure 13.3
D.O. Specialties Using ERAS, 2013

Anesthesiology	Neuromuscular Medicine & OMT
Dermatology (OGME-2)	Obstetrics & Gynecology
Diagnostic Radiology	Ophthalmology
Emergency Medicine	Orthopedic Surgery
Family Practice	Osteopathic Internship
Family Practice/Emergency Med	Otolaryngology & Facial Plastic Surgery
General Surgery	Pediatrics
Integrated Family Practice/NMM	Physical Med & Rehabilitation
Internal Medicine	Proctologic Surgery
Internal Med/Emergency Med	Psychiatry
Internal Med/Pediatrics	Public Health & Preventive Med (OGME-2)
Neurological Surgery	Traditional (Rotating Internships)
Neurology	Urological Surgery

letter, USMLE or COMLEX scores, and medical school transcript are scanned before they are transmitted to the ERAS PostOffice. (Note that, beginning in 2013, all USMLE/COMLEX scores will be sent directly to programs; you do not need to submit them again.) Each Dean's office (or the ECFMG for IMGs) has their own schedule for receiving and transmitting materials. Their built-in delays and your tardiness may make you miss some programs' application deadlines (they are all different). *It is your responsibility to know the schedule for your Dean's office, as well as the requirements and deadlines for each program to which you apply!*

The *MyERAS website* (http://services.aamc.org/eras/myeras) is your primary connection to the system. After you get your "electronic token" from your Dean's office, you can use this site to register for ERAS, receive your AAMC ID, and designate an ERAS password. (If you lose your password, go the MyERAS page and click "Forgot My Password." You should receive a copy of your password via e-mail in no more than two hours.) Once logged on, you can access virtually all the necessary parts of the system from any computer with Internet access. *MyERAS* is where you complete your online residency application, create and enter your personal statement, select the residency programs to which you want to apply, and specify which materials each of those programs will receive. Until you register, however, the Dean's office cannot submit any of your materials to ERAS.

Figure 13.4
M.D. Fellowships Using ERAS, 2013

Adolescent Med (Ped)	Oncology (IM)
Allergy and Immunology	Pediatric Cardiology (Ped)
Cardiovascular Disease (IM)	Pediatric Critical Care Med (Ped)
Colon and Rectal Surgery	Pediatric Emergency Med (EM)
Critical Care Medicine (IM)	Pediatric Emergency Med (Ped)
Endocrinology, Diabetes, & Metabolism (IM)	Pediatric Endocrinology (Ped)
Female Pelvic Med & Reconstructive Surgery	Pediatric Gastroenterology (Ped)
Gastroenterology (IM)	Pediatric Hematology/Oncology (Ped)
Geriatric Medicine (FP)	Pediatric Infectious Diseases (Ped)
Geriatric Medicine (IM)	Pediatric Nephrology (Ped)
Gynecologic Oncology	Pediatric Pulmonology (Ped)
Hematology (IM)	Pediatric Rheumatology (Ped)
Hematology & Oncology (IM)	Pediatric Surgery (GS)
Hospice & Palliative Medicine	Pulmonary Disease (IM)
Infectious Diseases (IM)	Pulmonary Disease & Critical Care Med (IM)
Interventional Cardiology (IM)	Rheumatology (IM)
Maternal-Fetal Medicine	Sleep Medicine
Medical Genetics	Thoracic Surgery
Neonatal-Perinatal Med (Ped)	Vascular Surgery (GS)
Nephrology (IM)	

The **ERAS PostOffice** is the computer network at the AAMC to which your application materials are sent. From there, they are forwarded to the designated residency programs. Using the *Program Director's Workstation [PDWS]*, residency programs download, collect, sort, review and evaluate these documents, and then rank the applications. Applicants can find out when their Dean's office uploaded their documents and when each residency program downloaded each document by accessing the *Applicant Data Tracking System (ADTS)*.

Registration
U.S. M.D. medical students/graduates. Applicants receive MyERAS electronic tokens (passwords) from their school's Dean of Student's office beginning in mid- to late June. This allows them to register for and access the MyERAS website starting on July 1. Each school establishes its own procedures for

distributing MyERAS electronic tokens and for processing ERAS applications and other materials.

Osteopathic students/graduates should be able to get this material from their Dean. D.O.s also need their NBOME ID number. Applicants can apply for Osteopathic programs starting on July 1; applications for allopathic programs will not be accepted until September 15. **Canadian students** should follow the directions from their Dean of Students, since they will usually apply via the Canadian Resident Matching Service (CaRMS). **Military applicants** should contact their military counselor for any special instructions, since the Military Match is in December, prior to both the Osteopathic Match (February) and the NRMP Match (March).

ERAS and International Medical Students/Graduates

To participate in ERAS, IMGs request their MyERAS electronic token (a 14-digit alpha-numeric code) from the ECFMG's On-line Applicant Status and Information System (OASIS) at https://oasis2.ecfmg.org/. The fee ($100 in 2012) is non-refundable and must be paid prior to receiving the electronic token. This fee includes transmission of the ECFMG Status Report, which lists your passing score(s) on any tests administered through the ECFMG, to all residencies to which you apply. The ECFMG will accept ERAS applications only from individuals who have an eight-digit USMLE/ECFMG Identification Number. This number is given to individuals when they apply to take their first examination through the ECFMG. (**Note** that the token is for *residency* applications only; fellowship tokens are obtained from the ERAS Fellowships Documents Office.)

Once you have your electronic token (password), you can go to MyERAS to register. After you have received your AAMC ID number through MyERAS, download the ERAS Document Submission Form (DSF), which can be completed and printed online using OASIS. Submit it with your documents to ensure direct delivery to the ECFMG's ERAS Department. Be sure to identify each of your documents with your AAMC ID or USMLE/ECFMG Identification Number and the document type (e.g., 0-123-457-6, MSPE/Dean's letter, page 1). Write this identifying information on the *back* of your color photograph. After the ECFMG gets your MSPE, color photograph, medical school transcript, and letters of recommendation (LoRs), they will scan them into your file. Some LoRs can now be entered directly using the ERAS LoR Portal. Also, your ECFMG certification status will now be automatically transmitted to ERAS.

Your LoRs and MSPEs must be original documents, manually signed in ink by the letter writer. If your original medical school documents are not written in English, send only a high-quality copy of the translation. Be prepared to show program directors both the original language documents and the translator's certificate at your interviews. Keep copies of all documents you send. Documents that the ECFMG submits to ERAS are stamped "Duplicate for ERAS use" and are shredded after they are scanned. Be sure to keep copies to use during the "scramble," in the event that you don't get a position in the Match. The ECFMG has a "Return of Document Service" (RODS) that will send requested documents back to the applicant for $25 per ERAS application year, plus shipping costs if it is being sent internationally or via a method other than the U.S. Mail. They will not return LoRs for which the applicant has opted to waive his or her right to view the letter. You must make RODS requests through OASIS.

If you use the ERAS system the following year as well, you are a Repeat Applicant, and thus may reuse your MSPEs, medical school transcript, photograph, or LoRs. As of 2011, however, only those LoRs that were transmitted in the previous year through the ERAS PostOffice can be reused. You will have an opportunity to choose previous LoRs from a list after you receive your token through OASIS; once you save your selections, you cannot go back to the list, but must resubmit any LoR you did not save through ERAS Support Services.

Note: *All IMGs must obtain ECFMG Certification before starting a post-graduate training program.* For questions about IMG applications through ERAS that are not answered on the website, contact: eras-support@ecfmg.org. The ECFMG also sends out a free e-newsletter, *ECFMG-ERAS News*, with updates that can be accessed or subscribed to at www.ecfmg.org/eras/erasnews.html. Technical questions about ERAS should be sent to the AAMC's website (www.aamc.org/eras).

Submitting Your Profile and Application

After you obtain your ID and password, you are ready to create your personal "Profile." This contains your basic information, including contact information, social security number, NRMP Applicant Code, USMLE ID, and AOA (honorary) status. IMGs list their visa type and ECFMG Certification status. For residencies, IMGs apply through the ECFMG's "OASIS" (see Chapter 15). This information can be entered piecemeal at any time during the application process. It *should be updated* with revised information, such as new phone numbers/addresses, AOA (honorary) induction, or changes in your visa status.

Once your contact information is entered, you can click on "My Application" at the MyERAS page to begin completing your "Common Application Form" (CAF). The information in your CAF is used to compile a standard résumé that is sent to program directors. This ensures that each residency program receives a résumé that contains the same information, displayed in exactly the same way, from each applicant.

Most applicants suggest that you print out the "MyERAS Application Worksheet (CAF)," fill it in off-line and check it for accuracy. This will make it much easier to complete your online CAF. Check all information carefully *before* you "certify" your CAF; once you certify it and submit it to the ERAS PostOffice for processing, it cannot be changed.

IMGs may indicate on their CAF that their medical school might not provide a MSPE/Dean's letter or a transcript to the ECFMG.

Supporting Documents

The "My Documents" area of ERAS is used to create personal statements and a list of recommendation letter writers, and also to authorize the transmission of USMLE transcripts.

ERAS Personal Statement

Formatting the personal statement in ERAS can be tricky. Since the ERAS program only accepts basic computer formatting (ASCII text), any special fonts, characters, or formatting (such as italics, bold, apostrophes, quotation marks, and hard returns) will be deleted and often cause strange characters to appear in your ERAS personal statement. Many residency directors have received personal statements containing random letters and characters, truncated sentences, or one-word lines.

To produce the best-looking ERAS personal statement, first create it using a text editor (.txt). The AAMC recommends using Microsoft "Notepad." Those with Office or Windows usually can access it on the "Start" menu or in the list of programs under "Accessories." It allows you to select a font, but little else. Also, the program does not check spelling or grammar—both vital components in producing a professional document. So, you may want to use a word processor. If you do, save it as a "plain text," "text-only," or an "ASCII text format" file. (The file name will appear with the extension ".txt".) Only after performing this step should you cut and paste the document into your ERAS application. An alternative is to type your personal statement directly into ERAS—that is a bad move.

If you produce more than one personal statement, give each one a unique title so you can remember which one accompanies a particular application. (The programs cannot see these titles.) This is particularly important if you are applying to more than one specialty or have different information you need to supply to different programs.

Once a personal statement has been transmitted to a program, it cannot be edited. If you later find typos or need to make corrections, you should create another personal statement with a different title. This new document can then be "assigned" to any program to which you apply. The old one can be "de-assigned," although the program may already have downloaded and printed a hard copy of your original document. Using the "Program Selection Report" (from "My Reports" or "My Programs"), applicants can see a list of the programs and which personal statement has been assigned to each.

ERAS gives you the opportunity to write a very long (up to 28,000 characters, or about eight pages) personal statement. Don't do this. *Limit your statement to one page.* While this may be difficult to do, no one wants to read more than one page from any applicant. If a program requires specific information that is not included in your transcript, CAF, or other materials, attach it as an addendum to the personal statement you send them. IMGs may want to add specific information about their visa, Fifth Pathway, or ECFMG Certificate status. IMGs should also explain the absence of a transcript if their school will not supply one.

Since ERAS does not have a separate place for a résumé that you generate, if you wish to include one, attach this file to the end of each personal statement. Many residency directors, however, specifically request that a separate résumé not be included on ERAS, since they feel that the ERAS application contains all relevant information.

When you have finished putting a personal statement onto ERAS, print a copy for yourself using the "Print Personal Statement" button in MyERAS. If you need additional help understanding the instructions, go to www.aamc.org/students/eras/support/ by clicking the heading "My Documents." Or see one of the short instructional videos listed at www.aamc.org/students/eras/resources/start.htm.

Note that ERAS and the AAMC look askance at plagiarism, whether it is from another applicant or a website. If discovered, they say that they will notify all residency programs to which you have applied. Consider yourself warned.

Letters of Recommendation

Beginning with the 2013 season, most letters of recommendation (LoRs) can be uploaded directly to the Web, using the new **ERAS LoR Portal**. You need to deliver or send a request to all the people you want to write LoRs on your behalf. To do this, you must enter their names in the section labeled "Letters of Recommendation." Even though the system will accept only *four* letters for each program, you do not need to limit the number of names you enter. After all, you may want to send different letters to different programs. The Dean's letter and transcript do *not* count as one of your four letters.

After you have entered all the names, you must finalize the LoRs in MyERAS. The system will then generate a unique Letter Request form for each author; print it out and give it to them. This form provides instructions to the authors, including how to submit LoRs via the ERAS LoR Portal or by mail. Be certain that you neatly fill in your identifying information on the form, if needed. These letters must be typed, so that they can be uploaded or scanned easily. All letters should be addressed to "Dear Program Director." The remainder of the format is up to the writer. Letter writers must return *both* their recommendation letter and the cover sheet you sent them as specified in their Letter Request Form. These letters must *not* go directly to programs participating in ERAS.

As with all recommendation letters, if they don't quickly appear in your Dean's office or on the ADTS list as being sent, check with the letter writer to see if he or she has returned it.

IMGs applying to California programs also need to submit a copy of the "Postgraduate Training Authorization Letter," often called the "California Letter," issued by the Medical Board of California (www.mbc.ca.gov/applicant/application_international.pdf). Getting this letter requires a separate application and fee. Obtaining the letter takes several months. List "California Letter" as one of your recommendation letters. If you do not yet have the "final letter" from California, submit the temporary document they send you. When you receive the final document, send it to the ECFMG with a note attached saying that it replaces the temporary document.

ERAS has a Letter Request Form for IMGs and special instructions for preparing a reference letter that you can download from its website. IMGs should make good photocopies of their recommendation letters to send to the ECFMG. Note that the ECFMG stamps every document with "Duplicate for ERAS use" before scanning it into ERAS. This notifies the programs that the ECFMG cannot verify whether the document came from the applicant, the letter writer, or directly from the medical school.

Fifth Pathway graduates (the program has been discontinued) should send their Certificate as one of their recommendation letters.

Résumé

ERAS will not easily accommodate a personalized résumé in the system, but will generate one based on the information you provide in the CAF. If you want programs to receive your personalized résumé, you must mail it to them, take a copy with you to the interview, or send it through ERAS as part of the Personal Statement or in place of a recommendation letter. (You can only do this if the program doesn't require that you send four letters, the maximum ERAS allows for each program.) However, sending it via ERAS is probably unnecessary unless you have a detailed history that ERAS information doesn't accurately reflect.

Photograph

While no longer required, a full-front view photograph is recommended "if you want your application to be complete." The photograph, which programs use as a visual aid, cannot be viewed by a program until you have been selected for an interview. You will probably be at a disadvantage if you fail to supply your Dean's office with a 2.5- by 3.5-inch (wallet size) color photo, with your ID number written on the back, for the application. The same requirements apply to digital photographs, which should be in the ".jpg" format. For more information on your photograph, see "A Picture?" later in this chapter.

Transcript & Dean's Letter/Medical Student Performance Evaluation (MSPE)

Your Dean's office will automatically send transcripts and the Dean's letter, which has been renamed the Medical Student Performance Evaluation (MSPE) to reflect its role as an evaluation rather than a recommendation, to ERAS for all registered residency applicants. These will be sent to all programs to which you apply: programs can download transcripts as they are posted. MSPEs/ Dean's letters for all applicants to ACGME-accredited programs are released by the ERAS PostOffice on October 1. MSPEs/Dean's letters for all applicants to Osteopathic internships are released on October 15.

International medical students/graduates must send a copy of their transcript and MSPE/ Dean's letter to the ECFMG. If these cannot be sent, either because your school does not produce them or because they are unavailable, indicate that on your CAF in the appropriate box. (At some non-U.S. schools, transcripts may be called mark sheets, time sheets, or hour sheets.) The documents must be no larger than approximately 8.5 inches by 14 inches (21 cm by 35 cm) so they will fit into the scanner. Also, the ECFMG will scan only about five pages. If your transcript is longer, number the pages according to their order of importance and they will scan them in that order. Send copies made on paper with a plain background. If they are on "security paper" with a background designed to make forgery difficult, the scanned image may be unreadable.

Add Programs

At "Programs," you can choose between "Selected Programs" and "Applied to Programs." *Selected Programs* are those that you have reviewed, selected, and are currently assigning documents to, but that have not yet been sent your application. You can add or remove programs in the "Selected" area at any time. You can select, but not apply to, programs before you submit your CAF.

Applied to Programs are programs to which you have sent your application. Before you send materials to a program, be certain that you want to apply there—and that they participate in ERAS. Once you click on this area, an invoice appears. Your final bill reflects the number of programs to which you apply. Check it carefully, because fees paid to ERAS are not refundable!

While reviewing the lists of residency programs on ERAS, those that are "grayed out" do not participate and cannot be selected. Applicants must apply directly to those programs, as well as to those in non-participating specialties. Some programs may be listed even though they do not participate in ERAS. It is *your responsibility* to ascertain whether a program is currently an ERAS participant.

When you click on "Transmit," your application materials are immediately sent to your "Selected" programs. Once you do this, your "Selected" programs become "Applied to" programs and cannot be removed. Your Dean's office receives a list of these programs and, according to their own schedule, also sends their information to the programs. If you wish, you can add programs to the "Applied to" category at a later date. If you have paid for more programs than the number to which you have actually applied (see Cost, below), there is no additional fee to add programs later.

Osteopathic graduates can use the Program tab to search for and select Osteopathic internships by location and by type.

Assign Documents

The identical CAF, MSPE/Dean's letter, transcript, and photo will be sent to each program you apply to, but you can vary the recommendation letters and personal statements that will be sent. You can also decide whether a USMLE and/or COMLEX transcript is sent.

A maximum of four recommendation letters can be sent to any one residency program. If there is a letter writer who might help you more in one program than in another (for example, if you are applying in more than one specialty), be sure to assign their LoRs to the appropriate programs. The same holds true for personal statements. You may want to individualize the statements for different programs based on their apparent interests, specialty, region of the country, etc. Some programs may also want specific information from applicants; the personal statement is where you can add it.

Once you press "Save," the LoRs and personal statement assigned to a program are sent and you cannot change those specific documents. If you need to do so, you can de-assign the original document and assign a new one in its place. Remember, however, that the program may already have downloaded a copy of the original document and put it in your file. If so they will have both the original and the new documents. (If you reassign documents that have not already been sent to them, they will not know.) Once a USMLE and/or COMLEX transcript is sent to a program, it cannot be de-assigned.

Applicant Data Tracking System (ADTS)

Use your ERAS ID number and password to access the ADTS through MyERAS to make sure your documents have been sent through the ERAS PostOffice. The ADTS report lists each program to which you applied, when your Dean's office uploaded your documents, and when each residency program downloaded each document. Your Dean's office also has access to ADTS, although residency programs do not.

Questions

MyERAS has a detailed "Help" section that is available when you log on. For further information, go to the AAMC's ERAS web page (www.aamc.org/students/eras/) and click on "Using MyERAS" for a breakdown of the process, or download the ERAS annual *Applicant Manual* under "Resources to Download." The support page also contains a path to breaking news about ERAS, which you can access by clicking on "Alerts."

If you can't find answers to technical questions, e-mail the ERAS support staff at myeras@aamc.org or call 202-862-6264 (8 A.M. to 6 P.M. EST Mon-Fri). For faster service, include your name, AAMC ID, designated Dean's Office, and return e-mail address. For the best response, include the exact wording of error messages (cut and paste, if possible), information about the type of computer being used (manufacturer, processor, amount of RAM, available hard disk space), the operating system (e.g., Windows XP, Windows 7), the Web browser you are using (e.g., Internet Explorer) and version number, and your ISP (e.g., Verizon, Comcast). International medical students and graduates can also send technical questions to the above address, but procedural problems should be sent to the ECFMG at eras-support@ecfmg.org. There is a useful FAQ page about ERAS on the ECFMG website at www.ecfmg.org/eras/index.html#15.

Computer Requirements

You do not need to own a computer, but you do need access to one that has 32 MB RAM and an Internet connection with at least a 56 kbps modem or network connection. The machine should have Internet Explorer 7.0, Firefox 8.0, or a later version of one of these browsers.

You also need a personal e-mail address to receive communications from residency directors, your Dean's office, ERAS (such as if you lose your password), and, for IMGs, from the ECFMG. You will need to check your electronic mailbox, including your "bulk mail" folder, frequently. Many program directors use e-mail to ask additional questions and to offer interview slots to applicants. Individuals who use any of the free e-mail accounts must remove *all* their spam and junk-mail filters.

Also, if you learn that most residency programs have downloaded your ERAS materials but you haven't heard from any of them, you may want to check to see if you received messages that your computer (or your ISP's computer system) rejected as "spam."

Cost

ERAS creates a "Processing Fee Invoice." Print this invoice only *after* you are ready to submit your application materials to programs, since the fee partly depends on the number of residencies to which you apply. *Once you pay your money, ERAS does not give refunds.*

U.S./Canadian medical students/graduates: For the 2013 cycle, the ERAS fee for medical students and graduates from U.S./Canadian schools was $92, which includes sending applications to up to 10 programs in a single specialty. Applying to between 11 and 20 programs costs $9 for each additional program, the next ten cost $15 each, and, if you apply to more than 30 programs, each additional application costs $25. If you apply to programs in more than one specialty or for both ACGME-accredited (M.D.) and AOA-accredited (D.O.) programs in the same specialty, you must pay an additional $92 plus the costs if you apply to more than 10 programs in either group. (When applying to military programs in multiple specialties, they count as applying to only one specialty, and cost $92 for up to 10 applications. Simultaneous civilian-program applications incur the standard separate fee.)

For example, 20 Emergency Medicine programs and 5 Preliminary Internal Medicine programs will cost $274 (Emergency Medicine = $92 + ($9x10); Internal Medicine = $92). If an Osteopathic student applies to 6 ACGME-accredited and 12 AOA-accredited Internal Medicine programs, it will cost her $202 (ACGME-accredited programs = $92; AOA-accredited programs = $92 + $18). Most students elect to have ERAS send all their USMLE or COMLEX (NBOME) transcripts to programs for a single $70 fee.

International medical students/graduates: Before they can register with ERAS, IMGs must pay an extra (and separate) $90 fee for the ECFMG to act as their "designated Dean's office." After they receive your money, the ECFMG will send your ERAS electronic token by e-mail, scan and transmit your supporting documents, and transmit your ECFMG Status Report. To complete the application process, you must also later pay the ERAS application fees (minimum $92), the fee for your detailed USMLE score report ($70 for an ECFMG-provided transcript), and the NRMP registration fee.

For those who are arithmetically challenged, ERAS automatically computes the fees. The fees can be paid only with a VISA or MasterCard credit card; ERAS no longer accepts checks. You can also print out the invoice and send the credit card information to the address on the invoice. Once the Dean's office transmits your file to the ERAS PostOffice via the Internet, all fees detailed on the invoice must be paid within two weeks to avoid canceling your application. ERAS never gives refunds, even if a program to which you've applied has withdrawn from their system.

Deadlines

Each residency program has its own deadline for receiving application information. Be certain that you know these deadlines and have your materials to ERAS before they are due. Once materials are in the ERAS PostOffice, they are normally sent to the programs within hours. Your Dean's office may take a bit longer to enter your reference letters and transcript into the system.

Transmitting & Receiving Information

Individual programs, rather than ERAS, set residency application deadlines. However, the ERAS PostOffice usually opens on September 15 and transmits new applications daily. All Osteopathic Deans' letters/MSPEs that have been received are transmitted on October 15; those from M.D. schools are released on October 1.

Get your photograph to your Dean's office as soon as possible so that it can be transmitted. Likewise, ask your letter writers to submit their LoRs promptly. As the application season progresses, the folks responsible for submitting your information may get swamped. The ERAS system also reportedly gets a bit slower with masses of application materials coming and going. If you have completed your online application as soon as possible, submitted your photograph, and had your recommendation letters submitted early, you should have rapid and smooth sailing. Even if there are glitches, they can be more easily fixed when both your school's ERAS staff and the folks at the AAMC have more time to work on them.

Dean's offices receive a confirmation that the application materials they send have been received. To learn when your application was transmitted to the ERAS PostOffice and the date each residency program downloaded your file, go to the Applicant Document Tracking System (ADTS). Like the ERAS PostOffice, it begins operating at the same time each year (usually September 15). If a program has delayed downloading your ERAS application, contact them directly to learn why.

The Résumé

Your résumé, also known as a *curriculum vitae* or *c.v.,* is a word picture of yourself. Writing it helps you to put your accomplishments "on paper" and identify activities needed to advance in your specialty. Once you have your résumé, you will update and use it throughout your professional career. You should provide a copy to:

- Individuals who will write your reference letters.

- Outside programs at which you want to do electives.

- Programs where you must mail or fax your application.

Try to tailor the information you provide to the specialty for which you are applying. For example, extracurricular activities and community service may be less important to program directors in Surgery than to those in Family Medicine.

While a good résumé will not guarantee that you get into a residency, a poor résumé will certainly eliminate you from consideration. For more detailed information, see also *Résumés and Personal Statements for Health Professionals,* 2nd ed., by James W. Tysinger, Ph.D. (Galen Press, Ltd.).

Misrepresentations

Only include true information in your résumé and personal statement. About 20% of residency applicants, and many more fellowship applicants, who list publications either falsely claim authorship on a real paper or list non-existent papers. One study, for example, showed that nearly one-third of Gastroenterology fellowship applicants misrepresented their academic accomplishments. Others have found similar distortions among Surgery, Psychiatry, Emergency Medicine, and Radiology applicants. Residency directors know this. Programs can (and do) easily use computer searches to check listed publications. Such "misrepresentations" are often unintentional, and can occur when, for example, a faculty member with whom you conducted research tells you "Our study was published, and I recognized your contributions." In fact, the faculty member may have acknowledged you in a footnote and not on the author line. Consequently, it is dangerous for applicants to list any activity unless they can verify it with original documents.

Sometimes applicants misstate their manuscript's status because they do not know how to properly cite it. The Council of Residency Directors (Emergency Medicine) suggests the following guidelines:

1. Published manuscript: give full citation.

2. Accepted manuscripts (in press): list acceptance date, and bring the acceptance letter to your interviews.

3. Submitted manuscripts: list submission date.

4. Research experience (or manuscript in progress): list research title/ hypothesis, time period for the research, and research mentors.

Take a copy of all published works, acceptance letters, submitted articles with the submission letter, and letters from research mentors listing research dates to all your interviews. For presented papers, take a copy of the published abstract or, even better, a copy of the meeting's program.

"Headhunters" (recruiters) estimate that about one-third of résumés include lies. Many applicants think that they will be forgiven for embellishing their résumé. At least for residency applicants, forgiveness is rarely granted, and doctors' résumés are part of a paper trail that follows them wherever they go. Aside from any moral question, lying on application materials may result in not getting your desired residency position. If discovered during your training, that lie puts you at risk for immediate dismissal.

A few people each year try to enter residencies despite never having graduated from medical school; some succeed. Because of the notoriety given such cases, residency programs and state medical boards increasingly check on applicants using databanks run by the Federation of State Medical Boards, the American Medical Association, the ECFMG, and the AAMC.

Résumé Layout

Those using ERAS will have their résumé information entered in a generic style. However, you can also provide programs and LoR writers with your own more-detailed and personalized résumé. Those not using ERAS must provide programs with a résumé.

When compiling your résumé, there are several rules to follow, and several pitfalls (Figures 13.5 and 13.8) to avoid:

1. **Emphasize your strengths.** Write the résumé so these aspects of your past are prominent.

2. **Be clear, concise, and accurate.** Unless you are extraordinary, one, or at most two, pages will suffice.

3. **Design your résumé to be pleasant to the eye,** clean, and unclut-
   tered. (See "Résumé Graphics," below.)

4. **Use action words** (Figure 13.6) wherever possible. As Mark Twain
   said, the difference between the right word and the almost-right word
   is the difference between lightning and a lightning bug.

5. **Follow the standard layout** recommended in the checklist in Figure
   13.7. Use the examples (Figures 13.9, 13.10, and 13.11) when you
   design your own résumé. These examples are chronological résumés.
   This is the type preferred by most residency directors.

6. **Print it on an inkjet or laser printer** that doesn't leave unsightly
   smudges.

7. **Do not put "Résumé" or "Curriculum Vitae" at the top** of the document unless you think that those reading it are idiots. Résumé formats
   are immediately obvious, and these words waste valuable space.

Some experts recommend that your first résumé is most easily organized
using 3- x 5-inch cards (or their computer equivalent). Simply label one card
for each of the topics in Figure 13.7 that applies to you. Then collect the
information on each card (including names, dates, addresses, etc.) that you
will need to complete the section. Put these cards in the order you want to see
them on your résumé, and type the information onto your résumé.

After printing a sample copy, check it carefully for spelling errors. One
medical student wrote, for example, "I am passed USMLE . . ." and "I would
like to know weather . . .." As you might expect, he had a difficult time getting
a position. Even if you are a native English speaker, have a literate person
proofread your materials before you send them.

Figure 13.5
Résumé Disaster Areas

- Poor organization
- Poor grammar
- Handwritten
- Poor photocopy
- Exaggerations
- Lack of name, address,
  telephone number

- Narrative, rather than outline
- Misspellings of any kind
- Unexplained time periods
- Unnecessary information
- More than two pages
- Insufficient information

Figure 13.6
Action Words for Your Résumé

accelerated	developed	introduced	recorded
accomplished	directed	invented	reorganized
achieved	discovered	launched	replaced
active member	distributed	led	represented
actively	edited	made	researched
adapted	effected	maintained	responsible for
adjusted	elected	managed	restored
administered	enlarged	modified	revised
advised	established	monitored	scheduled
analyzed	examined	motivated	selected
arranged	excelled	negotiated	served
assisted	expanded	obtained	set up
awarded	experienced in	operated	sold
built	focused	organized	solved
chairperson	formulated	participated in	streamlined
charted	founded	performed	strengthened
compiled	generated	persuaded	studied
completed	guided	planned	successfully
conceived	headed	prepared	supervised
conducted	identified	presented	supplied
constructed	implemented	produced	taught
controlled	improved	proficient at	tested
coordinated	increased	programmed	trained
counseled	influenced	promoted to	translated
created	initiated	proposed	unleashed
delivered	installed	provided	updated
demonstrated	instituted	published	won
designed	instructed	ran	wrote
determined	interpreted		

Only then should you decide on the graphic presentation you want. Once again, ask someone who knows you well to review it to be certain that you have portrayed yourself in the best possible manner. Figures 13.8 to 13.10 demonstrate some positive and negative examples. There is no perfect résumé style.

After further revisions, get some objective feedback, preferably from your adviser, your mentor, or the Dean of Students. If that is not possible, get someone to look at it who has experience with resident applicant résumés.

Figure 13.7
A Résumé Checklist

❏ Name[1]   ❏ Extracurricular Activities[3]
❏ Address(es)   ❏ Personal[3]
❏ Telephone Number(s)[2]   ❏ Birth Place & Date
❏ Objective   ❏ Marital Status
❏ Publications   ❏ Children
❏ Research   ❏ Work Experience[4]
❏ Presentations   ❏ Licenses & Certifications[5]
❏ Language/Computer Skills   ❏ Military[6]
❏ Honors & Awards   ❏ Education[7]
❏ Reference Statement   ❏ Medical School
❏ Applicable Jobs   ❏ Grad School
❏ Professional Memberships   ❏ Undergraduate

1. If you have changed your name, be certain that there is a clear statement explaining why your name differs on your transcript, licenses, diplomas, etc. If at all possible, it is best to keep one "professional name" throughout your career, even if you plan on changing your name in a social context.

2. Include all mailing addresses, telephone numbers, and e-mail addresses where you can be reached for the next six months.

3. Optional information. Include extracurricular activities only if they are extraordinary or applicable to medicine, such as working in a hospital, in a medical or research laboratory, with the Ski Patrol or a volunteer ambulance service. Personal information can be supplied at your own discretion.

4. Include the dates that you held jobs. Other than military service, include only those jobs that you held for long periods of time, were applicable to medicine, or were full-time positions.

5. List currently held health-related licenses, such as R.N. (give states and dates), and health-related certifications, such as EMT, ACLS, ATLS, and PALS (give expiration dates).

6. The type of discharge that you received is legally privileged information. If it was anything less than honorable, don't include it.

7. Only include undergraduate and graduate school, medical school, and any other medically related course. You have been out of high school a long time now, and no one is interested in that.

Figure 13.8
Sample Résumé, The Disaster

Don't you have a first name?

Isn't it obvious that this is your C.V.?

CURRICULUM VITAE

I. R. Smarte   *Phone/Fax/Cell phone numbers? E-mail address?*
405 Campbell Ave. Washinton, DC 20043 *← Dates at this address?*

Irrelevant in all circumstances

Citizenship: USA *← Assumed, unless otherwise stated*
Birthdate: October 27, 1967
    ← Who cares?
Spouse's name: Les Smarte, I.R.S. Agent *← This will really win points!*
Child: Matthew, age 4
Family:Mother: Helen S. Dingle, age 71, retired
       Sister: Jean Folks, age 45, Prof. Poly Sci

Undergraduate education: Univ. Of Arizona, 1993
    B.S. in Cell Biology   *Spelling!*
    Honors: Phi Beta Kappa, Cum Laud Graduate.
    Extracurricular Activities: Pep Squad,
       Marching Band, Biology Honorary, *← Which one?*
       Rescue Squad *← Which? Where?* *Written corrections are sloppy!*
                    Spelling!   *When?* 1997

Include only if your transcript is difficult to interpret

Post graduate ed: Univ. Of Cinti., 1987 Toxicology
    Honors: Munroe Scholarship *← What is this?*
    Research/Publications: ``The Effect of a Sub-
    freezing Environment on Cellular Metabolism   *When & where were these published?*
    in Rats.'' (Thesis); Simons, G., Smarte, I.R.,
    Sullivan, J.P. ``Cellular Inhibition of Rat Tail
    Growth in a Subfreezing Atmosphere.''
                    ← Spell out! *Capitalize!*
Med School-- U of MD, 2001
    Honors: Sherk Scholarship, Ama stud rep
    physiology, social/prventatave med, OB/GYN.
    Electives: forensic sci, experimental sugr lab
                        ← State that job was medically related
Employment: 93/95 US Air Force, Staff Sgt.;
    91-93: carpenter (part-time) *← Irrelevant*

Interests: Radical Student Alliance; Messianic *Irrelevant? Counterproductive*
    Religious Revival
                Spelling!
Why list references?
References: Fr. John X. Anlen: Our Lady of Sorrow, *Priest*
    31 Ensel Street, Baltimore, MD *Zip Code?*
       Michelle Rout, M.D., Radiology Resident, *Resident*
U. of AZ, 1501 N. Campbell Ave., Tucson, AZ 85724
       Sally Friendly: Director, Messianic *Friend*
Student Revival, 1 North St., Reuther, MD 20933

Counterproductive References

✱ *Sloppy! Inconsistent* ✱
Formatting

Figure 13.9
Sample Résumé, Style #1

──────────────── **IRENE R. SMARTE** ────────────────

405 N. Campbell Ave.   5573 Chillum Place, Apt. D
Washington, DC 20043   Reading, PA 19601
(202) 555-9087   (610) 555-1836
[Use: 8/11–10/11 & 4/12–6/12]   [Use: 11/11–3/12]

e-mail: IRSmarte@medstud.net

OBJECTIVE   Superior training in Radiology which will give me the basis from
                       which to practice in either the academic or the private sector for
                       the next forty years.

EDUCATION   M.D., University of Maryland School of Medicine
                           Baltimore, MD
                           Sept. 2008–June 2012 (anticipated)
                       M.S., University of Cincinnati
                           Cincinnati, OH
                           Major: Toxicology
                           July 2006–June 2008
                       B.S., University of Arizona
                           Tucson, AZ
                           Major: Cellular Biology
                           Sept. 2000–June 2004

HONORS/   *Medical School:*   Sherk Scholarship (Most promising student
AWARDS   in the sophomore class)
                                              Class Vice-President: Junior Year
                                              Student Representative, AMA, 2011-2012
                       Graduate School: Munroe Scholarship (2 years)
                       Undergraduate: Phi Beta Kappa
                                              Dann-Victor Scholarship (2 years)
                                              Cum Laude Graduate
                                              President, Biology Honorary, 2003–2004

MILITARY   Staff Sergeant, Medical Service Corps
EXPERIENCE   U.S. Air Force, 2004–2006; Honorable Discharge
                       Responsible for administering a 40-person Radiology
                           department at a regional hospital.

PUBLICATIONS   Simons, G; Smarte, IR; Sullivan, JP: Cellular Inhibition of Rat Tail
                       Growth in a Subfreezing Atmosphere. *Journal of Arctic Biology.*
                       2009;3(1):12-16.

RESEARCH   "The Effect of a Subfreezing Environment on Cellular Metabolism
                       in Rats." (M.S. Thesis) Primary Investigator: Prof. G. Simons, Ph.D.

ACTIVITIES   Member, Wheaton Rescue Squad (Ambulance and Heavy Rescue)

PERSONAL   U.S. Citizen; Excellent Health

REFERENCES   Furnished upon request

Figure 13.10
Sample Résumé, Style #2

This is a slightly different style than the résumé in Figure 13.9 above. Some information has been purposely omitted. Other information has been combined. Two new sections have been added for you to use as an example.

IRENE R. SMARTE

405 N. Campbell Ave.
Washington, DC 20043
(202) 555-9087
e-mail: IRSmarte@medstud.net

OBJECTIVE
Superior training in Radiology which will give me the basis from which to practice in either the academic or the private sector over the span of my career.

EDUCATION
M.D., *University of Maryland School of Medicine*, Baltimore, Maryland
    September 2008–June 2012 (anticipated)
    • Sherk Scholarship (Most promising student in the sophomore class.)
    • Class Vice-President: Junior Year
    • Student Representative, AMA, 2011–2012
M.S., *University of Cincinnati,* Cincinnati, Ohio
    Major: Toxicology, July 2006–June 2008
    • Munroe Scholarship (2 years)
B.S., *University of Arizona,* Tucson, Arizona
    Major: Cellular Biology, September 2000–June 2004
    • Phi Beta Kappa
    • Dann-Victor Scholarship (2 years)
    • *Cum Laude* graduate
    • President, Biology Honorary, 2003–2004

MILITARY EXPERIENCE
Staff Sergeant, Medical Service Corps, U.S. Air Force, 2004–2006; Honorable Discharge
Responsible for administering a 40-person Radiology department at a regional hospital.

RESEARCH & PUBLICATIONS
Simons G, Smarte IR, Sullivan JP: Cellular Inhibition of Rat Tail Growth in a Subfreezing Atmosphere. *Journal of Arctic Biology.* 2009;3(1):12-16.

PROFESSIONAL ORGANIZATIONS
    • American Medical Student Association
    • American College of Radiology, Student Member

LANGUAGES
    • Spanish (Fluent written and spoken)
    • Russian (Written only)

EXTRACURRICULAR ACTIVITIES
    • Member, Wheaton Rescue Squad (Ambulance and Heavy Rescue)

REFERENCES
Furnished upon request

Figure 13.11
Two Other Acceptable Résumé Formats

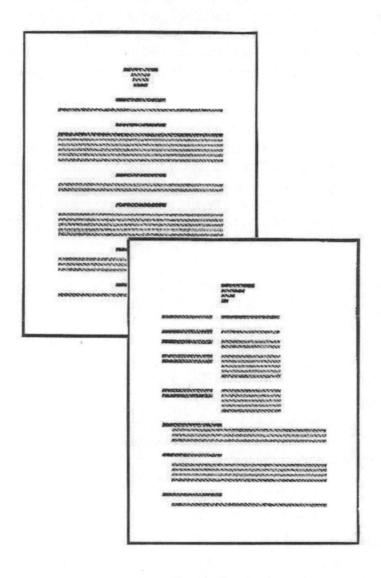

If you just can't get your act together, another option is to pay a commercial service to produce your résumé. You will, however, still have to provide the information, tell them how you want it organized, and proof it for accuracy. (Most of them will proofread it for the spelling of common words.) Résumé services can be found in all large cities, around most universities, and on-line. Their charges vary by location and the amount of work they need to do.

Résumé Graphics

Avoid having a résumé that looks like every other résumé in circulation! Your résumé must have a clean and distinctive appearance. Like all of your written communications, it must attract attention. Essentially, it must be more attractive than the competition. To accomplish this, you must pay attention to the paper size and appearance, margins and spacing, type size and style, and layout. The key to an effective résumé is to plan it carefully, and make sure the final product reflects the planning that went into it.

Paper
Most applicants use white bond paper. Your résumé will stand out if you use something different. Gray, ivory, or white paper with a textured or "pebble" finish will stand out among the throng of résumés. The weight of the paper is also important. Use 20- or 24-pound paper. If you plan to print your résumé on both sides of one sheet of paper, which is actually not a good idea, be sure that the paper is opaque enough so that the printing will not show through.

Paper Size
Again, most of the résumés received by residency directors are on standard 8½" x 11" paper. Several other sizes are available which may serve to help your résumé stand out. The most acceptable is the "Monarch" size of stationary (7¼" x 10½"). Another possibility is using an 11" x 17" sheet, which will fold over into an 8½" x 11" folio. You can then put your name, address, e-mail address, and telephone number on the outside cover.

Margins & Spacing
No matter how good your résumé is, it will look cheap, rushed, and cramped if you do not leave an ample margin. When using a standard 8½" x 11" sheet of paper, leave side margins of 1" to 1½". The space at the top of the page should be at least 1½", and at the bottom at least 1". If you will be using Monarch paper, leave ¾" to 1" margins on either side of the page. A minimum for the top and bottom margins is 1".

Type Size & Style

Type comes in different sizes, known as "points," which designates the number of characters per inch. Either 11- or 12-point is adequate for most résumés, since it is easily readable and available in most printer fonts. Type also differs in height.

Various styles of type (fonts), such as Ariel and Times Roman, are available. Some variety can be added to your résumé by altering these type styles appropriately. This technique is most effective when used for the captions and subheadings. Make sure that all styles are complimentary to those used for the main body of your résumé. Boldface, underlining, italics, and asterisks or bullets (circles) can, if used sparingly, highlight important areas of your résumé. But don't get carried away and use too many font sizes and styles— they just distract the reader!

The Personal Statement

The personal statement that many residency programs request causes more anguish among applicants than almost anything else in the application process. A great deal of time and effort is often put into these epistles—and, in general, it is mostly wasted. Although some program directors (especially those in primary care specialties) carefully read applicants' personal statements, many use personal statements only to eliminate those individuals who clearly stand out as being: (1) relatively illiterate, (2) pompous or tactless, or (3) outside the mainstream of physicians in the specialty or institution.

The key to writing a good personal statement is to *be honest, but not shy* about trumpeting your virtues. If possible, relate an interesting story about yourself that highlights your attributes. Many students find this hard to do. The elements of a "safe and sane" personal statement include:

Section 1: Why do you want to go into the specialty? Briefly explain what has drawn you to the specialty. If there was one particular event that stands out, describe it. Your trait analyses from Chapter 4 may help you out. Do not state that you are interested in the field primarily because of either the monetary rewards you anticipate or the way in which it fits your lifestyle. These reasons are evidence of a shallow personality and a sloppy decision-making process.

Section 2: What do you intend to do during your career in the specialty? Be general. For community hospital programs, it is always safe to say that you are planning on a primarily clinical career with some clinical research and teaching. This question may be difficult to answer in some high-powered academic centers where there is a palpable rift between the researcher–physicians and the physician–occasional researchers. You may want to tailor this part of your personal statement to the institution to which it is being sent, as well as to your particular interests. Do not state, however, that you want to be a small-town practitioner if you are applying to a high-powered research program, or vice versa.

Section 3: Other interests. What else do you do with your time? Be brief. Discussing your family, sports, and community activities is safe. This section of your statement should be the shortest.

Additional points that you may want to address in the statement include explanations of any major problems, deficiencies, or questions that might arise after a review of your application or transcript. You might want to mention something particularly outstanding from your undergraduate career or your life outside school. *Avoid discussing politics or religion.* Neither has any place in any of your application materials. Tysinger's *Résumés and Personal Statements for Health Professionals* (see *Annotated Bibliography*) contains special instructions for addressing these issues, as well as numerous examples of personal statements.

The personal statement format (Figure 13.12) is now constrained by the limitations of ERAS (unless you apply to a specialty or program that does not participate). But you can still make it interesting, and even enjoyable to read. One applicant, for example, had a five-paragraph statement, each paragraph beginning with a key phrase that had been said to her and that related to her specialty of choice (e.g., "Aren't you scared to take care of all those really sick people?"). There are many other interesting ways to write the personal statement. The keys are to make it:

- short enough to read easily
- in readable English without spelling or grammatical errors
- based on one or more stories that illustrate your life
- interesting

As with all other materials you send to programs, review your statement for content and format before you type the final copy. Just as with the résumé, there is no one perfect style.

Occasionally, students ask whether they should try to make their personal statement unusual enough to stand out. Literate and witty are the best ways to make a personal statement get noticed. One applicant, for example, vividly wrote, "Activity is my oxygen." The faculty remembered her!

Figure 13.12
Format for Personal Statement

One page

Product of a clean (no smudges) laser or inkjet printer

Proper grammar, spelling, and composition (Have someone else
    look over your work.)

Generally though, you take a big risk by writing a very unusual personal statement. Remember that physicians, in general, are conservative animals. Anything odd or unusual will ordinarily be viewed negatively. Readers normally define a personal statement as "unusual" if it is cute, flippant, or crass. That is not the impression you want to create. Of course, some applicants have gotten interviews and even positions based, in part, on unusual personal statements. But it is rare. Unless your life story itself is unusual, stick with standard and boring.

Most personal statements will be in simple paragraph format and printed in the ERAS application, which allows little flexibility. Those not using ERAS may want to use an alternative format for their statements. Figures 13.13, 13.14, and 13.15 give examples of a poorly written personal statement, a good statement in a standard format, and a well-done statement in an alternative format.

Reference Letters

The reference letters that you have sent to residency programs are reflections of you in other people's eyes. They play an important part in getting you a residency position. Obtaining good reference letters, however, takes advance planning, hard work, and initiative. If you are willing to make the effort, the steps outlined below will help you to get the best possible reference letters. They will also help you make the most of the ones you do get.

Figure 13.13
Sample Personal Statement, Poor

This poorly written personal statement simply recites facts, in rudimentary English, that are available on the candidate's résumé. He doesn't appear to appreciate General Surgery or his time with the Air Force. He has apparently not learned spelling or grammar. His seemingly misogynist attitude doesn't help, either.

MAXWELL I. SMARTE

My plan is to get into a great residency to help sick kids by becoming a pediatric surgeon. I met one in med school, and he was a great guy. Right then I knew I wanted to be eexactly like him. It will also let me use the OR skills I learned in the USAF.

I desire to enter a surgery program where the faculty can help me get into pediatric surgery. Five years seems like a long time to learn the basics, but I'm willing to do that since it seems to be the only route into the specialty.

My background is pretty typical for Minnesota farm boys. No one expected me to go to college so at 18, I joined the USAF. I was a surgical tech and than OR supervisor. I had 1 tour in Japan, one in Afghanistan, and the rest in the US. Finally, I got out (after 4 years wearing the "blue suit") and entered college on the GI bill. Preferring numbers and ideas too writing, I majored in Chemistry and did real good. I graduated in 3 years.

Med school was pretty easy, given my background. I didn't have to study to hard to score a 212 on USMLE Step 1 and, since its clinical medicine, score 220 on Step 2. I also got honors in surgery and pediatrics, but not in the areas I don't plan to enter. During school I got to work with a woman pediatric surgeon whenever I was not busy. I got to go to the OR and work with her in the ED.

I'm not too interested in doing research, but will do it if necesary. I'd like to teach and work at a teaching hospital when I'm done. Students and residents need good role models, and I think that I'd be a really good one.

I'm planning to get married (again) next summer and have some kids of my own. However, that shouldn't interfere with my training, since my wife will stop her career as a pharmacist to care for them.

Finally, I would like to ask you to consider my application to your general surgery residency so that I can continue along my steady career path towards my worthwhile goal of being a pediatric surgeon.

Thank you.

Figure 13.14
Sample Personal Statement, Good

This personal statement catches the reader's attention immediately with a well written personal anecdote. The candidate expresses clear, reasonable goals and expectations, discusses the reasons for those goals and clearly describes his ultimate career goal, academics. He also acknowledges the importance of General Surgery.

MAXWELL I. SMARTE

As I cradled the infant in my arms, I only hoped that our surgical team could repair the internal damage that an improvised explosive device had done. On an unusually still night in Afghanistan, I was the senior NCO on the surgical team, and was directing my team to rapidly prepare the OR for pediatric surgery while I attempted to comfort the baby. Amazingly, a Pediatric surgeon had been assigned to our unit, although he was really only expected to operate on our adult soldiers. He scrubbed; I agonized. The child, too injured for our help, died before we could begin.

I have no expectation that I can save every child, and certainly could not have saved the child I held that night. But, as I saw throughout both my U.S. Air Force Medical Service and my clinical work in medical school, there are countless children who need the ministrations of an excellent Pediatric surgeon. In addition, medical students and residents need excellent teachers in this surgical specialty. I plan to be one of the few who get the opportunity to both do and teach Pediatric Surgery, most likely through a tertiary academic center.

With a clear goal in mind, it was relatively easy to excel in undergraduate school, and I finished in only three years with a Chemistry degree. Medical school allowed me to combine academics with clinical work. I did very well on the USMLE (Step 1, 212; Step 2, 220) and achieved honors in both Surgery and Pediatrics. For enjoyment and motivation, I spent many evenings working with one of our Pediatric surgeons when she was on call.

Although my ultimate goal is Pediatric Surgery, I recognize that to be great in that field requires an in-depth knowledge of the special skills possessed by General Surgeons. Having worked in the OR and in outpatient surgical settings over many years (since soon after joining the U.S.A.F. and continuing through medical school), I know that I have both the mindset of a surgeon and the necessary technical finesse. What I seek is great teachers and substantive clinical experience.

My hope is that you will consider me for a position in your General Surgery residency program, since I believe that it fits my desire for an excellent educational experience.

Figure 13.15
Alternative Style Personal Statement, Good

MAXWELL I. SMARTE

hard working   I grew up in Minnesota, spending summers on my parents' farm. It was here that I learned the value of hard work.

mature   At age 18, I joined the U.S. Air Force. Rising to the rank of Staff Sergeant, I experienced a period of personal growth. Four years in the service as a surgical technician and OR supervisor, both stateside and in Japan, gave me a more balanced view of life.

academic & clinical skills   After completing undergraduate school in three years with a Chemistry major, I entered medical school, where I scored 212 on Step 1 of the USMLE and achieved Honors in Surgery and in Pediatrics. I spent many evenings working with one of our local Pediatric Surgeons.

career goals   The latter activity convinced me that Pediatric Surgery will provide what I want from a career in medicine— to cure sick children, care for those with both acute and chronic diseases, and be involved in the broadest type of General Surgery.

After residency, I would like to work at a major tertiary care teaching hospital. There I could combine practice, teaching, and research. My choice of residency reflects these long-term goals.

summary   In summary, I am a hard working, mature individual who has a clear vision of a career in Pediatric Surgery. Both my experiences and training have reinforced my dedication to this dynamic and exciting field of medicine.

Sincerely,
Maxwell I. Smarte

Figure 13.16
Information in MSPEs/Dean's Letters

Type of Information	Percent with this information
Discuss student's enthusiasm & motivation	98%
Basic science years' narrative	97
Matriculation date	97
Expected graduation date	94
Clerkship narratives	92
Adequate grade information (comparative data)	75
Comparative data for student*	74
Repeated courses/Remediations	71
Adverse academic actions	63
Gaps/Leaves/Absences	58

* May appear in an Appendix to the letter.
Adapted from: Shea JA, O'Grady E, Morrison G, Wagner BR, Morris JB: Medical student performance evaluations in 2005: an improvement over the former dean's letter? *Acad Med.* 2008;83(3):284-91.

MSPE/Dean's Letter

Each year, medical schools send about a quarter of a million MSPEs/Dean's letters, costing each school from $25,000 to $50,000. This averages out to more than 17 letters per student, although some students request that more than 100 letters be sent! Each school has a standard format for these letters. Most M.D.-granting schools follow the AAMC's format, although how much of the suggested information they contain varies (Figure 13.16). Osteopathic schools' Dean's letters are relatively long and detailed, with varying types of information.

MSPEs usually include some personal background information about the student, with reference to his or her undergraduate experience. They then detail the student's preclinical and clinical course work. Most letters include direct quotes from the student's performance evaluations.

Many schools create charts based on the AAMC's guidelines (Figure 13.17) that show a student's performance on clinical clerkships compared with that of his or her classmates or with a compilation of several recent classes. Some also include the student's results on the Objective Structured Clinical Examination (OSCE), a standardized measure of clinical performance now being used at nearly all U.S. medical schools.

Figure 13.17
AAMC's Template for Medical Student Performance Evaluation

Template

Medical Student Performance Evaluation
for

_____
Student's Legal Name

_____
Month, Date, Year

Identifying Information

_____is a fourth-year student at_____in_____.
Student's Legal Name   Medical School   City, State

Unique Characteristics

(Provide narrative information about distinguishing characteristics exhibited and any significant challenges or hardships encountered by the student during medical school)

Academic History

Date of Expected Graduation from Medical School:

Date of Initial Matriculation in Medical School:
_____
Month, Date, Year

_____
Month, Date, Year

Please explain any extensions, leave(s) of absence, gap(s),
or break(s)in the student's educational program.   or ❏ Not applicable

For transfer students: ❏ Not applicable
Date of Initial Matriculation in Prior Medical School:
_____
Month, Date, Year
Date of Transfer from Prior Medical School:
_____
Month, Date, Year

For dual/joint/combined degree students: ❏ Not applicable
Date of Initial Matriculation in Other Degree Program:
_____
Month, Date, Year
Date of Expected Graduation from Other Degree Program:
_____
Month, Date, Year
Type of Other Degree Program:
_____
Degree, Major

Was this student required to repeat or otherwise   ❏ No
remediate any coursework during his/her   ❏ Yes - Please explain:
medical education?

Was this student the recipient of any adverse actions(s)   ❏ No
by the medical school or its parent institution?   ❏ Yes - Please explain:

Figure 13.17 (continued)

Academic Progress

Preclinical/Basic Science Curriculum:
(Provide narrative information about overall, not course-specific, performance)

Core Clinical Clerkships and Elective Rotations:
(Provide a narrative evaluation about each core clinical clerkship and elective rotation taken in chronological order)

Example I
(when school policy requires that students complete all core clerkships prior to enrollment in electives)

Example II:
(when school policy permits interspersal of core clerkships and electives)

Clerkship 1:	Clerkship 1:
Clerkship 2:	Clerkship 2:
Clerkship 3:	Elective 1: (Provide location if an "away" elective rotation)
Clerkship 4:	Clerkship 3:
Clerkship 5:	Clerkship 4:
Clerkship 6:	Elective 2: (Provide location if an "away" elective rotation)
Elective 1: (Provide location if an "away" elective rotation)	Clerkship 5:
Elective 2: (Provide location if an "away" elective rotation)	Clerkship 6:

Summary

(Provide a summative assessment, in narrative format, of the student's comparative performance, relative to his/her peers, in medical school, including information about any school-specific categories used in differentiating among levels of student performance)

_____
Signature of School Official

_____
Name of School Official

_____
Title

_____
E-mail address

Figure 13.17 (continued)

For purposes of illustration only; school-specific course and clerkship names, grading systems, and categories of overall performance will vary by school.

Appendix A
Graphic Representations of Comparative Performance in Preclinical/Basic Science Coursework

Appendix B
Graphic Representations of Comparative Performance in Core Clinical Clerkships

Appendix C
Graphic Representations of Comparative Performance in Professional Attributes
(Final recommendations expected by 2006)

Appendix D
Graphic Representations of Overall Comparative Performance in Medical School

Figure 13.17 (continued)

Appendix E
Medical School Information Page

_____
Medical School Name

_____
City, State

Special programmatic emphases, strengths, mission/goal(s) of the medical school:

Special characteristics of the medical school's educational program:

Average length of enrollment (initial matriculation to graduation) at the medical school:

_____
Years   Months

Description of the evaluation system used at the medical school:

Medical school requirements for successful completion of USMLE Step 1, 2 (check all that apply):

USMLE Step 1:   USMLE Step 2:
- ❏ Required for promotion   - ❏ Required for promotion
- ❏ Required for graduation   - ❏ Required for graduation
- ❏ Required, but not for promotion/graduation - ❏ Required, but not for promotion/graduation
- ❏ Not required   - ❏ Not required

Medical school requirements for successful completion of Objective/Observed Structured Clinical Evaluation (OSCE) at medical school. OSCEs are used for (check all that apply):
- ❏ Completion of course
- ❏ Completion of clerkship
- ❏ Completion of third year
- ❏ Graduation
- ❏ Other:_____

Utilization of the course, clerkship, or elective director's narrative comments in composition of the MSPE. The narrative comments contained in the attached MSPE can best be described as (check one):
- ❏ Reported exactly as written
- ❏ Edited for length or grammar, but not for content
- ❏ Edited for content or included selectively

Utilization by the medical school of the AAMC "Guidelines for Medical Schools Regarding Academic Transcripts." This medical school is:
- ❏ Completely in compliance with Guidelines' recommendations
- ❏ Partially in compliance with Guidelines' recommendations
  Exceptions:
- ❏ Not in compliance with Guidelines' recommendations

Description of the process by which the MSPE is composed at the medical school (including number of school personnel involved in composition of the MSPE).

Students are permitted to review the MSPE prior to its transmission:
- ❏ Yes
- ❏ No

There are multiple methods used to describe a student's position within her class. Most MSPEs include a histogram or other chart showing a student's grades in comparison with those of her classmates.

About 20% of the letters give the student's class rank, or at least the quartile of the class in which they fall. The lack of class ranking can hurt top candidates who apply for very competitive programs, since many residency faculty give top-ranked individuals from "average" medical schools preference over unranked students from "top" schools. Many more letters give a general description of a student's position in their class. To avoid the overblown syntax used in many recommendation letters, some schools now give a numerical breakdown of the rankings they use. For example, the top 10% of graduates (from this year or recent years) may be rated "outstanding," while the next 25% of graduates are rated "excellent." There is no question in anyone's mind where you stand (at the bottom of the class) if you get a "satisfactory" overall evaluation.

More than one-third of all MSPEs do not include information about a student's failing grades, marginal performance, leaves of absence, or even the need to repeat entire years of study. Official transcripts, however, often have this information, so the discrepancy simply reflects negatively on the letter writer and the school. That may be why residency directors generally consider MSPEs to be the least useful information they receive about applicants (see Figure 19.1).

While these letters usually carry the Dean of Student's signature, 41% of schools use multiple letter writers, including subsidiary deans, administrative personnel, faculty committees, and individual faculty advisers. It is helpful to know the system at your school in case you are allowed to supply additional information. Your Dean's office will be happy to explain the system they use.

As a matter of policy, as well as common courtesy, 88% of medical schools show students their Dean's letter before they are sent out. *Your first responsibility* in regard to your Dean's letter is to *review it carefully*. Check for mistakes. But more important, check to make sure that all good evaluations, special honors, awards, and activities have been mentioned. If there are problems or discrepancies in the letter, bring them to the Dean's attention at once. This letter will be used not only when you apply for a residency position, but also in the future when you are looking for post-residency fellowships or employment.

Virtually all residency programs require a Dean's letter before they invite applicants for an interview. The letters are not always a big help to residency faculty in screening applicants; however, they do serve as a gross measure of a student's achievements compared with his or her classmates. A group who reviewed Dean's letters from all U.S. medical schools felt that nearly half failed to provide either an adequate format for locating necessary information or the information itself.

The medical school deans and faculty who write the Dean's letters want all their graduates to match into the best possible residencies. They are also unreasonably threatened by a fear of tort litigation if they are too candid about a student's performance. The writer's underlying theme is the old adage, "If you can't say something nice, don't say anything at all." A letter to the *New England Journal of Medicine* once remarked that Adolf Hitler's Dean's letter might have read, "A natural leader . . . good communication skills . . . likes to find solutions to problems." The result is a bland, positive, often oblique and incomplete picture of a graduate.

Even with all the letter's drawbacks, experienced residency directors know that if they read between the lines, the Dean's letters may help them screen candidates. They first look for the word "good" used to describe the student. Translation: Below-average performance. They also look for words like "enthusiastic" (manic?), "organized" (obsessive-compulsive?), "colorful" (bizarre?), and "active social life." (flirt?). Letters that dwell on a candidate's dress and punctuality suggest that the author is hunting for something nice to say. They are rarely as explicit as the comments heard about applicants in conversation (Figure 13.18). Finally, the Dean's letter, in combination with a transcript and a telephone call, is a good method of eliminating any charlatans posing as medical students. (Yes, they really are out there.)

It is particularly disturbing when one or two schools each year cannot seem to get their Dean's letters out on time. In recent years, the schools where this has happened have been among the best in the country. Those who suffered were the medical students who did not get interview spots (most residencies have only a limited number) and therefore did not get to select from many of their top program choices.

Thus, your *second responsibility* in regard to your Dean's letter is to *keep track of when it is supposed to go out*. United States M.D.-granting medical school Deans have agreed to a uniform release date of October 1 (October 15 for D.O.-granting schools) for current medical students. No Dean's letters are to be mailed or sent via ERAS before this date. Some Deans bypass the spirit of this requirement by announcing that they are willing to supply verbal information to program directors prior to the letters' official release date. The October dates give the Deans' offices plenty of time to write the letters. Make sure that *your* Dean's letter has been completed and is ready to be sent by ERAS or mailed on the release date. (If you have already graduated from medical school, the rules permit your old Dean's letter to be sent whenever you request it.)

Figure 13.18
Disparaging Comments about Applicants
(but too witty for most faculty)

- "Works well when under constant supervision and cornered like a rat in a trap."
- "He would be out of his depth in a puddle."
- "Technically sound, but socially inept."
- "This young lady has delusions of adequacy."
- "He has the wisdom of youth and the energy of old age."
- "The nursing staff would follow him anywhere, but only out of morbid curiosity."
- "This student has reached rock bottom and shows signs of starting to dig."
- "When she opens her mouth, it is only to change whichever foot was previously in there."
- "He sets low personal standards and then consistently fails to achieve them."

Your *third responsibility,* if you are not using ERAS or CAS, is to supply the Dean with a correct list of program names and addresses in a timely manner. If you don't do this, it does not matter how good the letter is, or how timely the school was in getting it ready. If it cannot be sent for want of an address, you still lose.

Other Reference Letters

Whom to Ask

Most of the reference letters you will send to residency programs will come from those individuals you have personally asked to write them. It is essential for you to know whom to ask.

Residency directors know that these letters usually contain glowing references, so the more specific the authors can be—based on actually observing you or at least getting specific reports from other faculty or residents—the better the letters are viewed.

The Ideal Reference

The ideal reference letter is from an individual who is well-known to program directors in the field—a nationally recognized figure in the specialty of choice, who: (1) has worked with you clinically, (2) thinks you are a "star", and (3) came from at least one of the institutions to which you are applying. If the individual works at one of the specialty's residency programs, it is optimal if their letter says that you have been strongly encouraged to apply to his or her program. All this may be difficult to achieve in one letter. But you should think of such a reference as the "gold standard."

Other Clinical Faculty

Other good reference sources are faculty with whom you have worked clinically and who thought you did a great job. Look for those clinical rotations where you did "Honors" work to get these letters. But don't stray too far from your area of interest. Getting letters from a Psychiatry attending will not be too effective if you are applying for a Radiology position. If you have cultivated a mentor early on, whether or not he or she is in your desired specialty, it might be useful to have him or her write a letter for you. If your mentor has worked with you clinically (and if they haven't it is *your* fault), his or her opinion will often carry a great deal of weight.

Preclinical Instructors

How about your preclinical instructors? Weak! Unless you are applying to Pathology, Public Health, or a very heavily research-oriented program, these letters should be used only in addition to any required reference letters. Everyone can tell how well you did in Anatomy by your grade. The clinical programs want to know how well you treat live patients.

Researchers

"But I've done research," you say. "Can't I get a letter from my research preceptor?" Again, unless you are going into an area where this particular research will be central to your training, such a letter should be considered only as additional support. In general, medical students participating in research are used as "scut puppies." They frequently contribute very little except brute labor. Often they actually have little contact with the research director, and consequently, that individual may know very little about their clinical abilities.

Counterproductive References

Do not get letters from residents, friends, relatives, the clergy, politicians, or patients. You think I'm being funny? Not a bit. I have personally received reference letters for residency applicants from individuals in all these categories. Letters from these sources normally do not help your application. They will probably be detrimental. Residency directors are interested in how well you will do in their program. They want consistent information from reputable, knowledgeable sources. That means your teachers. "If she can't get these letters, there must be something wrong with her," they say. Don't make them think that!

When to Ask

Don't be a wimp! If you want a letter from a particular individual, ask for it. But ask at the right time and in the right way. When is the right time? If you are on a clinical service with the individual, ask while you are on the service, or soon afterwards. Don't wait until six months or a year later. No matter how great a job you did, the faculty member's memory of you will fade with time. Ask if the letter can be drafted now, saying that you will give him or her the ERAS cover sheet or list of programs (if not using ERAS) at a later time.

If it is from a mentor or adviser, ask for a reference letter during a counseling session. If someone has arbitrarily selected your adviser, first think about whether he or she knows you well enough to write a letter.

If the letter you want is from a faculty member in your desired specialty, you will get it either because you have been working with the individual for some time (volunteer, clerkship, etc.) or because of your performance during a clinical rotation. If it is due to the former, just ask. If the latter, do some investigation before you start any clinical work in the department. With whom will you be working? Does this individual meet the qualifications you need for a reference? If not, is there a way of switching the schedule so you can work with someone who will be a good reference? Once you select the individual or individuals, let them know early in the rotation that you are interested in their specialty and would like them to write you a reference letter if they think you have done an excellent job by the end of the rotation. This motivates both of you. You will know that additional scrutiny is coming your way from the faculty members, and the faculty members will pay extra attention to your performance.

How to Ask

Several years ago I received a scrawled letter from a student who had rotated through our department some months before. Addressed to "Residency Director," it asked, "Dear Sir: Please write a letter of reference to:" and proceeded to list a number of programs. There was no return address. Seeing no way to refuse, and personally feeling that the student had done, at best, an adequate job during his rotation, I wrote the following letter: "Mr. Student did a clinical rotation with us in July. He performed adequately." This, if you haven't guessed, is a very negative letter. I don't know if this particular student ever did match in our specialty, but his discourtesy, not to mention lack of insight and poor clinical aptitude, certainly did not help his chances of getting the residency he desired.

Don't send blind letters or coded messages. Ask for a reference letter directly. But phrase it in such a way that neither you nor the faculty member will be saddled with either a negative or a neutral (read: "negative") letter.

One way of doing this is to ask if the faculty member "would feel comfortable writing me a strong letter of support?" If the answer is anything other than emphatic "Yes," look elsewhere. Before he retired, one of our wisest and most experienced faculty members, Dr. Douglas Lindsey, offered to write letters for every medical student. He wrote them honestly and then showed the student the letter. It was up to the student to decide whether it was sent. This was an excellent policy of a great teacher. Unfortunately, very few physicians make it a policy to send copies of the reference letters they write to the individuals for whom they write them. In the business world, this is standard practice and common courtesy. Too bad it isn't yet a widespread practice within the medical profession.

One way of circumventing the problem of a poor reference letter is to ask for a copy of the letter for your files. This gambit is somewhat tricky. If you firmly believe that the individual you have asked will write a superlative letter but will not give you a copy, go ahead   at some risk. If the individual agrees to give you a copy of the letter, then you stand a good chance of, at least marginally, upgrading the quality of the letter by discussing the content with the writer.

Once a faculty member has agreed to write a reference letter for you, hand them a nice folder containing:

1. A copy of your personal statement.

2. A copy of your current résumé.

3. Any official forms that must be included with the letter (such as the ERAS Letter Request Form).

4. A list of reference letter components (see Figure 13.19).

5. A page with your name, the date you requested the letter(s), the address(es) of the recipient(s) [if you know them], and the date it is due.

6. Stamped envelopes for the recipient(s). If you are using ERAS or another computerized application service, you may need to address only one envelope—to your Dean's office. If you are applying to programs that don't use computerized applications, you will need an envelope for each program.

7. A stamped, addressed envelope for your copy.

Giving them this packet will make it easier for them to produce the letter and show them that you "have your act together."

Figure 13.19
Elements of a Reference Letter

It is very useful to include the following items in reference letters for applicants to residency programs:

A. Extent of Letter Writer's Contact with Student
1. How long and intense was the contact
2. Clinical or non-clinical
3. Give details of any specific incidents that stand out

B. Scholastic Record
1. Standing in graduating class
2. Course honors/awards
3. Other honors/awards

C. Medical Abilities
1. Interaction with patients
2. Ability to synthesize information (problem solving)
3. Diagnostic ability
4. Physical examination ability
5. Laboratory use/test interpretation
6. Technical skills
7. Use of pharmacological agents
8. Clarity of oral presentations
9. Clarity/completeness of charts
10. Knowledge of medical literature

D. Personal Characteristics (List strongest points first.)
1. Relations with peers, faculty, ancillary staff
2. Communication skills
3. Respect for others
4. Willingness to assume responsibility
5. Ability to recognize personal limitations
6. Dependability; consistency
7. Integrity; moral and ethical qualities
8. Initiative; industriousness
9. Motivation; interest; enthusiasm
10. Maturity
11. Flexibility
12. Sense of Humor

E. Overall Impression of Student
1. Rating compared with other students
2. Would you want him/her in your program?

If you do happen to get a reference letter that isn't glowing, don't panic. You have one card left to play. If the letter has not yet been sent out, don't give the author any program addresses to which he or she can send it. If you have followed the plan above, you should get a copy of the letter long before you yourself even know where you are going to apply. You will also have plenty of time to collect other, more complimentary letters. By the time you are ready to send out reference letters, you should have a file of copies of letters that have been written on your behalf. Select the best and ask these individuals to mail them to the appropriate individuals or programs. If you can pull it off, this is virtually a no-lose situation.

A few students have been asked to sign statements that they have not seen their reference letters. This is ridiculous and unenforceable. Don't sign. However, it is common practice for students to be asked to sign a waiver of their right to request to see reference letters. If you are forced into this type of situation, you may have to sign it and hope for good letters. If possible, you do want to see those letters before they go out.

The Format

While your MSPE/Dean's letter will follow the institution's format and will be professionally done on College of Medicine stationary, the same may not be true for your reference letters. It is almost unbelievable that faculty physicians send out reference letters that are not on letterhead, are printed on poor-quality printers, or are handwritten. This is a negative reflection not only on these individuals, but also on you. If you believe that any of the individuals from whom you have requested a letter will have difficulty producing a professional-appearing document, either offer to have the letter typed for them or just ask someone else. Physicians working for the federal government and those in solo or rural practice seem to have the most difficulty producing professional reference letters. It should be noted that the best format is typewritten on letterhead stationery with a handwritten note from the writer. That gets attention.

Although most medical school faculty send out many reference letters, they have never been taught what should go in them. They might find it useful if you give them a copy of Figure 13.19, Elements of a Reference Letter, when you ask them to write your reference letter. Individuals from outside your medical center whom you are asking for a reference would almost assuredly appreciate a format to guide them in writing the letter.

Some specialties and/or programs now use a Standard Letter of Recommendation (SLoR). Pioneered by Emergency Medicine, SLoRs are designed to improve communication about applicants. These can be more easily scanned into computers and analyzed than can normal reference letters, although many people still send both a regular letter and this form. The form includes key information, such as how likely the applicant is to match at the reference's residency program ("guaranteed," "very likely," "likely," etc.), how their grade compares with those of other students from the same year, and how the applicant measures up compared to other applicants for which the reference has written letters. Look for them to be used more frequently in the future.

Note of Caution

The ECFMG has advised IMG applicants that they have discovered numerous altered or falsified letters of recommendation. Often program directors spotted the problem. The ECFMG investigated and barred those individuals from ever having an ECFMG Certificate, meaning that they can never participate in an accredited U.S. residency program. Those already certified had their Certificates withdrawn.

Such "irregular" behavior undoubtedly occurs in the non-ECFMG application processes as well. Falsified resumes have been documented among residency and fellowship applicants. Severe consequences can result from using falsified documents—including *dismissal from programs after you have matched.*

A Picture?

Whether photographs should be a part of any employment application is questionable. Since requiring a photograph is illegal under civil rights legislation (it indicates race, gender, and age), ERAS has changed its procedures: It no longer requires a photograph, but suggests that the file will not be complete without one. The photograph is not visible to residency programs until after you have been accepted for an interview.

What kind of photograph do you include? As with everything you do in conjunction with your application, your photograph should look professional— especially because the first version they will probably see will be the black and white scanned version from ERAS. Have it professionally done. Don't use your camera phone, have your friend take it with her pocket camera, or use a passport photo. This is your career at stake.

Go to a professional photographer and explain that you need a portrait photo. Unless you are specifically asked for a black-and-white picture, get it in color. ERAS specifies that you must submit a color photograph showing a full front view of your head and shoulders with your entire face centered in the middle of the photograph. It must have a plain white or light-colored background and be approximately 2.5 by 3.5 inches and not more than 3 by 4 inches.

It may be less expensive to order extra copies of the photographs your school takes of students in the second or third year. But if you have noticeably altered your appearance since then, such as growing a beard or changing your hairstyle, get a new set of pictures. The benefit of using a professional photographer is that no matter what you really look like, you will appear much better in the professional's picture. Also, make sure that you look like a neat, clean professional. As you would in the interview itself, don't wear a fancy (party) hairstyle, informal clothes, or extravagant jewelry when your picture is taken.

You use the color photograph once you have been granted an interview. Especially if you didn't submit it with an ERAS application, have a photograph ready for the program to include with your application material. Actually, it is illegal for a program to request a photograph, even after you have been interviewed in person. But you are not going to wait for them to request it—you will arrive at the interview with the photograph in hand.

Why should you do this? For a very obvious reason: You want to be remembered. Do you really think that an interviewer will remember anything specific about Jerry Glover or Mary Smythe after seeing forty applicants? Probably not. They may even have trouble recalling applicants using the ERAS picture. But with a great color photograph to jog their memory during final selection, the good impressions that you left with the faculty will come flooding back.

Finally, before handing the picture to the residency secretary for your file, make sure that you put a gummed label on the back with your name, address, e-mail address, telephone number, and the date that you are interviewing.

Oh yes, remember to say "cheese."

The Transcript

Your official medical school transcript, which will be required by nearly every program to which you apply, is a coded summary of your progress through medical school. The key word here is "coded." Every transcript uses symbols, some of which are rather arcane. Familiar to most residency directors are such designations as "H" (Honors) or "A" for top grades. These symbols are widely used. Somewhat deceptively, however, some schools use "High Honors" for a top grade and "Honors" for the runners-up. Some schools, for their own reasons, use symbols that are distinctly different from those used in most transcripts. A few use "O" (Outstanding), "S" (Superior)—which indicates a less-than-Honors grade in some schools, but the top grade in others—or various numerical systems to designate a top grade. Those using numerical systems also tend to obscure the student grades with multiple columns of irrelevant data.

If you have done well in school, it is important that it be obvious to the faculty members who will review your transcript. No, the school's detailed explanation on the back of or accompanying the transcript does not help. If it needs that much explanation, the school needs to revise its method of recording grades. That, however, is something you cannot do anything about now. What you need to do is to include a separate page that summarizes your transcript with your application materials. This transcript summary page, which is *separate from your résumé,* should include all of the following:

1. A list of all courses in which you received "Honors." Clearly specify that the grade, whatever it is called on the transcript, is in fact the top grade given out at your school.

2. A list of all courses in which you received a "B" grade, if such grades are given out at your school.

3. An explanation of any unusual grades or symbols on your transcript. This means detailing why there was an "Incomplete" listed for Biochemistry. It is very important to do this. If it was because you turned in a required project late, it is far different from what is assumed otherwise—that you failed part of the course and had to make it up.

4. A list of courses you will take in the balance of the year, but whose grades may not yet have been received or recorded by the registrar. The purpose of this is to alleviate concerns caused by misinterpretation of the transcript. Some schools use a "P" (which generally means "Pass," the average grade) to indicate that a course is "In Progress." If this appears next to the rotations taken early in your senior year (which probably will include your specialty elective), it could mean curtains for any chance to get an interview unless you explain it.

5. An explanation of any leaves of absence taken during medical school. If this needs more than a few words, state that it is further explained in your résumé or personal statement.

6. An explanation of any awards listed on your transcript, including who gave the award and the achievement recognized.

7. Identify your class rank if your school notes this on the transcript, or if it will be to your advantage (if you are in the top half of your class) to do so.

Obviously, to intelligently write a personalized explanatory cover letter, it will be necessary for you to review a copy of your transcript. You can get this from the Registrar's office. Most individuals in these offices will be very happy to help you. Some even suggest that you come in and review your transcript periodically to ensure that they have not erred when recording your grades. Occasionally, however, some registrars may be reluctant to show you your transcript. In those cases, request help from your Dean of Students. After explaining why you want to review your record, you should have no difficulty in obtaining a copy for yourself.

Finally, you may get excellent grades in significant courses after sending in your initial transcript. It would serve you well to send, near the end of the interviewing "season," an updated transcript to the programs where you have interviewed. Make certain that the registrar has received and recorded late grades before the revised transcripts are sent out. Also, see if the Registrar's office can attach a note stating that this is an updated transcript. This will alert the programs to replace the transcript currently in their files with the new one that contains important, updated information.

A word now to those whose grades have not been stellar. An obscure transcript can often work to your advantage. You certainly do not want to call attention to it by enclosing the explanation of the transcript described above. Rather, you would like to have the transcript ignored as much as possible. It is still important, though, to explain in your résumé or personal statement any leaves of absence, failing grades, and courses-in-progress.

Finally, just as with the Dean's letter, make certain that your transcript is sent out on time if you are not using ERAS or CAS. Many students will be trying to send out transcripts simultaneously. This overburdens the Registrar's office. If your transcript is delayed, your work to get the right interviews might go for naught. Try to get your request in a little early. It is acceptable to forward a transcript before you have sent in, or even completed, the program's application. So get those addresses to the Registrar's office as soon as you can. Make sure that one of the addresses is that of your mentor. When he or she receives a copy (discuss this in advance), you will know that the programs should have received their copies as well.

Timing—It's Your Future at Stake

Now that you have spent a great deal of time getting your material ready, make certain that you send it all in early. The requirements for granting interviews stiffen as the "season" progresses. When the first completed applications arrive, most programs are rather liberal about granting interviews. Later, as the vast influx of applications arrives, applicants are compared against those who have already been granted interviews. The requirements, therefore, get more demanding with each passing week. Perhaps more important, nearly half of Pediatrics residency directors and about one-fourth of those in Family Medicine and Anesthesiology use a "first-come, first-served" basis for selecting candidates to interview.

Thus, it is vital to get your materials in as soon as possible. Once you have requested that everything be sent or you have actually sent it to the programs, you can safely sit back and wait for interview requests, right? Wrong! Haven't you ever received a birthday card in the mail two months late, even though it was postmarked before your birthday? Of course you have. Not that the mail is slow or prone to frequent errors. But if your career depends upon the programs receiving all of your materials by a specific deadline, then it behooves you to be sure that they get it. And most programs do have specific deadlines.

If you use ERAS, check your application's status by using their tracking system, ADTS, accessed through the ERAS website (www.aamc.org/students/eras/start.htm). If you don't use ERAS, keep a log of everything that is supposed to be sent to each program. When you think that all of your materials should have arrived at the programs, and if you have not received any e-mail from them, call and ask. You should also do this if you are applying to non-ERAS programs.

If a program indicates that your file is incomplete, ascertain exactly what is lacking. If the missing document has been sent to multiple programs, check with more than one program. The problem may actually be that the documents are filed incorrectly or that they have not yet downloaded your materials. But it may mean that you will have to send duplicates to some programs. Remember that for programs requiring a Dean's letter, the file for graduating students will not be complete until at least the first week of October (M.D. students) or mid-October (D.O. students), since these letters are not released by ERAS (or sent from the Dean's office to non-ERAS programs) until that time.

There is another method you can easily use to assure receipt of your materials for non-ERAS programs, including all Fellowships. You can enclose a self-addressed, stamped postcard with each application for the program to use to notify you when all your materials have arrived. The postcard, with a place to put a date, should say, "All necessary application materials have been received by the (name of residency program) Residency Program for (your name)." *You* should fill out the blanks before you enclose it. Attach a small note asking that the postcard be returned when all of your materials are received. Dropping something in the mail is far easier than sending you an email. Occasionally, even a detail as small as using this postcard will suggest something positive about an applicant. An example of one such postcard that our program received is shown in Figure 13.20.

In any event, once your file is complete, you should be able to e-mail the programs to find out whether you will be offered an interview. If you don't get a response in a reasonable time, call them. Calling, if you are pleasant about it, may get you an interview you might not otherwise have received. Some students use a priority mail or a courier service (FedEx, United Parcel Service overnight, etc.) to ensure that their material gets to the program (or to the ECFMG when they are acting as an IMG's Dean's office). Unless the materials are being sent from outside the United States or Canada, this is probably overkill.

The bottom line, then, is to plan ahead to get all your material to the residency programs on time—and then check to make certain it was received.

Figure 13.20
A Completed-Application Postcard

Date _____

Congratulations! Your application is now **complete**.

_____ Please call to schedule an interview.
_____ We will contact you to schedule an interview.
_____ Sorry, buddy. Ever thought about law school?

Thanks for all your help.

Program _____

Telephone _____

Contact _____

14

Special Situations

To be a bullfighter, you must learn to think like the bull.

Spanish Folk Saying

We hold these truths to be self-evident, that all men are created equal;
that they are endowed by their creator with certain unalienable rights;
that among these are life, liberty and the pursuit of happiness.

Thomas Jefferson

THE ARCHETYPICAL PHYSICIAN in the United States was, for a long time, a White, Anglo-Saxon male. But this has changed drastically over the last forty years.

There was a large influx of foreign-born, foreign-trained physicians during the perceived doctor shortage in the 1960s and 1970s. Advancements in the rights of women and minorities also were made during this time, and it gradually became easier for all qualified applicants to medical schools to equitably compete for entrance into the profession. This resulted in an increasing number of physicians who did not fit the classic male "WASP" mold. Soon after, these physicians began knocking at the doors of residency programs to get further training. Gradually, the once-barred doors of the specialties opened. However, many groups still have particular problems gaining entrance into residencies.

Of note is that the federal Equal Employment Opportunity Commission (EEOC) has ruled that once you have obtained a residency position, you are an employee. This means that you are specifically protected under Title VII from discrimination in employment based on race, color, sex, religious beliefs, or national origin. You are also protected under the Equal Pay Act and the Age Discrimination in Employment Act.

There are excellent resources for medical students who may encounter problems or who have special circumstances, including the American Medical Student Association's (AMSA) sub-groups and list serves for those students who are disabled; lesbian, gay, transgender, or bisexual; minorities; or women. AMSA publishes information about these groups on their website and in *The New Physician*.

Women

The first woman to earn a U.S. medical school diploma, Dr. Elizabeth Blackwell, graduated from the Geneva Medical College in upstate New York in 1849. Despite many obstacles, she graduated first in her class. Yet in 1921, more than 70 years later, only 8% of U.S.-hospital internships accepted women. Today, women account for about 48% of medical students and 45% of residents and fellows. Unfortunately, just 33% of medical school faculty members, and only 25% of the clinical faculty, are women. On average, there is only one woman department head per medical school, and only 10% of medical school Deans are women.

It is no longer unusual for women to constitute the majority of a medical school class; they comprised more than half of the 2012 entering class at U.S. M.D.-granting medical schools. In 1970, about one in 13 U.S. physicians (7.7%) was female; currently, one in three actively practicing physicians (34%) is a woman; the lowest percentage is in Idaho and Utah (~20%) and the highest is in Massachusetts (~35%). This is a significant advance from the 1890s, when the new Johns Hopkins Medical School, because of its need for the funds that women were raising, and then only under duress, agreed to accept qualified women as medical students. In 1977, there were no female residents in more than a third of all specialties. In 2012, women were training in every accredited area except for a few minor subspecialties that had a small number of total trainees; 11 specialties had more than 1,000 female residents in training.

Nearly all women physicians say that they are satisfied with their careers. Those most satisfied have more children, have less stress at home, are strongly religious, and feel in control of their work life. Nevertheless, many would choose a different specialty or another career if given the chance.

About 46% of female physicians under 35 years of age are in Primary Care, in contrast to only about 30% of male physicians in this age group. This gender disparity is similar for physicians who are from 35- to 44-years-old. Forty-seven percent of all women physicians specialize in General Internal Medicine, General Pediatrics, Family Medicine, or Obstetrics and Gynecology. However, only 66% of women physicians are Board-certified in their specialty, as opposed to 72% of men.

This does not mean that there is no longer discrimination against women trying to get residency positions. While the match rate for women is better than for men in Family Medicine, Internal Medicine, Anesthesiology, Emergency Medicine, and Diagnostic Radiology, the reverse is true in some other specialties. General Surgery, Orthopedic Surgery, Obstetrics and Gynecology, Pediatrics,

Psychiatry, and Pathology have consistently higher match rates for men than for women. In the last four of these specialties, it has been suggested that a form of reverse discrimination is occurring: Program directors may be giving preference to male applicants in an attempt to reverse the preponderance of women in those specialties (Figure 14.1).

One of the biggest discrepancies is in General Surgery, which is practiced by 5% of male physicians, but only 2% of female physicians. While there has been a marked increase in the number of female surgical residents, a noticeably smaller percentage of women matches as compared to male applicants. A survey of both male and female physicians cited General Surgery, Orthopedic Surgery, and Urology as the specialties that most restrict opportunities for women, although the percentage of women residents in these specialties has risen in recent years.

Respondents in this same survey cited Family Medicine, Obstetrics and Gynecology, Pediatrics, and Internal Medicine as having an equal or higher rate of opportunity for female physicians. Internal Medicine has a much higher percentage of women practitioners than men, despite having had subspecialty training.

Figure 14.1
Women's Representation in Selected Specialties

Specialty	% of All Physicians in this Specialty	% of Physicians in the Specialty that are Women	% of Residents in the Specialty that are Women
Internal Medicine	12%	33%	37%
Family Medicine	9	36	53
Pediatrics	6	58	63
Psychiatry	4	35	51
General Surgery	4	16	29
Obstetrics/Gynecology	4	32	77
Anesthesiology	4	23	34
Emergency Medicine	3	24	37
Orthopedic Surgery	3	6	12
Radiology	1	16	27

Adapted from: American Medical Association: *Physician Characteristics and Distribution in the U.S.* Chicago, IL: AMA, 2011 various tables; and Accreditation Council for Graduate Medical Education: *Data Resource Book*. Chicago, IL: ACGME, 2011, various tables.

Figure 14.2
Gender of Medical School Faculty, by Rank

Academic Rank	Men		Women	
	Number	Percent of All Faculty*	Number	Percent of All Faculty*
Professor	25,974	19.0%	6,299	4.6%
Associate Professor	19,250	14.1	8,157	6.6
Assistant Professor	33,957	24.9	24,766	18.1
Instructor	6,584	4.8	7,513	5.5
Other	1,577	1.2	1,577	1.2
Total	**87,342**	**64.0%**	**49,182**	**36.0%**

* Percentages may not total 100% due to rounding.
Adapted from: AAMC Faculty Roster System, 2009.

Greater awareness of federal laws prohibiting discrimination against women in hiring and during employment, as well as a change in social attitudes toward professional women, have made discriminatory practices more complex and subtle. These practices, often based upon irrational fears (such as about working with women as equals), are not only unfair but also arbitrary, and may be a reason for the under-representation of women on residency faculties. The percentage of women faculty members varies greatly by specialty. In addition, their academic ranks are lower than those of male colleagues (Figures 14.2 and 14.3).

One example of widespread discrimination is seen in the discrepancy between the average male and female physicians' income. Female physicians in practice (and not working for the federal government) still receive an average of 40% less annual net income than their male counterparts. This is only partially explained by differences in specialty, practice setting, age, and productivity. The exact amount varies by specialty, but this trend pervades medical practice.

Sexual Harassment

Sexual harassment, including physical harassment, sexual slurs, sexual advances, and educational inequalities based on sex, is common. The EEOC's definition of sexual harassment is:

Unwelcome sexual advances, requests for sexual favors, and other verbal or physical conduct of a sexual nature constitute sexual harassment when:
1. submission to such conduct is made either explicitly or implicitly a term or condition of an individual's employment;

Figure 14.3
Women M.D. Faculty in Various Specialties

Specialty	% of Faculty in Specialty that are Women	% of Women Faculty that are Full Professors	Ratio of Men to Women Faculty that are Full Professors
OB/GYN	53%	9%	3.0
Public Health	52	16	1.9
Pediatrics	51	12	2.5
Physical Med/Rehab	45	8	2.6
Dermatology	47	15	2.7
Family Medicine	45	8	2.9
Psychiatry	45	11	3.2
Internal Medicine	35	11	4.8
Pathology (Clinical)	37	20	3.4
Neurology	34	12	5.5
Anesthesiology	34	8	4.5
Ophthalmology	32	14	5.3
Emergency Medicine	30	5	5.9
Radiology	27	14	4.8
Otolaryngology	28	10	7.8
Surgery	20	12	10.7
Orthopedic Surgery	16	9	16.2

Adapted from: AAMC Faculty Roster System, December, 2011.

2. submission to or rejection of such conduct by an individual is used as the basis for employment decisions affecting such individual; or
3. such conduct has the purpose or effect of unreasonably interfering with an individual's work performance or creating an intimidating, hostile, or offensive working environment.

Unfortunately, nearly half of women physicians report having been harassed on the basis of gender, and more than a third report having been sexually harassed by patients, peers, or attending physicians. The frequency of both is about the same during medical school and training. (It decreases somewhat when the physicians enter practice.) It is experienced more frequently by women than men and, in residency, varies by specialty. Figure 14.4 lists those specialties with the highest and the lowest reported incidence of sexual harassment. Married women and those with children reported less harassment than single women.

Gender discrimination and sexual harassment affect specialty choices. The greatest impact occurs during core electives and elective clerkships. In addition, experiences during the residency selection process affect how applicants rank programs. Observing and hearing about such discrimination or harassment may affect applicants' choices as much as experiencing it.

Most women say they do not report harassment because they fear a negative impact and because they do not believe any action would be taken, even though virtually all teaching hospitals have policies regarding the sexual harassment of residents. Individuals who sexually harass residents generally have a higher professional status. One study showed that while lesbian physicians suffer no more harassment than their heterosexual peers, they report these offenses four times as often.

During the residency selection process, women are also often asked sexist, blatantly illegal questions. See "Illegal Questions" in Chapter 21 for more information.

Even without discrimination, women in medicine have unique personal challenges. The training period of medical school and residency cuts directly across the childbearing years. This results in women physicians having fewer children, and at a later age, than non-physician women. Only 60% to 70% of married women physicians have children, compared to 90% of their married male counterparts.

Figure 14.4
Relative Incidence of Sexual Harassment*

1. Urology
2. Family Medicine
3. Psychiatry
4. Emergency Medicine
5. Obstetrics/Gynecology
6. Internal Medicine–Pediatrics
7. Neurological Surgery
8. Neurology
9. Physical Med & Rehab
10. Internal Medicine
11. Otolaryngology
12. General Surgery
13. Pediatrics
14. Orthopedic Surgery
15. Radiology
16. Radiation Oncology
17. Dermatology
18. Transitional Year
19. Anesthesiology
20. Ophthalmology
21. Pathology

* Ranked from highest (1) incidence to lowest (21) incidence.
Adapted from: Baldwin DC, Daugherty SR: Distinguishing sexual harassment from discrimination: a factor-analytic study of residents' reports. *Acad Med.* 2001;76(10):S5-7.

Additional information for and about women in medicine can be obtained from the American Medical Women's Association (AMWA), (215) 320-3716; www.amwa-doc.org. This organization provides student members with educational loans, scholarships, and awards; use of a bed-and-breakfast program; and a bimonthly journal. Another source of information is Women Physicians Congress, American Medical Association, (312) 464-5622; (800) 262-3221; www.ama-assn.org/go/wpc. This section of the AMA serves as an information resource on issues relating to women physicians. Many individual specialties also have separate societies for women physicians. You can locate them through the main specialty society, AMWA, or the AMA.

Marriage, Pregnancy, And Children

The problems associated with adjusting to marriage and having children during medical training were once thought to be solely a woman's concern. Not any longer. While women do have unique biological concerns regarding pregnancy, both men and women physicians now frequently base career decisions, including choosing a residency, on how their family will be affected. The major concerns include maintaining the family relationship, coping with pregnancy, and caring for children.

Marriage

Half of all medical students marry during medical school or residency training, and more than 60% of physicians divorce within ten years after completing residency. One study showed that Psychiatrists have the highest divorce rate at 50%, followed by Surgeons with 33%. Up to 70% of medical marriages are dysfunctional, partly because physicians often hold a position of unquestioned authority at work and it can be difficult to relinquish this role at home. Residents' marriages are at particular risk for work-related difficulties, since they work longer hours, have more trouble "winding down" after work, are sleep deprived, and are often too tired to participate in social or leisure-time activities.

Does this mean that your partnership is doomed? No! All new professionals have the same stresses. One key to success is to lend your partner as much support for his or her career as you deserve for your own. Another is for both partners to recognize that, at least during residency, theirs will not be the idyllic marriage that balances a thriving career with a loving and active family life. Ultimately, residents with successful marriages cope better, remain more productive, and are happier than those whose marriages are foundering.

More than three-fourths of medical students' domestic partners play a significant role in deciding to which residency programs they apply, where they accept interviews, and how they rank the programs. Partners have more influence on these decisions than do medical school faculty, residents, other family members, or classmates. Many partners also travel to the interview sites and investigate job opportunities while there. Ultimately, while 60% of male and female medical students try to satisfy both their own and their partner's needs when selecting programs, nearly 33% of male and 20% of female medical students make their final selections based primarily on their own needs.

Traditionally, women have changed their name when they married, either taking their husband's name or using a hyphenated surname. Women physicians may want to reconsider this decision, especially for your professional life. Women physicians often find it easier to keep their maiden name for legal documents and official records, such as USMLE records, the Boards, medical school diplomas, residency certificates, and medical and controlled-substance licenses. When your name differs among these documents, it may generate a slew of additional paperwork every time you need to use them for relicensing, job applications, and other activities. During their careers, all physicians have to deal with these activities more often than you would ever have thought possible. If you have married another doctor, keeping your maiden name may help lessen any confusion about which "Dr. Richardson" patients are seeking. Additionally, using a separate professional name helps keep your home address and phone numbers private, maintaining more security for your family. If, in the future, you become divorced, widowed, or remarried, your professional identity would not be affected. Finally, if you plan to publish, you should keep a constant name so that your articles can be found easily.

Dual-physician marriages have their own difficulties. In physician–physician marriages, both earn less money individually than other physicians, and each person is less likely to feel that their career takes precedence over their spouse's. However, both usually feel as successful as other physicians in achieving their career and family goals, and they benefit more from shared work interests. Nevertheless, the women in these partnerships are more likely to make professional sacrifices for their spouses than are their cohorts who are married to non-physicians.

Balancing personal and professional goals, and the responsibilities accompanying each, can be a major challenge for both men and women—although women have more stressors. Significant social expectations on women physicians, apart from their medical careers, can create tension between their private and professional lives. This contributes to the fact that only 66% of female physicians marry, compared to 90% of both non-physician women and male physicians. In addition, since up to 70% of married women physicians are married to other physicians, the complications mount.

Compared with women physicians partnered with non-physicians (usually other professionals), the women in physician-physician relationships are more likely to bear the primary responsibility of caring for their children and home. Many do this by working fewer hours and subordinating their career to that of their partner. As many as half of all women physicians change their career plans because of marriage or family responsibilities.

In the end, however, marriage enhances well-being. Married men and women are generally happier and less stressed than single people. Men benefit more from marriage than do women. However, both show decreased stress, which can help to enhance physicians' lives—especially during residency.

Pregnancy and Family Leave

Among the most stressful personal situations that residents must deal with are pregnancy and child rearing. Increasing numbers of women are having children during their medical training. Before 1950, 24% of women physicians with children had them during medical training. Since then, more than half of all women physicians with children had their first child during residency. Approximately 7,500 current women residents (15%) will become pregnant at least once during their training. Many more residents will experience fatherhood.

A 2010 study found that a significant percentage of women residents delayed childbearing until after residency due to their belief that pregnancy was a risk to their careers. They reasoned that pregnancy during residency would extend their time in training, decrease their chance to obtain a fellowship, and increase their risk of pregnancy-related complications (it doesn't), and generally interfere with their career. While some of this may be true—such as extending the length of training—delaying childbearing until after residency risks "subfertility," since fertility markedly decreases after age 35. Compared to younger women, those over 35-years-old also have an increase in chromosomal abnormalities (Odds Ratio [OR] 4.0), miscarriages (OR 2.0), congenital abnormalities (OR 1.4), and caesarean sections (OR 1.6).

Maternity/paternity leave (often incorporated into "family leave") has lengthened over time, although women are still unhappy with the amount of time off they receive for pregnancy and childbirth. These policies have been problematic for at least two reasons. First, women residents who have been pregnant feel that the leave, if less than six-weeks-long, is inadequate. Second, because these policies only apply to a subset of residents (parents, usually mothers), extended leave can wreak havoc on schedules and on the baseline educational requirements that must be met for Board certification.

All leave policies are ultimately the responsibility of the sponsoring institution. The ACGME's *Essentials of Accredited Residencies in Graduate Medical Education: Institutional and Program Requirements* stipulates that residency applicants in all specialties must be informed, in writing, of parental leave policies and that this information must be included in a resident's contract. In addition, it states: "There must be a written institutional policy on leave (with or without pay) for residents that complies with applicable laws. The institution must provide residents with a written policy concerning the effect of leaves of absence, for any reason, on satisfying the criteria for completion of a residency program."

In reality, most programs deal with pregnancies on an *ad hoc* basis. Therefore, how individual programs interpret the requirements varies. *FREIDA* indicates whether a program has a written maternity, paternity, and/or family leave policy. It also frequently lists the maximum time allowed for each— although many programs list "NGO" ("negotiable"). As women become an even greater presence in medicine, longer pregnancy leave, greater flexibility within the residency programs, and increased availability of childcare for medical students and residents will become mandatory.

The Federal Family and Medical Leave Act, which took effect in 1993, applies to most residents. It requires employers with 50 or more workers to grant up to 12 weeks of unpaid leave each year to new fathers and mothers (including adoptive and foster parents) after they have worked at the job for one year. The same amount of leave time must be available for employees to seek medical care for themselves or to care for their spouse, child, or parent with a serious health condition. Sick leave, vacation, and personal leave can all be incorporated into this time period, so employees may be paid for some of their time off. Approximately three-fourths of teaching hospitals have a written parental leave policy. At these hospitals, maternity leave averages 64 days (range: 21 to 180 days), and paternity leave averages 46 days (range: 1 to 120 days). At many institutions, much of this time off is unpaid.

As evidenced by the relative paucity of adequate paternity leave policies (at least one hospital generously offers just one day off), male residents may have more difficulty than women getting time off to fulfill their parental responsibilities around the time of birth. More male residents will become parents than will women residents because there are more male residents, and most of them are married to non-physicians.

The 1978 Pregnancy Discrimination Amendments to the Civil Rights Act of 1964 state that women affected by pregnancy, childbirth, or related medical conditions are to be treated the same as disabled employees for all employment-related purposes, including being covered by fringe-benefit programs. A number of states also have laws governing the rights of pregnant employees.

Most women physicians who have been pregnant during their residency report inequitable treatment during the pregnancy, ranging from unconscious slights to actual harassment. To lessen stress, some women physicians suggest trying to plan pregnancies for the time between the second and third years or during the fourth year of medical school, during the senior year of residency (not a surgical residency), during a year off, or after residency. (Of course, pregnancies often cannot be "planned.") If you become pregnant, give your (hopefully supportive) colleagues adequate notice that you will be taking leave.

Pregnant residents usually have lifestyles that they would not recommend to their patients—long hours, rigorous physical activity, poor eating and sleeping habits, and exposure to disease. Fortunately, studies show that these stressors have little effect on the success of their pregnancies, although there appears to be a higher-than-expected incidence of preeclampsia and preterm labor (but not preterm delivery). Additionally, female resident physicians have fewer induced abortions than do their non-physician counterparts (Figure 14.5).

According to an AMA review, pregnant residents should take breaks every few hours; take a longer "meal" break every four hours; maintain adequate hydration; regularly vary their work positions by sitting, standing, and walking; and minimize heavy lifting, especially if associated with bending.

Up to one-third of women who were pregnant during their residency training would counsel others to avoid the experience. They found that the farther along they were in their residency, the easier the pregnancy was to manage, since their work schedules were more flexible and coworkers were more supportive.

The most obvious issue for women is fatigue, both during and after pregnancy. Consider whether the pregnancy, unexpected circumstances related to the pregnancy, or caring for an infant might delay your progression through, or graduation from, medical school or residency. In part, this will depend on your support system, especially at home. Also, consider the financial aspects of pregnancy. How much will *you* have to pay for your (and the baby's) medical care and for the delivery? You will also probably have to buy furniture, clothing and other baby supplies (toys, car seat, stroller, diapers, etc.).

If you are considering pregnancy during your training, you may want to look for large training programs that might have more flexibility to modify

Figure 14.5
Pregnancies and Complications

Complication	Non-Physicians	Physicians
Mean age at first delivery (yrs.)	25.2	27.0
Mean number of children	2.9	1.8
Stillbirths/1000 births	3.7	3.2
Spontaneous abortions (%)	12.5	12.7
Elective abortions (%)	13.1	11
Premature delivery (%)	7.6	12.4
Pregnancy-induced hypertension (%)	7	5.4
Diabetes (%)	1	1

Adapted from: Pinhas-Hamiel O, Rostein Z, Achiron A, et al.: Pregnancy during residency—an Israeli survey of women physicians. *Health Care for Women International.* 1999;20:63-70.

schedules for pregnancy leave, or to investigate training programs that clearly state their maternity leave policy in their application material. (It is becoming more common for these policies to be titled "Parental," "Family," or "Maternity/Paternity/Adoption" leave, rather than "Maternity" leave.) *FREIDA* includes a question about maternity and paternity leave for each program.

Children

Childcare can be an enormous burden for residents, especially if both parents work. Women carry most of the child-rearing burdens in our society, and cannot be both residents and parents without some help. Childcare facilities, although relatively common in the business world, have yet to appear in the medical field on a regular basis. Even when hospitals do offer childcare, it often is not available to residents' children. See the discussion of childcare in Chapter 11.

It is very difficult to find routine childcare services that can accommodate a resident's extremely long (and sometimes unexpectedly longer) hours. Start searching for childcare during pregnancy. Consider a nanny service, a live-in helper, a regular baby-sitter, or a day care center. Make sure that you have a back-up plan in case something unexpected happens at the hospital. Resources with helpful tips for men and women are listed under "Marriage and Parenting" in the *Annotated Bibliography*.

Couples Matching

Resistance to matching couples at the same institution seems to have succumbed to the reality of nearly 4,000 new physician–physician couples each year. However, matching couples into the same training program, which occurs much less often, may still pose a problem. This may be due to the faculty's concerns about the effect upon both the individual residents and the esprit de corps of the entire program if there is any strife between, or a breakup of, the couple. This concern is not at all assuaged by the marginal commitment to each other shown by some interviewing couples.

Using the NRMP Couples Match often reduces the strain in two-physician (medical student) marriages/relationships. In the 2012 Couples Match, 878 couples (an all-time high) participated; they had a match rate of 91.6% for both matching and 94.6% for at least one of them matching. Rather than being more difficult than individual matches, as might be expected, couples using the NRMP PGY-1 Couples Match actually have about the same match rate as do individuals who go through the regular NRMP Match (94.1%). Part-time, also described as "Shared-Schedule," positions are available in some programs (see below).

In most cases, problems revolve around the process of matching successfully as a couple. Most problems arise when the partners do not both use the NRMP Match, they are from different medical schools, or they are in different years of training. The latter is the only problem that will be addressed here. The others will be discussed in Chapter 23.

If you and your partner are in different years of medical school training, there are three viable options for you.

1. The senior partner goes through the Match for his or her specialty. The junior partner can then concentrate his or her efforts on programs in the geographic area compatible with their partner's Match results. However, this could mean separation for one or more years while the junior partner finishes school, which may be unacceptable.

2. The senior partner goes through the Match and then the junior partner transfers to a medical school in the same geographic area to complete his or her medical school training. Some schools, especially private schools that rely on income from tuition, make transferring out very difficult. For information about transferring schools, search "Transfer Policies for Applicants to Medical Schools" at www.aamc.org/students/

medstudents. On that site, you can search either by the type of transfer policy or by the school.

3. The senior partner limits selections on his or her rank order list to the geographic area of the junior partner's medical school and matches into a less desirable spot if necessary. When the junior partner graduates, both partners can enter the Match again, with the senior partner seeking an advanced position. In the past, this was accomplished by the senior partner first matching into a "Preliminary" or "Transitional" year—these programs are disappearing as residency funding tightens. In 2012, 6.2% of those in the NRMP Couples Match elected to have one partner remain unmatched when the other matched at a specified level on their ROL.

There is no question that the whole Match process causes a great deal of stress among physician couples. And, if programs are not chosen with care, the stress does not end there. Couples must find out how flexible the programs will be in scheduling both on-call and vacation time. Also ask for details about how to request time-off and schedule changes. With both partners in training, flexible scheduling may be necessary for you to see each other at all. Absence may make the heart grow fonder, but in excess it can devastate a relationship. Check for scheduling flexibility before you rank a program.

Part-Time (Shared-Schedule) Positions

A shared-schedule position is one in which two residents, who usually pair up before interviewing and applying to programs, agree to each spend less than full-time in a single residency slot. In essence, they share one position.

This can be done either by having each participant spend less time per day at work or, more commonly, by alternating the weeks or months worked. This requires a great deal of forbearance on the part of a lot of people. First, the partners must be willing to work together and be flexible. Second, the program must be willing to work within the agreed-upon format. At present, very few residency applicants apply for part-time positions; in some years, none apply.

In many ways, physicians seeking part-time residency training face similar problems to those encountered by couples trying to match—although *they are completely different arrangements*. Part-time positions came into their own in the late 1970s, when changes in attitudes resulted in a federal law (now lapsed) that required most programs to offer positions to physicians who were only willing to commit limited time to residency training. (That law specified that each resident work no more than two-thirds time for no less than half-time pay. You can try to figure that one out for yourself.)

No two shared-schedule positions are ever structured in exactly the same way. *The key is to obtain the arrangement with the program, whatever it is, in writing. Be sure you have it in writing before you rank programs for the Match.* If you require scheduling in a specific manner, then get this agreed to and spelled out in advance by both your partner and the program. Chapter 23 contains the special rules for entering the NRMP Match for shared/part-time positions.

Part-time programs appear to have worked well for those involved in them; however, only about 5% of programs offer "shared-schedule/part-time" positions (Figure 14.6). Most are in Family Medicine, General Internal Medicine, Pediatrics, Preventive Medicine, and Psychiatry. The national societies and Boards in other specialties may be unfamiliar with this type of program, even if some of their residencies offer it.

The number of part-time residency positions varies by geographic region. Less than 1% of residency programs in the Mountain States (AZ, CO, ID, MT, NM, NV, UT, WY) offer part-time positions; in the northern Central region (IL, IN, MI, OH, WI) 18% of programs offer these positions. Less than 1% of military and Puerto Rican programs offer part-time positions. In reality, few residents take part-time positions.

A trainee's need for a part-time residency position often results from other pressing needs, including family considerations, the simultaneous pursuit of another profession or training program, and significant involvement in outside activities. Individuals in this type of program spend less time in any single year working, but, by the time they finish, they will spend as much or more total time in training than do full-time residents.

Usually, two physicians, both entering the same year of training, agree to split one residency position. The individual method by which a split position is achieved varies greatly from program to program. There are several keys to success:

1. You must find a flexible partner to pair with you, preferably *before* you begin to look for programs. This will often be a spouse, significant other, or good friend from school.

2. You must find a program willing to work with you to arrange a part-time position. Both *FREIDA* and the AMA's *GMED Companion* list programs that have said they will accept shared positions. The percentage

Figure 14.6
Shared-Schedule/Part-Time Positions Offered by Specialties

Specialty	Number of Prog. with Shared/Part-Time Positions	Percent of Prog. with Shared/Part-Time Positions
Allergy & Immunology	8	9%
Anesthesiology	5	4
Colon and Rectal Surgery	1	4
Dermatology	1	<1
Emergency Medicine	2	2
Family Medicine	29	8
Internal Medicine	28	10
Medical Genetics	7	14
Neurological Surgery	2	<1
Neurology	4	3
Nuclear Medicine	2	<1
Obstetrics & Gynecology	2	1
Ophthalmology	3	2
Otolaryngology	1	<1
Pathology, Anatomical & Clinical	3	2
Pediatrics	30	17
Physical Medicine & Rehabilitation	1	<1
Preventive Medicine (all areas)	24	27
Psychiatry	37	24
Radiology, Diagnostic	3	1
Thoracic Surgery	1	<1
Transitional	3	4
Urology	0	0

Data derived from American Medical Association; *Graduate Medical Education Library 2010–2011*. Chicago, IL: AMA, 2011; and *FREIDA*.

of programs with shared-schedule/part-time positions varies widely among major specialties. While no General Surgery programs offer part-time positions, they are offered by 27% of Preventive Medicine programs and 24% of Psychiatry programs.

3.   During the application process you and your partner will have to work together closely and interview together. This will emphasize to the program that you are applying as a team.

4. Get an agreement *in writing* from each program about how their part-time position will work *before* you list it in the Match. Otherwise both you and the program will be going blindly into a nebulous arrangement from which it is unlikely that *any* party will emerge happy.

Shared-schedule residencies do work, but the amount of preparation that is necessary to make them work successfully is enormous. Getting a good partner, choosing the right program, and making certain that all parties understand and agree to the details from the beginning are the keys to success.

Gay, Lesbian, Bisexual, And Transgender Applicants

Lesbian, gay, bisexual, and transgender (LGBT) medical students and physicians are a largely invisible minority, although they are becoming more visible within the medical profession as our society becomes more accepting of diversity. Maturing societal attitudes now recognize diverse sexual orientations and gender identities, and many individuals feel more comfortable identifying themselves as gay, lesbian, bisexual, or transgender. LGBT medical organizations have thousands of dues-paying members, and membership is growing. The AMA has established the LGBT Advisory Committee, and has partnered with the Gay and Lesbian Medical Association to launch a nationwide survey of physicians' knowledge and attitudes about the unique health care needs of LGBT patients.

As mentioned in other sections, however, medical practitioners generally have conservative attitudes toward their life and work, as exemplified by the difficulty that many national physician organizations have approving resolutions banning discrimination on the basis of sexual orientation. Two national surveys found that 40% of General Internists and 50% of Internal Medicine residents had witnessed homophobic comments in their workplace. In 1996, about 10% of physicians said that they would oppose openly gay and lesbian physicians seeking residency training in Obstetrics and Gynecology, Urology, and Pediatrics; and 10% would not refer patients to them no matter what their specialty. Another study of Psychiatry residents and faculty and Family Practice residents found that one-third were homophobic.

Therefore, LGBT residency applicants face difficult and, ultimately, very personal decisions regarding their sexual orientation or gender identity. Is this an aspect of your life you want to be open about during the interviewing process? Should you include some of your gay-identified activities and affiliations on your application or CV? What happens if those activities become part of your interview? Many applicants simply choose to avoid the topic and its possible negative impact on getting a residency spot.

As one medical student, Lydia Vaias, wrote in *JAMA*, "Interviews are uncomfortable, scary processes for everyone. They are particularly terrifying for lesbian and gay people, because we must grapple with telling who we are, without revealing an integral aspect of ourselves." Moreover, a medical school's respect for diversity may stop short of transgendered applicants. For support around these issues, consider joining a LGBT medical student list serve.

Becki Legg, a Stanford medical student, wrote: "I invented a male fiancée so that I could have some means of talking about my partner whom I had left back in my home state of Arizona. I was so afraid that my gayness would hurt my career that I lied to everyone, including my roommate and best friends. The energy it took to do this was enormous and I know it interfered with my class work." She later decided to "leave my LESBIAN forehead sticker at home when I start a new clerkship." When applying to residencies, her decision was "not to mention my gayness in my written applications, but in interviews I will probably out myself if I get the chance." She reasoned that she didn't "want application reviewers to form an erroneous first impression" before they met her, but also didn't "want to take a chance on ending up in a homophobic program so [she wanted the interviewers] to know what they could potentially end up getting."

There is an additional problem for gays and lesbians: Except in a few states or hospitals, your partner will not qualify for "spousal" benefits. Since these benefits are worth a substantial percentage of your income, this may be a significant loss.

One national group lends assistance and support to gays, lesbians, and bisexuals in medicine: the Gay and Lesbian Medical Association, (415) 255-4547; www.glma.org. The AAMC's website (www.aamc.org/members/gsa/glbt) provides resources to educate straight medical students and patients on LGBT issues and includes institutional self-assessment tools. The Gender & Sexuality Committee of AMSA (www.amsa.org/gender) provides news about LGBT projects and conferences, as well as a directory that rates medical schools and residency programs on LGBT-friendliness. And the AMA's GLBT Advisory Committee posts links to additional resources at www.ama-assn.org/ama/pub/about-ama/our-people/member-groups-sections/glbt-advisory-committee/glbt-resources.shtml. There are also a number of local groups in larger cities, and specific groups within some medical specialties.

Psychiatric Illness

Some medical students require psychiatric interventions, due either to pre-existing illnesses or to new conditions that appear during medical school. Why should this distinguish them from others needing medical treatments?

Some medical boards ask for complete psychiatric records of all physicians who have had psychiatric treatment when they apply for or renew their medical license. In those states that require residents to have a medical license, this includes individuals accepted to residency positions.

Residency director Norman Fost, M.D. (also a bioethicist) dealt with such requests by leaving this space blank when completing forms. Instead, he attached a note stating, "All of our residents and faculty have emotional problems. Some are sensible enough to seek professional help. If I believed Dr. X's problems interfered with his/her ability to perform duties of the position he/she is applying for, I would tell you."

Perhaps your Dean of Students can treat these requests the same way.

Underrepresented Minorities

The term "underrepresented minority" is based on government definitions of those groups that have fewer physicians than would be expected from the groups' population. The AAMC defines those "underrepresented in medicine" as "those racial and ethnic populations that are underrepresented in the medical profession relative to their numbers in the general population." Generally, this term refers to Blacks (African-Americans), American Indian/Alaskan Natives, Native Hawaiians, Pacific Islanders, and individuals of Hispanic Origin (Cuban/Mexican-American/Puerto Rican/Other Hispanic). Although there certainly are other minority groups facing many of the same problems, these are the groups with the largest number of U.S. medical school graduates that appear to be underrepresented in residency programs—especially in the subspecialties. A group that doesn't fit neatly into any category is "multiple races." They also appear to be an underrepresented minority, although the group is so diverse as to make comparisons difficult.

A survey of graduates from the class of 2009 at M.D.-granting medical schools demonstrated a decrease (since 2005) in the percentage of all underrepresented minorities except Hispanic (5.7%). However, the number of first-year minority enrollees to medical school increased by 9% from 2009 to 2010; ranging from a 2.9% increase for Blacks to a 9.1% for Hispanics. Hispanic male enrollees had the most significant growth (17.1%). These increases are viewed as encouraging given the increasingly diverse U.S. population.

Figure 14.7
Minority Representation on Medical School
Faculties in Various Clinical Specialties*

Department	Native American**	Black	Mexican American	Puerto Rican	Other Hispanic	Multiple Races	% of Specialty's Faculty* that are URM
OB/GYN	0.4%	7.0%	0.7%	1.5%	3.0%	2.0%	14.6%
Family Med	0.2	5.1	1.3	1.4	2.7	1.4	12.0
Phys Med/Rehab	0.3	3.4	0.3	1.5	2.0	2.3	9.8
Pediatrics	0.3	3.4	0.6	0.9	3.2	2.1	10.5
Public Health	0.3	6.7	0.3	---	3.2	0.8	11.3
Anesthesiology	0.3	3.4	0.4	0.6	2.8	2.4	9.8
Emergency Med	0.2	4.8	0.6	1.3	1.8	1.8	10.5
Internal Med	0.3	2.9	0.5	0.8	3.0	2.2	9.6
Surgery	0.3	3.2	0.6	0.8	2.9	2.4	10.2
Dermatology	0.1	2.5	1.1	1.0	2.0	1.9	8.4
Ophthalmology	<0.1	1.9	0.4	0.3	2.2	2.0	6.9
Psychiatry	0.2	2.6	0.5	0.6	2.9	1.3	8.1
Pathology (Clin)	0.2	1.4	0.4	0.4	3.1	2.4	7.9
Radiology	0.3	2.1	0.4	0.7	2.6	1.9	7.9
Otolaryngology	0.2	2.2	0.2	0.4	2.6	2.4	7.9
Neurology	0.1	1.2	0.5	0.1	2.9	2.2	7.0
Orthopedic Surg	0.3	2.7	0.5	0.4	1.8	1.9	7.5

Abbrev: URM = underrepresented minority
* Percentage of all medical school faculty in that specialty. Totals may vary due to rounding.
** Includes Alaskan and Hawaiian natives.
Adapted from: AAMC *Faculty Roster System,* December 2011, Table16.

In recent years, underrepresented minorities comprised about 21% of practicing U.S. physicians and 12.5% of all physicians in U.S. residency programs (Black, 6.3%; Hispanic Origin, 9.9%; Native Hawaiian/Pacific Islander, 0.6%; American Indian/ Alaskan Natives, 0.3%).

Underrepresented minority physicians are more likely to enter a generalist specialty (Family Medicine, Internal Medicine, and Pediatrics) than are physicians from other racial or ethnic groups. Among those entering generalist specialties, they are four times more likely to practice in socio-economically deprived areas than are other physicians.

Although there has been an increase in the number of minority physicians in all specialties, relatively few of these specialists are on the faculties of medical schools (Figure 14.7). Approximately 10% of full-time medical school clinical faculty are minority physicians: many of these are at the three predominantly Black schools and the three Puerto Rican schools. The faculty at these six minority schools comprises less than 2% of the total medical school faculty in the country.

Minority faculty representation is important because these individuals provide role models for minority medical students. Their absence creates an enormous void that is hard for other faculty to fill. Because this absence is especially acute in many of the non-primary care specialties, some minority medical students feel considerable social pressure to enter primary care and "return to their communities." If they do enter a subspecialty, they often are made to feel like traitors since many subspecialists' services are not readily available to minority communities.

A higher percentage of minority medical students plan to enter Family Medicine, Internal Medicine, Pediatrics, Psychiatry, Obstetrics and Gynecology, and General Surgery compared to their classmates. They do not plan to go into the smaller specialty and subspecialty areas in comparable numbers. Because role models are not available to show them alternative routes for their careers, they may feel that their options are more limited than those of the majority of medical students.

As Dr. Freeman Favors, a Black Emergency Physician, said, "Many minority students think to themselves 'I don't see minorities in this specialty, so why try to get in?'" This becomes a self-fulfilling statement. It keeps many minority students from even applying to many specialties, and thus they accept only a handful of minority residents. Dr. Favors wasn't intimidated, and he has done very well in his chosen field. He exhorts minority students to be courageous when setting their professional goals. He also suggests that minority students who desire to enter hard-to-match-with specialties look for regions of the country where their minority is underrepresented. As he says, "They can be at a competitive advantage by being a 'rare gem' at such programs and institutions."

No matter what specialty minority medical students want to enter, it appears that they consistently do worse in obtaining residency positions compared to other students. Many reasons have been given for this. While racial and ethnic barriers have fallen in some specialties, there still appears to be an "invisible quota system," due to reluctance by some to rank too many minority candidates for the Match. This may be because some faculty members still feel uncomfortable having more than one or two minority residents in a program. Given the uncertainty of the Match, ranking a lot of minority candidates could result in several such students matching with their program. This is probably equally true in those programs using a non-NRMP matching process.

During the past decade, programs with the highest percentage of minority residents and fellows have been those in municipally owned hospitals, those in the western United States, those with major university affiliations, and those at hospitals with 700 or more beds. Programs with the smallest number of minority residents and fellows (as a percentage of total residents and fellows) have been in small hospitals (399 or fewer beds) that are university-owned, those run by the Veterans' Administration, and those in the southern United States.

Pressure is being put on medical schools to increase the number of both minority faculty and minority residents. Grants to encourage minority faculty's education and research provide strong incentives, as do the embarrassing statistics published by the AMA, the AAMC, and the federal government about minority representation in each school and specialty. State governments that fund health-related positions also look at these numbers: If you are a minority student, this could work to your advantage. To get a good position, however, you still have to be as good as, or better than, the competition—and be able to demonstrate that to interviewers and selection committees. This is one reason why you are reading this book: to learn how to do exactly that.

Of particular concern is one study that showed that 20% of Blacks and Hispanics (including Puerto Ricans) were not in a residency program three years after graduation from medical school. At present, the reasons for this are unclear, but these findings suggest that these physicians enter medical practice, probably in primary care, at a disadvantage when compared to their fully trained colleagues.

Harassment

About one-third of underrepresented minority residents felt that they had suffered ethnic discrimination during their first year of residency. In most cases, this is expressed as racial or ethnic slurs, favoritism toward other groups, poor evaluations, and denied opportunities.

Minority women physicians experience harassment based on their ethnicity at a rate six to nine times that of white women. Black women physicians have the highest rate; 35% of those less than 50-years-old experienced harassment during training and 32% experienced it in their practice. Forty percent of Muslim women had experienced ethnic harassment.

Native American Applicants

Physicians identified as Native Americans make up less than 0.5% of all U.S. physicians. One must be at least one-eighth Indian to be considered a Native American or an Alaskan Native. Most of these physicians practice in the West and the South. There are only about 55 Native American physicians per 100,000 Native Americans in the population. This is the lowest ratio of any ethnic group's physicians to their population in the United States. It is, therefore, unlikely that a Native American medical student will come across a role model either in his or her home environment or at medical school. Recent studies suggest that about half of all current Native American physicians are in primary care specialties. Only about 0.9% of all residents are either Native American or Alaskan/Hawaiian Natives.

It is not always apparent that one is a Native American. Listing membership in the Association of American Indian Physicians on your application is an unobtrusive way of mentioning that you are a minority candidate. All other things being equal, this might give you an edge. For more information about and for Native Americans in medicine, contact: Association of American Indian Physicians, (405) 946-7072; www.aaip.org.

Black Applicants (African-Americans)

Today there are approximately 90 Black physicians per 100,000 Blacks in the population. Of these physicians, about 25% graduated from one of the three predominantly Black medical schools: Meharry Medical College, Morehouse School of Medicine, and Howard University Medical School. Only about 5% of all physicians in residency programs are non-Hispanic Blacks.

Approximately 25% more Black physicians choose primary care specialties than does the general population of physicians. There are usually role models available for Black medical students, either at their medical school or in the community. Most medical schools have some Black faculty members, albeit not in all specialties.

Yet discrimination does exist within the medical fraternity. One study showed that if a residency program uses USMLE Step 1 scores to screen applicants for interviews, Black applicants suffer disproportionately. As you expand your horizons to search for the ideal training program, be aware that you may have to do more to prove yourself than other candidates. And unfortunately, this reality may persist throughout your training, as well as afterwards. For more information, contact: National Medical Association, (202) 347-1895, www. nmanet.org; or the Student National Medical Association, (202) 882-2881; www.snma.org; e-mail: snmamain@msn.com.

Hispanic Applicants

Hispanic applicants should know that many interviewers are unaware that the term "Hispanic" represents a diverse classification category. "Hispanic" includes persons of Cuban descent, Puerto Ricans, Mexican-Americans (Chicanos), and those of Latin American or Central American descent. Federal government guidelines do not consider all of them minorities; in medicine, some definitely are not minorities. Cuban-Americans, for example, are represented in medical schools to a greater extent, as a percentage of population, than nearly any other subgroup in the United States.

However, even including all Hispanic physicians, there are only about 80 Hispanic physicians in practice per 100,000 Hispanics compared to approximately 202 white physicians per 100,000 whites in the population. But 61% of Puerto Rican physicians have graduated from one of the three medical schools in Puerto Rico. Partially due to language and cultural barriers, relatively few of these graduates apply to mainland training programs.

In recent years, about 2% of new interns were Puerto Rican, 1.8% were Mexican-American, and 1.8% were "other Hispanics."When surveyed, 9.9% of all physicians in residency programs classified themselves as Hispanic. As the U.S. Hispanic population grows, fluency in both Spanish and English will become a definite plus for any applicant. If you have this skill, promote it in your application materials. For more information, contact: the National Hispanic Medical Association, (202) 628-5895, www.nhmamd.org.

Physically Impaired Applicants

The subgroup of physically impaired medical students is unique. The individuals in this group are singular both among medical students, for their tenacity and drive to overcome the obstacles to get where they are, and among the physically impaired, since they are able enough to complete medical school's clinical requirements.

There are about 3,000 practicing U.S. physicians with major physical disabilities. (Estimates of the number of physicians with disabilities range from 2.5% to 4%.) Of those medical students with known physical impairment (only about 0.25% of all medical students), approximately 25% have visual disabilities, 42% have neurological or musculoskeletal impairments, 8% have an auditory disability, and 14% have learning disabilities. While some residency programs may hesitate to take a physically impaired individual, this attitude is normally due to ignorance.

Educate these educators! Explain to them that you have been able to do what was necessary, with only "reasonable accommodations," in each of the clinical settings to which you were exposed. You may have to not only tell them in detail, but also show them. For, while federal legislation protects an individual from discriminatory questioning, such as being asked about the extent of your disability, it is permissible for interviewers to inquire about, and even to test, your ability to perform the job for which you are applying. Don't worry about this. If you did it in medical school, you can do it anywhere. Show your stuff!

As an example, after being denied admission to more than two dozen medical schools in the early 1990s, James B. Post IV, a quadriplegic since age 14, graduated in 1997 from Albert Einstein College of Medicine in the top 15% of his class. Upon graduating from medical school, he had little trouble getting an Internal Medicine residency position. A Physician Assistant, whom he paid for, helped him. He now practices Nephrology. Einstein had previously graduated a paraplegic who became a Pathologist. In the past decade, there have been up to ten quadriplegics in U.S. medical schools at any one time. In December 2004, a blind medical student graduated near the top of his class at the University of Wisconsin-Madison, where he was also completing a Ph.D.

In the past, a physician's disability usually influenced his or her specialty choice if it occurred before or during medical school. Severely handicapped individuals usually entered Physiatry, Psychiatry, Pathology, or Anesthesiology. Those with disabilities that occurred later tended to stay in their original specialties, if they could. Many severely handicapped medical students and physicians now employ sophisticated medical assistive technology that helps them use necessary equipment or interpret clinical results. Three of the most common devices are rising electronic chairs that enable paralyzed practitioners to stand over an OR table, voice-activated or "reading" computer programs, and the "Optacon" that converts EKG images into vibratory signals for the visually impaired.

Under the Americans with Disabilities Act of 1990, "disability" is defined as a physical or mental impairment that substantially limits one or more major life activities (e.g., caring for oneself, performing manual tasks, walking, seeing, hearing, speaking, breathing, learning, and working). Under the Act, persons are considered disabled if they have a record of such an impairment or they are regarded as having such an impairment. The Act requires potential employers to make "reasonable accommodations" for disabled job applicants and workers, as long as the accommodations do not impose "undue hardships" on their business operation. If you are a disabled residency applicant, that applies to you. In addition, if you are not currently disabled but become disabled once you are a resident, they must make reasonable accommodations for you.

While having a contagious disease (such as tuberculosis or HIV) is considered an impairment, the excessive use of drugs (both illegal and legal), alcoholism that interferes with job performance, sex-related behavior and disorders, and certain behavioral disorders (including pyromania, kleptomania, and compulsive gambling) are *not* covered by the Act.

If you believe that your impairment will hinder you when taking the USMLE or COMLEX, be certain, well before the application deadline, to contact the examining agency: NBOME for Levels 1 and 2, National Board of Medical Examiners (NBME) or the Educational Commission for Foreign Medical Graduates (ECFMG) for Steps 1 and 2, and the state or territorial licensing authority for Step 3 or level 3. They will tell you what documentation to submit so that they can arrange the special accommodations necessary for you to take the test. Special accommodations that they can make include granting extra time for the test or extra rest breaks, providing a reader or recorder, and using visual aids or enlarged-print examinations. If you test under any special conditions, your score reports and transcripts will include a note to that effect.

One caveat for those who do not think that they have a physical impairment that could keep them out of a training program: At least one-third of the Ophthalmology programs, all Aerospace Medicine programs, and a smattering of other programs test applicants for color vision and stereognosis. This is perfectly legal if all applicants are screened and they can show that the requirement is job related. Some applicants, especially men, fail such tests. You may want to find out whether you have this physical impairment prior to setting your heart on one of these specialties.

For more information about the American Disability Act applied to healthcare professionals, see the AAMC's (free in pdf) *Medical Students with Disabilities: A Generation of Practice* (search for it at https://services.aamc.org/publications/) or contact the U.S. Equal Employment Opportunity Commission, (202) 669-4900; TTY: (202) 669-6820; e-mail: info@ask.eeoc.gov; www.eeoc.gov.

Osteopathic Physicians

As an Osteopathic physician, you have one of two problems in getting a residency position, depending upon how you intend to approach your training: The limited number of Osteopathic specialties to choose from or the intransigence and constantly shifting rules of some Osteopathic licensing bodies.

Between 1970 and 2012, the number of D.O. students increased more than 900%, and the number of Osteopathic schools increased from 9 to 26. By 2012, there were nearly 4,000 D.O. graduates each year. However, D.O.'s can be certified by an Osteopathic specialty Board only in the following specialties:

Anesthesiology	Orthopedic Surgery
Dermatology	Otolaryngology-Head
Emergency Medicine	& Neck Surgery
Family Medicine	Pathology
Internal Medicine	Pediatrics
Neurology & Psychiatry	Phys. Med. & Rehab.
Neuromuscular Med/OMT	Preventative Medicine
Nuclear Medicine	Proctologic Surgery
Obstetrics/Gynecology	Radiology
Ophthalmology	Surgery

All these graduates could not enter D.O. internships if they wanted to: the approximately 2,500 funded Osteopathic first-year training slots are insufficient to meet their needs, and most aren't even in the specialties that these new physicians want to enter (Figure 14.8). This means that many Osteopathic graduates must look to the M.D. side of the profession for their training. The American Osteopathic Association's (AOA) Intern/Resident Registration Program (the "Match") and the Military's matching program are the only ways to get AOA-approved training (see Chapter 23).

AOA-approved first-year training provides three "Options" for D.O.'s, depending on the specialty involved. The Option required by each specialty is noted in Figure 14.8. (Always double-check with the AOA, as these requirements may change.)

OPTION 1 (OGME-1R, Resident) The first year of training is an integral part of the residency, and is considered to be the first year of residency training. Graduating students to match directly into the specialty's residency programs. Residents receive credit for an AOA-approved first year of training. This system is similar to that used for most ACGME-approved specialties.

OPTION 2: These specialties require a designated preliminary first year of training (OGME-1P). Students will match to the specialty residency program, and that program will ensure that students have the necessary AOA-approved OGME-1 training. Students match to one program. Currently used for Diagnostic Radiology, Neuromusculoskeletal Med/OMT,

Figure 14.8
Osteopathic Internships and Residencies*

SPECIALTY	Number of Programs	Total Approved Positions	Funded 1st-year Specialty Training Positions	Filled 1st-year Positions
Anesthesiology[†]	12	107	27	27
Dermatology[§]	20	123	41	31
Diagnostic Radiology[#]	14	133	20	19
Emergency Medicine[†]	43	979	216	214
Emerg Med-Family Pract[†]	5	59	7	7
Emergency Med-Internal Med[†]	12	130	18	10
Family Pract[†]	184	2,341	707	380
Family Pract-Neuromusculoskeletal Med[†]	7	49	10	9
Internal Medicine[†]	88	1,320	448	304
Neurological Surgery[†]	11	97	13	11
Neurology[†]	7	61	13	11
Neuromuscular Med-OMT[#]	27	100	11	10
Obstetrics/Gynecology[†]	31	370	72	69
Ophthalmology[#]	12	57	9	8
Orthopedic Surgery[†]	31	465	93	79
Otolaryngology/Facial Plastic Surg[†]	19	132	26	21
Pediatrics[†]	17	225	58	51
Physical Med & Rehab[#]	3	28	6	5

Preventive Med/Pub Hlth§	1	1	3	0
Proctologic Surgery†	2	1	5	<1
Psychiatry†	9	28	95	19
Surgery, General†	41	104	536	104
Radiation Oncology#		No Programs		
Traditional Rotating Internship	N/A	561	N/A	171
Urological Surgery†	11	19	123	19
Other Specialties/Fellowships**	143	109	511	105
TOTAL	**606**	**2,509**	**7473**	**1,580**

* These numbers are constantly changing. In May 2011, there were 2,553 funded 1st-year positions, of which only 1,640 had been filled.

† Students can match directly into these specialties, officially called the "OGME-1R Residency (Option 1)."

Requires a "Preliminary Internship," or OGME-1P Preliminary Internship (Option 2). Matching assures entry into both the preliminary year (OGME-1) and the residency years (OGME-2).

§ Requires a traditional rotating OGME-1 year, called OGME-1T, Traditional Internship (Option 3). Application to residency programs is done during the intern year.

** Of this number, there are 84 programs and 335 total positions in Internal Medicine subspecialties.

Information from: American Osteopathic Association, www.osteopathic.org/inside-aoa/Education/, May 2012 and October 2011.

Ophthalmology, Pathology, Physical Med/Rehab, and Radiation Oncology.

OPTION 3 (OGME-1T, Traditional) is a rotating internship used by individuals who have not yet decided on a specialty, who do not plan on going into a residency, or who wish to enter a specialty that does not go through the Match and requires a separate application. (Dermatology and Public Health/Preventive Medicine.)

Osteopathic graduates say they "jump ship" to M.D. programs because they believe these programs provide better training, pay higher salaries, and include specialty training that is unavailable in Osteopathic programs. That is not surprising since there are only 13 Osteopathic teaching hospitals with more than 300 beds in the United States. Osteopathic educators see AOA-approved postgraduate programs as a haven for D.O.'s interested in surgical or other non-Internal Medicine and non-Family Practice specialties.

Said one D.O., defending students who do M.D. residencies, "Students do not see anything distinctive in what Osteopathic graduate medical education training programs have that would differentiate them from [M.D.] programs . . . these choices may be the result of enlightened decision making and not necessarily an indication of disloyalty." If you intend to pursue ACGME-approved (M.D.) training, as did nearly two-thirds of recent Osteopathic graduates (including government and other joint AOA-ACGME-approved programs), you will have to deal with both the American Osteopathic Association (AOA) and the programs themselves. Also, beginning in 2014, you may find your choices restricted by the ACGME. See "Proposed ACGME Changes to M.D. Program Requirements," below.

As of 2012, about 11% of all residency programs in the United States had both AOA and ACGME (D.O. and M.D.) accreditation. About 11% of Osteopathic medical students plan on entering one of these programs. See Figure 15.2 for match rates in selected specialties. Another 47% plan on doing an M.D. residency, and 10% plan on entering a federal government-sponsored residency. About 32% plan on entering a residency approved by only the AOA.

"Dual" Programs

In the past, the AOA made it difficult to pursue training in ACGME-approved programs. As a D.O., you cannot get a medical license in four states (FL, MI, OK, PA) if you have not completed an AOA-approved internship. Some states may also require completion of an AOA-approved residency. Yet, faced with the increasing numbers of Osteopathic graduates and the small number of funded internship positions in many specialties, the AOA has created policies that allow for approval of some ACGME training programs.

These are known as "Dual" programs (Figure 14.9) and, as of January 2012, are pre-approved by both the AOA and the ACGME. In these programs, both D.O. and M.D. residents are fully integrated into the clinical and didactic parts of a single training program. (This is in contrast to the decreasing number of "Parallel" programs, AOA- and ACGME-approved programs that exist side by side in which D.O and M.D. trainees rarely interact.) However, this may change in 2014. See "Proposed ACGME Changes to M.D. Program Requirements."

In a survey of senior Osteopathic medical students about why they planned to enter dual programs, 43% said that a dual program "would allow ABMS Board certification"; 39% said it "would offer better educational opportunities"; and 34% said it "would offer more training opportunities."

Figure 14.9
Comparison of Selected Dual and AOA-Only Programs

Specialty	Dual Programs	Available Dual Positions	Filled (%)	AOA-Only Positions	Filled (%)
Child Psychiatry	1	6	50%	2	50%
Emergency Med	3	83	56	719	66
Family Practice	90	1,008	33	1,088	38
Internal Medicine	26	309	27	812	35
Internal Med/Peds	1	10	100	8	0
Neurology	1	6	67	33	52
OB/GYN	3	18	47	342	42
Occ/Environ Med	0	0	0	0	0
Pediatrics	14	180	49	27	48
Phys Med/Rehab	2	22	82	6	67
Psychiatry	4	39	62	33	18
Sports Medicine	3	9	56	33	27

Adapted from: Burkhart DN, Lischka TA: Dual and parallel postdoctoral training programs: implications for the Osteopathic medical profession. *JAOA*. 2009;109(3):146-53.

Individuals who complete dual programs have the option of taking either or both specialty Board exams (i.e., AOA and ABMS). If you want to do an ACGME-approved (M.D.) residency that is not a "dual program" and (a) plan to get a medical license in Maine, Michigan, Vermont or Florida; (b) become certified by an AOA specialty Board; or (c) do an AOA-approved residency, you will need to get the ACGME (M.D.) residency approved by the AOA or else later go through an onerous process with the D.O. licensing board.

AOA Approval of M.D. Programs

To get an M.D. program approved, use the rules under AOA's *Resolution 42* (A/2000—Approval of ACGME Training as an AOA-Approved Internship). This allows Osteopaths in (non-dually approved) ACGME internships or residencies to apply for AOA approval for their training. Only 12 out of 1,818 applicants have been denied approval since the resolution was enacted in 2000. The 4-part process is more fully described at: www.osteopathic.org/inside-aoa/Education/.

Basically, applicants must:

1. Be AOA members in good standing. Other than AOA membership fees, there is no cost for processing this application.

2. Complete the two-page application found on the AOA website.

3. Provide the AOA with a comparison of your clinical rotations with those required in the same AOA-approved internship. Your rotations must be completed during your first year of training and be equivalent to the standards listed on the AOA's website.

4. Complete one of these approved "educational activities":

   a. Attend the AOA Annual Osteopathic Medical Conference and Exposition.

   b. Attend the annual meeting of the relevant Osteopathic specialty college or AOA-affiliated divisional society that grants 8 CME Category-1A credit hours.

   c. While still in residency, prepare and conduct an Osteopathic clinical presentation to your ACGME residency program, or to the relevant Osteopathic specialty college, and/or submit a manuscript from this presentation and a verification letter from the program director for review.

Osteopathic physicians who are currently in, or who have completed, Federal or Military internships may apply for AOA review. Training programs will be approved on an individual basis. The AOA's procedures for approving Federal/Military PGY-1 training can also be found on their website. Applicants must be AOA members and provide a copy of their military or government orders. In addition, they must submit a copy of their clinical rotation schedule; the training must include all "core criteria" listed on the AOA website. Since not all programs will fulfill these requirements, the AOA suggests using elective time to complete as many of these requirements as possible.

The Program and Trainee Review Council (PTRC) meets in April, July and November. Applicants for approval receive written notification of the PTRC's action within 10 days after the meeting. Less than 1% of these exemption applications are denied. Call the AOA with any questions: (800) 621-1773, ext. 8276.

Information on M.D. Programs

More Osteopathic graduates are entering ACGME-approved training programs each year. Between 1986 and 2012, the number of D.O.'s entering PGY-1 positions in M.D. residency programs increased 250%. However, for whatever reason, ACGME-approved training in some specialties is almost completely off-limits to Osteopaths (Figure 14.10). Chief among these are various surgical specialties, such as Neurological Surgery, Hand Surgery, Ophthalmology, Orthopedic Surgery, Otolaryngology, Pediatric Surgery, Plastic Surgery, Thoracic Surgery, and Urology.

If you apply to ACGME-approved programs, make certain that you explain, in detail, exactly what your COMLEX scores mean (unless you took the USMLE—a smart move), what your curriculum consists of, and what the grading scale on your transcript signifies. (It might help to review "Comparing COMLEX and USMLE Scores" in Chapter 8.) Remember that these may be significantly different from the scores, curricula, and grading scales seen in applications from M.D. students.

Also, be careful about your Dean's letter. While most Deans of Osteopathic medical schools send out respectable letters that are comparable to those sent out by M.D. Deans, some send out almost cursory statements. One wonders if these are sent only to ACGME-approved programs, in an attempt to "keep you in the fold"?

While you may encounter problems when entering ACGME-approved programs, if that is the training that will meet your future needs, by all means, go for it!

Proposed ACGME Changes to M.D. Program Requirements

If you are planning on training in an M.D. (ACGME-approved) internship, residency, or fellowship, you may face even more challenges in the future. The ACGME has proposed two changes in its program requirements which, if implemented, will restrict D.O. entry into ACGME programs.

First, while the ACGME will continue to accept Osteopathic medical students into ACGME programs through the NRMP Match as before, starting in 2014, the ACGME plans to discontinue awarding credit for completing an AOA-approved first year of training. This would limit AOA-trained D.O.s' ability to enter a second year of ACGME training. This change would primarily affect residents who anticipate living in one of the four states (FL, ME, MI, and VT) requiring an AOA-approved first year of training for state licensure and wish to enter into ACGME training.

Second, beginning in 2015, the ACGME plans to discontinue recognizing completion of AOA-accredited residency training for entry into an ACGME fellowship program. This policy would restrict D.O.'s in AOA-accredited programs from direct entry into ACGME fellowships.

This proposal has created havoc among D.O. students. As this book goes to press, the AOA leadership has been in communications with ACGME leaders. The Osteopathic specialty colleges, AACOM, and many allopathic organizations are advocating against these changes. It is possible that the proposed policies may be withdrawn or changed. Osteopathic students and residents can find updated information on the AOA's Inside AOA website.

Common Questions

As an Osteopathic medical student or graduate, can I participate in the National Residency Matching Program (NRMP)? Yes, you participate as an "Independent Applicant." For additional information, see Chapter 23, *The NRMP and Other Matches*. Note that most programs now use the Electronic Residency Application Service (ERAS; see Chapter 13).

Should I take the USMLE or the Osteopathic licensing exam (COMLEX)? As an Osteopathic student, generally, you will want to take *both* the USMLE and COMLEX, since comparative results show that the COMLEX is a little easier to pass than the USMLE. The main reason to take the USMLE is that residency directors at M.D. programs can more easily judge your qualifications against other applicants. If you take only the COMLEX and apply for an M.D. residency, be sure to explain how the test is scored. If possible, send them copies of the official information sheet that came with your scores. Also, attach a small "cheat sheet" summarizing your performance.

What options do I have if I am in or have taken an Osteopathic internship? You have three options for residency training. First, you can directly contact Osteopathic or M.D. residency programs with openings and apply to them. (See "Not Using A Match" in Chapter 23.) Second, you can apply to an M.D. residency program through the NRMP Advanced Match, either as a senior student or during your intern year. Finally, you can simply enter the NRMP Match during your intern year to begin an M.D. residency at the PGY-1 level. The option you choose depends upon your personal situation and on the competitiveness of the specialty you want to enter. However, be sure to read "Proposed Changes to ACGME Program Requirements," above.

Is there discrimination against D.O.'s among M.D. residency directors? To deny that many M.D. residency programs discriminate against D.O.'s would be foolish. As Frederick Boling, D.O., who has practiced for 50 years, wrote in the April 2010 issue of *JAOA*, "I am fully aware that my D.O. degree is equal to any M.D. degree, but, unfortunately, most allopathic physicians and allopathic societies, colleges, academies, and other institutions do not understand that fact. The Osteopathic medical profession has made a great deal of progress in resolving this situation, but much remains to be done."

Indeed, many residency directors do not understand that Osteopathic training parallels that of M.D. schools. This discrimination, however, varies by the area of the country and by the specialty. In areas with many D.O.'s in practice and established Osteopathic medical schools, there is minimal discrimination. Where there are few D.O.'s, ignorance abounds. As for specialties, General Surgery and its subspecialties continue to be the major areas whose residency programs automatically reject most D.O. applicants.

Older Applicants

Many students now enter medicine after they have raised a family or as a second career. In the last decade, the number of students over 28-years-old entering medical school has doubled. This group now comprises about 34% of all graduating students; 10% are at least 30-years-old. Older nontraditional students may have some unique problems in medical school, and they may face some obstacles when applying for residency positions.

First, because older students may have more debt and more financial responsibilities than younger students, they may be tempted to jump into the most lucrative practice they can in the shortest amount of time. Many

Figure 14.10
D.O.'s in ACGME-Approved Residency & Fellowship Programs

Specialty	Number of D.O.'s in Training	% of all Available M.D. Positions
Allergy/Immunology	11	4%
Anesthesiology	463	9
Cardiovascular Disease	98	4
Child/Adolescent Psychiatry	57	8
Colon & Rectal Surgery	2	3
Critical Care Medicine (All)	49	14
Dermatology	17	2
Emergency Medicine	504	11
Endocrinology	34	6
Family Medicine	1,374	15
Gastroenterology (IM)	70	5
Geriatrics (IM & FP)	320	6
Hand Surgery (All)	0	0
Hematology/Oncology (IM)	46	3
Infectious Diseases (IM)	34	4
Internal Medicine	1,296	6
Internal Med–Pediatrics	100	7
Neonatal-Perinatal Medicine	33	6
Nephrology (IM)	49	6
Neurological Surgery	4	<1
Neurology	114	7
Nuclear Medicine	4	3
Obstetrics & Gynecology	388	8
Ophthalmology	12	1
Orthopedic Surgery	31	1
Otolaryngology	4	<1
Pain Medicine	40	18
Pathology	128	6
Pediatrics	656	8
Pediatric Surgery	0	0

Figure 14.10 (continued)

Specialty	Number of D.O.'s in Training	% of all Available M.D. Positions
Physical Med/Rehabilitation	301	25%
Plastic Surgery	4	1
Preventive Med/Pub Hlth (all)	20	8
Psychiatry	377	8
Pulmonary Disease (IM-All)	86	6
Radiation Oncology	9	2
Radiology, Diagnostic	172	4
Rheumatology (IM)	25	6
Sleep Medicine	8	8
Sports Medicine (All)	154	15
Surgery, General	208	3
Thoracic Surgery	2	1
Transitional Year	40	4
Urology	12	1

Adapted from: Brotherton SE, Etzel SI: Graduate medical education, 2008-2009. *JAMA.* 2009;302(12):1357-72.

may decide to bypass specialties in which they have a real interest but whose training takes longer. Bad move! If you have invested time, lost income, and endured the stress to get through medical school, you should aim for the goal you really want. Apply to the specialty that most interests you. The extra year or two of training will pay you back immeasurably in the satisfaction that you (and your family) have in your work during your career.

The second difficulty older applicants face is the negative attitude of some residency faculty members. They may perceive the older applicant as possessing maturity, but not enough stamina and energy to complete a demanding residency. Spending time with the program faculty, either in a clinical setting on a formal rotation or in educational rounds, may overcome their hesitation. During your interviews, describe your high energy level within the context of other answers. One example might be, "I stayed by her bedside all night in the ICU, monitoring her status and adjusting her medications. It was exhilarating." Finally, many older applicants come to medicine after other life experiences to truly serve humanity. Many faculty will respond positively to a heartfelt description of why you made such a difficult life decision. Tell them.

Physicians who are making a mid-career switch—changing specialties—are a subgroup of older applicants. The most common reasons physicians give for changing specialties, either during residency or after they are in practice, are: (a) they become enlightened or (b) they become disillusioned with their prior specialty. While about 40% of those who change specialties are generalists, 60% are specialists. Of those who change specialties late in their career (40- to 69-years-old), the most common profile is a woman international medical graduate with a hospital-based practice in an Internal Medicine subspecialty, Emergency Medicine (probably not residency-trained with this profile), a Pediatrics subspecialty, or Pathology.

Some physicians are forced to change specialties due to physical disabilities. Others need to change specialties, often to a primary care specialty, to find a job where they want to live. Residency directors may be reluctant to accept these applicants unless they can adequately demonstrate that they have come to terms with making the specialty change. Programs are not looking for applicants who do not really want to be in their residency.

The first question residency directors ask is "Are you seeking to enter our specialty or simply running away from the one you are in?" That is a darn good question—one you need to ask yourself before starting the process. Why do you really want to do this? At the least, it will cost you extra time, decrease your income, and alter your lifestyle or where you live.

If your extensive qualifications are used as a reason to not hire you as a resident, note that a New York Federal District Court ruled that an employer declining to offer a position on the grounds that the candidate is "overqualified" may be violating the Age Discrimination in Employment Act. According to the court, the term "overqualified" may simply be a code word for too old.

Physicians face multiple problems in making such a change. The most obvious problem for those going back to residency after being in practice is the resultant change in lifestyle. Going from a practicing physician's salary to a resident's salary can be a rude experience for both the physician and his or her family. Ego damage can also be a problem. The shift from the role of omnipotent attending to lowly resident can be quite a blow—especially when some of the residency's faculty are younger than you (or sometimes, your children).

Occasionally, physicians who have left clinical practice for administration or research decide to reenter the clinical world. This may be a daunting step. As one returnee noted, "My greatest fear was my ignorance—the amalgam of what I had forgotten combined with what had been added to the realm of practice since I had last been there." The key is to choose a supportive program that will provide a curriculum tailored to your individual needs. This may be harder to find than you assume.

The specialties that most commonly receive trainees who previously were in other specialties are Anesthesiology (sometimes called "the Foreign Legion of Medicine" for all the escapees from other specialties in its ranks), Diagnostic Radiology, Emergency Medicine, Family Medicine, Internal Medicine, and Neurology. Practitioners most commonly leave Internal Medicine for other specialties.

The keys to successfully making a mid-career switch are to adequately prepare yourself and your family for the changes, to carefully investigate what you are getting into, and to make contact in advance with potential residency directors. If you plan to take training in the town where you practice, attend some teaching conferences and make arrangements to observe or participate clinically with some of the attendings. Knowledgeable residency directors will see an applicant who comes to residency training with prior clinical experience as a real bonus—if you can show them that you know what you are getting into and that you want to be there.

Military/Public Health Service

Two basic questions come up when discussing your involvement in military residencies. First, what is involved in a commitment to the Armed Forces medical system? Second, how is playing this game different from competing in the normal application and matching processes?

There are several factors to consider when looking at military residencies. The most obvious is financial. If you are in the School of Medicine of the Uniform Services University of the Health Sciences (USUHS), you are obligated to do a military residency. The military is obligated to find you a first-year training slot. You have saved a great deal of money, and will pay it back with the years you commit to the service at much lower pay than your civilian counterparts receive.

If you have enrolled in the three- or four-year Armed Forces Health Professions Scholarship Program (HPSP), the military will pay for your tuition, expenses, and required books. They will also give you a stipend for living expenses. In return, you owe them four 45-day active-duty tours during each year of medical school, four years of active duty as an Armed Forces doctor, and four years of inactive reserve duty. If your residency lasts more than four years, you will owe more time. You have, of course, avoided a large debt by obligating yourself to military service. In addition, if you train in a military residency, you can expect a higher rate of compensation than if you were in a civilian residency. But you don't get something for nothing. Your colleagues will normally make up the difference in salary after they finish training and begin their medical practice, although most will also be saddled with a large educational debt.

Military residencies typically involve a greater time commitment than civilian residencies, and you can be pulled out after the first (internship) year to fill General Medical Officer (GMO) openings, tours that can last two to three years. This is most common in Navy programs. These GMO tours as a "sick call" doctor provide unique opportunities, and these years are subtracted from your time commitment. After the tour, you will continue your specialty training at the second-year level. After you have completed your active-duty obligation, you will become a member of the Independent Ready Reserves (your "inactive" duty). Be aware that as a member of the Reserves, you can be called up at any time, including while you are building a practice. Finally, since the September 11 attacks, the military reserves the right to keep you in the service in times of crisis. So, even if you have served your contracted time, you could be prevented from leaving until the crisis is resolved.

Military medicine is changing rapidly as the Armed Forces are being heavily used in multiple wars, thus requiring more physicians to serve abroad and for longer periods of time. Simultaneously, battlefield medicine is going "high tech," with many cutting-edge developments to assist military physicians in the field. On the domestic front, military medicine is being downsized and the medical care of military dependents is being outsourced to the civilian sector.

As noted above, Osteopathic medical students might want to consider military residency training. The AOA is usually willing to recognize as valid any residency that is done in the military. This provides Osteopathic graduates a chance at what may be a more intense and varied residency experience than they could obtain in the civilian world. Additionally, successful completion of a military residency generally allows the Osteopathic physician to apply for both M.D. and Osteopathic specialty Boards. Make sure, however, that the individual program has been approved by the AOA *before* you start your training. Also read the section titled "Proposed Changes to ACGME Program Requirements", above.

Finally, if you have your heart set on entering the specialty of Aerospace Medicine, you will normally need to join the Air Force or the Navy to get a residency position. And you usually will not be able to enter the residency directly from school or even after your internship. These programs routinely require applicants to have some experience, as well as to have passed short courses in Aerospace Medicine offered through the military. However, there are two civilian residency programs in Aerospace Medicine: one at Wright State University School of Medicine in Dayton, Ohio, and the other at the University of Texas in Galveston. If you are interested in training for Undersea and Hyperbaric Medicine, you will normally have to join the Navy.

If you want to do a military residency, how do you obtain a position? All U.S. Army and most Navy residency programs (all specialties) use the Electronic Residency Application Service (ERAS), although each branch also has its own application. (Chapter 13 has more information about ERAS.) According to former U.S. Army Surgeon General Ronald R. Blanck, the Army, Navy, and Air Force fill their first-year residency positions with graduates of the Uniformed Services University of the Health Sciences, medical students with an individual military commitment (often through HPSP), and those in the Reserve Officers' Training Corps. Only individuals on active military duty can participate in Armed Forces residency programs.

The military's selection system for matching applicants with programs is similar to the NRMP Match in that both applicants and programs send in rank order lists. However, representatives of the military teaching hospitals meet, exchange information about the candidates, and make the selections, rather than having it done impartially by computer. Priority is given to those on active duty at the time of selection and to graduates of the F. Edward Hebert School of Medicine, Uniformed Services University of the Health Sciences (military medical school) in Bethesda, Maryland. The selections are then finalized. There are generally many more applicants for military residency positions than there are available slots.

The military match occurs early in the senior year. Therefore, competing in the military match means you have to make career decisions very early. Finding out about military training programs is often more difficult than getting information about civilian programs. Your best sources of information, aside from the "Green Book" and *FREIDA*, are military residents, military physicians, and your military branch's Medical Personnel Counselor. These latter individuals vary greatly in quality and interest. Be certain to cross-check any information they give you.

Early planning and preparation are very important. Military residencies are extremely competitive, and the number of open spots varies from year to year depending on the military's needs. The residencies and subspecialties offered are also based on projected military needs, so if there are sufficient personnel in a particular specialty, acquiring training in it may be extremely difficult. To verify what has been approved each year for the Air Force, check the "Specialties" Table on their HPSP website at http://ci.afit.edu/cimj/specialties_table.asp. Neither the Navy nor the Army has a comparable website.

You should be able to get a good idea of the programs you wish to attend, since military specialties have only three to five residency programs each. To get into the specialty and the military residency program you desire, you are highly encouraged to do your "away" rotation (subinternship) in that specialty and at that site during or immediately after your third year of medical school. Arranging for this rotation can often take six months or more. Your activities during this subinternship are not much different than those described for a civilian subinternship. Be sure that both the residency director and the department chairman know who you are and are impressed with the job that you do. Try to set up your residency interview during your rotation. Also secure a letter of recommendation from a military doctor as one of your two letters of recommendation for the Match—not required, but certainly helpful.

You must submit applications to military residency programs the summer before your senior year. Interviews start shortly thereafter, and ROLs are due in mid-September, while civilian students are still interviewing. Be sure to wear a well-fitting, clean and starched Class A uniform to your residency interviews. Military bearing is important, just as it is during your clerkships. Health Professions Scholarship Program (HPSP) students should also interview at some civilian programs and enter the NRMP PGY-1 Match. However, if there are spots open in a military training program, you will not receive a deferment to a civilian program unless (a) your service decides it needs more physicians in your chosen field than its own training programs can provide or (b) you are a highly competitive student. With fewer students applying for HPSP scholarships, it is highly likely that you will do a military residency, particularly in the Army, which has more openings and more specialties than the other services. Nevertheless, you will need to apply to civilian programs as a backup. If you do match with the military, you must drop out of the NRMP PGY-1 Match. But your money won't be refunded.

One important note: If you owe an obligation to serve in the military or PHS, but either did not match with a military program or there is no military program in your specialty (e.g., the Air Force does not have a Neurological Surgery program), you will need to do a civilian residency. No civilian program will want you as a resident if they cannot be assured that you will be around for the duration of the program. The Navy, for example, has had an atrocious record of pulling their people out of training after the PGY-1 year to go on sea duty. Therefore, civilian programs will want to see *a written commitment* from the service allowing you to complete your training before going on active duty. There should be no difficulty in obtaining this before it is time for the civilian training programs to make up their rank lists for the Match.

The military services also sponsor some physicians during their civilian training programs. Residents in this program receive officer's pay, some benefits, and a salary bonus. The military obligation is equal to the time sponsored, with a minimum of two years.

Your active duty begins when you finish residency, unless you are given permission to go into a fellowship. Be aware that permission for fellowship subspecialization, an increasingly attractive option for many students, is often declined: You may serve your time, for example, as a general surgeon, instead of receiving more training in a Cardiothoracic Surgery fellowship. Military fellowships are highly competitive, and you may be given preference if you have seen active duty or plan on a military career, which makes the investment more worthwhile for the military.

Any moonlighting you do, either during your residency or while practicing medicine in the military, is subject to the approval of your commanding officer; most institutions have standard forms to request permission. While moonlighting, you are not allowed to care for (or at least charge) patients covered by the Military Health System, since you are already being paid to serve this community.

Students in the *National Health Service Corps' (NHSC) Scholarship Program* are required to enter (and complete) an approved primary care residency program; failure to do this will result in severe financial penalties of up to *three times the amount of the scholarship*, plus interest. Acceptable programs include those in General Internal Medicine, Family Medicine, Internal Medicine-Pediatrics, Internal Medicine-Family Medicine, General Pediatrics, Obstetrics/Gynecology, and General Psychiatry. D.O.'s must complete a Transitional/Rotating year before beginning one of the above residencies. The NHSC must approve your completed *Deferment Request Form* and your educational plan, although not the specific program, in advance. Note that military residencies are not acceptable.

In general, physicians who have completed military residencies strongly recommend not making a decision to go into military medicine based on financial need or on recruiters' glowing promises, but rather on a desire to participate in the Armed Forces. As one person put it, "The best advice I *never* heard while contemplating signing up for military medicine is that it is a good thing to do only if you if you think you would enjoy being in the military anyway. If you have concerns about deployment, spending several years living in undesirable places far from family, or the unique aspects of military medicine, do yourself a favor and do not sign up." Make certain that this option is for you and you understand the obligations involved before you sign on the dotted line.

An excellent guide for those considering the Armed Forces Health Professions Scholarship Program is available online at http://lukeballard.tripod.com/HPSP.html. The author wrote this unofficial guide, with lots of inside tips and good advice, while in the Air Force HSPS. For information on physicians in military and federal service, contact the Association of Military Surgeons of the United States, (800) 761-9320 or (301) 897-8800; www.amsus.org.

15

International Medical Graduates

If you really want to do something, you'll find a way;
if you don't, you'll find an excuse.

Anon.

INTERNATIONAL MEDICAL GRADUATES (IMGs), often referred to as foreign medical graduates (FMGs), include all those who have graduated from any of the more than 1,000 medical schools outside the United States, its possessions, and Canada. In January 2010, the AMA's Dr. Nyapati Rao summarized the issues facing IMGs:

> Among all advanced nations, America is the most welcoming country to IMGs. Nonetheless, the presence of IMGs in America has raised questions about the soundness and adequacy of IMGs' medical education, the quality of the medical care they deliver, their contribution to increasing the physician supply and deepening the physician misdistribution and finally, causing brain drain. On the other hand, IMGs often feel perplexed, overwhelmed and discriminated against, although they also feel appreciative of the opportunity to receive world-class medical training.

IMGs functionally break down into two subgroups:

1. **U.S. IMGs (USIMGs):** Individuals who are currently a citizen or permanent resident of the United States, but who received their medical degree outside the United States, Puerto Rico, or Canada. About a third of IMG physicians who have obtained U.S. residency slots in recent years are in this category. (Permanent Residents or "Green Card" holders are treated as U.S. citizens during the residency application process.)

2. **Non-U.S. citizen IMGs, also called Foreign National IMGs (FNIMGs):** Non-U.S. citizens who received their medical degree from a medical school not approved by the LCME, usually located outside the United States, Puerto Rico, or Canada. Such individuals are in the United States only temporarily as Exchange Visitors (with J-1 or, occasionally, H-type visas) to study, teach, or do research. Individuals in this group must have a firm offer of a residency position before applying for their visa.

Note that foreign nationals who now attend or who have graduated from U.S., Canadian, or Puerto Rican medical schools (with a visa) are not considered to be IMGs, so do not need to obtain an ECFMG Certificate. However, they may need to get another visa to remain in the United States to do a residency. Otherwise, these individuals go through the same process as any other U.S./Canadian medical school graduate. However, they must demonstrate to residency directors that they will have the necessary visa before starting training.

International medical graduates account for 29% of physicians in residency training; they comprise only about 22% of PGY-1s. Most non-U.S. citizen IMG residents come from India (21%), the Philippines (8%), Mexico (6%), and Pakistan (5%). The balance is relatively evenly divided among the other nations. About 40% of IMGs train in New York or California, with nearly 60% training in Internal Medicine or a Medicine specialty. Close to 27% of all primary care residency positions are filled by IMGs. Nearly 33% of IMGs pursue post-residency fellowships, while only 27% of U.S. medical graduates do so. Women comprise 31% of all IMGs in U.S. residencies, with half of them in primary care (compared to one-third of male IMGs).

While in 1963, IMGs represented slightly more than 10% of the U.S. physician workforce, by 2011, they constituted nearly 26%. IMGs' practices tend to be medical, rather than surgical (Figure 15.1). In 2011, about 78% of IMGs worked in patient care, with 72% in office-based practice (nearly one-quarter of all office-based U.S. physicians). Half of all IMGs work in New York (14%), California (11%), Florida (8%), Texas (6%), New Jersey (6%), and Illinois (6%).

The Negative Image

Even though IMGs comprise such a large percentage of residents and practicing physicians in the United States, residency faculty often have a negative image of IMGs. An article in *Academic Medicine* described residency faculty members' perceptions of why IMGs experience problems in U.S. residency programs. Among these are:

- Difficulty with medical or non-medical English.
- Differences in medical education.
- Length of time since graduation from medical school and last clinical experiences.
- Older, with more family and financial obligations.

Figure 15.1: IMGs Practicing Medicine in Various Specialties

	Number of IMGs in Specialty	% of Physicians in Specialty that are IMGs	% of all IMGs*
Internal Medicine	60,272	38%	32.0%
Nuclear Medicine	561	38	0.3
Pulmonary Diseases	3,659	34	1.9
Psychiatry	13,016	32	6.8
Pathology	6,288	33	3.3
Physical Med/Rehab.	2,556	30	1.3
Cardiovascular Disease	6,929	30	3.6
Neurology	4,960	30	2.6
Anesthesiology	11,567	27	6.1
Pediatrics	20,662	28	10.9
Child & Adolescent Psychiatry	2,150	29	1.1
Gastroenterology	3,475	27	1.8
Medical Genetics	149	26	0.1
Allergy & Immunology	1,007	24	0.5
General/Family Medicine	23,601	25	12.4
Colon & Rectal Surgery	275	19	0.1
Thoracic Surgery	972	21	0.5
Radiation Oncology	752	16	0.4
General Surgery	7,256	19	3.8
Obstetrics/Gynecology	7,309	17	3.8
Radiology (All)	1,661	18	0.9
Urological Surgery	1,497	14	0.8
Gen. Preventive Med	152	11	0.1
Neurological Surgery	749	14	0.4
Occupational Medicine	367	14	0.2
Plastic Surgery	812	11	0.4
Public Health	152	11	0.1
Otolaryngology	884	9	0.5
Emergency Medicine	2,752	9	1.4
Ophthalmology	1,364	7	0.7
Aerospace Medicine	32	7	<0.1
Orthopedic Surgery	1,563	6	0.8
Dermatology	615	6	0.3

* Column may not total 100% due to rounding.
Adapted from: American Medical Association. *Physician Characteristics and Distribution in the U.S., 2010.* Chicago, IL: AMA, 2010, Tables 3.1, 3.2.

- Cultural differences in their approach to and beliefs about gender roles, communication, authority, interpersonal relationships, and a physician's role or status.
- Traumatic experiences as persecuted minorities, new immigrants, or refugees.

Large numbers of IMGs continue to practice and train in the United States despite a lot of negative press. Over the past several years, IMGs have had much lower scores on USMLE Steps 1, 2CK, and 2CS than U.S. medical students and graduates (Figure 8.2). These widely reported results only reinforce the negative image of IMGs within the medical community.

Several incidents, including "worthless" medical degrees granted by some Caribbean medical schools, led the ECFMG to establish the Credential Verification Service (www.ecfmg.org/cvs/index.html) which allows residency directors, among others, to quickly verify ECFMG Certification. The incidents also led three jurisdictions (Maryland, Pennsylvania, and Puerto Rico) to ban IMGs from taking clinical clerkships in hospitals in their state. (Texas grants an exception for rotations if the hospital has an accredited residency in the same specialty.) Thirteen other states (AR, CA, CT, DE, FL, MD, MA, ME, NJ, NY, PA, PR, and TX) regulate IMGs in clinical clerkships. New York reportedly has the toughest regulations (and most expensive process) to certify non-U.S. medical schools to send their students for clerkships. In addition, AAMC rules preclude U.S. medical schools from "co-mingling" their own students with those from non-U.S. schools during required clerkships. (Some hospitals get around this by using "separate-but-equal" ward teams.) These restrictions, however, attack the mechanism through which foreign-trained medical students demonstrate their clinical competence and subsequently get residency slots and become licensed. (Twenty licensing boards evaluate the quality of a clinical clerkship when deciding whether to grant a license to an IMG.)

Licensing, Funding, and Residency Positions

While about 7,000 new medical licenses are granted to international medical graduates every year, there are thousands of IMGs in the United States who have not been able to obtain a license to practice medicine. In many cases, this is because residency programs will not accept them for training: *all jurisdictions in the United States require at least one year of postgraduate training in the United States or Canada for licensure* (Figure 8.9).

Twenty jurisdictions require IMGs to have at least two years of training for licensure and 28 require three years. This exceeds what most jurisdictions require from U.S. graduates. In addition, 22 licensing boards maintain lists of state-approved foreign medical schools whose graduates are eligible for a medical license. However, 23 U.S. licensing boards allow IMGs to take USMLE Step 3 before obtaining graduate medical education in the United States or Canada. Thirty-nine states will endorse the Licentiate of the Medical Council of Canada (LMCC) for a U.S. license when held by an IMG.

Residency programs, especially those that train large numbers of IMGs, are also concerned about changes in Medicare laws that severely restrict the programs' and hospitals' reimbursement for training non-U.S.-medical school graduates. These residency programs often operate on a shoestring as it is; threatening to further restrict their funds has had the desired effect of decreasing the training opportunities for IMGs.

When selecting potential residents, program directors look at the past performance of different groups of IMGs in residency programs. For example, IMGs, especially those who enter residencies outside a matching program, have a higher attrition rate than U.S. graduates. Also, IMGs pass some specialty board examinations, such as that of Internal Medicine, only about two-thirds as often on their first try as do U.S. graduates. Since residency programs are judged, in part, on their graduates' pass rates, this is important to residency directors.

Despite the unfavorable press and the tough requirements, the number of IMGs in U.S. residency positions increased from just over 12,000 in 1989 to more than 29,000 in 2012. The number of non-U.S.-citizen IMGs seeking first-year residency positions increased over this same period from 2,689 to more than 6,828. The 2012 PGY-1 match rate for this group was 40.6%—the lowest of all applicant groups.

USIMGs (U.S. citizens/permanent residents) make up just 8% of all first-year residents, but 43% of first-year IMG residents. There were 4,279 USIMG participants in the NRMP PGY-1 Match in 2012; 49% matched.

In the 2012 NRMP Match, IMGs made up a large proportion of those entering Family Medicine, Psychology, and Categorical Internal Medicine (Figure 15.2). However, a significant number of IMGs obtain positions outside the Match; in 2012, for example, 4,886 IMGs obtained PGY-1 positions through the NRMP Match, but about 7,300 IMGs entered PGY-1 training for 2012–2013.

The AMA's International Medical Graduates Section tackles licensure, discrimination, and visa issues on behalf of IMGs. For information, go to the AMA's website at www.ama-assn.org/go/membergroups and select the Section by name.

Figure 15.2
Types of Applicants (Percentages) Filling PGY-1 and
Advanced Positions through NRMP Match*

Specialty	% Filled by U.S. Senior Students/ Grads	% Filled by Osteopaths	% Filled by USIMGs, Fifth Pathway, & Can. Grads	% Filled by FNIMGs	% Total Positions Filled thru NRMP
Anesthesiology	81%	10.4%	5.5%	3.3%	97.4%
Emergency Med	84	10.3	4.1	1.5	100.0
Family Med	54	12.5	20.0	13.4	94.5
Internal Med (C)	58	6.8	11.6	23.7	99.0
OB/GYN	77	10.9	6.6	5.9	98.6
Orthopedic Surg	98	<1.0	<1.0	<1.0	100
Pathology[†]	63	9.2	7.3	20.6	89.4
Pediatrics (C)	72	10.4	7.7	9.9	98.7
Psychiatry	60	11.5	15.7	12.7	96.6
Radiology, Diag	85	5.8	4.3	4.9	92.3
Surgery, Gen (C)	87	3.1	5.2	5.0	100.0
Transitional	87	3.1	4.0	5.6	97.2
Total Unmatched[§]	**4.9%**	**25.3%**	**51.0%**	**59.4%**	—

* Numbers in the columns for percent of graduates matching within a specialty may not add up to total percentage matched due to rounding.
† A significant number of entry-level positions (PGY-1 or above) are offered outside the Match.
§ This percentage is for PGY-1. Note that between 2% (U.S. Seniors/Grads) and 48% (all IMGs) of the candidates either withdrew before the Match or did not submit a Rank-Order List.
Derived from: National Residency Matching Program. *Results and Data 2012 Main Residency Match.* Washington, DC: NRMP, 2012, Table 2.

ECFMG Certification

International medical school graduates must get an ECFMG Certificate to be eligible for: (a) acceptance into an ACGME-accredited residency or fellowship position in the United States; (b) a visa for entry into the United States as a medical trainee; (c) a medical license in all states except California and West Virginia; and (d) an application to take USMLE Step 3 (Figure 15.3). (Fifth Pathway students do not need an ECFMG Certificate.) The ECFMG issues about 10,000 new Certificates annually; 23% are issued to U.S. citizens and

23% to Indian citizens. About 55% are issued to men and 45% to women. The ECFMG charges a fee of $50 to submit an Application for ECFMG Certification

Note, however, that 14 states have additional requirements for appointment to a residency position (apart from an ECFMG Certificate) for IMGs. These are Alaska, Arizona, California, Connecticut, Kansas, Kentucky, Louisiana, Michigan, Minnesota, Missouri, Nevada, New Jersey, Pennsylvania, and Vermont. Their requirements can be found on each state's Medical Board website and in the AMA's *State Medical Licensure Requirements & Statistics*, available in most medical libraries.

To qualify for an ECFMG Certificate, you must be either a *student* attending a medical school listed in the current edition of the *International Medical Education Directory (IMED)*, published by the Foundation for Advancement of International Medical Education and Research (FAIMER), or a *graduate* of a medical school that is listed in this directory (your graduation date must be within the "Graduation Years" listed for the school). In 2013 the IMED will be combined with the World Federation for Medical Education's *Avicenna Directory* to produce the *World Directory of Medical Schools*, a listing of more than 2500 schools that offer undergraduate medical education worldwide. Beginning in 2023, the ECFMG will require physicians applying for certification to have graduated from a medical school that has been accredited through a formal process, such as is used by the LCME. They hope that this will spur efforts to develop globally accepted criteria for international medical education, thus improving health care worldwide.

If you have graduated, you must document completion of the educational requirements to practice medicine in the country in which you received your medical education. This must include at least four years of medical study for which credit was received. If the transcript received by the ECFMG is not in English, they will charge a translation fee (check ECFMG's website for the current fee). For medical diplomas, you must send the original-language document and an official English translation, or they will not be accepted. Foreign-national physicians must also have an unrestricted license or certificate to practice medicine in their own country. The specific credentials accepted for each country are listed in the annual *ECFMG Information Booklet* (see below). Individuals licensed only in stomatology, ayurvedic or homeopathic medicine, and those awarded only the diploma of Physician-Epidemiologist-Hygienist, Physician-Cyberneticist, Licensed Medical Practitioner, Physician-Biophysicist, Physician-Biochemist, or Assistant Medical Practitioner are not eligible for an ECFMG Certificate.

Figure 15.3
Requirements to Practice Medicine, Do Post-Graduate Training,
or Be a Clinical Research Fellow in the United States (Patient Contact)

	USMLE	ECFMG Certification	Applicable Visa
U.S. Citizen/Permanent Resident: Graduate of LCME-accredited U.S., Canadian, or Puerto Rican medical school	✓		
Foreign National: Graduate of LCME-accredited U.S., Canadian, or Puerto Rican Medical School (EVIMG)	✓		✓
U.S. Citizen/Permanent Resident: Graduate of Foreign Medical School (USIMG)*	✓	✓	
Foreign National: Graduate of Foreign Medical School (FNIMG)	✓	✓	✓

*U.S. citizen/permanent resident IMGs who entered the Fifth Pathway Program before July 2009 do not need to get an ECFMG Certificate.

The ECFMG website (www.ecfmg.org) contains a wealth of information, including one of the most important resources for IMGs, the downloadable *ECFMG Information Booklet*. This publication describes the steps in the ECFMG certification process, lists the contact information and application requirements for the various items necessary to obtain an ECFMG Certificate, and lists the medical credentials that the ECFMG accepts from each country. The ECFMG website also has a downloadable *USMLE Bulletin of Information*.

For those who already have, or are about to get, their ECFMG Certificate, the site also provides entry into ERAS (acts as your Dean's office). The Credential Verification Service on the site allows program directors, hospitals, and other employers to verify that you do, indeed, have an ECFMG Certificate.

OASIS

Accessible via the ECFMG website, the Online Applicant Status and Information System (OASIS) is a very useful tool for ECFMG applicants and ECFMG-certified physicians. You can use OASIS to check the status of your ECFMG certification, including whether the ECFMG has received your medical education credentials, or to request permanent validation of your Certificate. Information on the status of your USMLE application, scheduling permits, score reports, and transcript requests is available as well. Exam results are available only in electronic format through OASIS; the ECFMG will notify you by e-mail how to download and view the results (this information is viewable for 120 days from the date of notification). If you are sponsored by the ECFMG, you can use OASIS to determine the current status of your J-1 visa sponsorship. Additionally, if you are eligible to participate in the IMG Advisors Network (IAN), you use OASIS to access this free service (see "Acculturation").

The system also allows you to verify that the ECFMG's information about you, including name-of-record, contact information, and the status of your ECFMG financial account, is correct. If the information is wrong, you can change address and other contact information on-line, but name changes must be submitted on a separate form. If necessary, you can also make advance payments to your ECFMG financial account through OASIS.

If you plan to participate in ERAS, you will use OASIS to request and pay for the ERAS "electronic token" (initial password) that you will use to gain access to the MyERAS website. (**Caveat**: this token is for residency applications only; fellowship application tokens are requested through the ERAS Fellowships Documents Office [EFDO].) Once you are in MyERAS, you will be given your AAMC Identification Number. You will then use OASIS to access and complete the online Document Submission Form, upload your digital photograph, and track when your supporting documents are received by ERAS Support Services. For more information, see "ERAS and International Medical Students/Graduates" in Chapter 13.

OASIS can be accessed 24 hours a day, seven days a week, by individuals with a USMLE/ECFMG Identification Number and a special password. More information about OASIS, including how to obtain a password for this service, can be found at https://oasis2.ecfmg.org/. Technical difficulties should be reported to: oasis@ecfmg.org.

Application Process

You must submit an application, pay the $50 fee, and send the required documentation to the ECFMG. It may take several months to process this application, since your medical school must verify your education credentials. To speed up the processing time on all paperwork, always use the same (formal) name that is on your medical school diploma. Once the ECFMG has assigned you a number, use that on any correspondence with the ECFMG, licensing bodies, and residency programs.

USMLE

If you are an international medical *student* with an ECFMG number, you can take the USMLE Step 1 at any time. You must have completed at least two years of medical school before taking either Step 2CK or Step 2CS. Eligible international medical *graduates* can take the USMLE Steps in any sequence. However, *everyone* must pass Steps 1, 2CK, and 2CS to meet the medical science examination requirement for ECFMG certification. The ECFMG recommends that students complete their core clinical clerkships, including patient contact, before taking Steps 2CK and 2CS.

IMGs can apply for Steps 1, 2CK, and 2CS of the USMLE through the ECFMG using the Interactive Web Application (IWA) on the ECFMG website. You can complete the online application in one sitting, or save it and return to complete it later. Alternatively, you can print a paper application. The ECFMG does not register or extend the eligibility date for an applicant until they receive verification from the medical school that the applicant has graduated.

Participating medical schools can check the applicant's status through the ECFMG Medical School Web Portal (EMSWP), which electronically verifies primary source documents. Students print and fill out the *Certification of Identification Form* (Form 186) from the ECFMG website; an authorized official then certifies the document and sends it directly to ECFMG. Ask your school for a list of officials that can do this certification. Once accepted, the certification is valid for five years. For those medical schools that do not participate in EMSWP, students print out a different form, the *Certification Statement* (Form 183); unlike Form 186, a new Form 183 is generated with each on-line application.

The ECFMG reports international students' USMLE scores to their medical schools. You must formally request, through IWA, that these results be withheld and the ECFMG must receive this request at least 10 days before the exam date. In that case, the school receives only your name and a note saying "Record withheld at the request of the examinee." If you later want your USMLE transcript sent to the school, you will have to request and pay for it through the USMLE.

The ECFMG administers USMLE **Steps 1 and 2CK** to IMGs at about 300 testing centers within the United States and Canada, and at more than 100 other locations worldwide (see www.prometric.com). You must select a three-month eligibility period and the ECFMG must receive your completed application by the twenty-fourth day of that period, or you will be assigned to the next three-month period. If you receive approval to take the exam, you will receive a receipt showing the date of the exam, the test center's address, and the cost. About four weeks before the exam, an official admission permit that includes the time and location of the test will be sent out.

Step 2CS is administered only in the United States at regional testing centers: currently these are in Atlanta, Chicago, Houston, Los Angeles, and Philadelphia. You must choose one of the centers before completing your application. If you are unable to obtain the appropriate visa to enter the United States to take Step 2CS, you may request a full refund of the examination fee.

Each test takes one day. For applications submitted after January 1, 2012, there are limits both on the number of times you can take any Step or Component of the USMLE and on the amount of time between each attempt. See the USMLE or ECFMG websites for more details. Some states also impose their own limits on both on the number of times a Step can be taken and on the length of time allowed to complete the entire (Steps 1, 2CK, 2CS, and 3) process. Also, note that IMGs desiring to enter the United States on an H-1B visa (work permit) must pass Step 3 before they can obtain the visa. (For more information about the USMLE, see Chapter 8.)

While there are rumors to the contrary, the USMLE Steps 1, 2CK, and 2CS are scored identically for all examinees. It costs more to take these exams outside the United States or Canada, however, since an "International Test Delivery Surcharge" is added. The current charges and cities with ProMetrics testing sites are listed on the ECFMG website.

To apply to take **Step 3**, an applicant must have obtained an M.D. degree or equivalent; passed Steps 1, 2CK, and 2CS; obtained an ECFMG Certificate or completed a Fifth Pathway program; and met any other specific requirements imposed by the state licensing board administering the test. Information about specific state requirements is available from the individual state board or The Federation of State Medical Boards of the United States, P.O. Box 619850, Dallas, TX 75261-9850 USA; (817) 868-4000; www.fsmb.org.

If history is any guide, those IMGs with the best chance of passing the USMLE are younger than 30-years-old, male, native English speakers, FNIMGs, and educated in countries with a low infant mortality rate and a high per capita income. Those with the least chance of passing the USMLE are those over 40-years-old, female, non-native English speakers, those taking the test more than 10 years after graduating from medical school, USIMGs, and those educated in countries with a medium-to-high infant mortality rate and medium per capita income.

ECFMG English Language Examination

Although applicants for ECFMG certification are no longer required to take the Test of English as a Foreign Language™ (TOEFL®) or the ECFMG English Test—*all IMGs must be fluent in spoken and written English*. As of June 2004, the ECFMG accepts a passing score on USMLE Step 2 Clinical Skills (CS) as evidence that an individual's written and spoken English is sufficient to practice medicine in the United States. However, the ECFMG does recommend that IMGs take the Test of Spoken English™ (TSE®), offered by the Educational

Testing Service®, for self-assessment before taking Step 2CS. They suggest that you should receive a score of at least 45 on the TSE: If you don't get that score, you probably need to get additional English practice before spending the money to come to the United States to take the Step 2CS exam.

Note: For those who have previously taken TOFEL or the ECFMG English Test, these tests are no longer subject to expiration. You can request a permanent validation sticker to put on your document.

Even if your ability to read and write English is excellent, your chances of obtaining the residency you want (or any residency in the United States) may be improved if you take a *conversational* English course. (This is also true for those native English speakers who are not familiar with American idioms.) Unlike a standard English course, this type of course prepares people to speak American English. It is a skill you will need as a resident, and later as a practicing physician.

Clinical Skills Assessment (CSA®)

The ECFMG Clinical Skills Assessment (CSA), a test of clinical and communication skills, has been supplanted by USMLE Step 2CS. (See Chapter 8, "USMLE Step 2.")

Applicants who have already passed the CSA are not required to pass Step 2CS to meet the eligibility requirements for Step 3 and for ECFMG certification. If students were certified by ECFMG and the CSA pass date on their certificate is June 14, 2001, or later, they may request a permanent validation sticker for their CSA date. A passing performance on the CSA before June 14, 2001, however, remains subject to expiration (three years from the exam date) for the purpose of starting a residency in the United States. Applicants who have *both* passed the *former* ECFMG CSA *and* achieved a score acceptable to ECFMG on an English language proficiency test (such as TOEFL or the former ECFMG English Test) can use these passing performances to satisfy the clinical skills requirement for ECFMG certification.

To request official copies of your CSA performance history, you must complete a *Request for an Official ECFMG CSA History Chart* (Form 297) on the ECFMG website and fax or mail it to ECFMG with the $50 fee (2012). Each form can accommodate 10 copy requests. Allow four weeks for delivery.

Tips For All IMGs

Several hints have been passed on to me from IMGs who used previous editions of this book. Some of the most useful were from Bill Groves, M.D., who got his first choice of residency program. He wrote:

> If you are in an interview and cannot remember anything at all, and your English is deteriorating rapidly [even if you are native English speaker, as is Dr. Groves], remember how many babies you have delivered, how many times you did CPR, and how many times you worked alone [in the clinic or hospital]. Your education may at times have lacked quality, machinery, or medications, but it did not lack vitality.

> If the program apologizes for having IMGs and the resident apologizing is from Bangladesh, there is a double standard here, and no doubt friction between the residents and administration.

> If a program director calls you and says that all the competing programs are dropping out of the Match, that all of his slots will be filled by early February, and that you need to sign onto one of his remaining two slots immediately, don't do anything precipitously. Call the Match to check on his story—it is probably untrue. Yet you might want to take his interest as a compliment and consider the offer.

> It may seem unfair that American graduates can take clerkships right up until they begin residency, while you are barred from any contact [with patients, which may represent a year of decay of your clinical skills]. Do not doubt, however, that the law applies to you and will be enforced. Your temporary license may depend upon adhering to state requirements. If necessary, work temporarily in another state, and write the AMA for information and help.

What Dr. Groves did not mention is that there may be an even greater image problem for USIMGs than for FNIMGs. While foreign-born physicians have a reason for training outside the United States, it is often assumed that USIMGs could not measure up to U.S. standards and so had to leave the country. While this may be true for some, the fact remains that many qualified applicants are rejected by U.S. schools simply because there are not enough positions. USIMGs, at least, do not have to broach the language or cultural barriers faced by their foreign-born counterparts.

Non-U.S./Non-Canadian Citizens (FNIMGs)

International medical graduates who are not U.S. citizens generally encounter the biggest problems in obtaining residency training positions. Many programs just will not accept such applicants. Often, they will not state this plainly for fear of legal reprisal, although some programs have begun stating in their program information that they will accept only graduates of U.S. medical schools as applicants.

While selection committees have some problems evaluating an IMG's credentials, the problem is not as grave as it was in the past. The USMLE has provided an even playing field to assess all medical school graduates' knowledge. Apples can now be compared directly with other apples (if you don't mind being an "apple").

Some U.S. residency programs actually prefer international graduates. Though this may seem paradoxical, they have good reasons. The medical system views residencies with a high percentage of international medical graduates as inferior—even if their training is just as good as any other program. This message is clearly sent to U.S. graduates. Therefore, only the poorest U.S. students apply to such programs. According to the directors of some of these programs, they prefer to take the high-quality IMGs who are applying to their programs.

As an FNIMG, the best way to get a residency position is to apply to a program that has a relationship with your medical school. Some programs have drawn excellent graduates from one or two specific foreign medical schools over the years. They have developed good contacts within the schools and are not afraid, as are many other programs, of encountering forged documents, inflated grades, or poor quality instruction.

Sometimes international graduates are forced to take residency slots that are unfunded. In some cases they are called externships; in others they actually count toward completion of a residency. It is not unusual to see offers of payment for a residency slot either from the applicants themselves or from a third party acting on their behalf. Proposals of $25,000 or more per year (plus any cost for salary, benefits, and allowances) have been offered for competitive positions. There is concern, however, that many of the individuals filling these positions are not treated as equals, do not get similar responsibilities, and do not end up with training equivalent to that of other residents in the same program.

A good method for evaluating whether you, as an FNIMG, have a reasonable chance of getting accepted into a program in a particular specialty is to check Figures 15.1 and 15.2, the NRMP's Data and Reports section online, or the charts in *JAMA's* annual "Medical Education Issue" to see how many foreign-trained residents are currently training in or entering that specialty. In addition, check with your school to see if there are any particular programs in the United States with which they have a working relationship.

Visas

Even if you get a residency position, you have to worry about your visa. About 45% of IMGs hold J-1 Exchange Visitor visas or H-1B visas (Figure 15.4). J-1 visas are limited to the time typically required to complete the advanced medical education program. This means the time required for board certification by the American Board of Medical Specialists for a specialty and subspecialty. The maximum time is seven years. This limitation mostly affects individuals who extend their program to include research or chief resident years and then want to do a fellowship. (The "residency/fellowship" time includes a practice year for those specialties that require a year of practice to qualify for the Board exam, such as Pathology and Occupational Medicine.)

Figure 15.4
Citizenship and Visas of IMGs

Citizenship/Visa Status	Resident Physicians	
	Number	%
Native U.S. citizen	4,366	14.8
Naturalized U.S. citizen	2,705	9.2
Permanent resident	5,965	20.2
B-1, B-2 temporary visitor visa	122	0.4
F-1 student visa	23	<0.1
H-1, H-1B, H-2, H-3 temporary worker visa	4,777	16.2
J-1, J-2 exchange visitor visa	4,152	14.1
Refugee /asylee/displaced person	84	0.3
Other	437	1.5
Unknown citizenship/foreign born	4,152	14.1
Unknown citizenship/unknown birth country	2,705	9.2

Adapted from: American Medical Association: *International Medical Graduates in American Medicine: Contemporary Challenges and Opportunities*. January 2010, Table 13.

The ECFMG is the sole designated sponsor of J-1 visa holders through their Exchange Visitor Sponsorship Program. During the 2008–2009 school year, 6,561 J-1 physicians were sponsored for clinical training, nearly half of them in Internal Medicine. Visas are typically given only to individuals in ACGME-accredited training programs. The ECFMG will sponsor IMGs who are in non-ACGME-accredited programs for Exchange-Visitor visas only if the subspecialty is recognized by the parent American Board of Medical Specialties (ABMS) board. See their website for the current list of nonstandard subspecialty disciplines and links to the specific ABMS boards. Once an Exchange Visitor has entered their third year of training, they cannot change their specialty.

Visa rules change often. Generally, to obtain a J-1 visa, individuals must first get a Statement of Need from the Ministry of Health of the country of their most recent legal permanent residence confirming the need for them to get U.S. medical training. In addition, the U.S. Citizenship and Immigration Services prohibits moonlighting by residents who hold J-1 visas.

After determining eligibility, ECFMG issues Form DS-2019 (Certificate of Eligibility for Exchange Visitor [J-1 Visa] Status), which authorizes a specific training activity and the associated financial compensation. A physician can also request the form for their dependents when applying for a J-2 visa. Although you can leave the United States at any time with a J-1 visa, if you plan to be gone for more than 30 days or plan to go to a non-contiguous country, you must qualify for Automatic Visa Revalidation to reenter the United States. As of 2010, you must present your passport, the sealed envelope containing your DS-2019, the Arrival-Departure Form I-94 reflecting your J-1 status, and Customs Declaration Form CF-6059. Citizens of certain countries (Cuba, Iran, Sudan, and Syria in June 2010) are not eligible for Automatic Revalidation and must have a valid J-1 visa for reentry.

J-1 visas normally require the holder to return to their *home country* for a minimum of two years after completing training. This requirement also extends to their relatives holding J-2 dependent visas. Occasionally, exceptions are made if the home country writes a "No Objection" letter, the IMG qualifies for a Hardship or Asylum waiver (rare), or a U.S. government agency requests a waiver because they have a need for the individual. In these cases, you will need a visa status change, such as to H (temporary worker), L (intra-company transferee), or U.S. permanent resident (Green Card). Visas and the laws governing them, however, constantly change, so always double-check any information concerning them.

The J-1 Conrad Waiver, begun in 1994 by Senator Kent Conrad, allows states to exempt IMGs from having to leave the country for two years once they have completed their medical residency as required by their student visas.

Instead, they may apply for a work visa if they agree to practice in a Medically Underserved Area or in a Health Professional Shortage Area (as designated by the Department of Health and Human Services) in the primary care areas of Family Medicine, General Obstetrics, General Pediatrics, General Internal Medicine, or General Psychiatry for at least three years. As of 2009, states can use at least five of their thirty exemptions for licensed-specialty physicians. If your country of origin paid for your J-1 program, you will need to obtain a "No Objection" letter from that country. The Conrad Waiver also exempts recipients from the up-to-six-year cap on H1-B visas (a non-immigrant visa used by the majority of IMGs seeking to work in the United States). However, obtaining an H1-B visa is increasingly difficult, as the number of applicants has risen and nearly half of the visas are granted for computer-related occupations.

For current information about visas for IMG residents, see the ECFMG's online *Exchange Visitor Sponsorship Program Reference Guide* (www.ecfmg.org/evsp) or contact the ECFMG/Exchange Visitor Program, P.O. Box 41673, Philadelphia, PA 19101-1673, USA; (215) 823-2121.

Acculturation

Living and working in a new country and a new culture can be a daunting experience. Recognizing this, the ECFMG developed their Acculturation Program (www.ecfmg.org/acculturation/index.html) to help IMGs transition to working and living in the United States. The program includes several free resources that describe the U.S. medical system and daily life in the United States. IMGs and the staff at training institutions can access these resources for their own use, and some can also be downloaded to use to train others.

While the ECFMG plans on adding new material, as of early 2012, the resources on their site included:

- *The IMG Advisors Network (IAN).* This is a free service for IMGs who are registered with ERAS and NRMP to help them choose mentors from a database of volunteers who are ECFMG-certified. These mentors can answer questions about U.S. GME programs and help address practical issues, such as finding housing, opening a bank account, obtaining a visa, and getting a driver's license. In 2010, 643 advisees were matched with mentors to facilitate the process of moving to the United States for study.
- *The Interdisciplinary Health Care Team (IHCT).* This section introduces the concept of teamwork in the U.S. medical system, and explains the functions of many non-physician team members.

- *The One Dozen Most Important Things You May Not Have Known, Understood, or Realized about American Medicine.* This series of videos, analyses, and discussion questions introduces topics such as the doctor-patient relationship, the role of the patient's family, the U.S. healthcare team, the U.S. GME system, and professionalism. Users can download text and videos for each module from the Downloads page.
- *Glossary of "Medicalese."* Defines terms commonly used in U.S. medical settings.
- *What's in a Name?* This is an interactive, self-paced tutorial on meeting/greeting patients and colleagues in U.S. hospitals and clinics.

U.S. International Medical Graduates (USIMGs)

Most of the problems described above also exist for U.S. citizens/permanent residents who have taken their medical school training outside the United States.

What you have going for you is that you are most likely (70%) a native English speaker who has received medical school instruction in English (90%), so you should have no trouble passing the English Language Proficiency component of USMLE Step 2CS. What you have going against you is that you did not have the experience of attending a U.S. medical school. In 2009, 38% of IMGs in U.S. residency training programs were U.S. citizens or permanent U.S. residents. Of the 4,279 USIMGs who completed the NRMP PGY-1 Match in 2012, only 1,884 (49.1%) obtained a residency position. This is compared to the match rate of 40.6% for FNIMGs.

The largest numbers of USMLE exam registrants in 2009 that were U.S. citizens were students/graduates from Dominica (1,669), Granada (1,157), Netherlands Antilles (1,136), Antigua and Barbuda (733), and the Cayman Islands (727). Also in 2009, 2,375 Standard ECFMG Certificates were issued to U.S. citizens who had attended 197 medical schools in 63 countries. The largest numbers of ECFMG certificates were awarded to U.S. citizens from schools in Dominica (603), Granada (472), Netherlands Antilles (363), the Cayman Islands (170), and Israel (100).

As the struggle for adequate training and distribution of healthcare providers, particularly in primary care, continues, USIMGs are feeling the impact of the restrictions being imposed on all IMGs. In the future, it may take more than just excellent grades and good examination scores for you to get any position at all, let alone in the specialty that you desire.

Transferring to a U.S. School

The best advice for getting into a residency is to do everything possible to transfer into a U.S. medical school prior to graduation, although that is getting more difficult. To accomplish this, you will have to do very well in your studies in the first two or three years of medical school, in addition to performing well on Step 1 and both parts of Step 2 of the USMLE as administered through the ECFMG. Doing well on the USMLE will be an impressive accomplishment, since USIMGs have consistently done worse on licensing examinations than their foreign-born counterparts. Perhaps FNIMGs take the test more seriously—you should too. Study!

In recent years, most students who have transferred to U.S. schools had high GPAs after completing at least two years of medical school, did very well on the USMLE, and transferred to private schools or to schools in states where they were official residents. (Note that you cannot "transfer" once you have received your medical degree.)

No one keeps a master list of which schools will accept transfer students from non-U.S. medical schools, although Deans of Students at international schools with large numbers of U.S. citizens do keep lists of U.S. medical schools that have accepted their students. To locate a school that might accept you:

1. Check the "Transfer Policies Search" database, searchable by policies and programs, at www.aamc.org/students/medstudents.
2. Contact U.S. medical schools directly to inquire about their willingness to take USIMGs. Do not be "picky" about their location.
3. Mail inquiry letters to the admissions offices of all U.S. medical schools. For any school where you have any kind of "tie" (such as birthplace, undergraduate school, long residence, parents' residence, etc.), specifically mention that connection.
4. If you have to limit the number of letters sent, concentrate on the non-Ivy League private schools. State schools will often accept only students who are considered residents.
5. Write to Osteopathic medical schools. They often are more flexible than M.D. schools.

Many medical schools in the Caribbean promise that students will receive their third- and fourth-year training in affiliated U.S. hospitals, mostly located in New York. If you are counting on this happening, be advised that the *New York Times* reported, in late 2010, that "New York State's 16 medical schools are attacking their foreign competitors" by aggressively lobbying the State Board of Regents to halt this practice.

Fifth Pathway Program (This program has been discontinued)

Up until July 1, 2009, if you could not transfer to a school in the United States, you might entered a *Fifth Pathway Program*, which allowed students in countries that require a year of internship or of social service before granting the M.D. degree (primarily Mexico) to take a year of supervised clinical training at a U.S. medical school. Finishing this program was a route to medical licensure that avoided the hassles of getting an ECFMG Certificate and dealing with its attendant requirements. More than 7,500 individuals have completed the Fifth Pathway Program since it was initiated in 1971, and in recent years, about 100 completed the program each year.

In June 2009, the AMA Council on Medical Education decided to discontinue the Fifth Pathway due to the vague eligibility criteria, lack of supervisory control, and no clear definition for successful completion of the program. *Those who hold a valid Fifth Pathway certificate, however, can still apply to meet USMLE Step 3 eligibility requirements through December 31, 2016.*

Although Fifth Pathway graduates who have passed USMLE Steps 1, 2CS, and 2CK are eligible for licensure in 52 U.S. jurisdictions (excepting Guam and the Virgin Islands) until December 31, 2016, individual states may apply their own requirements and restrictions. Mississippi and South Carolina, for example, accept Fifth Pathway graduates only if the applicant is also certified by an ABMS Board (in other words, has completed both a residency and Board certification). For more information about the Fifth Pathway program, contact: the Licensure and Certification Section, American Medical Association, 515 N. State St., Chicago, IL 60610.

A New Alternative to Fifth Pathway

To accommodate students needing the Fifth Pathway-type experience, the New York Medical College (NYMC) in Valhalla, New York, revised their Fifth Pathway program in July 2009. They now offer a year of supervised clinical training in a "Pre-Internship Program." This program, which satisfies the requirements for the Universidad Autonoma de Guadalajara, School of Medicine in Mexico, provides a Certificate of Completion to the student's medical school after a year of internship. That school then verifies the student's final degree to the ECFMG for ECFMG certification.

To qualify for this program, students must be U.S. citizens or have permanent U.S. resident status and have:

1. Completed their undergraduate premedical studies at a U.S. college or university with grades and scores acceptable for entrance into a U.S. medical school.
2. Completed all formal requirements except the internship and social service at a foreign medical school listed in the *World Directory of Medical Schools* published by the World Health Organization.
3. An academic record acceptable to New York Medical College.
4. Passed USMLE Step 1.
5. *Not* completed their internship/social service requirement.
6. *Not* received their M.D. degree.
7. *Not* met the ECFMG's certification requirements.

The NYMC program charges a $100 application fee, plus an additional non-refundable $500 reservation fee once the student is accepted. Download the application and instructions from their website (www.nymc.edu/Academics/ScoolofMedicine/ThePre-InternshipProgram/index.html) and send it to the address on the application; an interview will be granted if all requirements are met. Contact NYMC at (914) 594-4489 or (914) 594-3651; PreInternship@nymc.edu.

NYMC's Pre-Internship Program lasts twelve months, with starting dates in January and July. The clinical programs offered vary among the seven participating hospitals in New York and Connecticut. From this springboard, many USIMGs can obtain residency slots, applying through the NRMP Match as Independent Candidates. The school gives students a Step 2CK Preparation Course with the Falcon Physician Review Program and a Clinical Skills Standardization Patient Course to prepare them for USMLE Step 2 CS, and allows students to take time off to go for residency interviews.

Canadian Citizens

Canadian citizens are not IMGs, but the United States has a somewhat schizophrenic attitude toward graduates of Canadian medical schools. While the same association that accredits U.S. schools also accredits Canadian medical schools and there is no question that their training is excellent, there is still ambivalence in many sectors about considering Canadian applicants for U.S. residency positions. In part, this stems from the dissimilarity of the entire Canadian educational system and the resultant difficulties in comparing Canadian applicants with those from U.S. schools. This can be remedied, in part, by including as much explanation as possible about your training, grades, honors, etc., with your application materials.

However, aside from the problem of comparing applicants, there also is concern about the lack of reimbursement in the future if Canadians are taken into residency training programs. Some state monies have already been withdrawn from programs that have Canadian trainees. Therefore, it is wise for any Canadian considering training at a U.S. program to check to see if the program will seriously consider Canadian applicants.

Even if you want to eventually practice medicine in the United States, it may not be as important as it seems to do a U.S. residency. That is because 46 U.S. states and territories will issue a medical license by endorsement to graduates of accredited Canadian medical schools who hold a Licentiate of the Medical Council of Canada. Those that don't are Florida, Guam, Hawaii, Louisiana, New Jersey, Puerto Rico, and the Virgin Islands.

Nevertheless, increasing numbers of Canadian medical school graduates now seek residency training in the United States, although they still constitute less than 1% of physicians in U.S. residency programs. This increase may be due to several factors: Canada's medical education system now forces specialty decisions earlier than in the past, they have reduced the number of residency positions, and Canadian provinces now make it very difficult for physicians to change specialties, or even to get licensed in their own specialty in another province.

The Canadian government forcefully discourages Canadian graduates from taking U.S. residencies. Canadians wishing to enter a U.S. residency program must get a J-1 visa, which requires a letter of support from their province's Ministry of Health. For the most part, Canadian officials are reluctant to provide these letters if they need more physicians in your particular specialty in the province. For more information, contact your province's Ministry of Health.

Finally, to be seriously considered as an applicant, it will be necessary to get an immigration card approving your working in the United States before you apply. Otherwise, even if you match with a program, you may not be able to work there. Without an immigration card, no program will consider you.

16

Preparing For The Interview

Every new answer raises a new question.

Folk Saying

NO MATTER HOW IRRATIONAL it may seem, the ten- to thirty-minute interviews that you will have at the residency programs will count more, in most cases, toward getting you into the program than the total weight of your previous 3½ years of medical school. That's not just my personal belief. Several studies have shown this to be true. It is not only the most important part of the resident-selection process, but also the most costly and most time-consuming. So now that you are preparing to go for interviews, put your best effort toward doing a good job. This is where it all comes together!

The Mock Interview

How well will you do when you are actually sitting in the hot seat being interviewed for that residency slot you want above all others? Do not wait until you sit in the real chair to find out! When you think that you are prepared to go on the interview circuit, arrange for a mock interview. This practice instills confidence and stifles anxiety, makes you calmer and more organized, and helps you sound better during the real thing.

A mock interview is to an interview what near-drowning is to drowning. In both cases, you think that you are going to die, but in the former, you live through it. Your mock interview should closely imitate the actual interview. You must prepare for it in exactly the same way that you will prepare for your real interviews. Dress the same, carry identical materials with you, and go over your answers to the questions just as you will before interviews at the residency programs. If you don't feel anxious, you're not doing it correctly. This interview must be as realistic as possible so that you will get the most accurate and useful feedback.

Who should conduct the mock interview? Ideally, your mentor and a specialty adviser, if you have one, since they are probably used to interviewing residency applicants. If not, the Dean of Students or another faculty member in the specialty with interviewing experience and your mentor should interview you. Tell them, if they do not know, that you want the mock interview to be as realistic as possible. You want them to ask you the "difficult" questions and treat you in the same manner they would treat any candidate—not as someone they already know. Then you want feedback on the way you presented yourself, the manner in which you were dressed, how you handled the questions, and an overall assessment of areas to improve before you hit the interview trail.

One useful technique is to record the interview in audio or video. Would you hire the person you hear or see? What seems wrong with the applicant (you)? How can you improve your interview performance next time? As with all other parts of the application process, this takes a little extra effort. Experience has shown that it pays off in a big way.

Besides the formal mock interview, it also helps to go over interview elements in your mind during those times when you are commuting, waiting for others, or holding retractors. Review potential questions and situations, as well as those from previous interviews. To remember the areas you want to review before the real interview, use the mnemonic "SHOWTIME."

- **Self:** What do you know about yourself? Have you adequately assessed your own knowledge, skills, and desires?
- **History:** How did you decide to enter this specialty and this program? Which aspects of your personal history can help you relate to an interviewer in this specialty, and this interviewer in particular?
- **Originality:** What makes you unique? What have you accomplished, experienced, or set as a personal goal that sets you apart from the crowd?
- **World view:** What do you believe in? Why are you striving for this particular goal? What will it mean in your life? How does this program fit into these goals?

- **Tell:** How are you presenting yourself? Remember that the impression you make begins at the moment you first interact with hospital and residency personnel and extends through every contact. For the interview itself, practice effective verbal communication, including looking alert and interested, appearing organized, and listening carefully.
- **Illustrate:** Practice non-verbal communication, including maintaining eye contact, sitting forward, gesturing effectively, and smiling—when appropriate. This is vital, since more than half the message may be delivered through nonverbal cues.
- **Manage:** Use well-placed questions and time-awareness to manage the interview. Be sure to get your key message across while fully (but not endlessly) answering the interviewer's questions.

- **Engage:** Throughout the interview, try to discuss those areas about which you are enthusiastic so that your conversation is animated and stimulating for the interviewer. If you enjoyed the interview, it is likely that the interviewer did also.

The "SHOW" part should not be recited as a litany, but rather used when questions arise in any of the applicable areas. Two things you probably want to memorize, or at least get down pat enough so that they sound smooth, are your opening introduction to the interviewer and a two- or three-sentence summation of your message (your strengths and desire to come to the program). The "TIME" elements are how you convey your message. Practice both.

Give the right nonverbal signals. Use a strong handshake to communicate energy and drive. Maintain eye contact. For successful eye contact, you must hold the interviewer's gaze for three to five seconds or until a thought or sentence is complete. Don't glance around the room; this indicates that you are bored. Avoid nervous mannerisms such as doodling or tapping your fingers. Smile often. Avoid slouching and other forms of bad posture that make you seem to lack confidence. Send a positive message. For example, lean forward in the chair to show interest and alertness.

Don't sweat over past interviews; just think about how they could have gone better. This frequent review will keep you ready to face the next interview without needing too much last-minute preparation.

Timing

Applicants always have many questions about the timing of the actual interviews. Because there is very little information or guidance offered to applicants, they must wallow through the morass of scheduling, traveling, and interviewing on their own. The most common question is whether to do an interview close to home or at the bottom-choice program first as a trial interview, thereby getting an idea of the interview process. That is not a good move.

As discussed above, you should learn how to go through the interview process by participating in a mock interview with your mentor and specialty adviser prior to embarking on your first trip. If you can avoid it, do not waste any real interviews on "practice." The programs that you consider weak based upon their written material may surprise you with their strengths when you visit them.

Ratings Inflate as the "Season" Goes On

A number of studies on interviewing show that programs' ratings of applicants become more favorable as the "season" progresses. Although one emergency medicine study showed no relationship between the date interviewed and the match list position, this may not hold true for all specialties—or even for all programs within a single specialty.

While early applicants have an easier time getting an interview when the composition of the entire applicant pool is uncertain, candidates interviewed early tend to have less-positive evaluations. This is, in part, because early interviewees are being compared to a hypothetical "best applicant" (see Chapter 19, The Perfect Applicant) rather than the available applicant pool. As reality sinks in, interviewers tend to raise their ratings to more accurately reflect a candidate's true position in comparison with his or her cohorts. This suggests that it is better for you to interview in the second half, if not near the end, of the interview season.

Last Interviewed Are Remembered Best

Unless you are among the last applicants interviewed, the impression you make will tend to fade as faculty members interview other applicants. When they make their selection decisions, the faculty will best remember those individuals who are interviewed last.

The difference in the selection rate between candidates interviewed in the second half of the season and those interviewed in the first half is only a few percentage points. But don't you want those points to work for you rather than against you? If so, plan to interview late. If you can manage it, schedule your interview on or near the last available date that each program offers. This can often be done easily if you get your materials to the program early. You will be offered an interview when there is still a wide choice of available dates. Scheduling your interviews at the end of multiple programs' interview schedules may not be as difficult as you might imagine, since various programs end their interviewing at different times.

After you schedule your interviews, send each program an e-mail or letter confirming your interview date, time, and location. Keep a "hard" copy for your records—in case your computer or smart phone crashes—and take it with you as a reminder on your interview trip.

Not My Top Choice

What should you do when your "bottom" program offers you an invitation to interview and you have yet to hear from your "top" programs? As they say, "A bird in the hand...". Schedule interviews at those programs that offer you an interview and *where you would actually be willing to go as a resident*. This should logically be all the programs to which you apply—unless you get additional information after you submit your application. Do this for three reasons:

1. You may find that one or more of these "bottom" programs actually perfectly meets your needs when you visit.

2. You may not hear from any other programs, so you need to make certain that you have an opportunity to train in the specialty that you have chosen.

3. Residency programs know that applicants will face this dilemma and, especially late in the interview season, expect a certain percentage of applicants to cancel their interviews.

Hopefully, you will eventually interview at some of your top choice programs, but you may not like them as well as the programs where you have already interviewed.

Time Off—Arranging the Senior Schedule

You must have the necessary time off to go to interviews. The average senior medical student spends eighteen days away from school on the interview circuit. However, over one-fourth spend more than twenty-one days on the road. This requires a little advance planning.

When should you go for interviews? If you are applying to a specialty that has a non-NRMP Match for PGY-2 positions right out of medical school, such as Urology and Ophthalmology, you will interview in November and December. If you are applying to programs through the standard NRMP PGY-1 Match (most of you will be in this group), interview season generally runs from November through early February. Some programs interview during only a portion, often the mid- to latter parts, of these time periods.

There are two ways to arrange for time off to interview; you can either take vacation or take an elective or research block that will allow you to obtain the time off you need. While attractive, this latter option must be investigated carefully. If you make a mistake, and cannot get the time off once you are on such a rotation, you may miss some important interviews. You cannot afford this. If possible, talk with the faculty member responsible for the rotation in advance. Find out if you will be able to have days off for interviews. If you know the specific dates or blocks of time, write them down, give the faculty member a copy and have him or her sign the copy that you keep. This way their faulty memory will play no part in determining your future.

By the way, if you have followed the schema proposed in this book, you should have plenty of vacation time available. While the interview circuit is usually no holiday (though it can be, see the next section), taking vacation time at this point may ease some of the pressures that can exist if you are trying to sandwich interviews among other responsibilities.

Wait-Listed?

If you get a letter from a residency program saying that you are "wait-listed" for an interview, do not despair. Residency programs sometimes send such letters when they think that there is little chance that an applicant really is serious—such as someone from the other end of the country.

Write a short email and letter thanking them and saying that you are still interested. One applicant who did this almost immediately got a reply from the program, which was her top choice, offering her an interview. She later matched with that program.

Travel Arrangements

The extensive traveling that you undertake during the interview process may be the most that you have ever done. It may be your first real chance to see many other parts of the country. For many applicants, it will also be a rude introduction to the frequent delays, cancellations, and sardine-can-like accommodations of our nation's air travel system.

Simply traveling to many parts of the country, packing and unpacking in hotels, and finding your way around strange cities will be very tiring—not to mention costly. More than 60% of all senior medical students find the cost of interviewing burdensome—the average student spends more than $1,600 on travel. There are, however, some methods to decrease your fatigue and to make traveling the interview circuit more tolerable, if not actually pleasant.

Clustering Interviews

The first method to consider is clustering your interviews. This can be done either chronologically (to use available blocks of time) or geographically.

It is not unusual for some applicants to fly back and forth across the country several times, as well as to make many side trips, for interviews. Clustering interviews geographically, however, saves both time and the considerable effort that is involved in traveling great distances. It also, of course, saves money. Clustering reduces your interviewing costs by lessening your time away from home (usually spent in hotels) and the amount of traveling you do. These costs, aside from the clothes you bought for the interview, can run anywhere from nothing to $5,000 or more. It will depend upon the geographical range in which you evaluate programs, the level of your accommodations, and your success in clustering interviews to use available transportation in the least expensive manner possible.

To cluster interviews, it is essential that you have both luck and flexibility. The harder you work on the problem, the luckier you will become. Flexibility results from getting your materials to programs early. This will allow you a maximum number of interview dates to choose from. Luck is involved with being offered interviews at the right programs in time for you to arrange clusters. Work with the residency secretaries to try to arrange these clusters of interviews. Most of the time, they understand your situation and are willing to try to help you out.

Some obsessive-compulsive individuals will try to schedule multiple interviews day after day for a period of time. This is very dangerous. They will eventually become stressed out, and may have fewer options if they encounter transportation delays. Remember, bad weather shuts down many of the nation's major airports during the interview season. In addition, they will have too little time to digest the information obtained from one interview before getting involved in the next one.

One method some applicants have used to obtain additional insight into a program is to informally drop by the hospital the evening after the interview, or the next morning, to talk with residents. This provides an opportunity to get a better perspective on the information gained in the midst of hectic interviewing. Some applicants also take time to get a feel for the community in which the program is based while they are there. If you plan to do this, build in enough extra time, particularly if you are clustering your interviews.

Special Fares

Another way to save money is by using special fares available from airlines, railroads, and bus companies. Often, these allow you unlimited travel during a specified period of time. With the deregulation of the travel industry and its resultant fierce competition, the rates, rules, and special offers change with dizzying frequency. Check with several travel websites until you are satisfied that you are getting the best possible value for your money. Remember, the only people paying full fare for transportation, especially air travel, are those having someone else pay for their trip. And the savings can be astronomical. Frequent-flyer/hotel programs, AAA membership, and sometimes your insurance company can also save you money by providing discounted car rentals, airline tickets, and hotel accommodations.

While getting low airfares has become more complicated, there are some specific strategies you can use. Once you know which cities you will visit for interviews, determine the standard 21-day advance-purchase fare. Then, if you find a fare that is 45% to 50% less, book it immediately. Such discounts are usually available only for limited times and there may be only a few seats available at that rate. You can also save by flying one of the no-frills, low-cost carriers.

The cheapest airfare may be to a lesser-used airport or to an adjacent city; if so, you will have to rent a car or arrange other transportation. But ticket prices may be low enough that even with increased transportation costs, the total cost may be less. The best airline deals may be found on the Internet, where many airlines post their lowest fares. You may also want to bid for tickets at one of the online auctions or contact one of the discount agencies available through the AAMC, AMSA, and similar groups. These are often listed in *The New Physician.*

If you buy a full-discount, restricted ticket (as you probably want to do), always check the rules first. Most are non-refundable, charge a fee to change flights or dates, and cannot be changed to a lower fare, even if it is later advertised. Still, it may be worth it.

If you must rent a car, the average daily rate varies depending upon which basic plan you choose. Generally, the pricing packages are (a) a daily rate with a mileage charge; (b) a daily rate with a limited number of free miles per day; (c) a daily rate with unlimited mileage; and (d) a rate that has free mileage over an extended period. Rates also vary according to the size and the style of vehicle, and additional fees (such as drop-off fees) can increase the cost. Special promotional rates are often available, especially over weekends, but should be specifically requested in advance.

Check several rental companies. Local car rental agencies and those not located at the airport (but who will pick you up at the airport) often have much lower rates than the national companies. You can get their telephone numbers from their websites. If you drive to your interview, always check ahead to find out where to park. At many medical centers, visitor parking can be almost impossible to find.

Surviving Air Travel

Most residency applicants fly to lots of interviews. Traveling for business is a vastly different experience than flying for pleasure. As a business traveler, you must do everything possible to save time and fly comfortably. Figure 16.1 lists suggestions gleaned from thousands of business travelers on how to do this.

You may get "bumped" from your flight, meaning there is no room for you even though you have a confirmed reservation. Sometimes, the airline may ask for volunteers to give up their seat for a negotiated sum. In some cases, they also add free tickets—so volunteering to be bumped may be a good deal if you have time to spare.

But, if you arrive at the gate on time and are bumped without volunteering, the airline may owe you a required fee that depends on how long you will be delayed and what you paid for the ticket. If the airline can get you to your final destination within one hour of the original arrival time, there is no compensation. If they can get you there between one and two hours after your original arrival time, the airline must pay you the one-way cost of your ticket up to $400. If they cannot get you there within two hours of the scheduled time or if the airline does not make any substitute travel arrangements for you, the compensation doubles to a maximum of $800.

Avoid checking your bags, if at all possible. If you have to check a bag, make a list of what is in it and take a picture of it to show them what it looks like. If your checked bags are damaged or lost, maximum reimbursement is only $1,250. If they lose it, file a claim with the airline's baggage claim department on arrival, and keep your baggage claim receipts. They will normally get your bag to you (if you stay in the same city) by the next day.

Ask the residency program you are visiting for the best and the cheapest (they may be different) ways to get from the airport to the hospital. Trains will usually be the cheapest and fastest transportation method—but may not be the safest method at certain times of day. Also, you may have to lug your baggage a distance to get to the train. A useful alternative is an airport shuttle. Remember to get the cheaper round-trip ticket. Taxis are for those who don't have to watch their budget and cars are for special situations or for additional sightseeing in the area

Alternative Transportation

Many applicants cut costs by using cars, trains and busses to visit residency programs. A car works well for nearby programs; trains and busses work well in certain major transportation corridors, such as along the east coast. The trick will be to find the transportation method that is the fastest, the least expensive, and the most convenient way to get to your destination. What you select will depend on what is available, your personal finances, and the time you have to make the trip.

Figure 16.1: Air Travel Made Easier

- Take early morning or late-night flights; there may be fewer delays then. (Late-night flights may also be less expensive.)
- Go a day before you must arrive—but not on the last flight of the day. Interview season occurs during the worst travel weather of the year, so your flight may be canceled or delayed.
- Keep your booking service's email, web URL, and toll-free telephone number handy. If your flight is canceled, call them to rebook you, rather than standing in line.
- Take a copy of that month's *Official Airline Guide* (or the relevant pages) to help reschedule flights. Check on the Internet, at your library or ask some of the more-traveled faculty for a copy.
- If you arrive at the airport early, try to get on an earlier flight.
- Know the security rules about what you cannot carry on the plane. Pute all metal objects in your carryon bag, take out your computer, and remove your shoes before getting to the security x-ray machine.
- Board the plane as soon as possible to make it easier to find space for your carryon bags.
- Sit in the front of the plane to be one of the first off the plane.
- Get an aisle seat. You can get to the bathroom easier and get off the plane faster. (You may be disturbed by the "inside" passengers climbing over you to get out.)
- If you are right-handed, sit on the right side of the plane so that people passing you in the aisle won't jiggle your arm when you work or eat. If you plan to sleep, get a window seat so other passengers won't crawl over you to get out. Seats in the exit row have more legroom, but on some planes those seats don't recline.
- Carry foam ear plugs or a small music player with earphones if you want to sleep or you fly on a small plane. Carry eyeshades if you want to sleep. Consider carrying a blow-up neck or lumbar pillow.
- Join the airlines' frequent flier clubs. You may board earlier and get special perquisites. Use one airline and its hotel and car rental partners to maximize benefits. Also join hotel and rental company's clubs.
- If you will fly a lot on one airline, consider joining their airport club. The relaxation between flights may be worth the cost of a one-year membership.
- Use a carryon bag with wheels and/or a garment bag that clips onto it.
- Dress comfortably. Unless you will go directly to your interview, carry your interview clothes and dress casually for the flight.
- Pack a snack and a small bottle for water. Many airlines no longer offer meals, and flight delays often prevent travelers from eating between flights. Fill your water bottle *after* you go through security screening.
- Order special meals, such as vegetarian, low-calorie, or kosher, if meals are serve on the flights. They are usually fresher than other meals.

Figure 16.1 (continued)

- Do exercises on the airplane:
  Neck Stretch: Flex and extend your neck 5 times anteriorly-posteriorly (toward the chest) and 5 times laterally (toward the shoulders). Then rotate your head from side to side 5 times; hold at full rotation for 3 to 5 seconds.
  Shoulder Stretch: Link fingers and hold them in front of your chest. Lift arms above your head (breathe while stretching), and hold your breath and position for 3 seconds. Bring your arms behind your head while breathing out. Hold your breath and position for 3 seconds.
  Arm Isometrics: Push down on the armrest for the count of 5 and then pull up on the armrest for the count of 5. Repeat 5 times.
  Lower-Back Stretch: Clasp your knee with both hands, pull it to your chest, and hold it there for the count of 5. Repeat with other leg.
  Leg/Foot Stretch: With your shoes off, press firmly with your palms on both knees. Dorsiflex your foot so your heels are touching the floor and your toes are raised as high as possible. Then plantar flex so that your toes touch the floor and the heels are raised. Repeat quickly 8 times.
- Use the airplane restroom before landing. This may save up to 20 minutes on the ground if you are first to the taxis or car rental counters.

Cheap Housing

The American Medical Association Alliance, in conjunction with AMA Medical Student Section and AMA Resident/Fellows Section, runs the Physicians-In-Training Host Program to help students reduce interviewing costs, get to know the community surrounding their potential residency program, and introduce them to local medical society and Alliance members. Using volunteer hosts, they will try to fulfill requests for housing for one- or two-night stays for up to three interview dates. Requests must be received at least two weeks prior to the expected stay. For more information and the application for housing, go to www.ama-assn.org/go/alliance and click on "In-Training" on the left sidebar and then, on the left sidebar on the next page click on "Housing for Resident Interviews." If you have trouble, call the Alliance at (312) 464-4470.

The American Medical Women's Association runs a Bed and Breakfast Program for its student members traveling to residency interviews (and also for physician members going to job or fellowship interviews or conferences). To use this program, choose the "Request a Host" tab on the program's homepage (http://www.amwa-doc.org/articles1-25/BedandBreakfastProgram). Read the term and conditions carefully before you electronically sign the contract. You must contact a prospective host at least 30 days before travel, as well as conform to other courtesies. After you enter the details of your trip, the AMWA national office will contact you with a list of member volunteers in that area; you should choose one and contact them to make arrangements. The program is operated on a volunteer, "first-come, first-served" basis. For information not on the website, contact AMWA's national student President-Elect at president. elect@amwa-student.org.

Another source for information about inexpensive housing is the residency program at which you are interviewing. If such information is not included in the material they send, call the residency's secretary and ask about good, inexpensive, and *safe* housing near the hospital. You will not be the first one to ask, and the program probably has a list of good places to stay. They may have arranged special rates for applicants at local hotels. Some programs even offer housing in a resident's or faculty member's home to applicants who request it. This is especially true if your host is an alumnus of your medical school.

If you decide to go it alone, make sure the location will allow you to get to the interview on time. Check out their security in advance—especially if it is in a crime-prone area, as are many locations around large teaching hospitals. If the establishment offers free services, such as breakfast, take advantage of them.

Get enough sleep. Before turning in, make sure that the curtains are tightly closed—and bring along some clothespins to keep them closed. Use a sleep mask for added darkness and a pair of soft earplugs (those made of wax are generally most effective) for quiet. Make sure to test the mask and earplugs at home to become used to them—and to be sure you can still hear your alarm clock. Check the room's alarm clock (bringing your own is even better) to make sure that it works. Then go to bed in time to get enough sleep and still get to the interview a little early, which will reduce your stress.

During your personal time, explore the local area, including the museums, sporting or cultural events, and shopping. To avoid the common feeling of isolation, stay in touch with friends and family via phone or e-mail. If you don't have a cell phone with lots of long-distance minutes, now is the time to get one. Also, exercise as you would at home. Check with your hosts or the hotel about safe exercise areas nearby..

Simultaneous Vacation

As mentioned, the interview circuit is no picnic. But in some situations, you can turn it into a real vacation. Try to chronologically cluster interviews but, if there is a break in your interview schedule, investigate vacation spots in the surrounding area. This can give you a relaxing break in the action—a needed rest period at a relatively low cost, since you are already nearby. If you have a spouse or significant other, he or she might want to meet you at this spot. A friendly face is sometimes a very welcome sight and helps to bolster the spirits. And having someone to talk to and to share your experiences with may add to the relief. Given the stresses of medical school and the anticipated heavy work schedule to come, you and your spouse or significant other (if you have one) probably need a vacation anyway!

Updating Information about the Programs

As the time for your interviews draws near, recontact the programs where you will be interviewing to request any new or updated information and re-check their websites. The material on their website or that you were initially sent was prepared the previous spring or earlier. Many things could have changed at the program. Some might even affect whether you still want to go to that institution for an interview. Other changes may affect your final program rankings.

The best time to ask about any changes in the program is when you arrange a date for your interview. If there is new written material, ask them to send you a copy. If it is not yet available, ask for as much information about the changes as possible.

Undoubtedly, you will be a more appealing candidate to the interviewers if you know up-to-date information about their program. If you don't, they will wonder why. So be sure to get the latest available information on the program before you leave for your interviews. Ask about changes once again when you are at the program—from the program director, the residency secretary, and the current residents.

Communicating with the Programs

Once you send your initial application packet, you will mostly communicate with programs by telephone and e-mail.

The first time you should contact the programs is about a month after you have requested that your material be sent to them. Find out if it has all arrived. If not, what is missing?

How you communicate with a program is very important. It is amazing that the nicest, most sophisticated individuals often have a terrible telephone "presence." Your voice over the telephone and your attitude on it will make a big impression on a program. Don't think that you can behave any way you want to on the telephone because you are *only* talking to the residency secretary! And don't express your extreme annoyance at being put on hold in rather crude terms.

As in many businesses, a secretary who interacts with applicants often has a major impact on who is selected—both for interviews and for final positions. Many residency directors ask their secretaries for input. And most take this input very seriously. Polish your telephone technique. Polish up those residency secretaries. They can be either your allies or your enemies. Make them think of you as a nice person, the kind that they want as a resident in *their* program.

E-mail is the modern way to communicate, and this also goes for residency programs. Increasingly, programs notify applicants via e-mail when they are selected for interviews. They also request that specific questions be forwarded either to the residency directors or to their assistants via e-mail. As with other correspondence, be certain that your e-mail messages to the programs are coherent, spell-checked, and grammatically correct. One way of improving your e-mail messages is to write them on a word processor and then paste them into your correspondence. As noted previously, be certain that your e-mail address doesn't appear sophomoric, such as "hotstuff@xyz.com."

17

Looking The Part: Interview Attire

In your town, your reputation counts; in another, your clothes do.

Talmud, Shabboth

I base most of my fashion sense on what doesn't itch.

Gilda Radner

THE KEY TO LOOKING GOOD at your interviews is to do what others do—but better. Yes, there is a "uniform" to wear. It is conservative, tasteful, and neat. It looks like upper-middle-class success. And it works. Of course, you wore blue jeans and sweatshirts during your first two years of medical school. Maybe you wore less as an undergraduate. You love to hang around the wards dressed in wrinkled scrubs, looking just like the residents. Don't imitate their sloppy dress; residents already have their training slots. Now is the time for you to shine—both literally and figuratively.

One interviewee, medical student Scott Fishman, described this uniform as "remarkably drab . . . a ridiculous costume . . . a rite of passage." He went on to say that, "sitting there waiting for our turns outside the interviewer's office, we all look like we are going to a funeral." Perhaps. But better to wear the uniform and appear to go to a funeral than not wear it and attend your own.

No, you don't have to go out and spend lots of money that you don't have on clothes you can't afford. Just do what you can to get into the uniform. Ideally, interviewers should not be aware of your clothes; you want them to remember you, not what you wore. The proper dress for residency interviews is essentially identical, no matter where in the country you are applying. Appropriate dress can help you a little. The wrong outfit will destroy you.

Remember that in the first seven seconds, interviewers make decisions based on your visual cues: your clothes, grooming, walk, stance, etc. After that, they begin evaluating you through your verbal skills.

Men

The Suit

A suit is the standard dress for an interview. It should be solid or pinstripe, navy or gray. "The men who run America," says John T. Molloy, author of

Dress for Success, "run it blue, gray, and dull." Do not wear a suit with bright or avant-garde colors or designs. "If you try to spruce up the look," Mr. Molloy continues, "you're in trouble."

The suit doesn't have to be expensive or in the latest style, but it should be tailored and well-made. If you don't have or cannot afford a suit, wear a navy-blue sport jacket with matching pants. If you don't have these either, it is time you visited a clothing store. Charge the bill to your future. Serious and solid is the image you are looking for in your outfit. And *before* you show up at your first interview, make sure that your clothes fit well. Few things distract an interviewer more than an applicant fidgeting with his tight collar.

The Shirt
Wear either a white or pale-blue solid-color shirt. Long sleeves are in order if you plan to remove your jacket. Avoid stripes, loud colors, or any weird designs. Shirttails should be long enough to keep the shirt tucked in, even when you raise your arms. With the top button fastened, your collar should fit snugly, but not so tightly that your eyes bulge.

The Tie and Belt
Wear a tie—even if you are a laid-back individual. An open-neck shirt and gold chain just won't cut it. Your tie should be solid, have repeating stripes (rep), small polka dots, or repeating small insignias (club). Avoid gaudy bright colors, large patterns, and black. The "power colors" are red and navy. Knot the tie so its tip meets your belt and put the back of the tie through the label, so the ends stay together. Do not wear a bow tie. It gives the impression that you're odd and out of touch with this decade.

Wear a plain, dark leather belt with a small buckle. It should go with your suit and be the same color as your shoes. Make sure the belt is neither too long (droopy end) nor too short (squeezing you to look like a blimp).

The Shoes and Socks
Wear black or very dark brown conservatively designed shoes. Make sure that they are in good repair and shined. Dirty shoes are male applicants' most common clothing error. Also make sure that there are no holes in your soles; if there are, keep your feet flat on the floor. Wear calf-length plain *socks* that match your suit.

Accessories
The key here is sedate. Limit *jewelry* to a watch and wedding band (only if you are married). If you wear a watch, avoid anything unusual such as a dive

watch or one with a picture of Spider Man on the front. No lapel pins, no ID bracelets, no tie clasps—and definitely, *NO EARRINGS OR OTHER IMPLANTED JEWELRY!* No matter what the protestations, that little flash of gold will cost you big points. Save it for later. Inappropriate or too much jewelry will elicit very strong negative responses.

If you wear an *undershirt*, a crew neck looks best, since it doesn't show through a shirt. If you wear *suspenders*, be sure that they button to your pants. If you carry a wallet or cell phone, they shouldn't bulge out of your pocket.

If you wear *glasses*, make sure that they the frames are standard: No initials on the lenses or unusual colors. It's best not to wear tinted or photo-gray lenses, since they place a barrier between you and the interviewer. Also, keep the lenses clean.

The *pen* and *pencil* you carry should look classy. They do not have to be gold, but they should not look like you got them from hospital stores or the local drug rep. And don't stick them in a shirt-pocket protector. To look the part of a serious candidate and have a convenient place to make notes and store papers, carry a small, zippered leather-covered *notepad* with the materials you need. If you use an electronic device (don't use anything larger than a pad-sized device) to take notes, make sure that you can use it to make your notes quickly; otherwise, revert to a pen and paper.

Grooming

As for personal grooming, be neat, squeaky clean, and conservative. Your *hair* should be short and a natural color. If it's shorter than you like, it's probably close to the right length. Ask your mentor (if he or she is over 35-years-old), a parent, or close (older) friend to advise you on this. Definitely avoid ponytails and other unusual haircuts. Make sure all hair has been recently trimmed and washed. Invest in a good haircut about one week before the interview; haircuts look best after one week. If you wear facial hair, it should be neatly trimmed. Avoid goatees and handlebar mustaches as these have strong negative connotations. Keep any tattoos covered. Trim and clean your *nails*. Remember, you are about to be a physician, putting your hands on, and in, patients.

The *odor* the interviewer perceives should be minimal—and then only that of deodorant or nervousness. Avoid after-shave; you are not going on a date. If you are concerned about your breath, carry breath mints. And above all, no alcohol (and, if possible, no tobacco use) within 24 hours of the interview. There are enough perceived and anticipated problems with drug abuse among housestaff. You do not have to show the interviewers that you could be part of the problem.

The bottom line is that you want to look as much like a successful upper-middle-class physician as possible. Wear the garments symbolizing the successful individual in our society. You certainly did it to get into medical school. It's time to do it again. There is no need to flaunt your lifestyle in your dress. Leave your personal preferences out of this. They can only harm you.

Women

The Suit

Although styles are changing in the workplace, the standard dress for a woman going to an interview remains the *suit*, preferably a skirted suit. A good suit suggests that you are an upper-middle-class professional—just the image you want to project. Don't be led down the path to destruction by following fads or fashion. The classic suit is the uniform of success. Find out what woman accountants or lawyers who work for large firms wear. This will be the "classic" style.

In purchasing a suit, choose wool or linen, or a synthetic that simulates either. The fabric should be solid, tweed, or plaid. For solid suits, the three best colors are gray (a couple of shades lighter than charcoal), medium-range blue, and dark maroon. Stay away from bold, flashy patterns. The skirt should extend to just below the knee (best); it should be no shorter than just above the knee. You should feel comfortable sitting in it. The matching jacket should be a blazer cut with long sleeves.

Two alternatives to the suit are a tailored dress or a skirt worn with a jacket. Neither is as powerful as the suit, but if you do not feel comfortable in a suit, these are two reasonable substitutes.

Many women have stated that they prefer a suit with pants. However, experts are unclear as to the effect of pants suits, so you probably want to opt for one of the other choices.

The Blouse

The *blouse* should be simply cut, not too frilly or lacy, and the neckline must not be too low. If it's equivalent to a man's shirt with one button open, it will be acceptable. The blouse should be cotton, silk, or a look-alike synthetic. Usually it will be white, cream, or pastel—not red or fuchsia. In general, it should be in a solid color that complements the suit.

The Shoes

Shoes should be simple pumps, closed at the toe and heel, and not brand new. They should be in a dark or neutral color that is compatible with your suit.

The heels should not be more than 1.5-inches high. Do not wear boots. Most residency applicants will be doing a lot of walking around the hospital; be sure that you will survive in the shoes you wear.

Accessories

Although a scarf is not as essential as a man's tie, it can be eye-catching if used properly. Wear silk or a look-alike synthetic and tie it in an ascot, necktie, or scout style. If worn, a scarf must have simple lines and no frills to detract from the center of attention—your face. Hosiery should be skin-colored.

As with men, the less jewelry you wear the better. Aside from a simple watch and wedding ring (if married), be careful about what other ornaments you wear. While a brooch or a simple necklace is often very suitable, multiple rings, bracelets, or anything ornate or gaudy is not. Very simple earrings or gold studs should be limited to one per ear. The appropriate watch is plain gold or silver. Wear nose studs only for religious reasons.

If you need to wear an overcoat, make sure that it is long enough to cover the bottom of your skirt. Multiple coat styles are acceptable; furs are not. If you wear gloves, make them leather. They should be the same color as your coat.

Do not carry a purse. Carry a leather zippered case, attaché case, or leather-bound zippered notebook with any necessities, including any electronic devices. This connotes power and authority. Put everything that you need in it, but do not overstuff it or keep it sloppy—you may have to open it during an interview. Some students have written that the zippered notebook is less awkward when carried to lunch, labs, or on ward tours. If using an attaché case, include a small leather-covered notepad. Avoid the drug company pens you use on the wards.

Grooming

As for the more *personal items*, such as hair, makeup, and perfume, just remember that you are going on a job interview, not on a date. If the interviewer is aware that you are wearing perfume, you are wearing too much. Similarly with makeup—it works best when it is not obvious. Be especially careful to avoid obvious eye shadow or eyeliner. Nails should be manicured. Your hair should be clean and conservative in appearance. If it is long, it is often a good idea to put it up to keep it from looking sloppy. Many consultants recommend that women should avoid hairstyles that cover either eye, and that their hair should be pulled away from the jaw line and ears so they will look more serious.

The bottom line is that you dress for the interview in a uniform. Although there is considerable variation allowed, for maximum success, applicants should adhere to the standard style. As one woman physician who did very well in her resident interviews said about the wardrobe, "sophistication and maturity are the keys to success."

Clothing Tips

Clothing as Camouflage

Clothes can hide real or perceived problems. For those "Doogie Howser" types who think they look too young to be taken seriously, dressing conservatively will age you a bit. Wearing glasses, even if you normally wear contacts, also helps.

Some people are self-conscious about their weight. Clothes can help disguise those extra pounds. Both men and women can wear slightly longer, or hip-length, suit jackets, and women can wear a loose jacket over a business dress or flared skirt. The key is to be certain that your clothes fit well. Even thin people look heavy if their buttons are popping out or their collar is too tight. Also, if you have tattoos, hopefully, your clothes can hide them.

Wear the "Uniform" Stylishly

Now that you have acquired the uniform, make sure that you get the most out of it. Your clothes must be clean and pressed. Do *not* travel in your clothes and show up five minutes before the interview looking like a Raggedy Anne doll that has gone through the washer. If possible, travel in your normal attire and arrive at the interview city the night before. You will get a good night's sleep and put on your freshly pressed uniform the next morning to go to the interview. Be sure to have the appropriate garments, such as overcoat, umbrella, etc., to protect your uniform in case of inclement weather. When you get to the interview site, slip into the restroom and give yourself a last-minute inspection.

Once you have dressed for your interview, forget about your clothes. They should be a natural part of you. Think of these clothes like new hiking boots. You don't want to go 20 miles in a new pair without breaking them in first. If you aren't comfortable in these fancy duds, wear them a few times before you hit the interview trail.

Packing

When packing for interviews, the motto should be "less is more." That will often be the only way to get all the necessities into the allowable size and number of bags. This is especially important now that the airlines are charging for checked bags. Two simple techniques for doing this are either to limit the time you have to pack to 20 minutes per city you will visit, or to put out everything you want for your trip—and then put half of it away.

Sophisticated travelers decrease the amount they carry by making sure that all their clothes go with everything else, by packing clothes that can serve more than one function, and by avoiding the tendency to pack for each potential "what if?" that could happen on the trip. Wear the bulky items. You can always stow a heavy coat in the overhead bin.

Packing lists ease pre-trip anxieties. Once you make a decision about what to take with you on one trip, use the same packing list for subsequent trips. That way you won't forget anything. Keep the list with you to serve as a record of your belongings in case your bags are lost.

How to Pack a Suitcase

Whether you use a large suitcase or a smaller carryon, the goal is for your clothes to arrive intact and as pristine as possible. To accomplish this, place your trousers, skirts, dresses, shirts, blouses, and jackets (all zipped or buttoned, and folded along their natural seams) in the suitcase, alternating side to side. Frequent travelers know that if suits, skirts, and dresses are neatly folded and placed in a plastic cleaner's bag, they will stay neat and pressed. You can even roll them up and they will remain pristine! (I know it seems bizarre, so try it out at home to prove to yourself that it works.)

Only after all items are partially in the suitcase should the remainder that are outside the suitcase be folded in, one garment over the other (Figure 17.1). Each item will then cushion the others and help prevent creases. Pack shoes, stuffed with toiletries, rolled-up socks, belts, etc., along the hinged side of the bag. Finally, stuff rolled T-shirts, undergarments, sleepwear, and sweaters in any available space to cushion the contents and keep them from shifting. When you unpack, the result should be neat and clean clothing.

On multi-day trips where you won't unpack and stay at the same location, put the items you will wear together on the same layer, so you can simply reach in and pull them all out at the same time. Put smaller items for each day, such as underwear, in plastic bags. To reduce the stress of residency interview trips, take along a memento of home, such as a family picture, a favorite book, or even a pillow (if you are not traveling by air).

Figure 17.1
Packing a Suitcase

Before packing, every garment should be buttoned, zippered, belted, and folded along natural creases.

- Place slacks, skirts, dresses, shirts, blouses, or jackets in your suitcase, alternating from side to side. (1-3)
- Line up the waistband or collar with the edges.
- "Interfold" the extensions left hanging over the sides.
- Fold one garment over the other, smoothing wrinkles as you go. (4)

Each item will cushion the other, helping to prevent creases.

What To Do If Your Suitcase Doesn't Show Up

Use Carryon, If Possible

A danger when flying is that your checked baggage won't show up—at least not in time to do you any good. The fact that it appears back at your home the day after the interview is little consolation for being forced to dress in "low camp" style for the interview at your most desired program. The solution, especially if you are only going to be away from home for one or two days, is to use a carryon garment bag and another small carryon bag that fits under the seat. This often provides sufficient packing capacity and will alleviate any worry about your uniform not showing up. (Depending on the current airline rules, it may also save you from paying additional money to check luggage.) And, since you don't have to retrieve your bags, it also saves you a lot of time at the airport.

It is essential that you carry with you the interview schedule, flight confirmation/schedule, travelers checks, credit cards, driver's license or other ID, jewelry, hotel/auto rental confirmations, and medications, as well as the telephone numbers and email addresses for your travel agent or website, your airline, and interview contacts. I have seen many distraught applicants whose air carrier lost the checked bag containing their interview materials and clothes.

Be careful when choosing your carryon bags. Each airline, and even each model or configuration of seats on a particular plane, has different allowable space and different rules for carryons. These days, traveling with as little baggage as possible is the best bet. Most airlines now limit you to one carryon bag and a personal item such as a purse or a briefcase. A few also charge for some bags. It is wise to look on the airline's website to avoid bringing bags that won't fit in the overhead bin or under the seat. If possible, get a carryon with wheels so you can roll it—your back will thank you.

Honesty Works

Okay, so you weren't able to use the carryon method—and now your baggage is somewhere between here and Outer Mongolia. You have an interview in three hours and are wearing hand-me-downs from a backwoods orphanage. What should you do?

First, don't panic. Any faculty member who will be interviewing you has undoubtedly had a great deal of airline travel experience. And anyone with that amount of experience has also had the airlines lose checked bags—often more than once. However, you need to make some show of good faith. First, badger the airline's representative. If you present a good enough sob story, they might front you money for a decent shirt or blouse and tie. You will need at least this much. Then, when you get to the interview, apologize to everyone you meet for your appearance. The "airline-lost-my-luggage" story never fails to both get the sympathy (or empathy) vote and keep that applicant in the interviewers' minds. A good story and a good attitude may actually win you some points.

Tax Tip

Since you may have just spent substantial sums on phone calls, travel, and transportation, you may be asking yourself whether these expenses are tax deductible. The answer is yes and no.

Most applicants are medical students who have no substantial income. Without income, they pay no taxes, so there are no deductions. In any event, students will be applying for their first job in medicine, so Uncle Sam would not allow the deductions anyway.

If, however, you are already working as a physician and are now applying for a residency or fellowship position, keep a careful record of your expenses (including postage, copying, telephone calls, travel, and lodging). These may be deductible as job search expenses if you itemize your income tax return.

18

The Visit

Hiring decisions are made in the first 30 seconds of the interview—
the balance of the time is used to justify the decision.

An axiom in the personnel field

Illusions are comforting; just don't rely on them.

Folk Saying

OKAY, SO YOU HAVE YOUR INTERVIEWS set up and you are ready to go and "knock their socks off." Remember that it is not only your interview performance but also how you conduct yourself throughout your entire time at a program that will determine whether the faculty ranks you highly. So here are some last minute tips to help you smooth out any remaining rough spots in the way you will present yourself.

Timeliness

To mangle an old saying, "Timeliness is next to Godliness." You will make a major impact on all interviewers, a significantly *negative* impact, if you are late for your appointments. Excuses may be fine for your mother, your spouse, and, sometimes, your friends and teachers. But they work poorly on prospective employers. Faculty's time is valuable, and they have set some of it aside to interview you. Don't waste their time, or yours, by being late.

Of course, unavoidable delays do occur. Unexpected bad weather and transportation breakdowns are the two most common causes, especially during the interview season—with the worst weather of the year. If you run into difficulties that will cause you to be late, have the courtesy to call ahead. Even if you only think that you *might* be delayed due to these or other valid factors, let the program know early. They will then be able to reschedule people and, possibly, to work you in at a later time or on a later date. Do not leave them wondering what happened to you. Even if you do not care about that program, leaving them hanging is extremely discourteous and unprofessional, and it may cost you a position at another program. Remember that many academics know each other—and they do talk about applicants when they get together. *The key is to show up on time, ready for action!*

Confirm Your Interview

Although you are expected to be on time and at the correct location, either you or the program may have made a scheduling error. Mistakes happen, especially when there are dozens or hundreds of individuals interviewing at the same program during a short period of time. It is embarrassing for an applicant to show up on the wrong day for a scheduled interview. Occasionally there is a disaster at the residency program that mandates that interviews be postponed or rescheduled. The professional way to avoid complications is to call to confirm your interview a day or two before traveling to the program. That way you stand little chance of making a wasted trip or being embarrassed by a scheduling error.

Know the Schedule

If you can get your interview schedule for each program before you arrive, so much the better. Have them e-mail or fax it to you. You will then know how to pace yourself throughout the visit. You will also be able to plan specific activities for any "free" blocks of time. Use this time to visit the library, the wards, and the other teaching hospitals in the program if they are nearby. Also, visit the cafeteria. Since this could be the food you eat for the next several years, how bad is it?

If you cannot get your entire schedule, at least find out what time you begin. Recheck your information the afternoon before to make certain that it is correct. You cannot afford to be late. It usually helps if you are *early*. Even if you have never been early for anything in your life, this would be an excellent time to start.

Once you get started on your interviews, it is up to the interviewers themselves, and the residency secretary, to keep everyone on schedule. Many interviewers have a bad habit of running over their allotted time. Do not let this make you uncomfortable. However, when you get to the next appointment late, apologize immediately and explain that you just got out of your last interview with Dr. X. If it happens to you, it has happened to others—and faculty members will understand and not count it against you. They probably are already aware of their colleagues' foibles.

Leave Some Time Flexible

Now that you have gotten the interview and have worked hard to make a good impression, do not ruin it all by running out early. Would you leave a fancy dinner party before dessert? Of course not. Scheduling departing flights out of town without giving yourself enough flexibility to "eat dessert" is the same situation. If you book yourself too tightly, you will not have any leeway in case your interviews run overtime. When they do, it will usually be because one or more of the faculty has an extra interest in your candidacy. This is a golden opportunity; don't blow it.

Also, you may find you have a greater interest in a program than you initially thought you would. In that case, you may want to investigate that program's and the city's finer points while you are there. You will need some extra time to do this. Remain a little flexible.

Attitude

SMILE! It doesn't cost you anything. Of course you are prepared to be on your best behavior with interviewers. But astute program directors are just as interested in how you act outside the formal interview setting as in how you act in it. This tells them more about how you will act during day-to-day program activities, how you will interact with your peers, and whether you will be able to get along with the ancillary medical staff.

Be pleasant to everyone, and be cheerful at all times. This does not mean you must fawn over the residents and bow down to the secretaries. It does mean, at the least, that you should not ignore them. They are real people. Treat them as the friendly individuals they probably are. Try to interact with them warmly. This also holds true for other applicants. When applicants are observed as a group, those who get along with others can be clearly identified. Having the other applicants enjoy your company is a very positive point in your favor. And working well with a team is a key ingredient in being a successful resident.

The bottom line is that sources other than the interviewers provide input that is often considered when programs decide which applicants will be offered residency positions. Always act as if you are under observation the entire time you are interacting with anyone at the program. The show doesn't stop until you walk out the hospital door at the end of the day, and it continues with every phone and written contact you make with the program.

One point worthy of mention is that reviewing your own medical school file may help you prepare for these interactions. The narrative part of your file usually contains a wealth of information from faculty and residents concerning how others perceive you. Take time to read through it before your interviews. Insights that you gain could lead to more positive interactions with the interviewers, as well as improvements in all your personal relations.

Uniqueness

Interviewers, like all individuals, receive only a small portion of the information directed at them. There is a great deal of "noise" between the sender's encoded message and the receiver's decoding of that message (Figure 18.1). Receivers take this information and change it to fit their preconceived ideas. It is from this information that they make decisions. As a residency applicant, you battle three communication devils.

Selective Exposure

People are constantly exposed to a tremendous amount of stimuli. They really notice only exceptional deviations from normal patterns. These deviations can either be positive (beneficial to you) or negative (counterproductive to you). It is essential that you be noticed—and noticed positively.

Selective Distortion

People tend to interpret data in ways that support, rather than challenge, their preconceptions. These preconceptions of you will, most likely, be based upon the written material that you have supplied to the program. It is your job to add to the positive feeling you have already worked so hard to create.

Figure 18.1:
Elements in the Communication Process

Selective Retention

People forget much of what they learn. And they forget it quickly. Your job is to make sure that they remember you.

Knowledge

About the Specialty

You have worked hard to get interviews for a position in your chosen specialty. Be certain you know a great deal about that specialty before you arrive at the programs. This does not mean medical knowledge; you will acquire that during your residency. It means that you should know about the specialty's culture.

- What do the practitioners in the field really do?
- What types of procedures do they perform?
- What level of reimbursement should they expect?
- How do other specialists perceive them?
- Do they have opportunities for subspecialty training?
- What are the requirements to take the specialty's Board examination?
- What is the outlook for the specialty in the future?

These are the types of questions that you should have asked yourself while making an informed decision about which specialty you wanted to enter. Faculty members want to know that you have made the effort to learn about their specialty before committing your entire professional life to it.

If you do not have this information, you may not have fully thought out your decision, and could later be very unhappy. Unhappiness is bad for both the resident and the faculty. It leads to depression, anger, and poor performance. It can also cause a resident to drop out of a program before graduation. Therefore, demonstrate that you have seriously thought about your career choice. Know about the specialty. Read the specialty journals and newsletters concerning pending changes within the field. The latter, if you can get copies from your specialty advisor or the specialty's organizations, are the most current. Read the editorials to know about the specialty's "hot topics." The more you know about a specialty, the more committed to it you will appear. And commitment is one of the most important qualities interviewers seek.

About the Program

Just as you must know the basic information about your chosen specialty, you also need to know about each program you visit.

You initially received a lot of information from their website and from *FREIDA*. If you were as careful as you should have been, you also have received additional updated written or oral information. Review this information before going into the interview. No matter whether this is your first interview or the twentieth, it is a major *faux pas* to confuse basics about the program where you are currently interviewing with information from another program. Be sure that you have the facts about the current program firmly in your mind before you set out in the morning. If you, like most people, have a little trouble keeping the details straight, write yourself some notes for reference.

Another way to get additional information about a program is to run a MEDLINE search (www.ncbi.nlm.nih.gov/pubmed/) on the faculty. Looking at articles written by the faculty will give you an idea of their medical interests. It may also provide some insight into questions they might ask you or subjects they might like to discuss. In any case, the more you know about a specific program before going into the interview setting, the better the chance that you will leave highly regarded and will be remembered.

Many programs use more than one hospital for training. If possible, see them all, even if you are only scheduled for interviews at one or two of them. They may not want to show you the other institution(s) for a very good reason—you would not rank the program if you saw them!

Talk to Residents for the Real Story

If you haven't talked to the current residents, assume that you really do not know very much about the program. Be very wary of any program that either does not give you the opportunity or that does not insist that you talk to some of its residents. Residents often see things quite differently than the attending physicians. And their perspectives, while not necessarily the same as those you might have in the same situation, may be much closer to yours than those of the faculty. These talks are usually informal, and because of limitations on the residents' time, may occur in a group setting. Nevertheless, the residents' opinions, viewpoints, and insights about the program should strongly influence how you will rate it for each of the factors on your "Must/Want" Analysis.

If there is a senior medical student on rotation in the department while you are there, try to talk to him or her. You cannot afford to miss this valuable perspective. One other source of information might be a graduate from your medical school who is currently training at that institution. Even if not in the same program to which you are applying, he or she will have intimate knowledge of the institution, and may even know something about your prospective department. Graduates from your *alma mater* may also feel some loyalty to you—and give you otherwise "forgotten" information. You will probably be able to locate such graduates through either your Dean of Students or your school's Alumni Office.

Basic Rules

Once you actually get to the interview site there are some very basic things that you need to do, aside from answering any questions in a satisfactory manner. In fact, questions and answers may, in some cases, be merely window dressing for the actual interview process.

The "behavioral interview" is becoming more common as laws increasingly limit the questions that interviewers can ask. Behavioral interviewers are much more interested in whether you look and act like you would fit into a job rather than whether you can answer any specific questions. They look for communication skills, physical presence, motivation, truthfulness, and how suited each applicant is to be a resident in their program.

All good interviewers look for small, but important, details. Some of these are discussed below.

Show Enthuslasm for This Program

It is important to show your enthusiasm for the specialty. But being enthusiastic about entering the training program *at which you are currently interviewing* makes interviewers rate you even more highly. Base your eagerness on the strong points that you gleaned from the program's information packet. Generally, the areas of which the program is most proud are highlighted on their website. So basing your interest on these areas will get the best results.

An amazing number of applicants arrive at programs with the attitude either that: (1) they are browsing and will not reveal that they really *want* a position at the program, or (2) the interest in the program that they show while interviewing will not influence their selection as a potential resident. Both approaches are wrong. Show enthusiasm! If you cannot work up any enthusiasm for a program, perhaps you should not be interviewing there. Also, if you can't garner enthusiasm for the program and specialty now, you won't be able to do it when you are working your third 30-hour on-call stint in a week. (Yes, that can still happen in some specialties, even under the ACGME's 2010 rules.)

Know How To Pronounce Your Interviewers' Names

How do you say Dr. Llnoyphthg? You don't know? How could that be when he will be interviewing you in five minutes? It may seem petty, especially with some of the difficult or unique pronunciations of names in the medical world, to expect you to know how to pronounce, on the first try, all the names of the people that you will meet. But it is expected. So you should know how. Remember that, above all else, a person's name is a unique part of him or her. Mispronouncing an interviewer's name can, even if subconsciously, leave a negative impression of an applicant.

At the start of the day, ask the residency secretary how to pronounce any difficult or unusual names among those listed on your interview schedule. As she tells you, write each down phonetically so you will be able to repeat it correctly when necessary. If this is not possible, listen carefully when the individual introduces him- or herself to you. If it is a difficult name, repeat it and ask if you said it right. Don't slip up on this simple point of etiquette.

Enter & Depart in a Polite, Assured Manner

Look confident! Walk into the interview with your head up, shoulders squared, looking poised. If you slink into an interview like a scared rabbit, how are you going to look to an interviewer? Certainly not like one of the people likely to get a spot in *their* residency program. Remember that initial impressions are very important. In the first minute, interviewers determine whether applicants meet their expectations. Let your body send a message of confidence, calmness, and control.

Greet interviewers with a firm, but not bone-crushing, handshake. This goes for both men and women. A dainty, dead-fish handshake connotes only meekness and a lack of authority. Avoid it like the plague. Extend your hand to the other person with the thumb up and out. Make sure that the web between your thumb and index finger meets the other person's web. Try to shake hands from the elbow, not the shoulder or wrist. It is also desirable to have reasonably dry hands. If your palms have a tendency to sweat when you get nervous, dry them off just before meeting each interviewer. One solution to sweaty palms is to sit, before interviews, with your palms exposed to the air rather than stuffed in a pocket or lying face-down in your lap.

Also, greet the interviewer with an enthusiastic voice and manner. When you begin speaking to an individual, the actual words you speak are much less important than the manner in which you say them. The first thing an interviewer notices is your tone of voice. You will also be judged by your enthusiasm, facial expressions, gestures, and posture. Therefore, try to act as if you are really pleased to have an opportunity to talk with the faculty and residents. Practice this with some critical observers at home. You must not sound forced or pretentious. If you do, you will do yourself more harm than good. Sincere enthusiasm will greatly enhance your entire visit.

During the interview, sit comfortably straight, leaning slightly forward in the chair. This demonstrates your interest through nonverbal cues. You can prove this to yourself. Have a friend (trying to keep a neutral expression in both instances) first face you, sitting forward in a chair. Then have the individual lean back in a relaxed posture. If you were the interviewer, which candidate would interest you more?

Other negative body-language traits include resting your head on your hand, tilting your head to one side (the coy look), and fiddling with your beard, hair, mustache, or earrings. Keep your head upright and your hands away from your head. Likewise, don't fiddle with your clothes, pen, or anything else.

Look your interviewer in the eyes. Applicants who look away when they answer questions suggest either that there is something less than honest about their answers or that they are afraid of the situation. Those who look away when the interviewer is talking (a true kiss of death) indicate that they do not care about what the interviewer is saying. Obviously, neither situation is favorable. Always try to look an interviewer in the eyes. Some experienced interviewers suggest looking at a person first in one eye, then the other. The recipient gets the feeling that the listener is listening intently; the listener avoids a glazed look some people get when they look at a person only in one eye (a common behavior). If you plan to try this, practice ahead of time; the first few times you do this you may be distracted and not hear what the speaker is saying.

Acknowledge what the interviewer is saying by nodding, and with brief verbal phrases such as "I see," "of course," or "yes." Try not to use expressions such as "wow," "awesome," or "cool," which convey something other than professionalism. It helps to vary the expressions you use so that you don't sound wooden or monotonous.

Your exit from the interview must also be graceful and enthusiastic. As speechwriters know, the last thing heard will be remembered best. Shake your interviewer's hand and say again how glad you are to have had a chance to talk with him or her. Offer to provide any other information he or she might desire about you. You will rarely, if ever, be taken up on this offer. State that you look forward to working with him or her. This should take less than 15 seconds and appear very smooth. It would not hurt to practice this one little segment so you don't appear awkward. As you can see from some television interviews, even the best speakers and the most intelligent individuals often look like dolts when terminating an interview. Don't let this be your downfall.

You Are Not Selling a Medical Student—
You Are Selling a Promise

Forget that you are a medical student. In the interview scenario, you are the promise of a bright future. You will be the specialty's finest clinician, a noted researcher, a diligent healer of indigent patients, and a solid member of the medical community. You will achieve this because you are an extremely hard worker who is compulsive, intelligent, responsive to teaching, happy in your work, and no trouble to the faculty.

That is the promise you are selling. To get into your chosen program, you must project the ability to make this promise a reality. How can you make a contribution to this program? You are the salesman. You are the product. Go forth and sell.

Materials for the Interview

Although it may seem rather silly to detail what you need to take with you to interviews, it is surprising how many applicants seem to forget some of the necessary basic materials. In addition to the basics, I suggest that you bring two forms: *Interview Notes* (Figure 18.2) and your *"Must/Want" Analysis* for that program (see Figure 11.1 for a blank copy) as part of your standard interview equipment. These will aid you later when you evaluate each program and write your follow-up letters.

General Materials

The first two items that you need to bring with you are the *directions to the interview site* (even with the address and a GPS, you may need directions within the medical complex) *and the telephone numbers* to contact the program if you get lost or are delayed. Next, carry along a printout of *key information from the program's website* and whatever *additional information you have received from the program*. You should review it immediately prior to setting out for the interview in the morning, as well as consult it during the interview day to refresh your memory or recheck questionable points brought up in conversation. Even if you have this information on your computer or smart phone, it helps to have a backup paper copy in case your "electronic brain" fails.

Of course, you should have a *list of questions* that you want to ask at each program (see Chapter 20), as well as a pad of *paper* and a *pen* to record the answers. Test your pens to make sure that they work. Bring a *photograph* of yourself to give to the residency secretary when you arrive. Also, if you have any additional credentials or paperwork that will be vital for the program to have, such as a written military deferment for training, be certain that you bring these with you.

Finally, bring *something to read*, be it a specialty journal, a news magazine, or a newspaper. You probably don't want to bring a book: No matter what you are reading, someone may have an issue with it. At most programs, you will spend a lot of time waiting. If you have something to occupy your mind, it will make you more alert and less cranky. However, *do not listen to an MP3 player* while waiting: Aren't you interested in what's going on? And don't forget to turn off your cell phone or pager!

Interview Notes

The Interview Notes form (Figure 18.2) is designed to give you an organized method for remembering key information obtained during interviews. Whether in paper or electronic (you can type it into your electronic device) form, this will prove to be extremely useful. For one thing, it provides a place to note specific materials or additional information to send to individual interviewers. You can also write the phonetic spelling of the interviewers' names on this form.

Some students have written that they took the elements from the "Must/Want" Analysis that were key to their decision making and abstracted the information onto a separate form. They then used that form to take notes during the interview day. If this serves your needs, go for it.

Your "Must/Want" Analysis as an Interview Checklist

The "Must/Want" Analysis you previously completed (see Figure 11.1) can now act as an interview checklist (see Figure 18.3 for an example). Its use both simplifies your evaluation of each program and helps you discriminate among them. The factors on your personal "Must/Want" Analysis and the weights you assigned to each one will remain constant for all the programs you visit.

Immediately following your visit to each program, score on a 1 to 10 scale (10 is perfect) how well the program does in each category. Even if you have previously given some items "Scores" based on written materials, those "Scores" should be considered tentative until confirmed during the site visit. Then multiply the "Weights" by the "Scores" for each factor to obtain the factor "Total." Adding the values in the "Total" column will give you your personal ranking for the program ("Program Evaluation Score").

Figure 18.2
Interview Notes

Program _____

Address _____

_____

Secretary _____

Telephone _____

E-mail _____

INTERVIEWER   NOTES

1. _____   _____
   _____   _____
                          _____

2. _____   _____
   _____   _____

3. _____   _____
   _____   _____

4. _____   _____
   _____   _____

5. _____   _____
   _____   _____

6. _____   _____
   _____   _____
                          _____

OTHER NOTES:

_____

_____

_____

_____

Figure 18.3
"Must/Want" Analysis used as an Interview Checklist, Example

Program #2 Mako General Hospital   Date Interviewed January 30

	WEIGHT	x	SCORE	=	TOTAL
Clinical Experience					
On-Call Schedule	5		6		30
Patient Population	2		5		10
Responsibility	14		8		112
Setting	7		8		56
Volume	10		8		80
Geographic Location					
Part of Country	1		2		2
Specific City	1		1		1
Reputation					
Program Age and Stability	2		5		10
Faculty					
Availability	5		4		20
Interest	7		7		49
Stability	3		3		9
Curriculum					
Number of Conferences	1		7		7
Special Training	6		9		54
Types of Conferences	2		5		10
Esprit De Corps	8		7		56
Research Opportunities/Training					
Knowledge	5		3		15
Materials	2		8		16
Time	7		8		56
Facilities					
Clinical Laboratory Support	1		2		2
Library/On-Line Journal Access	2		6		12
Safety/Security	3		5		15
No Restrictive Covenant	MUST		Yes		OK
Health Benefits					
Health Insurance	MUST		Yes		OK
Hospitalization	MUST		Yes		OK
Non-Health Benefits					
Childcare	MUST		Yes		OK

Figure 18.3 (continued)

	WEIGHT	x	SCORE	=	TOTAL
Disability Insurance	MUST		Yes		OK
Educational Leave:					
Funding Available	1		**8**		8
Time Off	2		9		18
Liability Insurance	MUST		Yes		OK
Vacation	1		7		7
Moonlighting	2		**2**		4

TOTAL OF ALL WEIGHTS =   100

PROGRAM EVALUATION SCORE = 659

This "Program Evaluation Score" can later be compared to those calculated after you visit other programs. In some cases, of course, your ratings may suffer from the same problem that interviewers face; early ratings will tend to be lower because they are compared to an ideal, whereas later ratings will tend to be higher since they are being scored in comparison to programs you have already visited. If this is taken into account, you should have no difficulty in correctly interpreting the scores.

The numbers in Figure 18.3 are based on the "Weights" given by our hypothetical applicant from Chapter 11. If you compare Figure 18.3 with Figure 11.8, you will note that some of the "Scores" (in boldface) and "Totals" for this program have been changed based on information obtained during the site visit and interviews. The applicant now has a more complete picture of this program; its "Program Evaluation Score" is now 659.

Behavior At Lunch

Applicants often go to lunch with the program's residents or faculty members. Several rules apply to this experience, as well as to any business lunch—for that's exactly what it is.

- *Stay away from alcohol!* You need to be on your toes, not under the table. Even if you don't lose your wits after imbibing alcohol, your afternoon interviewers may be teetotalers, and thus discount you as a viable candidate if you have been drinking.
- *Be polite.* Say "please" and "thank you" to the servers, and, at the end of the meal, to your host.

- *Do not eat too much.* The postprandial tide is a very effective soporific. Go easy on the carbohydrates. You don't want to sleep through the afternoon's activities, do you?
- *Use good table manners.* If you have never learned them before, now would be an excellent opportunity. You will need to know how to eat in a reasonably civilized manner throughout your medical career. Start this behavior at the interview lunch. Common errors that cost people jobs include: holding your fork like a knife, talking with your mouth full, not putting the napkin in your lap, not breaking bread before you eat it, and pushing food onto the fork with your thumb. Even in the hospital cafeteria, some table manners are necessary. If you need help, ask a civilized friend.

Pitfalls abound during meals. For example, a tale is told of Admiral Rickover, the father of the U.S. nuclear submarine service, who personally interviewed every officer applying to be a sub captain. If a person salted his food without tasting it, he was eliminated as too rash a decision-maker. Be wary.

If you go to a restaurant, don't order the most expensive items. Order food that is easy to eat: avoid any food that you cannot control. If you aren't skilled at twirling "strand" pasta, don't order it—it will be too messy. Shellfish that requires squeezing and digging, ribs, corn on the cob, and fried chicken are all difficult to eat with aplomb. Also, avoid foods that can cause accidents and embarrassment. Soups, creamy dressings, desserts, and greasy hand-held foods, such as tacos, can easily end up on your brand-new clothes. Onions and garlic can make even the most stalwart interviewer want to avoid you.

Never eat all the bread in the basket, and if it is in front of you, pass it around before you take any; same with the butter. Once you get it, tear your roll gently; don't saw it with a knife. And don't butter all your bread at once. You also don't want to blow on the soup; you may splatter it on others. Cut and take only one bite of food at a time—and always use your knife (not the fork) to cut your food. In a fancy restaurant with lots of cutlery, use the outer silverware first, reserving those above your plate for dessert. Also, if there are bread plates and extra glasses on the table, remember that your solid foods (e.g., rolls) are on your left and liquids (e.g., water) are on your right.

Sit up straight in the chair without hovering over your plate or leaning backward on the chair's back legs. Keep your elbows off the table and, as your mother said, never talk with food in your mouth. If you are asked a question just as you are about to put something in your mouth, go ahead and eat it, and think about your answer while you chew. To acknowledge the question, look at the person and nod. If you feel a bit of food between your teeth, swish silently and unobtrusively. If you notice someone else with food in his or her teeth, mention it unobtrusively. Don't do as one interviewee did at a Chinese restaurant: She popped an entire fortune cookie into her mouth, then removed the paper fortune and read it to her dining companions!

Don't share another person's appetizer or dessert unless invited to do so— and then, ask the waiter to split it for you. As for the napkin, rest it in your lap; never use it as a bib. When you finish your meal, don't place your napkin in the center of a dirty plate—put it on the table next to the plate.

During the conversation, generally avoid discussing religion, politics, and sexual preferences. The best advice is to use lunch to ward off true hypoglycemia. Consider that meal as simply another part of your interview. Do your real eating after you have left the program for the day and can relax.

19

The Perfect Applicant

How do you make silk purses out of a sow's ear?
Start with silk sows.

Samuel P. Martin III, M.D.

Perfection is in the eye of the beholder.

Proverb

BY NOW, AS YOU PREPARE to go for your first interviews, you are probably wondering just what residency directors are looking for in an applicant. There is no precise answer, but here are some program directors' thoughts on the subject.

The fundamental rule is that there is no perfect applicant. Although program directors constantly search for the beast known as the "perfect applicant," they know that this hunt is very similar to the quest for the Holy Grail, a fruitless endeavor. And yet, just as with the Holy Grail, the search continues.

As an applicant, you are probably paranoid enough to want to compare yourself against the perceived ideal of residency selection committees and program directors. While the ideal candidate varies from specialty to specialty and from program to program, there are some basics that seem to hold true for all.

A residency director in a competitive specialty once told me that his perfect applicant would be "a minority woman who graduated from Harvard Medical School at the top of her class, got honors in all her required third-year clinical rotations, had been elected to AOA, had a Ph.D. with a record of significant research and funding, scored in the 99th percentile on USMLE Steps 1 and 2, acquired superior reference letters from top colleagues in our specialty with whom she had worked closely and who said they wanted her in their program, had a dynamite personality, knew a lot about and loved the specialty, and had the energy of a 13-year-old."

"Why," I asked, "are you looking for these criteria?"

He explained that women and minorities have been generally under-represented in medicine and, if possible, he wanted to help correct this. Election to AOA, top class ranking at a good medical school, and high U.S. Medical Licensing Exam (USMLE) scores were the only standard criteria across all medical schools he could use to measure candidates. "Of course the USMLE

Step 1 has little to do with clinical medicine, but what else is there?" he asked, rather frustrated.

The answer is that excellent performance in third-year clinical clerkships is another, although less accurate, measure of performance. Since medical schools vary so much in their grading schemes (many do not have grading systems discriminating enough to obtain class ranks), it is often very difficult to know what a particular grade means. The courses also vary in their levels of difficulty and intensity. The closest thing to uniformity among medical schools comes in the third-year required clinical clerkships. Excellent grades in these courses usually suggest at least a modicum of clinical knowledge and ability.

Letters from colleagues in the field, especially those who have worked with the applicant, who want the applicant in their own program and who are available to honestly answer questions over the telephone are often the most significant part of an application package. Unlike the typical Dean's letter (officially known as the MSPE, or Medical Student Performance Evaluation), where every student appears to "walk on water," this is the closest thing to an honest appraisal one can get.

"But why include the other criteria?" I asked.

"No matter how good an applicant is," he continued, "he or she has to fit in with our program's residents and faculty. This is where our opportunity to talk with and interview the applicant comes in. And, because our program is so intensive, we need people with a great deal of energy and enthusiasm. The Ph.D. and research are there to be certain that I never get an applicant who meets all the criteria. If I did, I would probably be disappointed."

I asked him if he had ever met anyone, applicant or not, who met these criteria. Smiling, he replied that of course he hadn't, but he could still look for her.

What this residency director is seeking in applicants is little different from what the vast majority of program directors seek when deciding whom to interview. One survey showed that the most common traits that program directors look for include: grades in required and elective rotations in the specialty, grades in other clerkships, class rank, USMLE Step 2 scores, and AOA membership (Figure 19.1).

Figure 19.1: Relative Importance of Academic Criteria When Selecting Residents in Various Specialties

	Ortho	Gen Surg	OB/ GYN	Ophthal	Peds	Fam Med	Int Med	Emerg Med	Psych	PM & R	Path	Rad-Onc	DX Rad	Anesth
Grades, req. clerkships	3	11	1	3	1	41	1	3	1	4	8	5	1	2
Reference Letters	6	3	6	1	2	6	7	2	4	3	1	1	7	5
USMLE Step 1 score	2	2	3	2	9	7	9	8	8	5	3	3	3	1
Sr. specialty elective grade	5	8	7	6	3	5	8	1	5	1	2	6	8	4
Number of clerkship honors	4	4	5	3	3	8	2	5	7	8	10	8	2	6
Audition electives	1	12	9	12	6	3	9	4	3	7	5	4	15	9
USMLE Step 2CK	12	7	4	10	5	2	3	6	6	2	4	11	5	3
Class rank	8	9	10	73	8	12	5	7	11	9	7	9	4	8
USMLE Step 2CS -Pass	12	5	2	15	7	1	4	9	2	6	5	15	10	7
AOA honorary membership	7	5	12	5	10	15	6	12	15	15	13	12	6	10
Med. school's reputation	15	11	8	11	13	10	119	10	9	10	9	7	9	13
Med. sch. academic awards	9	14	13	8	14	14	13	145	13	14	10	10	11	12
Published research	11	13	16	9	16	16	16	151	11	164	14	1	13	16
Grades, preclin. courses	10	10	14	14	15	13	15	16	16	11	10	12	12	11
Other Sr. elective grades	14	16	14	12	12	9	14	11	13	11	15	12	12	14
MSPE (Dean's Letter)	16	15	11	16	10	11	11	13	10	13	16	14	16	

Adapted from: Green M, Jones P, Thomas JX Jr.: Selection criteria for residency: results of a national program directors survey. *Acad Med.* 2009;84(3):362-7.

While program directors in individual specialties differ slightly in which criteria they value the most, Figure 19.2 provides a summary of how the criteria are valued. Note that although students are very concerned about what appears in their MSPE, unless it contains negative information, program directors find it the least valuable of all selection criteria.

Most program directors have a good idea of what they are looking for in a resident. If they really know what they're doing, they have written criteria (an ACGME requirement) that are known to the other department faculty, and all interviewers should have a copy. As an applicant, you should be able to determine what programs are seeking based on what they highlight in their written materials, how their program is structured, and the institution(s) in which they reside. Make a list of the top three or four criteria you believe each program is seeking and stress, in the interviews, your qualities that match these criteria.

What residency directors *really* want are residents who will perform well clinically in their program without causing the faculty too much agitation or grief. Basically, they want an individual they can "plug and play": one who will fit easily into the program, will require minimal coaching to do extremely well, and already has proven clinical skills and judgment.

Figure 19.2
Relative Importance of Information Sources to
Program Directors in Most Specialties

1. Required clerkship grades

2. USMLE Step 1 score

3. Grades, specialty's senior elective

4. Number of honor grades

5. USMLE Step 2CK scores

6. USMLE Step 2CS-Pass

7. Class rank

8. AOA honorary membership

9. Medical school reputation

10. Academic awards in medical school

11. Grades, other senior electives

12. Grades, preclinical courses

13. Published medical school research

14. Research experience in medical school

* In addition to the specialties listed in Figure 19.1, information from program directors in Urology, Dermatology, Neurology, Plastic Surgery, Otolaryngology, and Neurosurgery is also included in this data.

Modified from: Green M, Jones P, Thomas JX Jr.: Selection criteria for residency: results of a national program directors survey. *Acad Med.* 2009;84(3):362-7.

No matter what criteria are used, the system is imperfect. The best that can be said about election to AOA, high USMLE scores, clinical honors in medical school courses, high class rankings, and positive faculty interviews is that individuals who meet these criteria usually do not perform dismally in training programs. Their performance is, in fact, usually above average. Similarly, those who performed near the bottom of their class in medical school continue to do badly in residency. Individuals who seem to fare the worst during residency are those who took leaves of absence or had academic difficulty during medical school and those with below-average performance in their required clinical clerkships.

Residency directors have different levels of concerns about applicants, depending upon what they see and hear. Figure 19.3 shows the results of a study about how they feel about common things seen in residency candidates' histories. These attitudes are pervasive among employers that hire individuals with a graduate degree. (Although the study is somewhat dated, the results still hold true.)

Figure 19.3
Items in an Applicant's History That Worry Residency Directors

Very Concerned

- Received disciplinary action in medical school
- Treated for alcoholism
- Received failure in a required clerkship
- Took extended time to graduate for academic reasons
- Has learning disability
- Failed USMLE Step 1 prior to passing
- Passed USMLE with minimal scores

Worrisome

- Graduated in lower third of class
- Received a grade of "Fail" in a preclinical course
- Had mediocre preclinical grades but strong clinical evaluations

Concerned

- Has family responsibilities
- Did not participate in extracurricular activities in medical school

Adapted from: Wagoner NE, Suriano JR: Program directors' response to a survey on variables used to select residents in a time of change. *Acad Med*. 1999;74(1):51-8.

Applicants and residency directors seem to place different values on applicant qualities. Some studies have shown that directors most admire personal characteristics, while students believe that their knowledge and skills are more important attributes in getting a residency position.

Regardless of studies or personal opinions, however, program directors will give up neither their search for the ideal resident nor their use of measurement criteria for applicants. Their job is still to weed through the morass of applications to cull out a group of potential residents. And since precious little else is available to help them make this decision, these are the criteria they will use and by which you will be measured.

20

The Interview

A job interview is like being on trial for your life.

Russian Proverb

He who asks is a fool for a minute;
he who doesn't is a fool forever.

Chinese Proverb

BEFORE BEGINNING THE INTERVIEW, keep in mind some research-based information about the process. First, interviewers develop a stereotype of a good applicant and then try to match the candidates to it. By reading the program information carefully, you may get a hint of what they think the "perfect" applicant is. Also, see Chapter 19, The Perfect Applicant.

Most residency faculty members are unskilled at employment interviews and make many errors when evaluating applicants. A typical error is the "halo effect," when they are overly influenced by a single favorable or unfavorable trait. Unfortunately, unfavorable information carries more weight than favorable information, so the halo effect is more likely to work against you than for you.

Related to this, when several outstanding candidates have been interviewed in succession, the average candidate who follows them will look worse than he or she actually is because of the comparison. The reverse is also true: an average candidate will look better when following several poor ones. You can't control, these factors, but they are worth remembering as you head into the lion's den.

Know Your Questions

It is important to know not only the questions you want to ask, but also what you are searching for in the replies. You should be looking for specific answers, e.g., the percentage of residency graduates that have passed the specialty's board examination on the first try, as well as observing the interviewers' attitudes toward the subjects you raise. Also notice their attitudes toward you as a person and toward residents in general. Are they friendly and open? Or haughty and cold? This could make a big difference in how you rank the program.

Know when to ask your questions. You will rarely run out of questions before you run out of opportunities to ask them. Most programs try to allow applicants the opportunity to have their questions answered fully. They gain as much, or more, information about you from your questions as they do from your answers to their questions. But wait for the proper time. Let the interviewers ask their questions first. Wait for them to ask if you have any questions of your own (Figure 20.1).

When you ask your own questions, do so in a courteous, diplomatic manner. More than one applicant has "gone down the tubes" by trying to cross-examine interviewers. Doing so is crass and demonstrates immaturity. Ask your questions in a way that expresses enthusiasm for a positive answer. Rather than the question "What problems have you had with accreditation?", you might inquire, "There haven't been any accreditation problems, have there?" The first is accusatory, the second merely inquisitive. Get your information. But be nice about it.

Ask simple, straightforward, open-ended (requiring more than a "yes" or "no" answer) questions. Do not ask questions with multiple parts or that are too long to follow easily. If you ask these types of questions, you will not get the information you want, but you will make a negative impression on the interviewer.

Finally, ask the right people the right questions. At the start of your interview day, ask the residency secretary which individuals you will meet with and what their positions are within the program. Ask the residency or department director about changes in the program or the current status of prior residents. Do not ask them about the call schedule or resident *esprit de corps*. These are questions to ask residents.

Figure 20.1
Typical Interview from the Interviewer's Viewpoint

Print a list of your questions in advance so that you can easily refer to it (and read it) during your interviews. (It's better during interviews to use a printed list rather than fiddling with an electronic device.) What questions should you ask, and what should you look for in the answers? The list below is divided into questions you should ask the faculty and those that you will want to ask residents. Some you may want to ask of both groups, especially Question 23, "Could you give me (show me) an example?"

The List—To Ask Faculty

1. What is the program's educational philosophy?
Before you begin your interviews, review your notes about the program. Reread the statements from their website and written material about their educational goals and objectives. Some programs emphasize preparation for an academic career; most try to produce strong clinicians who will work in the community. Ask the residency director to clarify any vague points so that you can determine if their goals are consistent with yours.

This leads naturally to your next question: *What do you look for in a candidate to meet those goals?* You then have a golden opportunity to briefly list your qualities that match their needs.

2. How have your graduates done on the specialty's board exam?
Although the primary goal of residency training is to prepare you to practice in your chosen field, an important milepost during your career will be passing the specialty's board examination. In many cases, passing "the Boards" determines the type and level of position you can fill. How have this program's residents done when they took their specialty board exams? If they have all passed, was this on the first try? This can be asked tactfully, as in "Did any of them have to take their Boards more than once?" Did they fare as well on the oral exams (you should already know if they have these in your chosen specialty) as they did on the written exams?

Residency directors should know this type of information. Although information on specific graduates is confidential, the cumulative data should be available to all residency applicants. If it isn't, then there may be a problem.

You also want to know how residents have done on the specialty's in-training examinations. These national tests, given annually at nearly all residency programs in most specialties, mirror subsequent performance on specialty board exams. In addition, does the program have any conferences or special programs to help their residents prepare for the specialty's boards?

The information you glean from these questions indicates, in part, the amount of didactic teaching, reading time, and interaction with the faculty that you will receive at this program. As might be expected, graduates of high-volume, high-workload programs often have worse records on board examinations than do those from lower volume programs. However, this is not always true, so it is important to get the specifics from each program you visit.

3. Is there much faculty turnover?

Tread gently in this area—it may be very sensitive. But do tread. You need to know about faculty stability. It gives a strong indication about the staff's and, by extension, the entire program's esprit de corps. If there is a large or rapid turnover in faculty positions, it may indicate that all is not well, even if there is a pretty façade.

There are several ways to get this information. The easiest is to simply ask how many of their faculty members will still be there in July. Otherwise, you can ask if any faculty members have recently been added—"As replacements?" you ask not so naively—or if any of the current staff will be leaving in the near future. This last is the least favorable way to ask the question. If you hear (usually from the residents), however, that either the residency director or the department director is planning to leave, ask multiple interviewers about it for confirmation. These are two changes that can markedly affect the program's tenor.

You might feel that faculty turnover is their business, not yours. Wrong! Would you make reservations at an expensive French restaurant for your birthday celebration if you thought that the chef/owner was going on vacation—and being replaced by the short-order cook from the greasy spoon next door? Don't go hungry. Ask before you commit to a reservation.

4. How would you characterize faculty–resident relationships?

The answer to this question might provide an interesting insight into how the program really functions. Listen for overly positive answers, as well as those that are negative or express indifference about the relationship or about their residents. If you ask several faculty members this question, you may discern a pattern. Most important, you want to compare the answers from the faculty with those from the residents on the same topic (see Questions 25 and 27).

5. Do residents have non-clinical responsibilities?

Of course you will be doing clinical work, and you need to talk to the residents about this. But what other requirements are there? If you arrive at a program expecting nothing but clinical work and there are additional requirements, you may be upset. Find out about all your obligations ahead of time.

There are usually four categories of extra activities:

1. *Research.* The program (or the national bodies controlling training in that specialty) may require the development and implementation of your own research project or your participation in ongoing research.
2. *Projects.* The faculty may strongly encourage residents to participate in departmental projects such as medical student education or in specialty society activities.
3. *Writing.* Written case reports, abstracts, and book reviews may be mandatory.
4. *Administration.* Either the specialty's Board or a program may require spending time as chief resident. This usually includes a number of administrative duties, such as serving on departmental or institutional committees and arranging residents' schedules for work, conferences, and vacation.

These extra activities may demand a considerable amount of your time during residency training. They may also contribute greatly to your education. But to make a rational decision about which program to choose, you need to know what extra activities each program requires.

6. Is this program particularly strong or well-known in any special areas?

If you have learned of any special training the residency offers, you may want to ask for more details. You also want to know about additional special courses, some of which may be too new to list in their promotional materials or which have not yet started. These will be extra perquisites of attending this program, and the interviewers will generally be thrilled that you asked. This allows them to show off their program to its best advantage.

When evaluating the interviewers' answers, remember that programs in which you do not plan to participate are of no benefit to you. An example would be an international elective that you cannot schedule because you must care for your three young children. Even so, the nature of these programs may demonstrate the program's educational direction.

7. How is the training divided?

This question is useful primarily for individuals who are applying to a combined residency program, such as Emergency Medicine–Pediatrics, Pediatrics–Psychiatry–Child Psychiatry, or Internal Medicine–Pediatrics. Each combined program operates a bit differently, so you will need to inquire about the details for each. Specifically, you want to find out how long you will work as a *de facto* intern in each specialty and when you will begin to assume significant patient care responsibility. Ask the faculty and the residents from all parts of the program.

You also want to know if your predecessors have been made to feel they were a part of the programs both academically and socially. Were they seen as "outsiders" in one or all of the programs, or have they been welcomed and easily integrated into all of them?

8.   What types of clinical sites are used?

Residency programs generally use a variety of clinical settings, including private, public, and Veterans Administration/military hospitals; private-practice preceptors; and distant rotations for specialized training. Which settings does this program offer—or require? Is there a wide variety of both out- and in-patient facilities appropriate for your optimal education in this specialty? Or have the sites been chosen for other reasons, such as because they provide funding for some resident training? Do the types of clinical facilities mimic the medical practice you envision yourself having?

Logistical questions associated with this topic include: Are there rotations at facilities that are out of town? If so, are housing and transportation supplied? If the primary residency is in an urban area with good mass transit, you still may want to ask whether you will need a car for some rotations.

Since residents spend virtually all their time in clinical settings, this information is very important. Be aware that many older, poorer, and badly funded residency-associated hospitals and clinics don't have enough staff (you do the "scut" work), up-to-date working equipment (you make do using available materials), or the necessary variety of clinicians on-site (you must refer interesting patients to other facilities) to provide you with the quality experience you need.

Depending upon the specialty to which you're applying, it may be vital or, at least, important to know whether the program will train you in the latest diagnostic and therapeutic equipment. Do they have simulators to train in, for example, laparoscopic procedures? Do they routinely use state-of-the-art monitoring and diagnostic equipment when treating patients? Are animal and cadaver labs available to learn other procedures? If, however, you are interested in remote medical practice, you should also work at clinical sites with only "bare-bone" diagnostic and therapeutic interventions.

9.   What patient population will I encounter?

The patients you see during residency determine, in large part, the types of learning experiences you have. Ask about the mix of adults and children, the ratio of men to women (this is especially important in Veterans' Hospital-based programs), and the percentages of acute (including trauma) and chronic problems. Less obvious factors are the patients' social mix, including private versus public patients (often with differing expectations and stress levels); the different cultures of and languages spoken by patients; and the racial mix (this may suggest emphasis on certain diseases).

10. Is training offered in medical Spanish or in other languages?

Spanish is becoming the second language in medicine throughout the United States. Learning the basics is a skill that will help you throughout your career.

Some programs help their residents to learn at least basic medical Spanish so that they can communicate with their patients. In some areas of the country, you may need to know another language to communicate with patients. Does the program offer opportunities to learn these languages? More important, do they pay for the instruction? Are language lessons a standard part of the residency curriculum or an elective? And, if such classes are offered, does the department make it easy for residents to attend on a regular basis?

A similar skill that is being taught at some residency programs is how to do histories and physical exams using an interpreter. This is an invaluable skill, and you will undoubtedly need this in most residencies and throughout your medical career. Asking about this is especially important at programs with a multilingual patient population.

11. Are there elective opportunities?

Each of us has a unique view of what our professional life will be like. Some may envision a life in private or group practice, while others believe their career will involve research, teaching, or foreign travel. Since most residency programs are structured to fit the generic physician entering the specialty, you may need specific educational opportunities to learn something about particular specialty areas—either to gain expertise or to find out if that is the direction you want to follow. Does this program allow sufficient time and flexibility to sample these different environments?

The easiest way to determine this is to ask both how much elective time is built into the program and how it has been used. The answers describe the program's standard pattern.

Next, you want to know the program's official policy concerning electives, so it is best to ask the program director. Find out the specific scope of elective experiences that are permitted. Are there geographical restrictions on where you can go? Can you sample only certain clinical or non-clinical areas? Is there any funding for electives? Also ask about faculty contacts that will make it easier to arrange such electives, especially off-site.

Note that even if you are currently not interested in areas outside the specialty's mainstream practice, you may develop an interest during your residency. If so, having the option to explore different tracks will allow you to expand your knowledge and skills.

12. Are there research opportunities?

Some applicants may envision careers in academia or research. If you are one of them, you will certainly want to enter a residency that can provide you with the resources and guidance to do research.

Start with the question "What research projects are the department's faculty and residents working on now?" That will give you their range of interests and the level of activity. Then, if one of the projects interests you, focus on that. Could you get involved? Would you have a mentor? Is that person funded for his or her research? Is that individual amenable to working with residents? How fairly have residents been treated when working with faculty members on research projects in the past? (Have the residents done the work but been given secondary credit?)

Also find out about available research facilities, funding, time, and support staff such as statisticians. Does the department or institution provide these? Is research required, tolerated, or actively encouraged? In addition, if you do research and it is accepted for presentation at a national meeting, will the department pay your way there? Will they give you the necessary time off? Ask now to avoid disappointment later.

Finally, you will want to attend one or more of your specialty's national meetings while you are in residency. National meetings are excellent places to make job contacts, meet residents from other programs, and gain additional insight into the specialty, so going to them can be very important. Does the program allow residents time off to attend them? Do they provide any funding for these trips? If so, is the funding available only if you are presenting a paper or an abstract at the meeting, or is it available to all residents?

13. Are administrative, bioethics, and legal training available?

Although academicians have been slow to recognize it, medicine is also a business—sometimes a dangerous business. How much training in the administrative and legal aspects of medical practice will you get at this program? Will you have hands-on training dealing with insurance, billing, contracts, hiring, and similar problems? Or are you expected to learn it all at the "school of hard knocks" after you begin your own practice?

Will you receive in-depth training about the legal pitfalls now so common in medicine, or will this come only after your first malpractice suit? How about the ethical issues involved in your specialty? Does the program offer a formal bioethics course? As medicine advances, practitioners must more frequently ask, "Just because I can do it, should I?" Bioethics helps you deal with this and other difficult clinical and research dilemmas.

Although the requirements for residency training now include the areas of law, ethics, and socioeconomics related to medicine, most training programs do not offer instruction in these areas. If you find one that does, it indicates that they have a dynamic and forward-looking residency director.

14. Is there a mentor/adviser system? How does it work?

You expect to do well in your residency program. Problems can develop, however. Your first hurdle may be simply learning the rules and the culture of a new institution. Having an experienced person to guide you through this maze can work wonders. This may be a senior resident "buddy" or a faculty member, or both, that has been paired with a new trainee. Is there a formal system of assigning "mentors" for new residents? If so, how are these assigned: randomly, by mutual interests, by sex, or by race? If a mentor/adviser system exists, it suggests that the program is at least trying to ease your transition from medical student to resident. Later you may want to ask residents how well this mentoring system works.

Another recent innovation at some residencies is personal financial counseling. It's an excellent idea, since many residents carry an enormous debt burden and the repayment rules keep changing. Does this residency have such a program?

15. What types of resident evaluations are used? How often?

Interns struggle through their first year in one of two modes (sometimes alternating between them): they believe they are doing a dynamite job or, more frequently, they believe they are learning little and their performance is marginal. Neither extreme is usually the case. But in the strange world of neophyte medicine, it is hard to know where you stand without some feedback.

How often does the program supply this feedback? What mechanisms are used? In the past, many residents went through one or more years of training blissfully unaware that the faculty thought their performance was less than adequate, only to be suddenly dropped from the program. (This used to be common in Surgical training programs.) Residency programs must now demonstrate to reviewers their mechanisms for evaluation.

Many Internal Medicine programs use not only periodic formal evaluations, but also "Early Warning Notes" and "Praise Cards," developed by the American Board of Internal Medicine, to deliver feedback between formal evaluations. Unfortunately, most faculty members are not comfortable giving individual residents constructive feedback while they are working with them, so formal evaluations become very important in gauging how well you are doing.

Another evaluation method is the in-service examination given by many Boards. These measure "book knowledge," and are used to compare residents at the same level of training across the United States. Ask if such exams are available at the program. Will you be allowed time off to take the exams (including the night before so you won't fall asleep during the test)? How are the results used—to help the resident assess his or her strengths and weaknesses, or to eliminate "weak" residents? Does the program offer standardized evaluation examinations or other methods of self-assessment in addition to the national in-service tests? It is nice to know how you are doing compared not only to your peers locally, but also to all other residents with whom you will take your specialty board examination when you finish the program. These tests are one way of finding out.

By the way, you will only understand how much you have learned during internship when you work with the new interns at the start of your PGY-2 year. You will be amazed how little they know and how far you have come.

16. How has health care reform affected this program and institution?

This is far from an idle question: Changes during the last two decades have led to the most devastating and grievous insults to medical education in more than a century. Medicare rules and punitive actions (fining medical schools and residency faculties millions of dollars) have forced most teaching hospitals to seriously restrict many residents' clinical independence. And new changes in Medicare payments and marked decreases in Medicaid payments for medical education have changed many institutions' ability to fund residency positions.

In addition, the encroachment of managed care organizations has siphoned off many patients from hospitals' teaching services and clinics. Even when the patient census has remained stable, declining reimbursement has often decreased the number of ancillary staff, available services, and any amenities residents once had. What actions have this residency program and teaching institution taken to assure that trainees continue to get a quality clinical education? Are they financially stable? Have these changes adversely affected residents' and faculty's esprit de corps?

17. Do you anticipate changes in the program's curriculum?

This is another of those questions that you should ask the residency director. It is a safe inquiry and can be asked directly.

Are changes in the curriculum expected in the near future? Why? "Near future" is defined as your time in the program. Residency programs may anticipate changes based upon modifications of board requirements, alterations in the patient base, or new directions being taken by the specialty as a whole or the faculty in particular. These changes may make a difference in your evaluation of the program—either favorably or unfavorably.

In some cases, interviewers may be able to give only general ideas about anticipated changes. Usually the faculty is not dissembling, but rather demonstrating both their hopes for the program and the complexity involved in altering many training curricula. In any case, know that no matter what you are told, some changes most likely will take place during your training. No program's curriculum is chiseled in stone.

You can elicit this information from the faculty and residents by asking "What has changed since you came to this program?" This is an easy and non-threatening way to get a sense of the frequency and types of curriculum changes at the program.

18. What is the program's accreditation status?

This is another sensitive question. Does that specialty's Residency Review Committee accredit the program? (Actually, it is the Accreditation Council for Graduate Medical Education that accredits the programs, but let's not quibble.) This indicates that the program is certified to prepare residents for the specialty's board examination. There are four possible answers to this question.

The first answer is "No, the program is not accredited." If you go through such a program, which is not in the NRMP Match since it is not accredited, *you will not be eligible to take the specialty's board exam.* A negative answer to this question should, in virtually all cases, eliminate this program from your consideration.

The other possibilities all come under the "Yes" category. The simplest is "Yes, full accreditation." This means that the program has been accredited without restrictions for a number of years. This is as good as it gets.

Two other possibilities are "Yes, provisionally" and "Yes, on probation." The former indicates that the program either has not been in existence long enough to get a full accreditation or has had enough recent changes to warrant being considered a "new" program. The problems here, common to all new programs, revolve around the question of stability.

The response, "Yes, on probation," indicates that the program is having major problems and is in danger of losing its accreditation. If that happens, any resident in the program may be left in the lurch, struggling to find another program to enter in mid-training. That is neither a pleasant possibility nor an easy thing to do.

Although you can indirectly look for information about accreditation in *FREIDA* (since only accredited programs will be listed) and some programs may mention their accreditation status in the material available to applicants, it is worthwhile confirming this at the interview; things do change.

You should ask the residency director. The most diplomatic way to do this might be "You *do* have full accreditation?" This allows a complete answer. If the program does have full accreditation, there will be a simple answer. If not, the residency director will have an answer already prepared for you. Sit back and take it all in. It may "get a little deep" at this point and you may have to lift your feet off the floor part of the time.

19. Is this a pyramidal program?

Most often found in Surgery and Surgical specialties, a pyramidal training program is structured so that only a percentage, usually about 50%, of those starting in the PGY-1 year will be allowed to finish the entire program. This is usually because the program needs "bodies" to accomplish much of the clinical work, but only has enough significant procedures, such as major operations, to accommodate a few chief residents. If you plan to go into such a program, e.g., "Categorical" General Surgery, be prepared for intense competition with your peers. However, if you are applying only for a one- or two-year "Preliminary" position prior to entering a subspecialty such as Orthopedic Surgery, it might work in your favor. If you are accepted into the program, it will mean that fewer of the Categorical residents will have to be dropped from the pyramid. Make certain that you ask this question—the information, although very important to you, often will not be offered spontaneously.

ACGME's rules now prohibit pyramidal programs. Many residents, however, report that *de facto* pyramidal programs still exist.

20. Have any housestaff left the program before graduating? Why?

Residents leave training programs for many reasons. Most residencies have had residents leave, usually because of illness, family circumstances, or simply changing their minds about which specialty to enter. This information is not what you are after. You want to know whether any residents have left because they were unhappy with the program, the faculty, or the training they were receiving.

A way to ferret out these individuals may be to ask, "Have any of the residents who have left this program gone into another program in the same specialty?" These are usually the folks who were dissatisfied with the program. Simply ask why they left. Although you may not get specifics, the tenor of the answer may be enough to let you know if there is a potential problem for you.

21. Where are your graduates?

This question actually has three parts. The first asks, "Where are your graduates geographically?" Are they practicing in the vicinity of the program or spread throughout the United States? Are they primarily concentrated in major cities or in rural communities? This gives you a realistic perspective about the program's orientation. Training programs reflect the needs of the populations they serve. The places where residency graduates feel comfortable working reflect the training that they have received.

The second part of the question asks, "What types of jobs do your graduates have?" Are they working primarily in academic centers, in private communities, in group practices, in research, in administration, or in other specific areas? Or are they in many diverse areas of practice? Again, this is highly reflective of the scope and quality of the training the residents in a program receive.

The third part asks, "What percent of the program's graduates enter fellowships?" The answer to this is relatively straightforward. It leads, however, to an opportunity to ask about the faculty's interest in having residents who plan to do subspecialty training and how much help they might provide you in obtaining a fellowship. It also demonstrates that you have an interest in fellowship training. That may be good, unless you are speaking with a General Internist or Pediatrician, who may not be as enamored with applicants who desire to do something other than primary care.

Ask this question in a general manner. If one of the parts is not answered, follow up with a more specific question designed to get the missing information. You might ask to see the map on which residencies often post the location of their graduates. If you locate a graduate of that residency in your home area, you can gain valuable insight into the program by talking with this individual.

22. Do you help your graduates find jobs?

This may be a new question to many residency faculty. In the past, there was little problem finding work after residency training. Today, with a "doctor glut" in some specialties outside primary care, there are fewer choice jobs to go around. So you might need some help to find them, especially if you are interested in entering a difficult market, such as southern California. Ask if the program will help you.

If they say you are on your own, it indicates that they (1) have little regard for your future welfare and (2) have little understanding of what their job as teachers really entails. In either case, you are now forewarned.

If they do offer help to residents in finding employment after training, what have they done for recent graduates and current residents? Are there individual counseling sessions? Are faculty contacts used to get positions? Will the faculty review job offers and contracts with the residents?

These are but a few of the possible ways in which the program can assist residents in getting their first jobs. You are having a hard enough time getting into a residency. Ask this question now to avoid as many problems as you can when you finish your training.

23. Could you give me (show me) an example?

This is one of the most important questions you can ask during interviews. Ask it to supplement questions you ask of faculty and residents.

In the process of trying to ascertain whether you would fit into a program, you need to have some firm information, not unsubstantiated statements. "Our resident on-call schedule is very benign," says the chief resident. "Could you show me the current month's schedule?" you ask. After you see the schedule, you will know if it really is as easy as they claim it is. If it is just the resident's interpretation of what "benign" means, you will know that too.

Many answers to questions lend themselves to confirmation or explanation. This is a safe, pleasant, and enlightening way to get further information about important points. You can never ask this question too often.

The List—To Ask Residents

24. Would you choose this program again? Why or why not?

This is the key question to ask residents. It will most likely produce the answers that will best help you to determine your fit with the program. As always, ask this question in a non-confrontational, low-key manner. No doubt this is not the first time the resident has been asked—or contemplated—this question. There is usually a great variation in the answers among the residents. You are looking for general consensus (good or bad), rather than the opinions of "outliers" who love or detest the program for unique reasons.

Faculty members at weak or dysfunctional programs hope that you will not ask this question of their residents. Beware! Some may actually limit your access to residents so that you don't get this feedback.

Two natural follow-up questions are: Which parts of the program do you like the most? Which do you like the least? And, while free time may not be a large part of your residency existence, you do want to know whether the residents (and their significant others) like the city and the area. Listen closely. You may have to "sell" the city to your family before they consider moving there.

25. What contact will I have with the clinical faculty?

Okay, the program's website lists 42 faculty members. Did they mention how often you will have contact with all of them? With *any* of them? The faculty only helps you if you have direct contact with them. If faculty members hide in their offices or labs rather than attend in the clinics, wards, emergency department, or operating rooms, they might as well not be there.

So the questions that you should ask the residents are: "How often are the faculty members present?" and "How often do you want faculty input but find that it is not available?" You might also want to ask "Are they available on nights and weekends?" Certainly, as a resident, you want to be able to exercise some independent thought and judgment. But you need adequate guidance from knowledgeable faculty during residency training. Does this program really offer it?

Also, do the faculty and residents interact informally, such as at holiday parties or on basketball or volley ball teams? This often provides a way to make closer contact with faculty members who may then wish to help you develop your career.

26. What has changed since you came to the program?

How quickly and significantly does this program's curriculum change? By asking senior residents what has changed since they arrived, you can easily find out this information in a non-threatening way. This is a question to also ask the faculty.

Their answers will provide a picture of the frequency and types of curriculum changes at the program. For example, have there been changes (major or minor) in the program's curriculum, rotations, or electives? How about the program's overall structure? Have there been major faculty changes? Most important, have there been changes in the patient mix or resident responsibilities? Do they think that these changes have been good for the program and for their education?

27. Do residents regularly have an opportunity to formally evaluate faculty and the program? What changes have been made recently as a result of this feedback?

This question really asks, "How important is the educational mission?" Feedback on the faculty's performance is an essential part of all education.

If the residency is serious about education, it will have a good evaluation system. Virtually all residencies, however, will say that they have an evaluation system, since the residency review boards generally require it. What is really telling is if they can recite substantive changes that have been made based on these evaluations. That means that they not only have the system, but also value their residents' opinions.

When asking this question, you may also get information on the institution's or residency's grievance policy, such as that used for harassment. Listen closely. Is the resident telling you about problems they have had, or how they have used the system to avoid problems?

28. How much didactic time is there? Does it have priority?
If you don't already have this information from the program's website or other sources, find out how much time is spent in lectures, seminars, journal clubs, and other didactic activities. If a current monthly schedule is available, ask for a copy to peruse at your leisure.

The more important question that you need to ask of one or more residents (not the faculty) is "Which has a higher priority, attending conferences or performing clinical duties?" In most training programs, residents must, at least occasionally, attend to clinical duties while conferences are in progress. But if this is the norm rather than the exception, kiss good-bye to obtaining any meaningful information about the number of didactic sessions. If you cannot attend the teaching sessions, they don't exist. Remember that didactic sessions significantly affect your learning and your chances of passing your in-service training exams and specialty board examinations.

29. What type of clinical experiences will I have?
Residencies are supposed to teach physicians to be excellent clinicians. For that, they must provide adequate clinical experience. How many clinical experiences will you have and how diverse will they be?

In surgical or procedural specialties, will you be performing procedures, or mostly watching? Is there a struggle between services or among residents on the same service for some procedures? At what level do residents graduate to more advanced procedures? In General Surgery, for example, if third- and fourth-year residents are still doing routine appendectomies, there is a definite problem. Similarly, if senior Pediatric, Family Medicine, or Internal Medicine residents "hog" every tube and line placement, it suggests that they have not had enough experience doing these procedures. Have previous graduates felt comfortable performing all necessary procedures by the time they graduated? If not, you should question whether such a marginal program is right for you.

A special situation exists in Obstetrics and Gynecology. Few programs now teach their residents how to perform elective abortions. If you plan (or think you might need) to do these procedures in your practice, ask specifically whether this training will be available to you.

Aside from the easily recognized procedures, how much responsibility do residents at each level have for managing patients, that is, for making the crucial decisions? Note that it is usually more difficult to decide *when* it is appropriate to do a procedure than it is to actually do it. Making that decision is what being a doctor is really about. Will you have increasing responsibility for patient care, progressively making more decisions as you show that you have the requisite knowledge and ability? Or will you be "thrown into the middle of the pool" the first day without adequate supervision? Or, perhaps worse, will you be kept in the "wading pool" for most of your residency?

Some programs offer unique learning opportunities, for example, new diagnostic or therapeutic techniques (such as genetically based cancer therapy), older but rarely available methodologies (such as hyperbaric chambers), or special training in areas of faculty expertise. As a resident, will these opportunities be available to you?

30. What is the relationship between this program and other specialties?
While you may expect to learn medicine from your own faculty and co-residents, the truth is that you will often learn as much or more from attendings and residents on other services. How well do the various specialties get along at the program's teaching institutions? Is there cooperation, strife, or open warfare among them?

This is an important issue. For example, how will you be treated when you rotate on other services? What type of interactions will you have when calling for or doing consultations, or when treating patients in cooperation with other services? Good inter-service relationships can make residency a much less stressful and more educational experience.

31. Tell me about the on-call rooms, meal plan, cafeteria, library, computer access, and parking.
You've already experienced a variety of on-call rooms during your clinical years in medical school. That was only a taste. When you use the call rooms night after night, their ambiance (or lack thereof) can greatly affect your outlook on life and work. Not only should you be told about the call rooms, but you should also be given an opportunity to see some during your visit to the program and institution. That way you can evaluate and compare them.

No resident has ever died from hospital food. (At least, I don't think so.) But when you get a chance to eat, it's a lot better if the food is tasty, looks good, has some variety, is served in a setting with at least some semblance of quiet and a pleasant décor, and is inexpensive (or free). There is a huge monetary benefit, not to mention morale boost, if food is provided. Some programs even provide meals when residents are not on duty. More hospitals are finding that jazzing up their cafeterias improves their image with hospital staff, trainees, patients, and visitors. How do the cafeterias at the locations you will work measure up? Can you tolerate this food, setting, and cost for the duration of your residency?

The library is the bellwether of an institution's educational commitment. Is it stocked with useful and up-to-date materials, staffed with knowledgeable and helpful people, and open long (or all) hours? Does the library have audiovisual and computer materials to supplement printed material? How about access to on-line journals and databases? Can you access library information, including on-line journals, from the hospital and clinics, as well as from home? When you need to access material for tomorrow morning's grand rounds, are the library's facilities adequate?

Our world is computerized, and the medical field, although currently lagging behind other segments of society, is no exception. Practitioners need to be able to use the Internet or local networks as readily as their stethoscopes. Does the residency provide access to computers and use them for teaching? Is Internet access available in the clinical areas? Are computer labs or specialists available to residents? Do they use VOIP for consultations or conferences? Do they provide access to programs and applications such as Epocrates and Pepid? How about special computer courses? It's no longer enough to know how to take a medical history and do a physical examination. You also need to know how to access electronic medical records (EMR), lab results, bedside nurses' notes, clinic schedules, library materials, databases, and, eventually, billing records.

Finally, how about parking at the hospital and clinics? Is it difficult to find or expensive? If you drive to your residency interview, you may get a taste of end" what the parking is like. Is this the norm for residents, or just for visitors?

32. Will I have time to read?

Your educational reading reflects a personal decision about what is important to you. However, if residents consistently answer that they are too tired to read, it suggests a deficiency in the program rather than in any individual. Education in any specialty depends on supplementing clinical experiences with reading. You cannot learn all you need to know on the wards, in the emergency department and clinics, or in the operating room. Reading will be important to you. Find out whether you will have time to do it from those who know—the residents.

The answer to this question will also help to identify those departments that have residency programs primarily to fulfill their service commitments, rather than to educate.

Ask senior-level (PGY-2 and above) residents this question; nearly all interns will tell you that they are too tired to read. That is certainly understandable given their schedules.

33. What support staff is available? Are they helpful?

Residents commonly feel overworked because there are too few people to perform what are typically non-physician tasks. You owe it to yourself to find out how much "scut" work the residents at a program typically perform.

Who starts routine IV lines, draws blood, and does clerical work? Who pushes patients to x-ray or to radiation oncology for treatments?

Does the institution provide an adequate level of nursing and ancillary support? Is this staff supportive, or merely an obstacle to good patient care? Are there backup teams you can call when you are swamped with admissions?

Even if institutions have sufficient numbers of support staff, their quality and interest in helping you may vary based on personnel policy and tradition. What is it like at the institutions through which residents in this program rotate?

While faculty may be able to tell you about some of the available clinical support, ask the residents for the real answers. Don't complain after the fact. Find out in advance.

34. What is the call schedule?

There are two main things that directly affect your life during residency—and they both relate to the call schedule. The first is the amount of time you will actually work. The second is who arranges the schedule.

Ask the residents how much time they actually work at each level of training. All specialties have officially limited the number of hours their residents can work. Per ACGME requirements, residents must work no more than 80 "duty hours" per week, averaged over a four-week period (Figure 20.2). "Duty hours" means all clinical, academic, and administrative activities related to the residency program or patient care, including moonlighting and in-house on-call time. Every seven days (averaged over a four-week period), residents must also have at least one continuous 24-hour period free of all educational, clinical and administrative responsibilities. Residents must also have at least 10 hours for rest and personal activities between all daily duty periods and after in-house call. In-house call must be no more often than every third night. Taking call from home is not limited, although any time a resident spends in the hospital is counted toward their 80-hour maximum, as is any "in-house" moonlighting (e.g., moonlighting within the residency program, the sponsoring institutions, or the non-hospital sponsor's primary clinical sites).

Figure 20.2
ACGME Requirements for All Programs' Resident Duty Hours

- Maximum of 80 hours per week, averaged over a four-week period.
  - Includes all in-house activities and all moonlighting.
  - The Residency Review committee for a specialty may require all specific programs to have a maximum of up to 88 hours per week.
- Maximum Duty Period
  - PGY-1 residents: Duty period may not exceed 16-hours duration.
  - PGY-2 residents and above: Scheduled duty periods may not be more than 24-hours duration. Residents may stay longer "on their own initiative" to continue to provide care to a single patient, but may not be assigned additional clinical responsibilities after 24 hours.
- Call Schedule
  - No more than six consecutive nights of (in-house) "night float" duty.
  - PGY-2 and above residents: No more often than every third night in-house when averaged over a four-week period.
  - At-home call: Only limitation is that time called back to the hospital counts toward the 80/88-hour weekly maximum. No at-home call on duty-free days.
- Moonlighting
  - PGY-1 residents may not moonlight.
  - In-house and external moonlighting counts toward the 80-hour weekly maximum.
- Mandatory Duty-Free Time
  - PGY-1 and "Intermediate-level" residents must have 8 hours free of duty between scheduled duty periods.
  - "Intermediate-level" residents must have 14 hours free of duty after 24 hours of in-house duty.
  - "Final-year" residents may be exempted from minimum duty-free periods (but still must conform to weekly 80/88-hour maximum hour standard).
  - Minimum of one scheduled duty-free day every week, when averaged over four weeks. At-home call cannot be assigned on these free days.

Although there has been good compliance with the duty-hour standards, not everyone plays by the rules. Faced with ever-tighter budgets, many residency directors skirt the rules so the institution can avoid the cost of adding residents. Some of the worst offenders have been the private hospitals. Due to the nature of their practices, the Surgical specialties and Obstetrics and Gynecology continue to have the longest hours.

Not many years ago, an applicant got a Surgical internship after having, he thought, asked all the appropriate questions. He expected to work long hours, but was astonished when he found that in addition to taking call in-house on alternate nights, he had to take call from home every night he was "off duty"! Ask in advance so you don't get any nasty surprises.

At many programs, the residency director, the secretary, a chief resident, or some unnamed individual in a back office makes the schedule, leaving residents feeling helpless. Indeed, the lack of control over one's life is one of the biggest stressors among residents. Some programs allow the residents themselves to generate the call schedule (as well as conference, vacation, and off-service schedules). If a program offers this, your mental health will be better for it.

Also, find out if days off are built into the schedule. Although all residents are supposed to be allotted four days off over a four-week period, many programs do not explicitly build them into the schedule and then apply pressure on residents to work even on "free" days. This leads to rapid burnout, frustration, and disgust with practicing medicine and the specialty. Avoid this by asking whether days off are scheduled, and how many there are each month.

35. Do you have a plan for sick days?

A natural part of the on-call schedule is an arrangement for coverage in case of illness, injury, or personal crises within the resident staff. It will happen, if not to you then to some of your colleagues—and you will be affected. If there is a plan, and there probably is, what are the "payback" arrangements and who arranges the backup? The less onerous these arrangements are for the individual, the better.

36. Do I need a medical license?

All U.S. medical licensing authorities require residents to have educational licenses, permits, certificates, or registrations. Generally, the institution pays for this, and supplies the licensing Board(s) with a list of resident names. Some licensing agencies may require you to pay the fee, which ranges from free to $425 (Nevada). In thirteen states, residents must pass USMLE Step 1;

California, Mississippi, North Dakota, Oklahoma, and Utah require passing Steps 1, 2CK, and 2CS.

Thirty-nine licensing jurisdictions require new permits or licenses when changing residency programs within the state. Eighteen require full licensure at some point during the residency or fellowship, usually after three to five years of training. Since all this is state-specific information, ask about it when you interview.

37. What are your moonlighting rules?

Moonlighting—working outside the residency program for income and experience—has long been common. If you have dependents or large expenses, this extra income may be vital. The experience, depending upon the nature of the moonlighting, can be invaluable. At the least, it may be the first time that you feel like a physician, fully responsible for your patient's care. By itself, that is a worthwhile, enlightening, and often scary experience.

Questions to ask about moonlighting include: Does the program allow, tolerate, or encourage moonlighting? Are opportunities available nearby? How are they arranged? Is there a specific individual (often a senior resident) that coordinates them? Is moonlighting permitted both within and outside of the training facilities? Do current residents moonlight? If so, at what PGY level do they begin and what pay do they receive? How do they handle malpractice insurance for moonlighting?

The ACGME's resident duty-hour rules may limit moonlighting in programs that bump up against the maximum average-work-week limit. However, it's doubtful that many programs will be willing or able to stringently track such outside activity.

38. What is the patient population I will see?

Patients (their numbers and age distribution, the nature of their diseases, and who cares for them in what settings) are the basic element of all medical training programs. If the program lacks an adequate number of patient encounters, it doesn't matter what else it offers.

It is necessary to first ascertain how many patients the residents care for. But aside from this, you also need to know how much time is spent caring for private patients and how much autonomy residents have when seeing these patients. While some programs have many patients coming through their offices or hospital beds, private practitioners often care for most of them.

Find out about the patient population served and the distribution of disease processes. Some teaching hospitals have an overabundance of a few types of disease processes, such as penetrating trauma, tertiary oncology, or AIDS. A skewed distribution does not provide adequate training for clinicians who will eventually serve a more diverse population with more common diseases. Today, as more medical care is being delivered in outpatient settings, residents should be sure they are seeing enough patients in the clinics and outpatient surgeries.

Finally, ask if there are medical students on the service. If there are, ask if you will be responsible for teaching them. Whether you feel that this is a plus or minus for you, find out in advance what to expect.

39. Do the residents socialize as a group?

This is one element, or at least demonstrates one element, of esprit de corps. Are the social events program-wide or institution-wide? This may or may not be important to you. If it is, you may also want to ask about the ratio of married to single residents (in the program or institution), how many have children, and how often social events occur.

Does there seem to be any particular activity that is of special interest to the residents, or do their interests vary? Is socializing related to educational activities, such as journal clubs? Or are they separate events, such as volleyball games or picnics? Note that if the socialization is resident-organized, it may vary considerably from year to year.

Confirm Questionable Points

The answers to a number of the questions that you ask the interviewers may be critical. Which questions these are will depend upon your own "Must/Want" Analysis. However, you may not get straight answers to some of them. This may be because no one knows the answer at the moment. For example, in October no one may really know how many of the faculty will still be on-site next July. But you may be getting the runaround for other, more nefarious, reasons. If you ask the residency director about how much faculty interaction there is with residents and the hemming and hawing begins, then you will need to get the real story. This is where the technique of cross-checking facts becomes useful.

Whenever you have some doubt about the answer to an important question, repeat the question to another interviewer. Or better yet, if it is appropriate, ask a resident in the program. In fact, if the issue is extremely important to you, ask everyone you talk to the same question. But be sure not to do so within earshot of others you have already asked (or will ask) that same question—it will be taken as a sign that you doubt their honesty, which, of course, you do. Remember that the program is trying to sell its product to you at the same time that you are selling yourself to it. Not all salesmen are honest. *Caveat emptor!*

Things Not To Ask

There are specific questions that must not be asked during an interview, even though they are important to you. These questions basically involve four areas: salary, benefits, vacation, and competition. Let's discuss each one individually, so you will know what information to get from the *appropriate* sources.

Salary

The salary you will receive as a resident will, in large part, depend upon three factors.

1. The mean salaries of housestaff around the country in the previous year.

2. The type of institution in which the residency is located.

3. The region of the country in which the institution is situated.

Most institutions base their resident salaries upon a variation from the mean salary that residents are receiving nationally. The variations in many cases are based upon the cost of living in the region of the country where the institution is located. In addition, those programs that have a relatively difficult time attracting residents, such as community and non-university hospitals, will tend to have higher salaries. Those with very large numbers of applicants will generally offer lower salaries. But, of course, you would be more than happy to do the residency for free, wouldn't you? Probably not. However, this is the attitude to take during the interview process. Salary will keep you alive and pay your bills—but do not try to find out what it will be during the interview. What are you, money-hungry?

The only exception to this rule is if you have any hint that the position is unfunded. Despite rules to the contrary, these positions still exist. They are most commonly found in highly competitive fellowships (post-residency) and at some institutions whose residents are mostly international medical graduates. If this is the case, and you are still interested in the position, at least ask about the non-salary benefits offered.

Benefits

Benefit packages are very important to you as a resident—as they will be for the rest of your career. Virtually all such packages include malpractice insurance and some type of medical insurance. Other benefits may include food or housing allowances, uniforms, cleaning expenses, disability insurance, moving expenses, parking, tuition fee waivers for the affiliated school, and childcare, to name some common ones (Figures 11.4, 11.5, and 11.6).

Remember, if you can use the benefit, it counts as additional salary. However, if the program offers benefits that you cannot use, such as obstetric care when you are not planning any children for now, the value of this benefit is lost to you. Do make certain that the medical insurance is comprehensive enough to cover serious illness or injury without a substantial copayment. You probably are already in debt up to your eyeballs and cannot afford steep medical bills.

Asking a faculty member about the benefit package, however, is generally like talking to the wall. He will normally have no idea what his own benefit package is, let alone yours. Don't make your interviewer look stupid. Avoid this topic.

Vacation

If you don't think that vacation is important, wait until you have been up most of every night for a week. At that point, dreaming about an upcoming vacation may be all that keeps you going. Most interns have three weeks or less of vacation, while most residents in their second or higher years have at least three weeks of vacation each year. In some programs, the vacation can all be taken at one time; in others, it must be taken as one-week blocks. The latter obviously doesn't allow much time for travel.

Asking an interviewer about vacation is akin to inquiring whether you would actually have to do any work during the residency. While everyone understands that vacation—even a resident's vacation—is important, interviewers assume that during the interview you will concentrate on the great educational experience that they offer, rather than your time off.

Competition

Who is your competition? It doesn't matter! Asking about other applicants will serve no good purpose and only directs an interviewer's attention away from you. The key, as has been stressed throughout this book, is to put your own best efforts before the residency faculty and let them select you based upon what they see. Forget the others. Concentrate on selling yourself.

Okay, so where do you find out about salary, benefits, and vacation? First, look at *FREIDA* and then the program's or institution's website. Normally, you will discover most of the information there. If not, then two other excellent sources are the residency secretary and the staff in the institution's Graduate Education office. In fact, the latter site is the place where you can get the most up-to-date information and still remain relatively anonymous. If all else fails, email the director of the institution's Housestaff or Graduate Education office.

Things Not To Do

Just as there are certain questions that you should avoid, there are certain things that you should not do during the interview. The following are attitudes or actions that will evoke a negative response from an interviewer.

Show Discouragement

Be upbeat! This is your time to shine. One poor interview should not influence the rest of your visit. Remember that the interviewer may not have thought it was a poor interview at all. Looking "down in the dumps" will destroy any positive effect that your interview could possibly have made.

Stand up straight. Lift up your chin. *SMILE*—it won't break your face. If you cannot find the courage to smile through some adversity now, you are really going to be in trouble when you get into your residency.

Disparage Other Programs, Faculty, or Applicants

You might very well be asked about the other programs that you have visited. The question could be phrased as, "Tell me about the poorest programs that you have visited." Although this may be tempting—you may have interviewed at some really horrendous places—back up a minute to redirect the question. Say that you are not in a position to determine which programs are poor, but there may be some that do not seem to meet your needs. Then you can describe specific aspects of programs that you feel did not fully meet your expectations. But go easy. If you really berate a program that you have visited, the interviewer might wonder what you will say about his or her program when you go elsewhere.

Do not say anything derogatory about faculty at another institution. It should go without saying that you will not berate faculty at the institution at which you are interviewing. No matter what you think, academic medicine, especially within the confines of any one specialty, is rather close-knit. There is a good chance that the person you are describing is well-known to the interviewer.

Falsify Background

Although it may appear that you could say almost anything about your background during the interview and get away with it, you do so only at great risk. The first danger is that you will immediately be discovered.

Not many years ago, a residency applicant was eloquently describing his activities in the Emergency Medical System. He stated that he responded to calls frequently even while in medical school. It was quite an impressive achievement. Yet, as he went on with his story, it became obvious to the interviewer that he was being less than honest. For, while he was describing activities in the opposite end of the country, it just so happened that the interviewer was also from that area and picked up on major factual errors in the story. These were confirmed by a call to the applicant's medical school, negating any chance he had of matching in that program.

The second danger is even worse. If information that you provide when you apply for any job, including a residency position, is later found to be false, it is grounds for immediate dismissal. Thus, giving fraudulent information puts you in jeopardy throughout your residency. Stick to the truth. Make it appear as favorable as possible, but stick to the truth.

Inappropriate Humor

There is a place for humor in interviews. A good laugh can be enjoyed, but, unfortunately, rarely is during residency interviews. However, humor should not be offensive. Even if laughter ensues after you tell an off-color, sexist, or racist joke, you almost certainly will have lowered yourself in the interviewer's mind.

In fact, most administrators consider off-color or inappropriate humor to be the major breach of workplace etiquette. If you have an uncontrollable urge to tell these types of jokes, at least keep them out of the interview.

Drink Coffee, Smoke, Chew Gum, and Bite Nails

Four activities that you must not do during an interview are drink coffee, smoke, chew gum, and bite your nails. You may very well be offered coffee by each interviewer. They mean well. But do they also offer you a bathroom break in the middle of the interview? No! And if you are concentrating on a full bladder instead of the interviewer's questions, you could end up in deep trouble. Avoid diuretics.

There are three problems with smoking. The first is that it is unlikely that your interviewer smokes, since the habit is now relatively rare among physicians. The second is that smoking looks bad during an interview. So even if you are addicted, hold out until the interview is over—or you have left the program for the day. The smell that lingers on your clothes and breath, if you smoke, will not endear you to non-smoking interviewers. Third, interviewers may be biased against hiring smokers. As of yet, no programs have gone public with an explicit ban on hiring smokers, but it is likely that it would be legal. There is no protection under current civil rights legislation for smokers. This makes it legal for an interviewer to inquire whether or not you are a smoker. Note, of course, that if they inquire, it can only be a (un-Lucky?) strike against you. About 25% of personnel directors admit that if offered two equivalent applicants, they would hire the non-smoker.

Chewing gum (or, banish the thought, tobacco) is absolutely out. It evokes a sophomoric image that will destroy everything that you have worked so hard to achieve. If blowing bubbles is your "thing," hold out until you leave the hospital. No one is physiologically addicted to chewing gum (except, perhaps, nicotine gum—use patches during interviews). One stick of gum at the wrong time can cancel your chance for a residency slot that you really want.

Finally, even though you are nervous and your common response is to bite your nails, restrain yourself when at residency programs. It signals your neuroses to interviewers. For clinicians, it also demonstrates potentially dangerous, infection-producing behavior.

Stressful Interviews

Stress interviews were once very common. Interviewers asked questions to purposely make applicants confused, fearful, and hostile. Employers believed they could weed out applicants who couldn't handle stress. The applicants they actually eliminated were individuals with enough self-esteem to determine that they didn't want to work for people who treated potential employees like dirt. While the business world long ago learned not to use this method, some residency programs still use the technique. Others treat applicants shabbily because that is how they treat their residents.

Panel Interviews

The most common type of interview is the one-on-one serial interview, in which you go from interviewer to interviewer, with each asking his or her own questions. Occasionally, though, you will be faced with a rather unusual interview scenario—the panel or group interview, in which from two to twenty individuals will all be interviewing you at the same time. There is a reason business people call this the "gang bang." It is generally considered a rather poor interview technique, both from an employer's and from an applicant's perspective. However, it is still in use, primarily because it is thought to save the interviewers' time. Some people also believe this technique is useful for jobs that require sophisticated communication skills—such as that of a physician.

These interviews will generally be conducted using either a question or a scenario format. In the question format, each panel member asks his or her own questions. In the scenario format, you discuss one or more cases with the entire panel.

The best approach is to look at the individual who asked the question when you answer. In the case of the scenario, since it is a question from the entire group, look at all the members while answering. If an individual member asks you a follow-up question, look at that person when answering. Do not try to determine the most influential people on the panel and direct most of your attention to them. The others will feel slighted. When the panel members meet together later to discuss the candidates, your implied insult will damage your chance of getting a residency position.

A particularly nasty variation used at some residency programs is to sit the applicant between the wings of a V-shaped table facing the interviewers seated on both outside wings. They then pepper interviewees with questions, alternating sides to make candidates swivel their heads back and forth to answer each question. One applicant quickly adjusted by simply slowing down and completely turning to face each questioner when she answered. Her solution was to avoid getting flustered. You could also get up and move your chair back so the angle to view the interviewers is not so acute.

Even worse is another technique that is employed (thankfully) by only a few Gestapo-like programs. At the end of an interview day, they bring two students at a time into a roomful of faculty. They then rapidly ask the students the same questions at the same time. This is really an abuse of power; my suggestion, if this happens to you, is to stand up, thank them for their time, and leave without participating.

If you are faced with any type of panel interview, remember that it will be as unnerving an experience for everyone else as it is for you. So, keep cool and knock their socks off!

Non-Interview Visits

There is one type of program visit, still very rare, to which you may be invited. This is the non-interview visit, which is essentially the same as a traditional interview visit, but without the interviews. While it has the same implications as any other invitation to visit a residency, the programs handle it somewhat differently.

At present, only a few of the most highly selective programs use this type of visit. You are not rated on the basis of your performance during the visit (unless you act really obnoxious). Rather, the residency faculty screens applicants based on their past performance in school, on the USMLE, and on other written materials they feel are important. They then assume that all applicants they invite for a visit to their program would make acceptable residents.

Residencies use the non-interview visit primarily to show an applicant the program. During the visit, applicants normally have multiple opportunities to see the program's physical plant, didactic program, and social milieu. They are encouraged to interact with faculty and residents, and to take the time to have all their questions answered. Generally, they obtain a better picture of the program than would be possible during a more traditional visit. Applicants invited for these visits get the maximum possible information; this ensures that those ranking the program highly are doing so with a sound knowledge of what they are getting into.

There are several principles upon which this system is based. The first is that the interview system, especially when using physician-interviewers who are untrained in personnel selection, is as likely to give erroneous information as it is to be accurate. A second is that creating a program with happy residents is best assured by giving applicants as much information as possible about it ahead of time. The last assumption is that if you have qualified applicants, those that are happy to come to a particular program for training make the best residents and, therefore, the best program.

This system is, at best, considered avant-garde. You probably will not be exposed to it. But if you are, do not be put off by it. You should still handle yourself in the same manner described elsewhere in this book.

Silence

The most stressful time during any interview can be a period of silence. This is an invitation to reveal all of your twitches, nervousness, and insecurity. It is also an opportunity to show self-assurance. Be strong!

Silence occurs for several reasons. Rarely are physician-interviewers disciplined enough, or nasty enough, to impose a period of silence simply to test an applicant. Rather, they may remain quiet while they contemplate a question or your answer. They also may suddenly have remembered that they didn't turn off their headlights when they parked their car that morning. Don't feel that a period of silence is negatively directed at you.

Some people respond to silence during an interview by fidgeting. They brush their hair back, move around in their chair, straighten their clothes, or mutter to themselves. Others try to break the silence by repeating (or worse, contradicting) what they just said. Don't do it; sit still, be calm, and be quiet—it too will end. One way experienced individuals combat periods of silence in interview-like situations is to simply begin counting the time to see how long the period lasts. It will seem like days, but it rarely lasts more than fifteen seconds.

You too can occasionally use silence to demonstrate your contemplative side. If an interviewer asks a particularly deep or thoughtful question, you don't have to jump in immediately with an answer, even if you are prepared for it. Wait a few seconds as you "think" it through. Rather than appearing impulsive, you now seem to be a deep thinker.

Control The Interview—Gently

As you will see in the next chapter, it is often possible to steer the interview in a direction that is beneficial to you. You can mold your answers to interviewers' questions in such a way as to bring out some of your most favorable points. However, this must be done subtly. Some interviewers may see your pushing an interview in a specific direction as being impudent. This, of course, would be counterproductive. So, if you can, steer the interview in a beneficial direction—but do it so gently that the interviewer does not notice.

Reasons Why Interviews Fail

Inadequate Preparation

The first reason that interviews fail is that the applicant is inadequately prepared. This book helps you to prepare for the residency interview. In the end, however, it is up to you to know about the specialty, the program, the faculty, your own ambitions and desires, and the questions that you will probably be asked during interviews. It takes hard work on your part to get ready for interviews, but in the end it is worth it.

Not Listening To Questions

The second reason is because the applicant does not listen to the interviewer's questions. The result is discommunication, distorting the messages coming in and going out. This is what happens when you let your mind wander during an interview—and it spells disaster. Remember that an interview is a battle of wits. If your thoughts stray during this encounter, you lose!

Even fast talkers listen faster than they talk. We usually speak only 100 to 150 words per minute, but we process about 600 spoken words a minute. This provides a lot of time for our minds to wander—usually spent thinking about what we are going to say next rather than about what is being said. Since we can only listen or think, we may lose what the other person is saying. When we think and our eyes wander (even momentarily), the speaker knows that we are not listening. The epitome of ignoring the interviewer and the interview is the apocryphal candidate whose cell phone rings during the interview, excuses herself, and proceeds to answer the phone.

Use "active listening." This involves briefly summarizing what you think the speaker has just said. It shows that you are carefully listening, allows the speaker to correct any misimpressions you may have gotten, and helps the conversation move forward. Don't wait until the end of the interview to do this, but rather intersperse it several times during the interview. For example, after the interviewer has described some attributes of their program, say "As I understand it, this residency's strengths are…" You might then continue with "How about…?"

Since many residency interviews are conducted in busy offices, clinical settings, or even hallways, you may have to concentrate very hard on the interview to avoid the ever-present distractions, sometimes justifiably called "interview blockers" (Figure 18.1). This can be difficult, but your experiences working in noisy patient-care areas should help you to concentrate on the task at hand. And don't just listen to the question; listen to *how the question is asked*. Many times an interviewer will give the astute listener clues to the answer that he or she is looking for. Figure 20.3, "Guidelines for Effective Listening," should help you out.

When speaking, use your normal voice rather than the higher pitch that people often use when they are nervous. Avoid using "fillers" to pad a pause in the conversation, such as "um," "er," "ah," or "you know." Rather, simply pause or use "and," "or," or "but" to join your thoughts together.

Also, never mechanically "give your presentation," downloading your spiel in a rote manner. Rather, keep in mind an outline of your "message" and interject it at appropriate points in the conversation.

Occasionally your mind may go blank during an interview. It's okay. Just apologize to the interviewer and simply ask for a moment to think about the question or, second best, ask the interviewer to repeat the question. As Sam Donaldson, the former television newsman, said, "Even the pros get tongue-tied."

Figure 20.3
Guidelines for Effective Listening

1. Demonstrate attentiveness.
2. Listen for "what" and "why" questions.
3. Don't interrupt the speaker.
4. Don't waste time evaluating the interviewer.
5. Listen for key issues.
6. Mirror back the interviewer's message.
7. Ask clarifying questions.
8. Identify feelings and attitudes in the interviewer.

One caveat. If you have carefully read the questions and answers in Chapter 21, you may be planning how to answer what you think will be the next question. Or, you may be analyzing how you might interact during your residency with the faculty and residents you have met. Stop! Turn off that mental audiotape and listen to the interviewer. By now you should be able to answer questions without rehearsing, and there will be plenty of time later to analyze your visit. Concentrate on what the interviewer is saying.

If you really listen, and you still can't understand what an interviewer is looking for, ask for clarification. This might also work (once) if you miss a question completely—but it would be unwise to count on using it repeatedly. Remember that the most ego-gratifying thing you can do for interviewers is to listen to them.

If you are asked a question you just don't know how to answer, be honest and say so. Perhaps you can say, "I'll have to think about that. Can we come back to that later?" Normally, the interviewer will oblige. It is then your responsibility to return to the question before the end of the interview. At that point, if you still cannot come up with an answer, say that you will continue to think about it and get back to the interviewer by letter. Then, in your thank-you letter, give that interviewer an answer to his or her question. In these cases, honesty (and thoughtfulness in later responding by letter), rather than bluffing your way through an answer, may be your key to success.

Answering Questions Not Asked

A third reason for interview failures is that interviewers may get annoyed by having questions answered that were not asked. Many students, while attempting to highlight their strengths, routinely give answers that have no relation at all to the questions that were asked (much like politicians).

Figure 20.4
Factors Influencing an Interviewer's Behavior

- Age & stage in life cycle
- Cultural background
- Interests
- Prior experiences
- Goals/Aspirations
- Successes/Failures
- Mood
- Personality

Here, you are treading the fine line between guiding the interview and destroying it. Answering a question about your spare-time activities with a description of your medical school awards makes no sense. Rather, talk about the rock band you organized or the Internet bulletin board you established. These both answer the question and highlight your initiative and talents.

Similar applicant behavior that interviewers detest includes answering questions with questions, telling jokes to change the subject, and answering with gibberish. Like reporters, good interviewers simply repeat their original question until they get a straight answer. Also, because interviewers are human, answers that might work one day may not work on another. Many factors can influence an interviewer's behavior (Figure 20.4).

Rambling

A fourth way to wreck your interview is to ramble, thus providing superfluous information. Interviewers are easily bored—not surprising given the number of applicants they must often see in one day.

If you have a lot of information to impart in answer to a specific question, tell the interviewer the main points, and then ask if he or she would like you to continue. For example, if you are asked to describe your medical school rotation in your chosen specialty, give the highlights in several sentences and then ask if the interviewer would like to know more. Since you are watching the interviewer while you answer, you may note nonverbal cues indicating that you have said enough. In general, keep your answers brief, to the point, and interesting.

Giving Warning Signals

The fifth reason that interviews fail is that the applicant inadvertently gives warning signals to the interviewer that there may be an unstable personality lurking behind a deceptive smile. Trained interviewers seek specific warning signs (Figure 20.5).

Figure 20.5
Warning Signs for Interviewers

- Inconsistent answers during the interview.
- Inconsistencies between what is said in the interview and past performance.
- Abrasiveness or any other personality quirk that makes the interviewer uncomfortable.
- Evasiveness.
- A pattern of unhappiness in former jobs.
- Blaming others for all the applicant's problems.
- Dullness when responding to questions.
- A pattern of taking advantage of, or of deceiving, other people.

Adapted from: Perham JC. Spotting bad apples: the warning signals. *Dun's Business Month.* October 1986:54-6.

Very few faculty interviewers are sophisticated enough in the techniques of employment interviewing to consciously recognize these signs. Being good clinicians, though, they unconsciously assimilate clues and will give the applicant a poor rating. It would be a good idea to review the warning signs and make certain that you do not demonstrate any unintentionally.

Interview Disasters

Life is often stranger than fiction, and so are some interviews. One national employment agency described some of the more unusual occurrences during interviews for professional positions:

- At the start of the interview, the applicant sat down in the interviewer's chair and insisted that the interviewer sit elsewhere.
- When an applicant was asked about loyalty, he showed the interviewer a tattoo of his girlfriend's name.
- An applicant pulled out a tape recorder, saying that he taped all interviews.
- Another left the dry cleaning tag on his jacket, saying that he wanted to demonstrate just how neat and clean he was.
- When told to take his time answering questions, an applicant began writing out the answers before speaking.
- During the interview, an applicant received three cell phone calls.
- Another brought his five children and the family cat to the interview.
- At the end of the interview, the applicant asked if she could use the fax machine to send out some personal letters.

Hopefully, you won't make these types of errors. Just think, if this is how other applicants behave, you don't have much to worry about. Of course, most medical students are smart enough to avoid such crass behavior.

Sell Yourself

The bottom line during an interview is that you must sell yourself. At the same time, you also need to elicit information. To have the best chance of being ranked highly by the programs, you must do a good job of showing your own wares. Interviewers are looking for specific attributes in applicants (Figure 20.6). When talking with the individuals at each program, remember that interviewers rate these elements in the applicants they interview. Although every program has a different rating form for interviewers to complete, the essential items will always be the same (Figure 20.7).

It is your job to point out how closely you resemble the interviewer's ideal candidate by exhibiting the sought-after traits. Remember, if you don't sell yourself, no one else will do it for you!

Figure 20.6
Personality Traits Interviewers Seek

Personal
- Enthusiasm
- Motivation/Initiative
- Communication skills
- Chemistry
- Energy
- Determination
- Confidence
- Humility
- Emotional control
- Common sense
- Good interpersonal skills
- Adaptability
- Intelligence

Professional
- Reliability
- Honesty/Integrity
- Pride
- Dedication
- Analytical skills
- Listening skills
- Ability to get things done
- Initiative
- Good work habits/work ethic
- Good judgment
- Motivation to achieve
- Problem-solving skills

Figure 20.7
Interviewer's Rating Form

Applicant Name_____   Date_____

Scale: 1 = Very Weak   10 = Very Strong

General

_____ Physical appearance (dress, grooming)

_____ Character (reliability, honesty, integrity)

_____ Timeliness

_____ Knowledge about specialty

_____ Knowledge about program

_____ Computer literacy

_____ Energy

Intellect

_____ Mental ability   _____ Judgment

_____ Flexibility   _____ Communication ability

Emotions

_____ Work ethic   _____ Personality (fits program)

_____ Motivation   _____ Teachable

_____ Attitude   _____ Sense of humor

_____ Stability   _____ Outside interests

_____ Self-confidence

Record

_____ USMLE/COMLEX score   _____

_____ Class rank   _____

_____ Medical school   _____

_____ Quality of reference letters   _____

_____ Clinical performance (general) _____

_____ Clinical performance (specialty) _____

_____ Honors/Awards   _____

_____ Research   _____

_____ **Total**   _____ **Number of Scored Items**

                          _____ **Average of Scored Items**

21

The Questions—The Answers

Silence is the only good substitute for intelligence.
Folk saying

Judge a person not by his answers, but by his questions.
Voltaire

WHAT MUST YOU REMEMBER in the process of preparing for the interview? And what must you remember during the interview? Only two things: *prepare in advance* and *sell yourself by showing your best qualities.*

Interviews generally start with some simple pleasantries and then move on to the skills/attitude evaluation (Figure 20.1). In this part of the interview, no matter what the format or the type of questions asked, most program directors look for three qualities in applicants: *intellectual strength, energy, and personal compatibility* with faculty, staff, and current residents.

Interviewers don't really want "the truth." They want "correct" answers. If you believe there is no such thing as the correct answer to a typical interview question, you are sadly mistaken. Good interviewers know exactly what they are looking for in a resident. They know how to extract the needed information in a way that is disarmingly benign. Their questions are simply tools with which to hammer out an impression of the applicant.

Intellectual Strength
Program directors already know a great deal about your performance in this arena. Reference letters, USMLE/COMLEX scores, transcripts, and narratives of clinical performance have preceded you. That is what got you in the door for the interview. Now they want to find out if you can think on your feet. Can you apply what you know to new situations? Are you really interested in learning, or just in getting through a program so you can go into practice? Do you know about anything other than medicine? Was it your quick smile rather than a solid intellect that got you your good grades? Do you believe that you have very little left to learn? Basically, the interviewer is trying to determine what you know, how well you are able to use what you have learned, and if you really want to learn any more.

Energy

Residents spend the majority of their time attending to patient care duties. No matter where a program is located or what the specialty is, fatigue, stress, and depression are pervasive. This is especially true during the PGY-1 year. The less this manifests itself in a program's residents, the fewer the problems with which the faculty must deal and, consequently, the happier they are. Make them happy. Demonstrate that you have the good humor, self-confidence, and stamina to go the distance. But don't just say the words—show them by your actions during the entire interview process.

Personal Compatibility

Remember that you are being hired to join an established group of practicing physicians, albeit at a very junior level. You will be responsible for the care of the faculty's patients. You will be their representative to the medical and non-medical communities. They will have to live their professional lives with you for the duration of your training.

A "personality" already exists for the group, the residency, the department, and the institution. Will you fit in? Will they be comfortable with you? A little thought and a lot of care are necessary here. A hyper-aggressive image may work in some locales, but fail in others. Modify the image you project to meet the situation. But don't fool yourself. If you will not fit in with a group, it is better to find that out during the interview, rather than after you arrive for a several-year stint as a resident.

Presenting Yourself

Show Your Best Qualities

As you answer the interviewers' questions, remember to highlight your best qualities to *sell yourself!*

And do not sell yourself short! Know what your strengths are. Know what the residency is looking for. If you don't have an obvious opportunity to let the interviewers know how well you meet their needs, make an opportunity. This may come through answering questions—all questions—with different strength areas you want to demonstrate. Or it may come in the form of a "question" at the termination of the interview, e.g., "Is it true that many Orthopedic Surgeons have woodworking as a hobby? I have a workshop at home and have made prize-winning furniture." Remember, if you don't sell yourself, no one will do it for you.

Prepare

When getting ready for the interview, it is absolutely essential to *prepare, prepare, prepare!* How many hours have you spent studying, preparing for exams? A thousand? Five thousand? The interview is, perhaps, the toughest exam of your life. Make sure that you spend enough time studying for it. The steps to preparing for an interview are very straightforward: learn to talk about yourself easily, and learn the types of questions interviewers ask and what they hope to learn from your answers. Then combine these and formulate your answers in advance.

Talking About Yourself

Talking about yourself can be very difficult. Most people are loath to extol their own virtues. You must be ready to tell the interviewers your positive qualities so that they hear them loud and clear.

First, put yourself in the position of the residency faculty where you will be interviewing. What job skills and personal characteristics would you want in an individual applying to *your* program? You should be able to get a good idea from the material you have collected from the specialty societies, from the program, and from talks with residents and specialists in the field. Write these characteristics down. Then write out questions that you would ask an applicant to your program.

Second, list your strengths that match these characteristics. This step requires a good bit of objectivity. You may need some help from your adviser or a close friend. The following exercise will help you to get in the habit of thinking and talking positively about yourself.

Exercise

List *three accomplishments* of which you are proud and what each accomplishment indicates about you:

1. _____

   _____

2. _____

   _____

3. _____

   _____

Next, list *three abilities* you have that will make you valuable as a resident in the specialty for which you are applying:

1. _____

   _____

2. _____

   _____

3. _____

   _____

Now, can you use these accomplishments and abilities in a short narrative that describes you? If you can, you have made a good start toward a successful interview.

Finally, write some great answers to the questions you developed. Be sure to incorporate your accomplishments and abilities into your answers. But do not memorize them word for word—they will sound forced. Guests on television talk shows prepare by making a list of the ten questions they *don't* want to be asked—and then developing answers for each of them. Note that this process may change a bit as you gain interview experience. But the process gets easier each time you do it. And it is worth the effort.

It's said that the famous trial lawyer, F. Lee Bailey, doesn't believe that he has won so many difficult cases because he is any smarter than his opponents—it is just that he is more obsessive-compulsive. Preparation is his key to success. Your preparation will be your key to getting a residency position.

Types of Questions

Typical interviewers use only five types of interview questions, although they can be phrased in many different ways. Recognizing the type of question the interviewer asks helps you determine what information he or she is seeking.

Closed Question

Closed questions ask for specific information and a simple, definitive answer. "How many years were you an undergraduate?" for example, deserves merely a simple answer, such as "four years." Nothing deep here. Interviewers use closed questions to elicit information seemingly absent from the application materials.

Open-Ended, Informal Question

Open-ended, informal questions also ask for specific information, but require more in-depth answers. Such a question might be "What clinical experiences have you had in this specialty?" This type of question also gives the applicant a chance to speak and become relaxed.

Open-Ended, Attitudinal Question

These questions are used to determine how well an applicant organizes his or her thoughts before speaking. An example is "What do you think of physician advertising?" Most interviewers want to see if the answer is concise and to the point.

Probing Question

Interviewers ask probing questions as follow-ups to open-ended questions. They become especially useful after the applicant has given an answer expressing an opinion. An example of this type of question is "Why do you feel that way?" This forces applicants to defend and further explain their previous answer. It also allows an interviewer to control the direction of the interview.

Sometimes an interviewer will go back to an earlier answer, quote the applicant, and ask a probing question, such as "You said you felt this area of the country was more progressive medically than your medical school's area. Why is that?"

Leading Question

Interviewers use leading questions to direct applicants' answers or to see if they have the gumption to express their own opinions. Unfortunately, it is not always easy to tell what is expected. Such a question might begin, "Residents in our specialty should go back to an every-other-night call schedule," and be followed by, "Don't you agree?" The interviewer may be serious or merely prodding the interviewee into an untenable position. If the intent is unclear, a way to find out before answering is simply to ask, "What makes you think that?"

Interviewer Techniques

Interviewers have numerous methods to trap the unwary applicant. They may, for example, ask three questions together at the start of the interview. Are you cool enough to remember them without being prompted? One method to help you remember them is to repeat them back "for clarification" after they are asked.

The interviewer may also give conflicting opinions about the same topic, such as:

"Residents in many programs are overworked."

"Resident work-hour restrictions are harming training programs."
Interviewers do this to see if the applicant will simply agree with both. Wrong move! Don't be a wimp! Suggest to the interviewer that the opinions "seem to conflict, if I understand you correctly."

Some interviewers treat the interview more like a psychological test by asking interviewees to complete sentences. Examples might be:

"If I were 10% more assertive, I would…"

"I sometimes act inappropriately when…"

"If I could say anything I wanted right now, I would say…"

As for psychological tests, about half of all U.S. companies use them, and about a fourth give formal personality tests to job applicants as part of the interview process. This has not yet caught on among residency programs. Prospective employers use these tests to measure "The Big Five"—emotional stability, extroversion, openness to new experiences, agreeableness, and conscientiousness. These test results (which can be faked by knowledgeable test takers) can then be validated in the interview. Residency faculty think that they can get the same information without using these tests.

Some savvy residency directors interview applicants twice—although one time may be during lunch or in a more informal setting. They may ask some of the same questions again. The second time they are interviewed, applicants are generally more relaxed and may give more complete information, or even respond differently to the same questions. *Remember that you are being evaluated the entire time you are at the residency program.*

Now, what are some of the specific questions you are likely to be asked?

Questions & Answers

The following questions are those that residency applicants have been asked over the years. Following the prototypical question and a discussion of possible answers, I have listed similar questions that applicants have been asked. Some are much more thoughtful or original than classic questions—such as "Why do you want to be a [fill in the specialty]?"—which nearly all applicants get tired of answering. It is impossible, of course, to prepare for or predict every possible question. However, if you have prepared for the questions listed below, you will have the self-confidence to answer anything an interviewer asks.

Note that these questions are often used in strange ways by interviewers. One residency applicant reported that she had been asked the main questions from this list *in the order in which they appear!* Don't count on this happening to you.

1. How are you today?

What a pleasant way for an interviewer to begin. A simple ice-breaker, you think. Wrong! Sophisticated interviewers use this, and similar questions, as rapid and effective screening tools. "Gee, it's raining outside and I got soaked coming here," said one applicant. "I'm really frustrated that my plane was late and that I had trouble getting a cab," whined another. These are the wrong answers.

"Great!" "Wonderful!" or "Really happy to be here!" should always be your reply to this question.

Residency interviewers look for individuals whose demeanor stays upbeat even under adversity. The travails on the interview circuit are insignificant compared to those during residency. Simple opening questions delivered in an off-hand manner will often expose an applicant's true personality far better than the well-rehearsed "deep" questions that most applicants expect.

Most people find the first three minutes of an interview to be the most difficult. Breaking the ice has tripped up many excellent candidates. You can ease this awkward moment—and make many interviewers grateful—by asking a question about a photograph, book, or other object in the room. This way, the interviewer must answer the question, you get a little breathing space, and the interview starts on a warm, friendly note.

The point is there are no innocent questions!
- Did you have any trouble finding us or getting here?
- You're looking a little flustered. What's wrong?

2. Do you have any questions?

This is the "behavioral" interviewer's classic opening. The interviewee is expected to take the initiative right from the start. Many applicants respond to this by asking standard questions and, therefore, waste this opportunity. When the "any questions" opportunity begins an interview, ask questions that highlight your strengths and knowledge of the specialty. Get this information from reading recent "throwaway" journals or news magazines for this specialty, such as *Internal Medicine News*.

Use this question to show interviewers the special expertise you can add to their program, and that you are achievement-oriented. An example might be, "I recently read in *Family Practice News* that Family Medicine is very involved in sports medicine. I have a real interest in this area based on my work as a football trainer in college, and I have taught new trainers. Do other people at this program also have an interest in sports medicine?"

Faculty members actually may ask this question because they do not know what else to ask. Since many applicants report that this is the most common question they are asked, make a long list of your own questions to use as answers. Never answer "No," since, no matter what the situation, a negative answer indicates that you have a less-than-serious interest in that program.

- Do you know much about our program?
- If you were in my (the interviewer's) seat, what would you ask? Okay, now answer those questions.

3. *Tell me about yourself.*

This is the granddaddy of open-ended questions (although, of course, it isn't really a question). You have the opportunity to say almost anything you want. You can put your best foot forward or stick it right in your mouth. This question gives you, by design, no hint of how to answer it. You can go off on almost any tangent. And if the interviewer is any good, you will be able to talk for as long as you want. The longer you talk, however, the less chance there is that the interviewer will place you very high on his list of potential residents.

To answer this and similar open-ended questions, first respond briefly and succinctly to the single question, "What motivates you?" For example, you might cite your most applicable qualities by stating, "I am a hard worker with a real interest in ENT. I like both the diagnostic and therapeutic aspects of the specialty and seem to be good at the technical procedures that I have been allowed to do."

Then stop. Ask the interviewer if you should continue. This demonstrates that you understand the interactive nature of interviews and that you have consideration for the other person's role. When you ask whether you should continue, many interviewers will direct you to other areas to discuss further. This will help both you and the interviewer a great deal by allowing you to answer the questions that the interviewer really wanted to ask.

- Which three adjectives best describe you?
- Tell me a story about yourself that best describes you.
- If you were going to die in five minutes, what would you tell someone about yourself?
- If you died right now, what would you want on your tombstone?
- Of which accomplishments are you most proud?
- Do you have any hidden achievements or qualities of which you are secretly proud? What are they?
- What are your team-player/leadership qualities?
- What might give me a better picture of you than I can get from your résumé?
- Tell me about your adolescence.

- How have you changed since high school?
- What was the most important event in your life?
- What shaped you and got you to where you are today?
- What was the most difficult thing you have ever done?
- If you could be on the cover of any magazine next month, which one would it be? What would the caption say?
- What do you like to cook?
- How would your best-friend/roommates/relatives describe you? What negative things would they say?
- Why did you write . . . in your personal statement/essay?
- What do you recall about your day before you go to sleep at night?
- What one thing do you want conveyed to the residency committee?

4.   What are your strengths and weaknesses?

This question represents the "Tell me about yourself" question phrased negatively. It asks, "Tell me what's wrong with you."

Would you want to answer that question? Of course not. And it is extremely unlikely that you will ever come up against it. But an inquiry about your strengths and weaknesses, essentially the same question, is very common. Basically, the interviewer asks you to jump off a cliff of your own design. All you need to do is to redesign the cliff so you can climb rather than jump.

First, answer the question about your strengths concisely. The only danger is talking too much. Then work on the dangerous half of the question.

Everyone has weaknesses. "Each and every one of you has something that makes you a jerk," said a Lieutenant Colonel briefing a group of officers about to be promoted to General. "Get in touch with your 'inner jerk' and work on losing that ugly part of your personality." Okay, so a little bit of you is a "jerk." How do you respond?

You must turn your "weaknesses" into more strengths. What character flaws would the faculty in this specialty approve of? Is your weakness that you are obsessive about completing your work in an exacting manner? Or is it intolerance for clinicians who do not perform their patient-related tasks with a professional attitude? Maybe it is an inability to go home at night unless all your work is completed. These are, undoubtedly, the types of "failings" that the faculty will be interested in encouraging rather than disparaging. But in relating these faults, show at least a little remorse about having them. Don't be glib.

- Tell me about your "secret identity," the part of your personality that you don't share with strangers.
- Are there any skeletons in your closet that you want to tell me about?

- How well do you take criticism?
- What is your pet peeve?
- If you could change one thing about your personality, what would it be?
- What are your three strongest qualities?
- What are your two worst qualities?
- Have you demonstrated leadership in any extracurricular activities?

5.   *If you could be any cell in the human body, which would you choose to be, and why?*

This is not much different from the directive to "Tell me about yourself." It is, however, a bit more inventive and has been used by many interviewers, especially in Internal Medicine, ever since it found its way into *The New England Journal of Medicine* (1990;323:838). Unfortunately, you may have a hard time not being reminded of *Saturday Night Live's* Baba WaWa's similar question, "If you could be any kind of twee . . .?"

The neuron was overwhelmingly favored by applicants for Internal Medicine internships, and by those for Gastroenterology and Geriatric fellowships. Most applicants said they wanted to be neurons "to be in control, to be stimulated and stimulating, and to be the center of all things." Since you are now prepared in advance for this question, try to be original. Don't be surprised if this question pops up along the interview route.

- Do you see yourself as more relaxed/casual/informal or as more serious/ dedicated/committed?
- Which is more important, the ability to organize, structure, and prioritize, or the ability to be flexible, modify, and make do as needed?
- Which is more important, knowledge or imagination?
- If you could be any kitchen object, what would you be?
- If you could sing any one song beautifully, which one would you choose?
- What is the strangest Halloween costume you ever wore?

6.   *If your house was burning, what three objects would you save?*

Some residency interviewers really believe Freudian analysis will help them choose the best residents. While this may seem to be essentially the same type of question as the one above, think again. This question narrows the scope to a very concrete and personal level by asking, "What do you value in your own life?" How important are material objects to you? Are you "sensitive" enough to reach for your beloved's picture, or are you "sensible" enough to grab your loved ones, the car keys, and the credit cards?

There is no one correct answer to this question. The best answer depends upon the nature of the person asking the question. Often, the questioner actually wants to know whether you have planned ahead or can think quickly, since a fire is a real possibility in our lives—unlike turning into a tree or a cell.

An alternate form of this question is "If you had to repack your belongings, what wouldn't you have brought with you?" This question is even more concrete, at least for the majority of students traveling to interviews. The follow-up questions will certainly be "Why leave that behind?" and "Why did you bring it?" Pack carefully.

- If you had unlimited money and two free hours (one day, one week, one month) what would you do?
- If you had three wishes, what would they be? (Shades of *Aladdin!*)
- What in your life is most important to you?
- If you knew you only had 6 weeks to live, how would you spend the time?

7.   What kinds of people are your friends?

"Know my friends, know me," goes an old expression. People attract similar folks as friends. An applicant's description of his friends often gives interviewers deep insights into his personality. This type of question essentially asks you to talk about yourself in the third person.

Answer this question as if you were describing yourself. Interviewers often respond favorably when married applicants state that their spouse is their best friend. Describing a spouse's glowing personal attributes only serves to enhance the applicant, as long as these attributes are not used as a contrast to the candidate's own qualities.

- Describe your best friend/roommate/spouse and their life.
- How are you similar and dissimilar to your best friend?
- How would your friends or coworkers describe you?
- Has someone ever come to you for help with a major personal crisis? What have you done to alleviate their emotional pain?

8.   Who are your heroes?

Related to the question "Tell me about yourself," this is a deep probe into your psyche. It evaluates your self-image, direction, and goals. How the interviewer interprets your answer may, to some degree, reflect his or her own personality, age, and background.

This is perhaps the most difficult interview question to answer. In an age without obvious heroes, your choice will, by necessity, be very personal. There are several possible responses to this question.

One answer you may have already thought of is that you have no heroes. You have, however, just completed many years of schooling, during which you had many new experiences and met countless interesting people as teachers, friends, and patients. Viewed from that perspective, it would be an unusual, and perhaps very narrow-minded, individual who could not find someone to look up to as a role model.

Another possible answer is to cite a family member, friend, or personal acquaintance. The follow-up question, of course, will be "Why?" There should be some identifiable attribute this person demonstrates that justifies your distinguishing him or her as your hero. A parent, sibling, or spouse is usually a very good choice. It shows respect for your family and a firm commitment to your roots. If you choose a physician as your hero, be prepared to explain how you are trying, or will try, to emulate that person's attributes in your professional life.

Historic or public figures are perfectly acceptable answers. These heroes can be drawn from science, education, or many other fields. But tread lightly if your hero is a contemporary religious or political figure. An interviewer's bias may affect her evaluation if your choice of a hero exemplifies major philosophical differences between the two of you.

The worst answer is to name a contemporary star of television, the movies, or popular music. In that case, both you and your answer will probably be seen as very superficial.

- What is your favorite movie? Why?
- What is the last non-medical book you read?
- What do "success" and "failure" mean to you?
- If you could accomplish only one thing the rest of your life, what would that be?
- What do you believe?
- Do you have any Black/Hispanic/etc., role models in medicine?
- What physician characteristics do you admire most? Least?
- If you could dine with anyone from the past, present, or future, whom would it be?
- Among the people at your school, whose work or life do you admire? Why?
- Tell me about your father/mother.

9. What do you do in your spare time?

The primary danger here is in giving too long an answer. Everyone likes to talk about him- or herself and this is an invitation to do just that. But keep it brief. If you collect rocks, for example, you might say, "I am an avid rock collector and have been for about ten years. I have had the opportunity to travel across the United States and Canada pursuing my hobby." Then stop. If the interviewer wants to know any more, he or she will ask.

Your answer should show that you are not a couch potato (although a computer aficionado is okay). Do not describe activities that may cause injuries resulting in prolonged sick leave. Also, pick a non-controversial topic; avoid discussing hunting, guns, or religion unless you are certain that you will not raise the interviewer's hackles. In general, speak about community-oriented and people-centered activities. The focus of the rock collector's description might be the people she meets at collector's conventions.

The questioner usually wants to learn three things from this query.

First, does the applicant have any interests outside medicine? An interviewee with no outside interests sends a serious danger signal. Residents who have no outlet for the anxieties, stresses, and frustrations of residency training may decompensate—and become a problem for the residency faculty. If you have no overriding outside interest, simply mention what you do in your spare time. Yes, spending lots of time with your spouse and children is certainly an outside interest.

Second, is the applicant more enthusiastic about his or her avocation than about the prospect of training for and practicing in this medical specialty? The key here is to show equal enthusiasm for both.

Third, the interviewer is screening out those applicants who are so wrapped up in themselves that they will not be able to pay any attention to their patients, peers, and faculty. How do they spot these individuals? They are the ones who go on and on and on about their other activities with no prompting—even after the interviewer gives negative cues, such as turning away from the applicant, coughing, or even standing up. Answer questions about your outside activities, as you have answered the other questions—fully, briefly, and with enthusiasm.

- What are your favorite games and sports? Why?
- Have you done any volunteer work?
- Why did you choose these activities?
- If you had a completely free day, what would you do?
- What is the most bizarre thing you have ever done (or did in high school or in college)?

- What was the most unusual occurrence in your life in the past month?
- Do you think you can remain intensely focused on learning this specialty for the length of the program? For the rest of your professional career?
- Would you work if you didn't have to? Why?
- Besides your future medical accomplishments, what do you wish to be known for by your peers, friends, and family?
- Where have you traveled? Why?
- What non-medical magazines do you regularly read?
- What have you contributed to groups and activities in which you participated?
- What have you learned from your volunteer work?

10. Which social networking websites do you use?

Tens of millions of people now use web-based social networks as their main method of communication. In fact, most people you know probably use one or more such sites.

Which ones you use regularly can say a good bit about you. So, if you do use such sites, name the sites and say that you view them as a way to stay connected to friends and family. But don't seem too eager when discussing the sites, or respond "I can't bear to be without access." You don't want to appear to be a web addict.

As you are, presumably, a rational user of social networks, do point out their advantages to you, as well as how careful you are about what information you post on the site. Be prepared to discuss the personal and professional security issues related to networking sites and to the Web in general.

- How much time do you spend each week on social networking sites?
- Now that you're about to be a physician, are there any items that you will need to delete from the site? Why?
- How has the Internet changed medical practice? How do you think it will affect your medical practice?
- What experiences have you had with Electronic Medical Records?

11. It says on your résumé that . . .

You wrote that you have a particular skill or learning experience. That may have been one reason you got this interview. Okay, show us how you would apply it.

This request is not made in the abstract. Rather, the interviewer gives you a specific situation, usually associated with medical practice, and possibly with the residency, and asks you to show your stuff. You wrote that you had experience working in a medical clinic for indigent patients. They ask you how you would obtain necessary medications for a child whose parents did not have the money to pay for them. Or you wrote that you served as the student on your hospital's bioethics committee. What elements do you look for when doing a bioethics consultation, asks the interviewer.

In some cases, the request can be even simpler. The interviewer starts speaking to you in Spanish or Russian. Well, you said you could speak it.

Anything you put in your résumé is fair game for the interviewer, including your extracurricular activities, publications or research, ability in a foreign language, travel, etc. Don't embellish! You are certain to run across at least one interviewer who will want to speak to you in Serbo-Croatian if you said you speak it fluently. If you said you participated in a study of histamine in rats, an interviewer is sure to ask you to explain how you could study the chemical's role in headaches or toxic presentations during your residency.

Since you may be asked about them, bring any written materials, such as articles, book chapters, etc., listed in your résumé to the interview. Even if they haven't been published, bring a draft copy so you can show it to interviewers if asked.

This is called the "predictive interview technique." It is very effective when the interviewer can make a specific connection with something in the applicant's history. For interviewees, this can be either a wonderful or a devastating experience. Be careful what you put in your application materials.

- What did you like about Kuala Lumpur (to an applicant who said he had worked in a medical clinic there)?
- How would you design a study to test whether drug Z works in congestive heart failure (to an applicant who says she has done several drug-related studies)?

12. In what situations are you most efficient and effective?

Medicine, and especially residency, is best practiced by those who are time-efficient. Residency directors know that those who can manage their time well will often make excellent residents. Part of managing time, however, is knowing what makes you efficient. Have you thought about how you optimize your use of time? Do you know the strategies that help you accomplish tasks faster, more successfully, and in a timely manner?

A particular interest in some specialties is whether you can multi-task. That is, can you walk and chew gum at the same time? Or more to the point, can you successfully handle multiple patient-related tasks for multiple patients at once? This is essential to function well in emergency departments, busy clinics, and on hectic ward services.

- When are you least efficient and effective?
- How do you handle interruptions when you are busy?
- When are you most creative?
- What makes you procrastinate?
- Do you see time as your ally or your enemy?

13. To which organizations do you belong?

People join organizations that further their own agendas, be they recreational, spiritual, political, or professional. The organizations you belong to reflect your goals, background, and interests. The question here is: how much do you want to reveal?

Which groups you join reveals your religion, political or sexual orientation, and cultural heritage. Since prejudice exists in many guises, it may be best to simply discuss the professional medical organizations to which you belong. These should include the student arm of the specialty's national organization, and might also include the AMA, AOA, or AMSA.

Most interviewers now understand that pressing you for information about other organizations might violate state and federal hiring rules. Note, however, that anything you included in your application materials is fair game during interviews. If you list an organization on your résumé, the interviewer may ask you about it.

- Your name sounds Hispanic (Arabic, Italian, Vietnamese, etc.). Is it?
- How did you learn to speak (non-English language)?
- When was the last time you went back to (country of origin)?
- Why do you think you are a minority?
- Would you have any trouble working in this predominantly Catholic (LDS, Jewish, etc.) hospital?

14. What are your plans for a family?

You probably will be asked a variety of questions that are not only uncomfortable, but also patently illegal under state or federal statutes (such as some of those listed under Question 13, above). Such questions also provide ammunition for discrimination-in-hiring lawsuits. (These suits are rarely brought, however, because discrimination is hard to prove in court.)

The litmus test to see whether a question is illegal is to ask yourself, "Is it important to my job as a resident?" If it is relevant, then the question is probably justifiable. (The law, however, can be convoluted, see Figure 21.2.)

Questions about family, childcare, and birth control are most often directed at women applicants. Other candidates may hear inquiries about race, nationality, physical infirmities, religion, and other subjects that are illegal for employers to raise. (See "Marriage, Pregnancy, and Children" in Chapter 14 and also "Illegal Questions," below.)

How should you respond to such questions? This can be very tricky. There are several possible approaches. The most common one is to just answer the question in the most favorable manner possible. It is the most politic thing to do and will not eliminate you from the pool of potential candidates. For questions about family planning, you could simply state that you have no plans to interrupt your training to have a family at the present time. If you already have children, you might directly address the interviewer's concerns by stating that your past performance demonstrates that your family responsibilities will not detract from your work or affect your ability to show up on time. Directly answering such questions may be preferable to saying "I prefer not to answer." Just as when invoking your Fifth Amendment rights, the listener will often infer the most negative response.

You may not, however, want to answer such questions, either because of the answer that you would have to give or because your principles just will not allow it. You then have three choices.

The first choice, which will still permit you to remain a viable candidate, is to laughingly ask whether the answer to the question, or the question itself, is relevant to being a resident. If you do this lightly, the interviewer will be able to back off from the question without losing face.

If you derisively ask whether the question is relevant, or simply state that the question is illegal (your second choice), you will be on the interviewer's black list. Don't plan on getting into that residency program. But, if you do not get in and you still want to, you have the option of taking legal action against the program for violating your civil rights (your third choice). This has been done successfully in the business world many times. It is only a matter of (a short) time until these suits become frequent in the medical community. In fact, they may become commonplace enough that there will be much firmer control over the entire interview process in order to avoid legal entanglements.

Still, you should approach these illegal and uncomfortable questions in a relaxed manner. This will yield the best results.

A legal way to ask such questions might be "Is there anything about your personal life that may affect your performance in this demanding residency?" Your answer is "No."

- How important is your family to you?
- How do you plan to juggle marriage (relationship) and medical practice?
- What do your parents do for a living?

15. If you could no longer be a physician, what career would you choose?

Once again, let's see who is really hiding beneath the polished interview veneer. How deeply are you committed to medicine? Is it an interesting part of your life or is it the core of your existence? How easily can you come up with an answer that you find acceptable? How upset do you seem by such a prospect?

Very few people can fake a response to something this important. Interviewers, especially those who live and breathe medicine, use this question to find people who have the same level of commitment. Older interviewers may ask this more frequently, since many distrust the resolution of younger generations.

One other reason for asking this question is that some studies suggest that there is a high correlation between alternate career choices and certain specialties. Those going into Anesthesiology or Radiology, for example, usually select highly technical professional fields, such as engineering, research, the "hard" sciences, law, architecture, or finance-related business. Those entering Pediatrics tend to select teaching, other health-related professions, the humanities, the arts, or non-professional careers.

Variations of this question may also be used to test an applicant's grasp of reality. The interviewer may ask, "What do you think you will do when you stop practicing medicine (at the end of a career)?" Others will probe even a strong answer to see whether applicants have considered any alternatives if they suddenly cannot practice medicine, at least in their specialty.

- Why did you choose to be a physician?
- If your brain was the only part of your body that worked, what would you do with your life?
- What will happen if you develop a debilitating disease while in residency?

16. You seem really interested in research. How will you incorporate that interest into your residency and career?

Are you sure you want to go to *this* residency? If you are interviewing at a program within a research institution, the interviewer may simply be assessing the strength of your interest in research and, perhaps, how strong a clinician-researcher you might be. However, if the interview is at a program that is primarily or solely clinical, the question may be asking how well you investigated the program before applying, whether your goals are consistent with those of the program, or if you will be happy going through this residency. This is a very legitimate faculty concern. If you have research as a possible career goal, be sure to apply to programs that share this interest.

- What are the most important traits for a clinician/researcher?
- How will the research you have done alter scientific thought? Help mankind?
- Let's discuss the details of the research you have done.
- How did the idea come to you for any research you initiated?
- How might acupuncture work? Do we know enough about physiology and biophysics to determine that?

17. In what subspecialty would you like to practice?

It is perfectly reasonable to say that you plan on practicing the primary specialty. But you may already have your heart set on becoming, for example, a cardiologist or a neonatologist. Residency faculty know that a great many applicants, especially in General Surgery, General Internal Medicine, and General Pediatrics, plan to take subspecialty fellowships. Feel free to tell them that you are *considering* that course. Realize, though, that many residents change their minds about which subspecialty to enter once they get more clinical experience, so couch your answer with the reality that your future is not certain and you will make your decision at the appropriate time during your residency training.

If you do specify a subspecialty in which you are interested, be prepared to answer questions about that medical area. Also, you may be asked what you know about how well that subspecialty is represented at that residency's training institutions and program. Do you know who the subspecialists are? Do you know how much time you will spend with them during your residency? Given your interests, if that subspecialty is not well represented at their institutions, why did you choose to interview at their program?

- In light of the bleak future for subspecialists, why would anyone go into Cardiology or Gastroenterology today?
- Have you considered going into [insert the interviewer's subspecialty]?

18. How do you make important decisions?

As you discuss some very important life decisions you have made, the interviewer may wonder how you came to these decisions. Individuals vary in how they make important decisions. This reflects their personality and thought processes. Are they thoughtful, deliberate, and slow, or are they inattentive, impulsive, and quick? Or, does their decision-making method vary appropriately with the situation?

Be prepared to discuss your own decision-making strategies with interviewers. Think carefully before responding to this question, however. They may respond by asking if the method you describe matches the method you used to make your decisions to enter medicine and to apply for the specialty. Or they may inquire about how this process affects your ability to perform in specific clinical situations or to make other obvious life decisions, such as those revealed by your résumé.

If you use the Must/Want Analysis to help decide on the qualities you want in a residency, take a copy (without the program's ratings) to your interview and show it to any interviewer who asks you this question. They will probably be impressed with your logical and deliberate decision-making process.

- Are you a "risk-taker" or "safety-minded"?
- What made you choose your undergraduate major/minor?
- How did you select your undergraduate/medical school?
- What was the biggest obstacle in your life? How did you overcome it?
- What was the most difficult stand or position you ever defended? Why was it difficult?
- What was the most difficult decision you have had to make in your life? How did you make it?

19. What were the major deficiencies in your medical school training?

This is your opportunity to demonstrate some realistic insight into the past three-plus years of your life. How well did your basic science courses prepare you for your clinical rotations? What were the strongest elements in your training? Where were the holes that you need to fill? No one believes that any medical school is perfect; residency faculty know this as well as anyone. However, avoid taking major swipes at your school. You will be an alumnus of the residency program at which you train no less than you will be an alumnus of your medical school. While a rah-rah response is not appropriate, neither is downgrading the training that you have received. Remember, your medical school training has gotten you as far as this interview.

While mentioning any deficiencies in your training you have the perfect opportunity to talk about your plans to remedy the deficit. These may include taking extra work or courses during the balance of your senior year and electives you plan to take while in residency.

- Why did you choose your medical school? How satisfied are you with your decision?
- What preclinical (clinical) medical school courses interested you the most?
- Did you enjoy your medical school classes? Why?

20. How do you explain your ... (low grades? leaves of absence? poor clinical narratives?)

Not everyone who reads this book has an unblemished, stellar record. In fact, very few medical students do. Most have some areas of their records that require an explanation. Perhaps you failed a basic science course or a USMLE Step, and had to repeat it. Or maybe you had to take a leave of absence at some point in your training. You should expect to be asked about these deficiencies if the faculty members interviewing you are at all on the ball.

You already know what these issues are, and you need to be prepared to explain them. If there is a good justification for a questionable action, such as having to take time off due to a death in the family or a personal illness, explain. But if the poor grade or poor clinical performance on a rotation was, as is usual, due to your failure to put forth your best effort, just say so. Do not give excuses; they will sound lame to almost everyone except you. Your answer should be a variation of the terse military response, "No excuse, Sir." Say that you did not give the course, rotation, etc. your best effort. If you think you can get away with it, blame it on immaturity, ignorance, or youth. This works best if the problem occurred during your first year in school, especially if you can demonstrate that you have expended more effort in subsequent years. If you have any questionable areas hanging over your application, be prepared in advance to answer for your aberrant behavior.

- If you could begin your schooling again, what would you change?
- Have you ever dropped a class? Why?
- Have you ever quit or been fired from a job? Why?
- With these grade(s) in (medical school subject[s]), how did you even get an interview here?
- Do you smoke? Use drugs?
- Do you like to study? How do you study best? What motivates you to keep studying?
- What did you do during this (specified) period of time?

21. Have you always done the best work of which you are capable?

If you imagine that you can just answer yes or no to this question, you haven't gotten the drift of the interviewing business yet. The correct response to this question must not only show that you have put in a tremendous effort, but also demonstrate humility—by acknowledging that you could often have done a better job.

How to do this? Simply say that you have always striven to do the best possible job that you could, but the results did not always match your effort.

This again stresses that you are a hard worker, you are humble, and you understand your limitations—all positive attributes. And this is all nicely wrapped up in that one-sentence answer. Very elegant.

- What have been your biggest failures in life?
- What have you done to ensure that these failures won't happen again?

22. With which types of people do you have trouble working?

This question asks, "Why won't you fit into the clinical team that exists at this residency?" In essence, what personality problems do you have? Will Rogers, the famous American raconteur, said, "I never met a man I didn't like." Maybe so, but most people have some difficulties with arbitrary, obnoxious, and loud individuals. This is not, however, what you want to say. The correct answer, if you cannot honestly state that you usually get along with everyone, is that you generally have problems with those individuals who do not pull their own weight.

This is also the answer to the parallel question, "What qualities drive you crazy in colleagues?" Again, this emphasizes your interest in, and ability to do, hard work. At the same time, it will normally hit a responsive chord in the interviewer, who also probably dislikes picking up the workload for slack colleagues. No one, of course, ever recognizes this problem in him- or herself.

Some interviewers will attempt to get the names of negative references by asking, "Who didn't you get along with in medical school or in past jobs?" Luckily, this is an unusual request, if only because programs are besieged with too many applicants to follow up on the information. If you are asked for such references, your willingness to provide them and your ability to explain why you didn't get along with certain individuals will say a lot about your self-confidence, honesty, and insight.

- Describe the best/worst attending or resident with whom you have worked.
- Do you prefer to work under supervision or on your own?

23. Are you "culturally competent"?

"Cultural competency" is one of the current catchphrases in medical education. You are most likely to encounter this question when applying to programs in Family Medicine or at institutions with large patient populations that clearly differ from your own background.

Cultural competence is the ability to understand, communicate with, and effectively interact with people across cultures. It often is thought of as including: (a) an awareness of one's own cultural worldview, (b) knowledge of different cultural practices and worldviews, and (c) cross-cultural skills.

While understanding some of your own biases is possible, in-depth knowledge of and the skills needed to interact with all the cultures you will meet during your residency is impossible. So, the best answer to this question is "No." Qualify it by saying that you respect other cultures and do your best to understand and work with people whose backgrounds and beliefs differ from yours. And, of course, you're interested in learning as much as possible about the culture(s) of the patient populations commonly seen at this program.

- Do you have experience practicing medicine through an interpreter?
- Have you had international medicine experience? Do you plan to do so in the future?
- Do you speak other languages well enough to do a history and physical exam?

24. With which patients do you have trouble dealing?

The interviewer in this case is trying to determine whether you will generate multiple patient complaints—a situation that faculty and administrators abhor.

No one expects you to be thrilled when you have to deal with whining, abusive, demanding, alcoholic, or drug-seeking patients. Most physicians do not like to treat such patients. You should state that while there are certain personalities that irritate you, you attempt to recognize these patients and then try even more than usual to act in a professional manner during interactions with them. This demonstrates professional maturity, survival skills, and common sense.

If you really dislike dealing with certain racial, ethnic, or age groups, or with people in general, you should probably reconsider your decision to pursue a medical career.

- What are patients most afraid of when they visit a doctor?
- If I called the last patient you took care of, what would they say to me?
- What would you find most difficult to deal with if (when) you were a patient?

25. How do you normally handle conflict?

Hopefully, you can answer that your interactions with people rarely lead to conflict but, when there is conflict, you try to work the problem through to a reasonable and amicable settlement.

You may want to prepare an example of just such a situation that you faced and how it was resolved. Optimally, this example will demonstrate that the conflict was handled in a thoughtful and good-natured manner, with good will restored at the end. Your attitude, facial expressions, and body language when telling such a story will reveal much about your personality and your real ability to harmoniously work with others.

- How do you respond when you are having problems with a nurse, patient, another medical student, resident, or attending physician?
- What do you do if your senior resident or attending tells you to do something you know is absolutely wrong (medically or morally)?
- Have you ever challenged a teacher in class or a supervisor, resident, or attending physician at work? What were the circumstances?
- How do you handle disagreements with more senior colleagues, peers, nurses, and ancillary medical staff?
- How do you handle criticism, whether it's fair or unfair, from a superior, a subordinate, a peer, or a family member?
- What was the most useful criticism you ever received? Why?
- What was your most difficult/stressful life experience? How did you handle it?
- What frustrates you the most?

26. With what subject or rotation did you have the most difficulty?

Similar to the question concerning your strengths and weaknesses, this one asks you to incriminate yourself. You cannot plead the Fifth Amendment, so you need to know how to work through it. If you obviously had problems with a course, as evidenced by a poor grade or dismal narrative evaluations, you will have to address this. Do so in a direct manner. Otherwise, use the same strategy you used for the strength and weakness question. Pick "difficulties" that will exhibit some of the strengths that you want the interviewer to see.

For example, by stating that your Internal Medicine rotation was difficult because of the vast amount of information you needed to assimilate through extensive reading and clinical time, you will impress the interviewer with both your insight and your hard work. Discussing the time it took you to master some special suturing techniques on your Surgery rotation suggests to the interviewer that you have gained a clinical skill that is a prerequisite to training in the specialty. In general, you should emphasize that any trouble that you have had was the result of the long hours you spent (explanation, not a complaint) in the learning process. However, if you really did poorly in a course or on a clinical rotation, you are probably being asked to explain why you did so poorly (Question 20).

Commonly, the interviewer will have already spotted your problem area and will also ask, "How will that affect your performance as a physician?" Of course, your answer is that it won't affect your performance, since you already have (or plan to) overcome any problems in this area through hard work or extra training.

- Tell me about your first day in anatomy. How did it change you?
- What has been your greatest challenge?

27. Why do you want to go into this specialty?

This is probably the question most often asked of residency applicants. The question poses two dangers. The first lies in not having a good answer. If you have gone through the steps in this book, you will have no trouble answering the question. You initially found out what aspects of medical practice you enjoyed and then matched them to the specialty that encompassed most of them. Then, you talked with multiple specialists working in the field, read as much as you could about the field, and tested your choice by spending volunteer time working in the specialty. With this background to support your answer, you should have little trouble convincing the interviewer that you have firm and valid reasons for entering the specialty.

The second danger is that interviewers will ask you this question so often—sometimes two or three times at each program—that you will become bored with your own answer. This will be obvious in your response and will reflect poorly upon your candidacy. Since each interviewer tends to ask applicants similar questions, your response will be compared with the answers from the other candidates they have seen. Be enthusiastic when replying to this question—every time. Try to take a new tack when answering the question with different interviewers. This way you will avoid repeating the same phrases, which will sound stale and trite not only to you but also to the interviewers. You have an excellent answer to this question; make certain that your delivery is just as good.

- What would you be willing to sacrifice to become a (specialist)?
- What is the greatest sacrifice you have already made to get where you are?
- If (this specialty) did not exist, what would you do?
- How did lifestyle considerations affect your specialty choice?

28. Why did you apply to this program?

No specialty has only one training program. So this question comes up quite often in interviews. Having based your program selections on your personal "Must/Want" Analysis, you have some excellent answers to this question (pick the areas you value highly). Maybe the program is particularly strong in research or in a particular subspecialty that interests you. Or perhaps the faculty is outstanding. Your answer to this question should include whatever attracted you to the program. In addition, it never hurts to say that the program also got a strong recommendation from your specialty adviser.

Review all material you have about the program, as well as your personal evaluation of it, before beginning the day's interviews. If you remember to individualize your answer for each program, you should have no problem. Your knowledge about the program should include:

- Residency size
- Academic mission
- Key faculty names & special interests
- Patient volume
- Clinical training sites
- Elective opportunities

- Research opportunities
- Number of key procedures performed
- Patient population mix
- Percent of women, IMGs, or minorities admitted

If you don't have some of this information, that's okay. Make sure you ask for it at your first opportunity.

A more personal way of asking this question is, "Why are you willing to leave the West (or Northeast, Midwest, etc.) to come here to train?" Rather than obviously directing the question toward the program's educational elements, the question appears to be asking a more personal question. Without thinking, you may answer, "Well, I don't really want to live anywhere but the Boston area, but I heard this was a good program and I thought I'd take a look." Bad move! You have fallen into the interviewer's trap. It is not even worth considering you for a position, since you said you would be unhappy away from Boston. The better answer is to say (hopefully with some truth) that you are willing to move anywhere there is a fine training program in this specialty. Then tell the interviewer what you consider to be the program's fine qualities.

- What qualities are you looking for in a program/residency?
- What interests you most about this program/residency?
- What have you heard about our program that you don't like?
- Are you applying here because it is a familiar environment?
- What do you think you will contribute to our specialty or to your community?
- How can you be sure that (specialty) is the right career for you?
- You said (a statement) in your application essay. What did you mean?
- What would you want your patients to say about you?
- What can be done to ensure that physicians are in (specialty) for the "right" reasons?

- Why do you want to leave (city or state where you live)?
- What do you think will be the most difficult aspect of living in this city, coming as you do from . . .?
- Do you know what you are getting into? Have you talked with physicians about what a career in our specialty is really like?

29. What will be the toughest aspect of this specialty for you?

This is another way of asking you about your strengths and weaknesses. Only the most skilled interviewers usually ask this form of the question.

Every specialty has complex areas to master; each specialty has its onerous aspects. What do you foresee as difficult areas for you? Your answer may deal with your learning to master certain skills or with the vexing areas of the specialty's practice.

It would be unrealistic for you not to recognize some difficult areas of the specialty, and failure to cite some might indicate that you know little about the specialty, yourself, or both. A good way to answer this question is to note one or more small or commonly recognized difficult areas, such as physics training in Radiology, and describe how you intend to overcome any problems you might have. The fact that you envision only small problems will either placate the interviewer or lead to other questions to be certain that you haven't missed the big picture.

If the question is asked in the form of the "most enjoyable" part of the specialty for you, answer in the most specific terms you can. Cite examples of experiences you had while working in the specialty that excited you, stimulated you to read further, or suggested interesting research opportunities. The more specific you can be, the better your answer will be received, and the better the interviewer will remember you.

- How will you handle the least interesting or least pleasant parts of this specialty's practice?
- What qualities are most important in this specialty?
- What would you be willing to sacrifice to become a (specialist)?
- What is the greatest sacrifice you have already made to get where you are today?
- Are you willing to work graveyard shifts and all weekends for a month or more at a time?
- How long have you stood on your feet at one time?
- Have you ever noticed negative aspects of (specialty) physicians with whom you have come in contact?
- What negative aspects do you see to pursuing a (specialty) career?

30. Why should we take you in preference to the other candidates?

Danger! This is one of those questions designed to quickly lead you down the garden path to disaster. What is your first response? Most of you would attempt to defend yourself against attack, probably by trying to compare yourself favorably with other candidates whom you either know or imagine. Wrong move.

Start by acknowledging that you will not make the decision about who gets into the residency. State that you are not qualified to make that type of decision. In addition, acknowledge that there undoubtedly are many good candidates applying to the program. Then, state that you can really only describe your own qualities and ask the interviewer if he or she would like you to do just that. If the answer is yes, you have an excellent opportunity to tout your best qualities and finest achievements.

Obviously, to answer the interviewer's initial question, you will want to stress those qualities that distinguish you from other candidates. You should concentrate on some of the areas mentioned previously—*energy level*, the *desire to do and to learn*, and the *ability to get along with others* under all circumstances. Never disparage other candidates. Only stress your own excellence.

- What can you add to our program/residency class?
- What computer experience do you have?
- What are some of the qualities a good physician should possess? Do you possess them?
- How will your background in . . . be of any use in this specialty?
- If you were on our residency committee, what would you look for in an applicant?
- Why should I tell the residency committee to pick you?
- If we had one spot left in the residency class, what one of your attributes qualifies you more than any other candidate?
- What makes you unique?
- Give me your sales pitch.

31. I don't think you'd be right for this program/specialty.

Medicine has some pretty crass folks populating its ranks, but very few would actually invite you for an interview and really mean it when they tell you that you would not be right for their program, much less the specialty.

If you are told this, recognize it for the ploy that it is. The statement is meant to fluster and confuse an applicant. A rather nasty maneuver, used only by cruel interviewers, it can easily be sidestepped if you see it coming. This is a statement that can only be answered successfully with a question. That question is "Why do you say that?"

If you come out swinging to defend yourself, you lose. Put the interviewer on the defensive by asking the question in your nicest, most polite manner. This will throw him or her off guard, and you might even receive an apology.

- Describe your ideal residency program in this specialty.
- Idaho … Hmm … Isn't that where the separatist militias live?
- I see that neither of your parents graduated from high school. What does that say about your genetic background?
- How would you contribute to this residency's reputation?

32. What is your energy level like?

Although this may be an interviewer's standard question, watch out. Some only ask this of older applicants and those who demonstrate less-than-adequate energy levels during their interviews. If you feel yourself fading, pump out a little more adrenaline and beef up your act. Now is the time to show your energy level. If you can't do it now, what will it be like at 3 A.M. while you are on call?

A question about your energy level must be answered with an enthusiastic "Very high." A very brief anecdote of just how high it is would be appropriate. An example might be, "I was able to make rounds on all my Medicine patients and write notes each morning before the residents even arrived." Try to make your anecdote appropriate to the specialty for which you are interviewing.

- When do you work harder than you ordinarily do?
- How many hours of sleep do you require each night?
- How well do you function without adequate sleep?

33. How well do you function under pressure?

Every physician, at one time or another, has been under pressure while practicing medicine. Some specialties have frequent stressors, and the physicians in them seem to thrive under this stress. Asking you about your performance under stress is, therefore, a natural question. The interviewer wants to know two things. First, have you thought about the pressures inherent in residency training, as well as those peculiar to this specialty? And second, are you up to them?

Assuming that you have gone through all the right steps to select this specialty, your answer should indicate that you operate at peak performance under the type of stressful conditions encountered in the specialty. Cite specific examples of your past performance under stress. Be sure that the examples, however, do not show that the stress resulted from your negligence, procrastination, or obstinacy. Assure the interviewer that you are up to the challenges this specialty has to offer.

A potential curve ball here may be a secondary question dealing with the administrative stressors brought on by government and third-party payer interference with medical practice. This question may be raised because it is constantly, and annoyingly, on many practitioners' minds. If this topic is raised, either state that you are certain that you will learn to handle these problems during residency, or respond by simply asking the interviewer "What are the biggest problems you are facing in this area?" In all likelihood, the interviewer will be pleased to speak about the subject at length. Be a good listener.

- How do you handle stress?
- Can you handle stress without the resources you are accustomed to relying on?
- When was the last time you cried?
- Have you ever faced death? How did you handle it?

34. Tell me about the patient from whom you learned the most.

This is a favorite question of elderly professors, as well as smarter young interviewers. It examines your medical knowledge, your insight into the patient's condition, your ability to think quickly, your attitude toward medicine and learning, and your compassion. If an interviewer asks this question, the balance of the interview remains on the same topic. How, then, should you approach it?

To be able to answer this question satisfactorily, you must prepare at least two patient cases in advance. Try to choose examples at least somewhat relevant to your chosen specialty. Select patients in whose care you were intimately involved. These should be people you helped treat for a prolonged period of time—either during many concentrated hours or periodically over time. If they had a specific disease or injury, read about it in depth. If they had a multisystem disease, be able to describe its effect on the various organs grossly and microscopically, as well as clinically.

What was it that you learned from these patients? Was it just the nature of the disease? Normally, this will not be enough. Did you learn something about your own limitations as a physician, the patient's fears and perceptions of the medical system, or the workings of the health care system itself? If you did, be prepared to say so. Also, know the follow-up information on the patients. If they were discharged, review their medical records to find out how they are doing now. If they died, did you attend the autopsy? (Attending your patients' autopsies is a good idea throughout your training—it reveals to you both what you missed and what you were powerless to change.) If you did not attend, obtain a copy of the autopsy report and read it. Following up on interesting patients demonstrates both your concern for them and your excitement in learning.

If you have prepared for this question and have begun to answer it appropriately, the interviewer may interrupt with his or her own "war story." Sit back, listen, and enjoy. You did just fine.

Over the years, applicants throughout the country have consistently said that being prepared for this question was the best advance planning they did for their interviews.

- What were your most memorable experiences in medical school/ college?
- If you had to choose the single most valuable thing you have ever learned, what would it be?
- What was the (non-medical) situation in your life when you had the greatest responsibility?
- Tell me about the non-physician health care provider who most influenced you.

35. What error have you made in patient care?

This is very similar to the question above, concerning the patient from whom you learned the most. In fact, the case illustrating your biggest error may be the same as the one from which you learned the most. If it is, say so. This question is used to test your humility, to ascertain whether you were allowed to do enough on your own as a medical student so mistakes were possible, and to determine whether you can learn from your mistakes. Obviously, these are all significant issues. Make sure you have prepared your reply before you visit any programs.

- What is your greatest fear about practicing medicine?
- What is your greatest fear about entering this specialty?
- What was the worst thing that ever happened to you? Why?

36. Where do you see yourself in five (ten) years?

Some realism, as well as the ability to read what the program and the specialty desire, is required to accurately answer this question. The questioner is attempting to find out if you have some life goals—and if these are consistent with the training that the program has to offer.

Have you looked beyond your existence as a trainee? Are you realistic? Do you expect to be the Surgeon General of the United States within the decade following the completion of your residency? Or perhaps you propose to be a full professor and head of a department at a major medical school. Both expectations are, of course, not realistic in the near future. On the other hand, applying to a high-powered academic residency program as preparation for working part-time at a small neighborhood clinic also may not demonstrate much realism.

The problem of incongruent goals stems from your evaluation either of your own abilities or of the program's goals for its residents. Residency faculties usually have at least a general vision of what they would like most of their graduates to do with their careers. They want your goals to be consistent with those of the program. This is beneficial to both you and them. For example, if a training program has been designed primarily to produce academic physicians, residents who hope to become community doctors will be very unhappy in it, and the faculty may be very dissatisfied with those residents as well.

To answer this question, you should have previously analyzed the program's written materials. Do they promote goals consistent with your personal goals? If the two widely diverge, perhaps you should consider looking elsewhere. Do not, however, be too certain about your final career direction. Many, if not most, residents significantly change their career orientation during or shortly after training. This should not upset you; it is a normal part of learning and maturation.

So, answer this question by giving a general response while listening to the interviewer. Try to understand the diversity of learning experiences that exist within the training program. Leave enough latitude in your reply, however, to allow for other possibilities in your future. Also, always phrase your answer in terms of a probability that may change with training, experience, and age.

- In ten years, in what specialty and under what circumstances will you be practicing? Who will be paying for your services?
- What are your life goals? What have you done to accomplish them?
- How would you describe "success"?
- Draw a picture of yourself in ten years.

37. How do you see the delivery of health care evolving in the twenty-first century?

This can be a very tricky question. It tests your knowledge of current events and politics, as well as your humility in recognizing that you do not have the ultimate answer. The interviewer, though, may think that he or she does. Only people who already have definite opinions about the trends in health care will ask this question. They actually may want to use it as a jumping-off point from which to expostulate on their pet theory. Since people like to hear themselves talk, give the interviewer a chance to say what is on his or her mind while appearing interested and you will do just fine.

The strategy for you is to give a broad answer to the initial question, such as "I expect that there will be numerous changes, not only in the way medicine is practiced, but also in the way it is paid for." You can go on to add that you do not have any definitive answers. This will give the interviewer a chance to jump in and give you either the lecture that was lying in wait, or at least some definite hints as to what he or she is thinking. You do not want to stick your neck out without some guidance.

This question is probably the closest that you will get to a direct inquiry about your political views, which is illegal in pre-employment questioning. Listen closely, nod your head a lot, and do not go out on a limb without some support.

- Would you be willing to work under a single-payer (government-run) health care system?
- How little would your annual take-home pay have to be for you to leave medicine for another field?
- What are do you think about homeopaths, naturopaths, and herbal medicine?
- How will a socialized medical system affect medical progress?
- If you were made King of the United States, what one thing would you change about health care delivery? Why?
- What is managed care? HMOs? PPOs? Capitation?
- What is the biggest challenge facing health care delivery?
- What does "a cross-cultural approach to healing" mean?
- What will you do as a physician to curb the rising costs of medicine?
- What is the nurse's role and how much responsibility should a nurse be given for patient care?
- Where does the money go in a prepaid medical system?
- What recent newsworthy medical event or announcement would you like to discuss?
- What is your least healthy personal habit?
- What is currently the biggest challenge in healthcare delivery?
- What is the solution to the health care crisis?

38. *What challenges will our specialty face over the next five (ten) years?*
This question is an important variation on the question about health care in general. It provides an opportunity for you to take the broad concepts related to

changes in health care and direct them towards the specific specialty to which you are applying. Have you given the specialty's future any thought? Have you given your own future enough thought? The information you obtained to answer the general question (above) about health care in the next century should give you plenty of ammunition to carry on a conversation about changes that might occur in this specialty. Of course, your wealth of knowledge about the specialty will also come in handy here.

As mentioned in the question relating to general changes in health care, give the interviewer an opportunity to sound off if it seems like that is what he or she wants to do. Listen actively. Be ready to jump in gently with an idea or two of your own, but don't argue. Some interviewers may bait you to see if they can make you angry or upset. No matter what they say, keep your cool. Remember that at least one of you has to remain professional.

- What do you think is the number one issue facing our specialty today?
- What would have to happen for you to leave (specialty) for another type of medical practice?
- Will new technological developments change our specialty? For better or for worse?

39. How will "professionalism" affect you in your residency? In practice?

"Medical professionalism" is commonly discussed as a vital concept at medical teaching hospitals. It seems, however, that everyone has their own definition of what this means. When asked this question, which will inevitably happen during these interviews or during your residency, you can answer either by first asking "How do you define professionalism?" or by using the elements (listed below) from Swick's frequently cited article (Swick HM: Toward a normative definition of medical professionalism. *Acad Med.* 2000;75:612–6.) to describe your perception of the term. In either case, this may lead to an interesting discussion of professionalism. You'll make a great impression on your interviewer.

According to Swick, medical professionalism (note that the items spell out the mnemonic "SALVE CURE") means that physicians . . .

1. *Subordinate their own interests* to the interests of others
2. are *Accountable* for themselves and for their colleagues
3. exhibit a commitment to *scholarship and Learning* to advance their field

4. evince *core humanistic Values*, including honesty and integrity, caring and compassion, altruism and empathy, respect for others, and trustworthiness
5. adhere to *high Ethical and moral standards*
6. respond to societal needs with *behaviors reflecting a social Contract* with the communities they serve
7. *deal with high levels of complexity and Uncertainty*
8. *Reflect* upon their actions and decisions
9. demonstrate a continuing *commitment to Excellence*

- Do you always act professionally while in a medical environment?
- During medical school, which of your physician teachers was the most professional? Why?
- Have there been times when you could have acted more professionally?

40. If a patient just stabbed your best friend . . . ?

Honing in on one element of professionalism, many interviewers' favorite question is an ethics scenario. In virtually all cases, it involves a situation in which there is no single "correct" answer. However, as with all ethics questions, some answers are wrong.

The key to answering this question (the question itself is usually, "What would you do?") is to tell the interviewer that you need a moment to think about it. Then think through at least one answer that does not violate either your personal or general professional values. Relate this to the interviewer. It is best if you do not say that your responses are based upon your religion, even if they are. Generalities, such as protecting patient autonomy or avoiding paternalism, work best.

Do not appear dogmatic; state that you are sure that there are other possible options. The interviewer may want to discuss the problem. If so, listen to the options presented and discuss them. Do not argue! Try to see the interviewer's point of view, but do not escalate the discussion into a religious debate or a shouting match. There's an old saying which suggests that one should never discuss religion or politics with friends, or you are bound to lose them. That applies just as well to residency interviewers.

- What would you do if the housestaff had a "job action" (strike)?
- What would you do if you saw another resident or physician snorting cocaine at a nightclub? On the job?

- What do you think about using animals in medical research/teaching?
- Should physicians be involved in assisted suicide or active euthanasia?

- What ethical questions will the health care delivery system face in the future?
- Should applicants who say they don't want to treat (AIDS, hepatitis B, life-threatening plague, etc.) patients be admitted to our specialty?
- What would you do if you knew Dr. X was cheated on an in-service exam?
- Is health care rationing ethical?
- Would you treat a colleague and a patient, each coming to you with an unwanted pregnancy, differently?
- How would you respond if a resident or a colleague wanted to keep a therapeutic error a secret from a patient and the patient's family?
- What do you think of hospitals that refuse admission to patients without insurance?

41. What do you think of what is happening in the (economy, China, Congress)?

The interviewer is trying to find out if you have pulled your head out of your medical books in the past four years. It's wise to prepare for this question by reading weekly news magazines for a month or two prior to the interview season. It is also prudent to read the newspaper and, if possible, watch the morning news on the day of your interview.

As for the question itself, hope that it is on a relatively innocuous subject. If not, don't antagonize the interviewer by giving a polarized viewpoint. Try to take a balanced view, looking at both sides of the issue, e.g., "on the one hand . . ., but on the other hand . . .." This shows that you do not have your head in the sand and that you are a diplomat—both desirable qualities.

- What is the last non-medical book you read?
- Are physicians doing enough to improve public health policies?
- Are physicians doing enough for women's issues?
- What do you think is the largest problem facing American society on a statewide or a national basis?

42. Teach me something non-medical in five minutes.

This is now the question I use most often. It shows me a great deal about applicants, including how well many of them think on their feet. It is also more fun to start off an interview this way than with many of the routine questions most interviewers ask.

With this directive, applicants have a marvelous opportunity to discuss something in which they are an expert—and the interviewer has guaranteed that he or she will pay rapt attention. Pick a topic that you know really well and that you can explain a small piece of to a novice in five minutes.

But which topic is best? Is it something about your hobby, something unique you learned in childhood, something from a previous job, or something truly different, such as a lesson you learned through a difficult experience? The key here is to pick a topic that will interest listeners, that fascinates you, and that can be successfully taught in the allotted time. Among the topics applicants have discussed are how to tie fishing lures, how to write a simple computer program, and how to select a melon. Not that I always understood them, but they were always interesting. Often this directive leads naturally to further questions about the topic.

Many applicants and interviewers find this the best, and most productive, interview question.

- Without using your hands, tell me how to tie a shoelace.
- How are art and medicine similar?
- What is "beauty"?
- Why are manhole covers round?
- Why is it called "the practice" of medicine?
- If you were the residency directory, how would you evaluate your performance halfway through your first year of residency?
- Give an example of a problem you solved and describe how you went about solving it.

43. Does the reverse side have a reverse side?

The comedian Steven Wright has made a career of asking unanswerable questions. Many of the questions attributed to him are actually from anonymous sources. This type of question can rattle, provoke, or amuse residency interviewees, depending on the intensity of the situation, their ability to understand spoken English, and the interviewer's attitude.

If you recognize that you are being asked this type of question—and most interviewees immediately will—laugh. Giving any other response is ridiculous.

- When the light goes out, where does it go?
- Why are there five syllables in the word "monosyllabic"?
- How come Superman could stop bullets with his chest, but always ducked when someone threw a gun at him?
- When I erase a word with a pencil, where does it go?
- Why do we wait until a pig is dead to "cure" it?
- Why do we put suits in a garment bag and garments in a suitcase?

- How many ping pong balls fit in an airplane?

44. Tell me a joke!

Several residency applicants say that they have been asked to tell the interviewer a joke—and that it was their greatest interview challenge. Don't improvise. It may be prudent to have one or two hilarious jokes that are clean, non-sexist, non-racist, non-religious, etc. As a source for this type of material, you might want to check out *Reader's Digest*.

- Name as many words that start with the letter "F" as you can in 10 seconds. (Careful now!)

45. Where else have you interviewed?

This is many residency directors' favorite question. Don't become paranoid when you hear it. In most cases, they are not trying to test your interview choices. They are doing two things.

The first is determining whether you have selected programs in a reasonably sufficient quantity and of a quality to assure that you match with a program.

The second reason they ask is usually to find out current information about other training programs. Often, you are the best source of information that is available to them about other residencies. Interviewers will be interested in pumping you for facts. Give them what they want. Tell them about what is going on in the places you visited. You may have to review all of your notes before each interview. If you just do not remember some of the specifics, be honest enough to say so. The interviewer will appreciate this. Be enthusiastic. But, as mentioned before, under no circumstances should you say anything derogatory about other programs or other faculty. If you say negative things about other programs to this interviewer, what will you say about this program when you go elsewhere? Negative comments are a sign of immaturity. Avoid them.

46. What if you don't match?

Okay. Now let's see you sweat a little. This question is most often asked during interviews for residency positions in the most-difficult-to-match-with specialties and programs. If you are not prepared for this question, you may internalize it and consider that it is a backhanded way of suggesting that you had better make other plans, since you won't be getting into a residency in this specialty. Keep cool. That is not why applicants are usually asked this question.

The interviewer is trying to determine whether you have had the foresight to plan for contingencies. Planning ahead says something about your personality.

Not making alternative plans if you are applying to an Orthopedic Surgery or Ophthalmology program is just plain foolish. And people who do foolish things with their lives are not the people these programs look for as residents. They also do not want applicants who are so uncommitted to the specialty that they say, unconcernedly, that they will simply train in another specialty if they do not match in this one. Interviewers would like you to mention alternative plans that include methods for getting into one of the specialty's training programs.

One such plan may be that you have also applied to some one-year programs, such as Preliminary Medicine or Surgery or some Transitional programs, so you will have a training slot for the coming year if you do not match in the specialty. However, you will still be in a position to re-apply to the specialty in the following year.

47. Can you think of anything else you would like to add?

The answer to this question should always be "Yes." If the interviewer has neglected any critical area that further explains your qualifications for a residency position, mention it now. Even if nothing was omitted, use this opportunity to give an abbreviated summary of your sales pitch.

This is an alternate form of the frequent query, "Do you have any (other) questions?" that can be positioned at either the beginning or the end of the interview. This question can be a disaster at the end of a long interview day when you are tired, hungry, and sleepy—just like an intern. The wimpy response, "No, I think all of my questions have been answered," is not likely to score very many points with an interviewer.

Even if prior interviewers have already answered all your questions, ask one of them again. A very useful question, of course, is to ask for information that you wish to verify. Here you will have an opportunity to confirm or clarify the information. Another type of question to ask is one that will demonstrate your knowledge of the specialty's clinical or political activities. An example would be "What is your feeling about the new genetic treatment for glioblastomas reported last month?" In any event, do not leave the interviewer in the lurch when you are given an opportunity to ask a final question.

• Is there anything else I should know about you?

48. If we offered you a position today, would you accept?

You are just finishing the last interview. Sitting with the residency director or department chief, you are suddenly faced with this question. Your first thought is "They can't ask me this. It's against Match rules."

Figure 21.1
Illegal Questions–Sex Discrimination

1. What was your maiden name? (They can ask, "What name is on your transcripts, diplomas, licenses, etc.?")

2. Do you wish to be addressed as Miss, Mrs., or Ms.?

3. Are you married? Single? Divorced? Separated? A single parent?

4. I see that you are wearing an engagement ring. When is the wedding?

5. What is your spouse/partner's name? What does (s)he do for a living?

6. How does your spouse/partner feel about your having a career?

7. Do you believe residents should use birth control?

8. Are you planning to have children? Anytime soon? (They can ask, "Do you foresee any long-term absences during your residency?")

9. How will you take care of your children while at work? (They can ask "Is there any reason why you cannot be at work at 6 A.M. or stay in the hospital for in-house night call?")

Unfortunately, some programs disregard all rules, especially if they are desperate for good candidates. This question really puts you in a bind. If the program is clearly your top choice, you have no problem. If it isn't, or if you have not seen enough programs to know yet, what do you say? A perfectly reasonable response is, "I would love to accept a position in this program. I feel obligated, however, to keep the (six) other interview appointments I have made. I will be finished with these interviews in two weeks and could let you know then." Usually programs will accept this answer. Take care, though, to make sure you *really* do have a position guaranteed if you take them up on their offer (see "Don't Believe Anything You Are Promised," in Chapter 23).

Illegal Questions

Interviewers continue to ask many applicants, especially women, blatantly illegal questions (Figures 21.1 and 21.2). One survey found that 86% of residency applicants had been asked illegal questions. The most common of these are about marriage and family plans. Indeed, asking women about childbearing and childcare is the most common gaffe interviewers make. Besides implicitly

Figure 21.2
Other Questions—Legal & Illegal Forms

Legal Form	Illegal Form
• How well can you handle stress?	• Does stress ever affect your ability to be productive?
• Do you currently use illegal drugs?	• What medications do you currently use?
• Do you drink alcohol?	• How much alcohol do you drink per week?
• Do you have 20/20 corrected vision?	• What is your corrected vision?
• Can you perform as a resident with or without reasonable accommodations?	• Would you need reasonable accommodations to perform your job as a resident?
• How many days were you absent from school last year?	• How many days were you sick last year?
• To what professional organizations, clubs, societies, and lodges do you belong?	• To what organizations, clubs, societies, and lodges do you belong?
• What languages do you speak, read, or write fluently?	• What is your nationality? How did you learn to speak, read, or write a foreign language?
• If you are not a U.S. citizen, do you have the legal right to remain permanently in the U.S.? If "no": What is your visa status? and Can you provide proof of eligibility for employment if hired?	• Are you a U.S. citizen?

asking whether a woman has children, this assumes that she must be the sole person responsible for making childcare arrangements. (Wrong!) Also, if a female applicant inquires about the provisions for maternity leave, she is often written off as not being a serious candidate.

Another set of illegal questions relates to disabilities. Under the Americans With Disabilities Act, if an individual has a visible disability (for example, uses a wheelchair or guide dog) or discloses voluntarily that he or she has a disability, the interviewer may not ask about its nature, its severity, the condition causing the disability, the prognosis, or treatments. They may ask about the applicant's ability to satisfy essential functions or requirements of the position, as long as all applicants are asked the same questions.

Since illegal questions are still being asked of all applicants (why this is allowed to continue is uncertain), it is important for you to be prepared for these questions.

How Should You React to Illegal Questions?

If you are asked these questions, there are three possible ways to respond:

Refuse to answer the query, perhaps stating that it is illegal to ask such questions or that it is none of the interviewer's business. Such an answer, however, while it is perfectly correct and legitimate, is likely to ensure that you will not get a residency position at that site.

Finesse the question. One way to do this is to ask the interviewer whether this information is really pertinent to obtaining a residency position. This gives the interviewer, who probably has been poorly prepared to do this type of interviewing, a chance to back off and save face at the same time. However, finessing a question must be handled with skill. Smile and be very pleasant while you parry these pointed questions. If you handle it correctly, you will still be a viable candidate for the program.

Answer the question. Most applicants take this tack, both in the medical field and in other employment situations. You can use either direct or indirect answers. For example, if asked about plans for a family and children, the direct answer might be "I plan to have children near the end of my residency." Since you might find this option distasteful, you could use an indirect answer, such as "My training comes first." These answers usually will not jeopardize your chance of obtaining a residency training position. Also, the interviewer probably does not even realize that he (or she) is being sexist and is violating both federal and state civil rights codes.

22

Post-Visit Follow-Up

We despise no source that can pay us a pleasing attention.

Mark Twain

JUST BECAUSE THE INTERVIEW is over do not think that you have finished your visit. You still have some work to do to maximize the effort you have already expended. This includes writing thank-you e-mails and letters, providing additional requested materials, and adjusting and completing your "Must/Want" Analysis for the program.

Thank-You Correspondence

The key to using post-interview thank-you e-mails and letters effectively is to remember that "out-of-sight is out-of-mind." Your letters will reinforce the positive impression you left with the interviewers. Remember, you were not the only candidate interviewed that day. And, by the time the faculty gets your e-mail and letter, they will have met even more applicants.

Return yourself to the front of the interviewers' minds by sending them short thank-you e-mails followed by typed letters. But, there are some rules to follow to obtain maximum results.

You should send a thank-you note to each person that interviewed you during your program visit. Make sure that you save the list of names, with the correct spellings, of the people with whom you interview, eat, or tour the facilities. Ask the residency secretary for a list of their names and e-mail addresses or, better yet, get the information from the program's website.

What To Include In Your Correspondence

E-mail

Within 24 hours of the interview, send a short thank-you e-mail (Figure 22.1) to each individual who interviewed you or who escorted you on a tour of the facilities. Don't simply list their names in the "cc" box of a generic note, however. Make each person feel special by sending them an individual e-mail with, if possible, a specific note about something both of you discussed or experienced during your time together. It takes only a little more effort to do

Figure 22.1
Follow-up E-mail Format

To: [E-mail address. If it bounces, call the residency secretary to get correct address.]
Subject: Thank you!

Dear Dr. [Interviewer's Last Name]:

Paragraph 1: Thank the interviewer for the courtesy and consideration shown to you during your recent residency interview [today/yesterday].

Paragraph 2: Reaffirm your interest in the program. Mention anything you did not mention during the interview that enhances yourself as a candidate for their program and for the specialty. (Make it brief.)

Paragraph 3: Say that you will provide any requested information once you return home.

Paragraph 4: Use a simple, positive closing sentence, such as "I look forward to working with you in the future."

Sincerely yours,
[Your name]
[Address, Telephone number(s)]
[E-mail address]

---

this, since you can cut and paste the basic message from a word processing file and then simply add the personalized items. Doing it this way looks very professional.

Mention specific topics of mutual interest that were raised during your interview, e.g., "the exciting new neonatal transport program" or "the unique border medicine experience." Include enough personal information to ensure that the reader will remember your interview. Match the e-mail's formality to the tone of the interview you had. Don't go for wit or length; concentrate on making yourself memorable.

Definitely send the e-mails within 24 hours of your interview. If you are still traveling, use your computer, tablet or smart phone, or use a computer in the hotel, internet café, or airport.

Letter

Unlike your e-mails, direct your letter to the main interviewer—generally the residency director. But don't forget the other interviewers; mention all of the interviewers in the text. Many applicants who send thank-you letters ignore these folks, even though they often have a major say in deciding whether their program ranks a candidate.

In addition, send each interviewer a copy of the letter you sent to the residency director, but include a brief, personalized note at the bottom of each one. This note should be handwritten (print if your penmanship is terrible). Again, you want them to remember you, so mention a subject that you discussed with that person during your interview. Try to make it something that only you, and not other applicants, may have discussed. That way you will achieve the maximum effect for each stamp you lick.

One tactic to enhance these letters is to quickly peruse each interviewer's office and bookshelves during your interview to try to ascertain his or her personal interests. Look for something unusual or unique you can mention during the interview. This will provide you with a subject to use as a good memory jogger later on. Of course, you will need to make notations on your Interview Notes form (Figure 18.2) to remind you of what to write to whom.

Send typed letters. Figure 22.2 shows a suggested format for your letter. And be sure to actually enclose any requested information with the letter. A few applicants forget this important step and must send a second letter.

Also, with the capability of computers and laser printers to produce quality photographs, it might be useful to have your picture on each of these letters, to better remind the interviewers who you are. If you don't have access to a color printer, most copy or print shops can quickly do this for you if you bring along a photograph.

Try to send the letters within 48 hours of the interview. You might not even be home yet, and I know that trying to stop and produce these letters will be a major inconvenience. But it's worth the effort. Take materials with you and get your thank-you letters out expeditiously. Most applicants now carry tablet or notebook computers with them and visit a local print/copy shop to generate their letters before leaving the city where they interviewed.

Telephone Follow-Up

Although many job applicants follow up their interviews with telephone calls, calling a residency director is usually counter-productive. Physicians are busy and do not like having their time wasted by sales pitches (from anyone). Unless you need to provide or obtain urgent information, or unless an interviewer specifically asked you to call, confine your follow-up messages to e-mails and letters.

Figure 22.2
Follow-up Letter Format

Your name　　　　　　Your Phone number(s) (include Country/Area codes)
Your current address　　Your E-mail

[Interviewer's Name]　　　　　　　　　　　　　　　Date
[Interviewer's Position and Department]
[Interviewer's Address]

Dear Dr. [Interviewer's Last Name]:

Paragraph 1: Thank the interviewer for the courtesy and consideration shown to you during your recent residency interview. Mention the date you interviewed.

Paragraph 2: Reaffirm your interest in the program. Mention anything you did not mention in the interview or e-mail that enhances yourself as a candidate for their program and for the specialty. (Make it brief.)

Paragraph 3: Provide any information that you told this interviewer you would send, including additional documentation or answers to questions deferred during the interview. If you do not have this information with you, say that you will be sending the additional information subsequently. Offer to provide additional information the program or interviewer might need.

Paragraph 4: Use a simple, positive closing sentence, such as "I look forward to working with you in the future."

Sincerely yours,
[Sign your name]

Type your name

P.S. Don't forget a handwritten note!

Specific Information

Occasionally, you will receive requests for additional information, either during the interviews or from the residency secretary. Such information can include anything from additional reference letters to a copy of an article that you quoted during the interview. State in your thank-you e-mail that you will send the requested material as soon as possible. And then send it. It will, again, reinforce the interviewer's positive image of you.

If you have signed up for a military scholarship program (HPSP), be sure that the programs to which you are applying have your written deferment on file, even if it was not requested. Residency programs will not seriously consider ranking you unless you can supply it to them.

Analyze Your Visit

There are two tasks to complete when analyzing your visit to each program: Determine how well you performed and determine how well the program meets your needs. Let's discuss the personal analysis first.

The following questions will help you determine how well you did at the program, particularly in the interview setting. They are adapted from *The Robert Half Way to Get Hired in Today's Job Market* (1981). Your analysis will also highlight problem areas to modify prior to visiting the next residency program on your schedule.

1. Did I look as good as I am capable of looking?
2. Could I have known more about the program and the specialty?
3. Was I relaxed and in control of myself?
4. Did I answer the questions in a way that stressed my ability, enthusiasm, and suitability for that program?
5. Did I listen closely to the interviewers?
6. Did I unobtrusively steer questions toward points I wanted to stress?
7. Did I tailor my answers to fit each type of interviewer?
8. Did I present an accurate and favorable picture of myself to everyone that I met?

Your second task is to analyze how well the program did. Use your previously prepared "Must/Want" Analysis form (Figure 11.1) for the program. Fill it out immediately. Rate the program's strength for each factor you listed. Use the 1-to-10 rating scale, with "10" being perfect.

Once you have completed the score for each factor (for example, Faculty Availability), multiply its "Weight" by its "Score" to get a "Total" for that factor. Then add up the factor "Totals" to give the final Total ("Program Evaluation

Score") for the program. You may now put this sheet away until you have completed a similar form for each program that you visit.

Ranking The Programs For Success

Using the "Must/Want" Analysis

Once you have finished your interviews, you should have a file of completed "Must/Want" Analysis forms (Figure 11.1)—one for each program with which you have interviewed. Now you will see their true benefit. Rather than relying on a *gestalt* or gut feeling of your impressions, you can use your completed "Must/Want" Analysis forms to give you an accurate picture of how well each program meets your self-designated needs.

Rank the programs by using the "Program Evaluation Score" that you assigned to each program. Simply arrange the forms with the Program Evaluation Scores in numerical order to find out what your Rank-Order List (ROL) for the Match should look like. The program with the highest Program Evaluation Score should be at the top (listed first) of your ROL and the one with the lowest score at the bottom (listed last), if at all.

One key point, however. You may be somewhat depressed after first having ascertained what you want in a program and then interviewing. You probably found that no program meets every one of your expectations. Hey, that is what life is all about. *There is no utopia.* In looking for a residency, as with any job search, some compromises are necessary. You should choose the program that best fits your own needs. The "Must/Want" analyses help you do this.

A conceptual way of how to look at your evaluation of residency programs is provided in Figure 22.3.

List Enough Programs to Be Sure You Match

One of the keys to success in the Match is to rank enough programs. (It should go without saying that you must have interviewed at the programs that you list.) Several factors coincide to determine how many programs are "enough."

The first is the specialty that you are trying to enter: The number of applications submitted and the percentage of unmatched students in different specialties varies widely. By now you should know whether the specialty you have chosen is a "tough" or an "easy" match. If you still need some guidance, see the asterisk (*) ratings in Chapter 3. The tougher the specialty is to match in, the more programs you will have to interview with and rank. The number of applications graduates send to programs in their first choice of specialty is listed in Figure 12.2.

Figure 22.3: How Applicants Evaluate Residency Programs

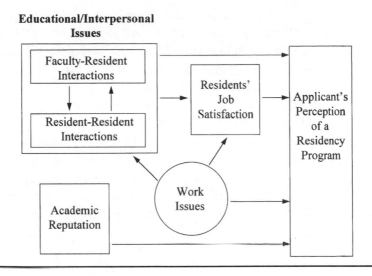

Geography also plays a part in the decision about how many programs to list. Some parts of the country are less desirable to medical school graduates than are others. In some cases, this may have to do with the quality of programs located there. But it also is related to the ambiance of the surroundings. The deep South, the Midwest, and large industrial or inner cities are locations that often have very good programs yet have fewer applicants than elsewhere. It might be to your advantage to rank programs in one of these locales if you are not the strongest of candidates.

Program match rates also depend upon the type of institution in which they are located. If you are looking mainly at university and major-medical-center programs, be prepared for stiff competition. While not necessarily the best, these programs are where most students apply. Of course, you want to meet your own needs, not those of your peers. Therefore, consider carefully the type of program you want. If you want a program at a big center, be prepared to do a little more interviewing and make a longer ROL.

Your assessment of your competitiveness really determines how many programs you rank. The greatest danger is that you will overrate yourself, interview at and rank too few programs, and then be left without a position. If in doubt, apply to a few extra programs. This will provide a greater chance of success, as well as more peace of mind, until you receive the Match results.

Hedge Your Bets as Necessary

Even if you have listed more programs than you think you will need to successfully match in your specialty, do not discard programs that you consider "sure bets" (i.e., weaker programs than those you have already ranked). Until you have a piece of paper in your hand stating that you have a residency position, nothing is certain.

Your best strategy, especially in the difficult-to-match-with specialties, is to list some "sure bets" at the bottom of your ROL, even if each of these is a slightly weaker program than others you have seen. Of course, if you think that the program is too weak, you may prefer not to match there. So, what should you do? Ask yourself, "Would I rather match at that program in the specialty of my choice, or not match in the specialty and take a chance in the Supplemental Offer and Acceptance Program (SOAP) during Match Week?" If you can answer that question, you will know how to fill out the bottom of your ROL.

Plan ahead for all contingencies. That means interviewing at one or two less-competitive programs and, possibly, for a Transitional or Preliminary Surgery or Medicine slot. This will give you the "stoppers" on your list to be sure that you match. But it is your choice. If you are willing to "guts it out" and risk participating in the SOAP rush to find an open slot, then the best of luck to you.

Go for the Gold

The preceding comments should not deter you from trying to secure the best residency position you can obtain.

As has already been mentioned, many of you will underestimate your own abilities and competitiveness; a few of you will overestimate your chances. Extend your sights and apply to the programs that you think will be the best for you. And, after you have applied and interviewed, make certain that you *rank your top choices first.*

Do not fill out your ROL in the order in which you think you will be selected by the programs. This will only decrease your chance of getting into the program you really desire. Put your prime program choices at the top of the list. Then rank the others in descending order of preference. That way, when Match Day rolls around, you can be confident that you have matched with the best program possible.

23

The NRMP & Other Matches

It is good to hope, but bad to depend on it.

Folk Saying

THE "MATCH," OFFICIALLY KNOWN as the National Residency Matching Program (NRMP), is how most medical students get their first-year (PGY-1, intern) training positions. Most of these positions are filled with the expectation on both the graduate's and the program's part that the entire training program will be completed.

In the 2012 NRMP Match, 24,034 first-year (PGY-1) positions and 2,738 PGY-2 positions were offered. The following are factoids from the 2012 NRMP Main Match:

Participants in the PGY-1 Match
- ~ 20,000 students and graduates from U.S. and Canadian M.D. medical schools
- 2,360 students and graduates from Osteopathic schools
- ~ 11,000 international medical graduates (IMGs)
    4,279 U.S. citizens from international medical schools
    6,828 non-U.S. citizens from international medical schools
- 1.05 PGY-1 positions offered per active participant
- 1.4 PGY-1 positions for each participating U.S. senior M.D. and D.O. student

Positions filled
- 68% by students or graduates of U.S., Puerto Rican, and Canadian M.D.-granting medical schools
- 20% by IMGs
- 6% by students or graduates of Osteopathic schools

Match Rates
- 95.1% of participating senior M.D. students from U.S. schools matched
- 74.7% of participating senior D.O. students matched
- 42% of participating IMGs matched:
    49% of U.S.-citizen IMGs matched to PGY-1 programs
    40% of non-U.S. citizen IMGs matched to PGY-1 programs

Unfilled Positions
- 5% were unfilled through the Match
- 50% of unfilled positions were for one-year Preliminary Surgery and Medicine slots (2011)
- 10.2% of applicants formally withdrew from the Match
- 8.1% of applicants failed to submit a rank-order list before the deadline

Separate Matches exist for Ophthalmology, Plastic Surgery, and Urology. See each specialty's listing in Chapter 3 for details about their matching program. There is negligible involvement in the NRMP Match by Nuclear Medicine, Preventive Medicine, and many Internal Medicine subspecialties.

While they can use the NRMP Match for M.D.-affiliated residencies, Osteopathic medical students match with American Osteopathic Association (AOA)-approved internships and residencies (other than those in the Military) through the *Intern/Resident Registration Program*. This matching program is run under the AOA's auspices by National Matching Services (see description later in this chapter; see also, Chapter 14).

The NRMP Match

In any competition, it is vital to know the rules *before* you play. This avoids having to learn through a process of trial and error. In as major an event in your life as the Match, learning as you go could be a disaster, so it behooves you to spend a few moments to become familiar with the way the system works.

When you need more information or application materials, you can get them from your Dean of Students or the NRMP, 2450 N Street NW, Washington, DC 20037-1127; (202) 828-0566 or toll-free at (866) 617-5838 (8:30 A.M. to 5:30 P.M. Eastern time); e-mail: NRMP@aamc.org; www.nrmp. org. Contact information is the same for Fellowship matches, except that the phone numbers are: (202) 828-6077 or toll-free at (866) 617-5834.

Why Have a Matching Program?

Prior to 1951, the matching of medical students to internship positions was a rather sordid affair. Appalling abuses of the system occurred, such as weak programs pressuring students to take less-than-optimal positions early rather than waiting for an offer from their top choice. And, while there was a purported uniform announcement date for several years, it proved to be unworkable.

As evidence of just how badly a new matching system was needed, in 1951, more than 98% of hospitals and 97% of students participated in the first Match. Organized by the National Student Internship Committee, the program was a huge success and led to the establishment of the National Intern Matching Program.

This organization's name and its sponsors have changed several times over the years. Currently, it is organized as the National Resident Matching Program (NRMP), and is sponsored by the Association of American Medical Colleges, American Hospital Association, American Medical Association, American Board of Medical Specialties, and Council of Medical Specialty Societies.

The original matching program used a card-sorting system, which was state-of-the-art in the early 1950s. This method, though it became antiquated, was not changed until 1970, when electronic data-processing techniques were introduced. But it was not until 1974 that the entire system was fully computerized. Currently, the entire computer program for the Match takes about six minutes to run. While the Match process has many flaws, as Winston Churchill said of democracy, it is "the worst [system] except all those other forms that have been tried from time to time."

In 2002, a lawsuit designed to destroy the NRMP was dismissed. The suit contended that the NRMP restricts competition, depresses salaries, and deprives residents of the ability to negotiate their salaries and work hours. The courts found that the NRMP was exempt from federal antitrust laws. This ruling was upheld in 2006; the U.S. Supreme Court subsequently declined to hear the case.

The key element in the Match is the "algorithm" (*see* "NRMP Algorithm," below). As a result of complaints, the NRMP changed their matching algorithm in 1998 from one that favored programs (program-optimal) to one that favors applicants (student-optimal). The algorithm treats all applicants (i.e., U.S. M.D. students, D.O. students, physicians, and IMGs) equally. (The San Francisco Matching Program [SFMP] also uses an algorithm in which applicant preferences always prevail.)

Of the U.S. seniors (from M.D. schools) participating in the NRMP Match in 2012, 56.5% matched with their first choice of program, 15.6% with their second choice, 9.5% with their third choice, and 5.7% with their fourth choice. The rest either matched with their fifth or lower choice of program or did not find a position in the Match. There were 815 participating U.S. M.D. seniors who did not match in 2012. Some most likely found a position during SOAP week. (In 2012, SOAP replaced the "Scramble" for unmatched slots.)

In 2010, of the 871 participating seniors who were unmatched, 194 still did not have a PGY-1 position after the Scramble; 179 of these students were considered "fully qualified" by their Deans. According to their Deans, the main reasons these qualified students failed to obtain a PGY-1 position were:

- Not competitive for their first-choice specialty, 45%
- Poor USMLE scores, 27%
- Rank-Order List (ROL) mismanagement, such as not ranking enough programs, 16%
- Difficulty communicating with programs in the Scramble, 10%
- Geographic reasons, such as ranking programs only in one city, 9%
- Overly aggressive ROL, such as only ranking more competitive specialties or programs, 7%
- Poor interviewing or interpersonal skills, 6%
- Professionalism issues, 3%
- Poor reference letters (LORs), 1%

The matching process has developed to the point where it can now accommodate all programs in all specialties that offer positions to senior medical students, regardless of the postgraduate level at which the program begins. However, many programs still do not participate in the NRMP Match.

"First-Choice" Residency Positions—A Warning

Medical students often boast about getting their "first-choice" of residency positions and medical schools proudly cite the number of their students who achieve this goal. These are misleading numbers, and you should be very wary of them in your own career planning.

Medical students are conservative by nature. But they also consistently underestimate their own worth. Hard to believe, but true! As a result, many settle for "safe" choices rather than aiming for their "dream" residency position. I speak with medical students from many medical schools, and the story is always the same: Even if they are AOA (medical school honorary), each student has what he or she feels is a valid reason why they are not as competitive as other students who are applying to what they consider the "best" residencies. So, they settle for something less than what they think will be optimal and they don't even apply to these "best" residencies.

Over the years, some medical schools have strongly encouraged their students to apply both to "sure bet" positions and to positions within their own hospital system. The cynic in me suggests that this is done to boost the rate of "first-choice" residency matches and also to make sure that their own residency programs are filled.

The best course is to not fall into these traps. Always strive to get the best residency position that you can. That said, the number of seniors that failed to match may indicate that they did not accurately assess their competitiveness.

Participating Specialties

Most PGY-1 positions are offered through the NRMP Match, and most of the programs in the NRMP Match require that you apply through ERAS. The majority of those not offered are military internships. However, PGY-2 positions in many specialties either are not offered through any Match (you have to negotiate directly with programs) or are offered through the specialty's own Matching program. The number of specialties and programs participating in the NRMP Match changes from year to year, as does the number of positions offered in each of these specialties. The best sources for current information about each specialty are listed in the "Specialty Descriptions" in Chapter 3.

Intern Positions

Some PGY-1 positions for medical students are classified as *"Categorical (C)."* These are in the broad specialties and do not require preliminary graduate training. They are designed for individuals who want to remain in the same program throughout their residency. Categorical positions exist in Family Medicine, Internal Medicine, Pediatrics, Emergency Medicine, Obstetrics and Gynecology, General Surgery, and Pathology. In addition, specialties whose Boards require a preliminary broad clinical experience can also offer Categorical positions if the individual program has made arrangements for this experience.

"Preliminary (P)" programs are designed for students seeking one or two years of broad prerequisite clinical experience prior to entering another specialty. They are available in Internal Medicine, General Surgery, and Transitional programs. While they are not designed to act as entry points for a full residency in either Internal Medicine or General Surgery, occasionally they can be used as just such a pathway.

PGY-2 and Above Positions

There are also positions available through the NRMP's Matches beyond the PGY-1 year. These are *"Advanced"* residency positions and *"Fellowships."* (Also see "Matching in Advance [PGY-2 and Above]," below.) Advanced residency positions are those positions above the PGY-1 level that are available to senior students. The presumption is that students will complete preliminary training before entering these programs. Fellowships, which are not available to students, are for individuals who have completed, or are about to complete, a residency in a primary specialty and desire more specialized training.

Figure 23.1
PGY-1 Training Accepted by Various M.D. Specialties

Specialty	Acceptable Training
Anesthesiology	Transitional internship with ≥ 6 months in any combination of in-patient IM, Peds, Surgery (or subspecialty), OB/GYN, Neurology, or FM, plus 1 or 2 months in EM and Critical Care.
Dermatology	Broad-based clinical year.
Neurology	Either ≥ 8 months in IM with primary patient care responsibility or 6 months in IM with primary patient care responsibility plus ≥ 1 month in two of the following: Peds, EM, FM, or other IM training.
Ophthalmology	Clinical training with primary responsibility for patient care (e.g., IM, Neurology, Peds, Surgery, FM, or EM) where ≥ 6 months are spent in direct patient care.
Physical Med & Rehab	Transitional Internship or ≥ 6 months in a combination of IM, EM, FM, OB/GYN, Peds, or Surgery.
Psychiatry (3-yr prog.)	Transitional Internship or PGY-1 training in IM, FM, Peds, or another clinical specialty requiring comprehensive and continuous patient care.
Diagnostic Radiology	Transitional Internship or training in one or a combination of: IM, EM, FM, OB/GYN, Peds, Neurology, Surgery, or surgical subspecialties.
Radiation Oncology	Transitional Internship or training in IM, FM, OB/GYN, Peds, Surgery, or surgical subspecialties.

Abbreviations: EM, Emergency Medicine; FM, Family Medicine; IM, Internal Medicine; Peds, Pediatrics.

Adapted from RRC requirements as listed in the American Medical Association's *Graduate Medical Education Library on CD-ROM* (2010-2011).

Advanced Residency Positions

Advanced programs offer positions *beginning at the PGY-2 or higher level* to senior medical students. The problem is that some programs offering such positions do not go through the NRMP PGY-1 Match. Applicants to these programs need to apply for the Advanced Position and also participate in the NRMP PGY-1 Match to fulfill their initial training requirement. This is especially true in Ophthalmology and Urology. The internships accepted as prerequisites for further training in other specialties are listed in Figure 23.1. The numbers (and types) of training programs and of positions available, as of 2012, are listed in Figures 23.2 and 23.10.

Figure 23.2
Medical Specialties, Programs, and Entry-Level Positions Offered

Neither the ACGME nor AOA has approved all the listed specialties.

Specialty	Total Number of Residency/ Fellowship Programs*	Number of Positions offered to Medical Students via a Matching Program†	Total Number of Entry-level Positions‡
Abdominal Radiology	11	0	45
Addiction Psychiatry	44	0	102
Adolescent Medicine	25	0	31
Adult Reconstructive Orthopedics	21	0	36
Aerospace Medicine	4	0	45
Allergy & Immunology	73	0	151
Anesthesiology	192	919	1,476
Blood Banking/Transfusion Med	48	0	74
Cardiology	181	0	2,465
Cardiothoracic Radiology	2	0	3
Chemical Pathology	3	0	4
Child and Adolescent Psychiatry	124	0	452
Child Neurology	71	99	146
Clinical Cardiac Electrophysiology	82	0	183
Clinical & Laboratory Immunology	1	0	2
Clinical Neurophysiology	90	0	263
Colon & Rectal Surgery	49	0	84
Cornea/External Disease§	64	0	73
Craniofacial Surgery§	19	0	19
Critical Care (Anesthesia)	46	0	91
Critical Care (IM)	33	0	179
Critical Care (Surg)	97	0	196
Cytopathology	85	0	152
Dermatology	112	23	363
Dermatopathology	54	0	91
Developmental/Behavioral Peds	22	0	21
Emergency Medicine	153	1,668	1,668
Emergency Med-Internal Med	11	26	26
Endocrinology (IM)	125	0	607
Endovascular Surg Neuroradiology	3	0	5
Facial Plastic Surgery§	37	0	38
Family Medicine	457	2,740	2,740
Family Med-Internal Med	2	4	4
Family Med-Psychiatry	8	12	12
Female Pelvic Med & Reproductive Surg *	24	0	24
Foot & Ankle Orthopedics	5	0	10
Forensic Pathology	39	0	82
Forensic Psychiatry	43	0	101
Gastroenterology	159	0	446

Figure 23.2 (continued)

Specialty	Total Number of Residency/ Fellowship Programs*	Number of Positions offered to Medical Students via a Matching Program†	Total Number of Entry-level Positions‡
Geriatric Medicine (FM)	42	0	72
Geriatric Medicine (IM)	107	0	301
Geriatric Psychiatry	58	0	71
Glaucoma§	54	0	62
Gynecologic Oncology	33	0	39
Hand Surgery (All)	73	0	154
Hematology (All)	87	0	162
Hematology & Oncology (IM)	132	0	475
Infectious Disease	145	0	366
Internal Medicine, Categorical	389	5,277	5,277
Internal Medicine, Prelim. (PGY-1 only)	307	1,861	1,861
Internal Med-Dermatology	8	9	9
Internal Med-Emerg Med-Critical Care	1	1	1
Internal Med-Medical Genetics	1	1	1
Internal Med-Neurology	2	2	2
Internal Med-Nuclear Med	2	0	0
Internal Med-Pediatrics	77	362	362
Internal Med-Physical Med/Rehab	2	0	2
Internal Med-Preventive Med	6	5	5
Internal Medicine, Primary	56	311	311
Internal Med-Psychiatry	10	20	20
Interventional Cardiology	123	0	283
Maternal-Fetal Medicine*	59	0	73
Medical Genetics	51	1	84
Medical Microbiology	12	0	17
Medical Toxicology (EM)	26	0	62
Medical Toxicology (GPM)	4	0	6
Mohs Micrographic Surgery§	50	0	51
Musculoskeletal Oncology	10	0	14
Musculoskeletal Radiology	28		54
Neonatology	91	0	221
Nephrology	151	0	374
Neurodevelopmental Disabilities	5	0	10
Neurological Surgery§	98	196	196
Neurology§	142	638	638
Neurology-Diag Radiology-Neuroradiology	2	0	2
Neuropathology	36	0	36
Neuroradiology	87	0	259
Neurotology (OTO)	12	0	10
Nuclear Medicine	56	0	102
Nuclear Radiology	21	0	38

Figure 23.2 (continued)

Specialty	Total Number of Residency/ Fellowship Programs*	Number of Positions offered to Medical Students via a Matching Program†	Total Number of Entry-level Positions‡
Obstetrics & Gynecology	251	1,240	1,240
Occupational Medicine	33	0	108
Oncology	16	0	57
Ophthalmology§	118	458	458
Ophthalmic Plastic/Reconstructive Surg	14	0	14
Orthopedic Sports Med	93	0	221
Orthopedic Surgery	161	682	733
Orthopedic Surgery of the Spine	16	0	27
Orthopedic Trauma	6	0	12
Otolaryngology	107	285	285
Pain Medicine (All)	94	0	312
Pathology (Anatomic & Clinical)	148	521	521
Pediatric Cardiology	50	0	102
Pediatric Critical Care Med	60	0	119
Pediatric Emergency Med (EM)**	11	0	21
Pediatric Emergency Med (PED)**	44	0	84
Pediatric Endocrinology	67	0	99
Pediatric Gastroenterology	51	0	69
Pediatric Hematology/Oncology	68	0	151
Pediatric Infectious Diseases	62	0	74
Pediatric Nephrology	39	0	50
Pediatric Neurosurgery§	16	0	20
Pediatric Ophthalmology§	40	0	48
Pediatric Orthopedics	23	0	33
Pediatric Otolaryngology§	20	0	26
Pediatric Pathology	28	0	41
Pediatric Pulmonology	48	0	60
Pediatric Radiology	46	0	75
Pediatric Rheumatology	22	0	24
Pediatric Sports Medicine	8	0	0
Pediatric Surgery	35	0	35
Pediatric Urology	18	0	19
Pediatrics, Categorical	190	2,475	2,475
Pediatrics, Preliminary	52	55	55
Pediatrics, Primary	13	67	67
Pediatrics-Anesthesiology	4	7	7
Pediatrics–Dermatology	3	1	1
Pediatrics–Emergency Med	3	7	7
Pediatrics–Medical Genetics	12	7	7
Pediatrics–Phys Med & Rehab	3	2	2
Pediatrics–Psychiatry–Child Psych	9	18	18

Figure 23.2 (Continued)

Specialty	Total Number of Residency/ Fellowship Programs*	Number of Positions offered to Medical Students via a Matching Program†	Total Number of Entry-level Positions‡
Physical Med & Rehabilitation	26	86	367
Plastic Surgery (All)§	57	101	121
Preventive Medicine, General	5	4	284
Procedural Dermatology	27	0	25
Psychiatry	189	1,118	1,121
Psychiatry–Family Med	6	10	10
Psychiatry–Neurology	3	2	5
Psychosomatic Med	14	0	21
Public Health	17	0	64
Pulmonary Diseases (IM)	21	0	117
Pulmonary Diseases & Critical Care Med (IM)	97	0	344
Radiation Oncology	78	171	171
Radiology, Diagnostic	188	1,111	1,111
Reproductive Endocrinology	29	0	32
Retina–Vitreous§	87	0	96
Rheumatology	108	0	198
Selective Pathology	22	0	88
Spinal Cord Injury Med	21	0	31
Sports Medicine (EM)	3	0	5
Sports Medicine (FM)	68	0	111
Sports Medicine (IM)	2	0	3
Surgery, General (Categorical)	242	1,146	1,146
Surgery, General (Preliminary)	291	1,221	1,221
Surgical Critical Care	84	0	170
Thoracic Surgery (All)	85	20	136
Transitional Year	110	941	941
Trauma Surgery††	26	0	42
Undersea & Hyperbaric Med (EM)	1	0	2
Undersea & Hyperbaric Med (GPM)	1	0	2
Urology§	120	9	277
Vascular Neurology	22	0	44
Vascular Surgery (All)	35	41	163
Vascular/Interventional Radiology	101	0	251

*Number of institutions participating. Some separate applicants into two or more "programs" based on whether they are applying as Categorical, Preliminary, Advanced, or Physician candidates.
†Positions at either the PGY-1 or the PGY-2 (Advanced) level available for medical student matching. Positions open only to physicians are not included.
‡All entry-level positions available (at various years of training) in accredited programs. Some must be matched with during internship or residency; others are only in the Military Match.
§Uses San Francisco or American Urological Assn. matches. Plastic Surgery uses NRMP only for PGY-1 year.
**Fellowship programs that follow residency. "Pediatrics/Emergency Med" is the combined residency program.
††Programs that meet the guidelines of the American Association for the Surgery of Trauma; this subspecialty is not recognized by the ACGME.
Numbers derived from: *FREIDA*, the NRMP, and the San Francisco Match websites, and other sources.

Note that all graduates of Osteopathic medical schools must complete an AOA-approved internship before beginning Osteopathic residencies (Figures 3.2 and 14.8), although the internship and residency are now combined for some specialties.

Combined Programs

Similar to doing a double (or triple) major as an undergraduate, these programs combine training in more than one specialty which, supposedly, are complementary. Examples include Internal Medicine–Pediatrics and Neurology–Psychiatry. Combined programs are in non-surgical specialties. Surgical specialties call their programs "Integrated."

Integrated Programs

Medical students can use the NRMP to match into "Integrated Programs" in Neurosurgery, Plastic Surgery, Thoracic Surgery, and Vascular Surgery. These programs combine the required training in General Surgery with training in these specialties. In contrast to the traditional fellowship path, the time needed to finish such a program is markedly shorter. However, graduates cannot take General Surgery Board exams. These specialties also offer fellowship programs.

Fellowships

Thirty-seven sub-specialty programs have fellowship positions available through the NRMP and 14 others use the San Francisco Matching Program (Figure 23.10). Participation in these Matches is limited to individuals who have completed or who are about to complete residency programs in the prerequisite specialties.

Nearly all fellowships require completion of the basic residency before beginning the program, although you should check their current rules, since some now allow entry before the end of the primary residency. Also see the Fellowship descriptions in Chapter 3 listed either under the parent specialty or separately (designated by an "F" following their name).

NRMP Match Rules—General

NRMP Algorithm

The NRMP Match algorithm is complex; this is a brief summary:
1. The Match handles each applicant in sequence.
2. An attempt is first made to place an applicant into his most-preferred program.

3. If this is unsuccessful, an attempt is then made to place the applicant into the second, third, etc., choices on their rank-order list.
4. This process continues until there is a (tentative) match or until the applicant's listed programs have been exhausted.
5. When subsequent applicants are processed, an attempt is first made to place them into their most-preferred program.
6. If a program they ranked highly has ranked them higher than applicants already tentatively matched, the new applicant gets the spot and the previously matched applicant goes back through the algorithm.
7. When an applicant is "bumped" from a spot and goes back through the Match, the process begins again with their first-choice program.
8. The Match is complete when all applicants have been matched with one of their choices or all the programs listed by applicants have filled their positions.

One element of this algorithm generally remains unstated: The NRMP allows several hundred hospitals each year to designate positions in one program that, if unfilled in the Match, can be transferred to positions in another program that can be filled.

Rank-Order Lists

The list in which you order and submit the programs is called your Rank-Order List (ROL). The programs complete a similar list of candidates. After you complete the NRMP worksheets (found on their website), you can enter your ROL into the NRMP's computer system from any computer with Microsoft Internet Explorer 6.0 or higher (best), Firefox version 3.0 or other Mozilla compatible browsers. JavaScript, Java applets, and cookies must remain enabled for the R3 (Registration, Ranking, and Results) System to work. (As of 2012, Safari for Mac users was not supported; download Firefox if using a Mac.) If you have a problem, check with NRMP's on-line User Guide to find the latest system requirements.

The ROL can be entered in one or more sessions and can be modified as often as necessary until the posted deadline, usually in mid-February. *To complete the process, you must certify your list; otherwise, the NRMP does not recognize it as having been sent to them.* It is best to finish using the R3 System a few days before the deadline, since the system becomes very slow (due to heavy use by procrastinators) during the last 24 hours before the deadline. You can enter your programs one at a time or ten at a time, from most to least desirable. Applicants are responsible for the correctness of their individual ROLs; use NRMP's search function to find the correct 9-digit program codes. You can print a copy of your personal ROL at any time by clicking on the

"Display/Print" button and then using your Web browser's "Print" button. The NRMP accepts ROLs only via computer. Do not mail or fax them your list.

Access is granted only to individuals with both an NRMP Code (which is also your AAMC ID) that is assigned when applicants register and a Password that applicants select at the same time. Participants can later change their password, if they wish to do so. Your password should be kept confidential and in a safe place.

Upon completing your ROL, "certify" the list by clicking on the "Certify" button and reentering your password. You can still modify the list after certification, but you *must recertify it* for it to be used in the Match.

IMGs can participate in the NRMP Match, even without an ECFMG Certificate, *if the ECFMG notifies the NRMP that all requirements for certification have been met* before the Match is run.

In 2012, the basic NRMP Match registration fee for all applicants was $50, payable online by VISA, MasterCard, or Internet check. This fee allows the applicant, without additional charge, to rank up to 15 different programs on the ROL, as well as a total of 20 different PGY-1 programs on one or more Supplemental ROLs. In the Couple's Match, each partner pays the individual fee and there is an extra $15 fee for submitting as a couple. This allows them to rank 30 different programs (including "Unmatched") on their primary ROL and up to 30 different programs on all Supplemental ROLs. Each additional program pair listed costs $15. Each additional listed program on the primary or supplemental ROL for individuals or for couples costs $30.

Before entering your final ROL, complete the *worksheets* on the NRMP website. You will use them to check the accuracy of your submitted ROL, which lists only the "NRMP Program Code." On the worksheet, list the program's "Rank Order" (number 1 through as many as you choose to list); "Hospital Name/City, State"; "Program Description" (specialty and type of program, e.g., Surgery–Categorical); and "NRMP Program Code" (from the current *NRMP On-line Directory*). The worksheet you use depends upon whether you are applying as an individual (including those applying for shared-schedule positions) or as a couple.

The *Supplemental ROLs* are used by students applying to one or more Advanced Programs for Students. The Advanced Programs are listed on the Primary ROL. For each Advanced Program or group of programs listed, you should enter acceptable associated PGY-1 programs on the Supplemental ROLs. Each Supplemental ROL will be designated by a letter (e.g., A through D). The same Supplemental ROL can be linked to more than one Advanced Program.

If, for example, you list six Advanced Programs, four of which are in widely dispersed locations and two of which are in the same city, then you will probably want to use one Supplemental ROL containing the PGY-1 programs for the two Advanced Programs in the same location. If you don't mind moving your residence between your first and second years, you can use the same Supplemental ROL for all the Advanced Programs to which you apply, no matter what their geographic location. If you match to the advanced program but not a first-year program, the Match still applies, and you will need to seek a PGY-1 position after the Match, usually in the Scramble. The basic NRMP fee allows applicants to rank up to 20 Advanced Programs and a total of 20 PGY-1 programs on their Supplemental ROLs. Each additional program listed costs $30.

Although there is no limit to the number of specialties (or programs) you can include on your ROL, it has been demonstrated that the individuals with the greatest success in the Match are those who rank only one specialty. However, if you are attempting to get into a highly competitive specialty, such as Orthopedic Surgery, this does not preclude you from listing some Transitional or Preliminary (Medicine, Surgery) programs at the bottom of your list.

Optimizing Your Rank-Order List

What techniques can you use to achieve the best possible outcome in the Match? There are two things to remember: *list your first-choice program first* and carefully *consider how many programs you should list.*

Applicants consistently do best if they list their top choice first. After listing the top choice, applicants might theoretically get better results if they listed programs based on knowing how all the other applicants rated programs—information which is unavailable. Therefore, *rank programs in the order of their acceptability to you*—not in the order in which you think you are acceptable to the programs. This will give you the best chance of matching with a program you think is optimal for you.

How long should your ROL be? If you apply to a highly competitive specialty (see ratings in Chapter 3) or to programs in an area of the country where matching is difficult, it's probably better to have a long ROL. If you apply to programs that are easier to match with, you may want to have a relatively short list.

The key to success is to consider, for each program you list, whether you would rather go to that program or whether you would prefer to be unmatched and take your chances in the rush of unmatched candidates for positions. Applicants who list a high number of programs on their ROL have a better chance of matching (Figure 23.3). For all applicants, a common reason for not matching is that they do not list enough programs. The same holds true

Figure 23.3
Average Number of Programs on Applicants' ROLs

Year	Number of Programs Applied to	
	Matched Applicants	**Unmatched Applicants**
1996	6.4	5.4
1997	6.9	5.2
1998	7.3	5.0
1999	7.4	5.1
2000	7.3	4.8
2001	7.4	4.7
2005	7.7	4.5
2010	9.3	4.5
2011	9.5	4.4

Adapted from NRMP information, October 2011.

for residency programs: those that fill list approximately 9.4 candidates for each position. Programs that don't fill list only about 4.9 candidates per open position.

No matter how competitive (or non-competitive) the specialty, list all the programs with which you would like to match. If this isn't a long list, or if you are applying to a specialty that generally has many positions open after the Match, a reasonable strategy may be to list fewer programs (only those with which you *really* want to match). See Figure 23.4 for a decision tree to help you decide whether to rank a program.

Confidentiality

Match rules do not allow programs or applicants to ask each other how they will be ranked. The ROLs from both parties are considered confidential. Either party can, if they so desire, release this information to the other. Any comments about what is (or will be) on a list, however, are not binding. Many students have been grossly misled by a program's faculty member who told them that they would be "ranked high enough to match." Of course, many did not match with those programs although the students had listed them in first place.

Programs are not supposed to offer contracts for appointment to applicants prior to the general announcement of NRMP Match results. To enforce this, applicants are expected to report any such offers to the NRMP, who will presumably take punitive action. In recent years, eight percent of students have reported that they were asked to make a commitment before a Match result, either the NRMP Match or a specialty match, was announced. So much for the ethics of academic physicians.

Match Results

Match results are released stepwise over the course of "Match Week" (Figure 23.5). All information is available to applicants through postings on the NRMP website; access requires both an applicant's NRMP code and their password.

Match Day is in mid-March. Applicants can find out *whether* they matched at noon Eastern Time (ET) on Monday of Match Week. At the same time, a list of filled and unfilled programs is released, but the locations are revealed only to unmatched participants who are eligible to participate in the Supplemental Offer and Acceptance Program (SOAP; discussed below). At noon (ET) on Tuesday of Match Week, the locations of filled and unfilled positions are posted.

Matched applicants can discover to which programs they will be going at 1:00 P.M. (ET) on Match Day (Friday of Match Week). Under NRMP rules, both applicants and programs are bound by the Match results just as if they had already signed the official appointment documents. Programs send those documents to new residents beginning on the day after Match Day.

Employment Requirements

Even after you match with a program, you may need to successfully complete specific pre-employment requirements, such as drug testing, to get the position. If there are such requirements, applicants should be informed of this, preferably in the material provided by the institution, before they submit their rank-order list.

Non-U.S. citizens must have a current visa allowing them to enter a residency program, otherwise they cannot begin their residency, even if they have an ECFMG Certificate and have matched with a program.

Illegal Behavior

The NRMP considers two actions illegal for an applicant or a program. The first is supplying forged credentials or letters of recommendation to programs. This is not only illegal in terms of the Match, but also may be either a misdemeanor or a felony in some states. It certainly could prevent you from ever getting a license to practice medicine.

Figure 23.4: NRMP Rank-Order List Decision Tree

Is this program first on your list? — **Yes** → Rank

↓ Yes

What is your level of interest in the program? — **High** → Rank

← Do not rank

↓ Moderate

Do the higher ranked programs on your list fill? — **Yes** → Rank

↓ No

Are you likely to match in higher ranked programs? — **No** → Rank

↓ Yes

do you prefer not matching to being matched in this program? — **No** → Rank

↓ Yes

Do not rank

Adapted from a similar algorithm produced by Christopher Leadem, Ph.D., Former Dean of Students, University of Arizona College of Medicine, Tucson, AZ.

The second is for a program to refuse to accept an applicant who has matched into that program (program illegality) or for an applicant who has matched to refuse to accept the position (applicant illegality). While in the past the NRMP took action if it received "credible evidence" that such activities had occurred, the NRMP now expects that the individuals and programs involved will settle any disagreements themselves.

Schedule of Events

For 2012, the uniform national date for *releasing the Medical Student Performance Evaluations (MSPE or Dean's Letters) at M.D.-granting schools was changed to October 1.* (In prior years it was November 1.) Although not all Deans play strictly by the rules (some offer to essentially read the letter to program directors over the telephone), most Dean's Letters go out on that date.

For the NRMP PGY-1 (Main) Match, the ROLs are due in mid-February and Match results are released in mid-March. Although it varies by specialty, "early" Matches require their ROLs to be turned in by early to mid-January, with Match results released in mid- to late January.

The exact dates for the events in the Matching program change from year to year. Figure 23.5 gives a list of the *approximate dates* for each milepost in the process. For the exact dates each year, check the NRMP website.

Institution

All programs at teaching institutions that participate in the NRMP Main Match may accept senior U.S. students from M.D.-granting medical schools into their residency programs at the PGY-1 level only through the NRMP or another national matching program. Unfortunately, the same does not hold true for the institutions' Advanced (PGY-2 and above) positions. Therefore, some Advanced positions may be offered through the Match, while others are matched in other ways. This practice leads to a considerable amount of confusion.

Name & Address Changes

The NRMP collects applicants' names, addresses, and e-mail addresses when they register. It is vital to keep at least your e-mail address current, since the NRMP and programs will first contact applicants using e-mail. Unfortunately, many e-mails sent to applicants are returned to the NRMP and the programs as "undeliverable." Also, add the NRMP's e-mail address to your 'safe' addresses, so that messages will not be put in your spam folder.

You do not want to miss a message from the NRMP or a program; it can seriously affect your career. Get a stable e-mail provider and make sure that they continue to host your address. Also, use an e-mail "handle" that conveys a professional image: "ImTooSexy@gmail.com" just might cost you an interview. If you need to change your e-mail address, you can do it instantaneously on the NRMP's website.

Withdrawal from the NRMP Matching Program

By signing the NRMP's contract to participate in their Match, you agree to withdraw from the Match only if you:

1. Accept an appointment from the military.
2. Decide not to pursue a PGY-1 training position in that year.
3. Otherwise obtain a residency position that begins in the current year.

In the last case, the program director must send a letter to the NRMP. (Matching through the Canadian Resident Matching Service [CaRMS] is not considered a withdrawal.) To withdraw from the Match, U.S. senior M.D. students need permission from their Dean. Independent applicants can withdraw themselves from the Match on the NRMP website.

Some students think that they can easily withdraw from the Match either by not turning in their ROL or by turning in a blank ROL. This is not true. Note also that the NRMP sends a list of all Match participants who have not turned in ROLs and who have turned in blank lists to their medical school Dean.

The NRMP automatically withdraws candidates who cannot verify their medical school attendance or graduation or who do not pay the required fees, IMGs who have not completed the ECFMG requirements, and Fifth Pathway students or graduates who have not completed USMLE Steps 1, 2CS, and 2CK or their equivalents.

Student Candidates

Schools

Although the majority of participants in the NRMP Match are students at U.S. schools granting M.D. degrees, you can participate even if you do not fall into this category. However, the rules change slightly depending upon the category into which you do fall.

LCME-Accredited Schools
Students from schools accredited by the Liaison Committee on Medical Education (LCME), which includes virtually all M.D.-granting institutions in

Figure 23.5
Important Dates For NRMP Applications, the Match, and SOAP

March–November: Students get information about residency programs by mail or from their websites.

Early July: Applicants register with ERAS (separate from the NRMP) and begin completing their application materials.

Mid-July: *NRMP Directory of Programs* is posted on the NRMP website and updated weekly. Programs start registering on September 1; most don't get their listings on-line until November or December. Until then, rely on *FREIDA* for information about which programs plan to participate in the NRMP.

September 1: *At noon (ET),* applicants begin registering for the NRMP's Main Match (for PGY-1 and Advanced positions).

November 30: *Applicants' early registration deadline is at 11:59 P.M. (ET).* After this date, there is an additional $50 charge. Applicants can technically register until the deadline for submitting their ROLs. Don't do that! Register early so programs will have your NRMP number when they want to rank you.

Mid-January to Mid-February: Applicants and programs enter their ROLs using the Registration, Ranking, and Results (R3) System on the NRMP website.

January 31: Programs must submit the final number of available positions.

February 22: *The R3 System closes at 9 P.M. (ET).* NRMP must have both applicants' and programs' *certified* ROLs, plus any other required information, by this time. Withdrawal deadline for Independent Applicants who have accepted a position via another matching plan or by outside agreement.

Monday before Match Week: NRMP sends recertification request to Deans and the ECFMG.

Wednesday before Match Week: 12:00 noon (ET) is the deadline for Deans and the ECFMG to recertify that applicants are eligible for SOAP.

Friday before Match Week: At 12:00 noon (ET), NRMP notifies all applicants of their SOAP eligibility. (This has confused many applicants. See "Eligibility" for an explanation.)

MATCH WEEK (Mid-March)

Monday of Match Week (4 days before Match Day): *Applicant and program results (matched/unmatched and filled/unfilled) are posted to the NRMP website at 12:00 noon (ET).* The locations of all unfilled positions are released *only* to unmatched and partially matched participants that are eligible for SOAP. At 1:00 P.M. (ET), unmatched and partially matched applicants may log on to ERAS (in SOAP mode) and create applications for unfilled positions. ERAS will begin sending applications at 2:00 P.M. (ET).

Tuesday of Match Week (3 days before Match Day): Programs with unfilled positions begin to enter their SOAP preference lists into the R3 System at 11:30 A.M. (ET). Program-initiated telephone interviews continue.

Figure 23.5 (continued)

Wednesday of Match Week (2 Days Prior to Match Day): Programs must enter their SOAP Preference lists by 11:30 A.M. (ET). Beginning at noon (ET), SOAP offers are made every three hours (noon, 3 P.M. ET) and are *valid for 2 hours*. Program-initiated telephone interviews continue; can add applicants to the bottom of their preference lists until 2:30 P.M. (ET).

Thursday of Match Week (1 Day Prior to Match Day): At 8:00 A.M. (ET), schools receive Match Results. At 2:00 P.M.,(ET), programs receive their Roster of Matched Applicants. SOAP offers are made at 9 A.M., noon, and 3 P.M. ET; they are *valid for 2 hours*.

Match Day (Friday of Match Week): Final Match results are posted on the NRMP website at 1:00 P.M. (ET). SOAP offers are made at 9 A.M., noon, and 3 P.M. ET; they are *valid for 2 hours*. At 5:00 P.M. (ET), SOAP concludes and ERAS' SOAP mode ends. An updated List of Unfilled Positions continues to be posted through May 1.

Mid-March to Mid-April: Programs/applicants mail and receive letters of appointment and contracts.

---

the United States, Puerto Rico, and Canada, enter the Match by permission of their Dean. For students in U.S. schools, the medical school's Dean decides which students are eligible to participate. To determine this, the question the Dean must answer is, "Will the student graduate this year?"

Canadian Resident Matching Service (CaRMS)

Canada has its own electronic application service (AWS) and resident matching program (CaRMS). Both can be accessed through the CaRMS website (www. carms.ca). The CaRMS Match takes place in two rounds, or "Iterations," held one month apart. The first round matches only graduates of a Canadian medical school who do not have any previous post-M.D. clinical training. Some provinces will consider students who are in their final year at an LCME-accredited U.S. medical school for the First Iteration, provided that they are Canadian citizens or have "Landed Immigrant" status. Information on individual province eligibility requirements can be found on the CaRMS website. All participants must have passed at least Part 1 of the Medical Council of Canada Qualifying Exam. Additional restrictions apply to non-U.S. international medical graduates and students (one is passing the Test of English as a Foreign Language, or TOEFL) and to graduates of Osteopathic medical schools.

Individuals may enter both the NRMP and CaRMS. However, since the CaRMS often completes the First Iteration of its match before the NRMP is run, candidates who enter both programs essentially rank all Canadian programs on their list higher than the U.S. programs.

Applicants must inform CaRMS, in writing, if they have applied to both the CaRMS and the NRMP. If an individual matches through CaRMS, the NRMP automatically removes that applicant's name from the NRMP lists *unless they are notified not to do so*. If an applicant is in the NRMP Match to obtain an Advanced position beginning at the PGY-2 level, that applicant *must tell the NRMP not to withdraw* their rank list if they are matched through CaRMS.

The second round of the CaRMS Match is for unmatched candidates from the first round plus independent candidates, including IMGs and physician candidates. Any applicant matched to a position in the United States through the NRMP Match will be withdrawn from the Second Iteration of the CaRMS Match.

In most provinces, participants must be a Landed Immigrant or a Canadian citizen to obtain postgraduate training in the funded residency programs. The requirements for each province are available from the Canadian Resident Matching Service, 171 Nepean Street, Suite 300, Ottawa, ON K2P 0B4, Canada; (613) 237-0075 or (877) CARMS-42; e-mail: help@carms.ca; www.carms.ca.

AOA-Approved Schools

Students from medical schools approved by the American Osteopathic Association may also participate in the NRMP Match. However, PGY-1 programs available through the NRMP Match do not fulfill the Osteopathic licensing requirements in some states. It is important that you check each state's Osteopathic Medical Board's rules *before* you decide to enter the Match.

If you want to participate in the Match, you do so as an Independent Applicant by logging onto the NRMP website. Your medical school will send the NRMP the required proof of your enrollment or graduation. Those applicants who enter both the AOA and NRMP matches must accept an offered AOA position and will be automatically withdrawn from the NRMP match.

Non-LCME-Approved Schools

Students at or graduates of medical schools not approved by the LCME, which includes virtually all medical schools outside the United States, Puerto Rico, and Canada and a very few within these jurisdictions (you already know if you are in this group), can apply to the NRMP Match only as Independent Applicants. This includes international medical graduates (FNIMGs and EVIMGs), U.S. citizens graduating from non-LCME approved schools (USIMGs), and Fifth Pathway students. (See Chapter 15 for more information.)

To participate in the Match, each applicant must furnish proof that he or she has either completed all the requirements for Examination Council for Foreign Medical Graduates (ECFMG) certification, or obtained a full and unrestricted license to practice medicine in the United States. While you can sign up for the NRMP Match and submit an ROL without being certified by the ECFMG, you must have completed all requirements for this certification by the time the ROL is due (mid-February). The NRMP will check with the ECFMG at that time. If you do not meet the requirements, you will not be allowed to proceed in the Match.

Couples Match

Because physician–physician couples were becoming more common, the NRMP instituted a Couples Match to assist couples in matching in the same geographic location. In recent years, couples' match rates have been comparable to those of students matching as individuals (Figure 23.6). The Couples Match is *not* only for those who are married or engaged. Any applicant pair can use this Match, including those who are dating, gay/lesbians, or even close friends. Independent applicants (Osteopathic students, graduate physicians, and IMGs) can also use the Couples Match. (Chapter 14 has additional information for couples.)

There are significant differences between going through the Match alone and going through as a couple. The initial step in entering the Couples Match is simply for each member of the couple to enroll in the Match and indicate in the R3 System that they want to be in the Match as part of a couple.

Unlike those in a shared-schedule position (described in the next section), couples apply to and interview at programs separately. They should, of course, try to select programs in corresponding geographic areas. For example, if one partner applies only in Washington, DC and the other only in San Francisco, they could not match with programs where they could live together during their residencies. However, if they both apply to programs in each city, there should be some compatible matches (*see* Figures 23.7 and 23.8).

Figure 23.6
NRMP Couples Match Results, 1991–2012

Year	Number of Couples	Number with Both Matched	Number with One Matched	Number with Neither Matched	Match Rate %
1991	377	349	17	11	94.8%
1995	499	433	33	33	90.1
1999	536	496	27	13	95.1
2001	561	518	25	18	94.6
2005	606	552	39	15	94.3
2010	808	730	50	28	93.4
2011	809	739	53	17	94.6
2012	878	804	54	20	94.6

Adapted from: NRMP Advance Data Tables, *2012 Main Residency Match*, Table 16, May 2012.

The special worksheet for the Couples Match can be found on the NRMP website (www.nrmp.org/res_match/special_part/us_seniors/couples_worksheet.pdf). After the partners apply to and interview at programs, each needs to evaluate the programs just as if he or she were matching as an individual. They then must work together to develop the combinations of programs to put on their Couples Rank-Order List Worksheet. Figure 23.8 is an example of one couple's list. Up to 400 pairs of programs can be listed without an extra charge. The programs are matched by rank order, and any combination of specialties and locations can be used. Note that PGY-1 choices on a Supplemental ROL are not paired in the Match. Therefore, any PGY-1 spots listed to accompany Advanced programs should be geographically compatible with the partner's paired choices.

In many cases, programs will be listed more than once. This may be especially true for the higher-ranked programs. It is also possible for one partner to elect to be unmatched against the other partner's selection. This option is normally reserved for the bottom of the ROL, where it is used as a "stopper" to attempt to prevent both partners from going unmatched.

When entering the ROLs on the R3 system, each partner enters his or her choices independently. Be careful that the numbers of the choices for both partners' lists match. One safeguard is that the partners are required to have the same number of listings, even though some of those listings may be "unmatched" (NRMP Program Code = 999999999). Both applicants need to know their partner's NRMP Applicant Code, not their R3 password, to enter an ROL in the Couples Match.

Figure 23.7
Example of a Couple's Worksheet

Partner 1	Partner 2
Washington, DC–Prog. A	San Francisco–Prog. 1
Washington, DC–Prog. B	Washington, DC–Prog. 1
San Francisco–Prog. A	San Francisco–Prog. 2
None	Washington, DC–Prog. 2

This is the way each partner independently ranked the programs at which they interviewed. They now need to work together to form combinations of these selections within each geographic area for their Couples ROL. (This is shown in Figure 23.8.)

Figure 23.8
Example of a Couple's Rank-Order List*

Partner 1	Partner 2
Washington, DC–Prog. A	Washington, DC–Prog. 1
San Francisco–Prog. A	San Francisco–Prog. 1
Washington, DC–Prog. B	Washington, DC–Prog. 1
Washington, DC–Prog. A	Washington, DC–Prog. 2
San Francisco–Prog. A	San Francisco–Prog. 2
Unmatched	Any Program Listed Above

*Based on the individual preferences in Figure 23.7.

Four important things to note: First, if one partner withdraws from the Match, the other partner will be ranked as a single candidate using the ROL he or she submitted. Second, couples are treated only as a single unit, meaning that if they do not obtain a match using any of their pairs of programs, the NRMP will not run their lists independently to find a match. Third, the NRMP is not your mother. It does not inquire as to how or why a couple is trying to match together. However, your Dean of Students will know that you are using the Couples Match. If you wish this information to be kept confidential, you may want to make a special appointment to talk to your Dean. Finally, if both partners match to Advanced programs, their Supplemental ROLs are not treated as a unit in the Match. The couple function works only for the couple's primary ROLs. The NRMP considers any Supplemental list individually and does not pair it with the partner's corresponding Supplemental list.

Even more complicated for some couples are the problems that occur when both partners are not going through the NRMP PGY-1 Match. For example, if one partner is interested in Urology and the other in Internal Medicine, major problems can develop. Since Urology is one of the specialties that sponsors its own Match, the NRMP's Couples Match will not work for them. In this case, the best solution would be for the pair to make a tentative list similar to that used by those going through the Couples Match. Then each partner should explain the situation to the program and department directors during their interviews. If you find yourself in this situation, ask them to make a commitment to you. If one residency position can be secured in advance, the partner can then attempt to match only with geographically compatible programs.

It is perfectly legal for program directors to make a commitment to you in advance. But programs participating in the NRMP PGY-1 Match are *not allowed to offer you a contract*. You, of course, have to place a great deal of trust in the program unless you are offered a contract to sign. Program directors cannot bind you to a commitment if they participate in the NRMP Match, and so they also need to trust you. Remember, if you do not deal honestly with the programs, the next couple to apply will have a much more difficult time.

Shared-Schedule/Part-Time Positions

A shared-schedule position, unlike the Couples Match, is one residency position held by two individuals. As explained in Chapter 14, the individuals involved want to do their training on a part-time basis, over a longer period of time than is normal. The NRMP provides a short description of their method for dealing with these positions at www.nrmp.org/res_match/special_part/us_seniors/shared_residency.html.

Programs that say they offer part-time (shared-schedule) positions are most frequently found in Family Medicine, Pediatrics, Preventive Medicine, Internal Medicine, and Psychiatry. There is a separate listing of all programs offering shared-schedule positions in the AMA's *GMED Companion: An Insider's Guide to Selecting a Residency Program,* published annually and available at most medical school libraries. This information is also available in the program descriptions on *FREIDA*. The NRMP website has a much shorter list of programs that have made the commitment to offer shared-schedule positions (click "My Reports" in the menu after you register).

To participate in the NRMP Match for a shared-schedule position, notify the NRMP directly at (202) 828-0566 or (Toll free) 866-617-5838. In reality, very few applicants choose to enter into this type of arrangement; most of those who contact the NRMP about part-time positions actually want to enter the Couples Match.

The NRMP issues shared-schedule applicant pairs a single NRMP Applicant Code to be used in the Match. In addition, a single combined name is used on the candidate list sent to the residency programs. For example, applicants Robert Smith and Mary Jones would be the candidate "Smith/Jones" for purposes of the Match. They would submit only one ROL, and could only be matched as a pair. If one of the pair drops out of the Match, the other must tell the NRMP whether he or she still wishes to participate as an individual. If so, the NRMP may assign them a new Applicant Code.

Physician Candidates

Physicians already in training or who have completed a training program can apply to enter the NRMP Match as Independent Candidates. Graduates of medical schools not approved by the LCME or AOA must furnish proof either that they have ECFMG Certification or that they have a full and unrestricted license to practice medicine in the United States. There are about 40 positions in fewer than 20 programs that are open only to physician candidates.

Military Appointments

Military medical training programs usually will accept only those individuals already obligated to do military service because they attend the Medical School of the Uniform Services University of the Health Sciences, participate in the Health Professions Scholarship Program, or have another type of prior commitment. There are usually too few military positions available to accommodate the number of individuals who apply.

In order to have the best chance of obtaining a position, you will have to participate in both the Military and the NRMP PGY-1 Matches. The military selects their residents before the NRMP PGY-1 Match (except for the Army and Navy PGY-1 slots that are in the NRMP Match), so those individuals who do not get military positions will still be able to get a residency position through the NRMP Match. The NRMP and the American Osteopathic Association are automatically notified when individuals match into a military position. For more information, see "Military/Public Health Service" in Chapter 14.

Don't Believe Anything You Are Promised

Several years ago, an applicant who our program had ranked highly called to say that she had not matched. That was surprising, since she was a very competitive applicant. Looking for a position, somewhat desperate, she admitted that she had listed only one program on her rank-order list. Why had she done this? Not for any of the common reasons related to family or other personal commitments. Instead, she had relied upon a promise from the residency director of a particular program, which was her first choice, that she would be ranked high enough to guarantee her a position. But that did not happen and she was left out in the cold. I have seen similar scenarios play out numerous times—often involving excellent students who had reason to believe that they would match with a particular program, only to find that they were either unmatched with any program or psychologically unprepared to go to their second-choice program.

The moral of such stories is that you should be extremely wary of any faculty member's promise to match you at a program. This holds true up until the point that either you get your Match results or you actually get a *firm and specific offer, in writing, from an individual authorized to make it.* (One student wrote saying he got just such a verbal offer and showed them this section of the book to demonstrate that he really did need a legitimate written offer. He got it.) If you fall for a specious promise, your dream of matching with the ideal residency may prove to be ephemeral.

According to surveys, residency programs contacted about two-thirds of applicants to inform them that they were being ranked highly. About one-third felt that programs lied to them, and one-quarter felt that programs made at least informal commitments to them. This doesn't portray medical educators as excellent role models.

As mentioned previously, couples with one or both partners applying to specialties outside the NRMP PGY-1 Match must take a calculated risk by asking for just such a commitment. In these cases, obtain the commitment from both the residency director and the department chairman, if possible. And make it clear that you are willing to sign a contract if it is offered.

Be aware, however, that *even a written contract for a position offered in the NRMP Match may not be valid.* The NRMP Match rules say that any contract for a position offered in the NRMP Match that is signed before the Match results are released is superseded by the results of the Match. Some specialties and programs, however, do not offer positions through the Match. If one of these programs offers you a position, they should simultaneously offer you a contract.

The AOA's Intern/Resident Registration Program states that programs can tell applicants that they are "very likely," "likely," or "unlikely" to be ranked in a top position for that program. Surprisingly, the only thing you can rely on is if they tell you that it is "unlikely." At least then you know not to buy real estate in that city.

What To Do If You Don't Match

On Monday of Match Week, all participants find out if they have matched. If, for some reason, you do not match, you will most likely be eligible for NRMP's Supplemental Offer and Acceptance Program or "SOAP" (which replaced the Scramble in 2012).

Being unmatched does *not* mean that you have failed; *matching is not the final measure of your worth.* You will certainly not be the first individual in history who did not match; about 6% of U.S. M.D. seniors have failed to match through the NRMP in each of the last five years (Figure 23.9). By going through the steps in this book, you are less likely to find yourself unmatched than some of your classmates. In addition, the preparation you have already done will not be wasted. It will give you an edge, even if you do end up without a position. The first rule is: DON'T PANIC!

You may first want to consider whether the specialty you chose is still what you want. Many students have second thoughts after making their initial commitment. You now have a chance to reconsider—but you must reconsider quickly. As soon as you hear that you haven't matched, you must be on the ERAS website to submit applications to unfilled programs. If you aren't sure about a specialty, one option is to pick one of the many Preliminary Surgery or Medicine slots that go unmatched. These may act as stepping-stones to PGY-2 slots in the new specialty of your choice.

If you decide that you still want to go into the specialty you initially selected, you will need to be geographically flexible. Training in the urban ghetto or the rural hinterlands (sites with many unmatched positions) may not be so bad after all; you will get a chance to expand your horizons, and you may even grow to like it. If you are flexible, you are almost sure to get a reasonable position in most specialties. (A few specialties, like Orthopedic Surgery, rarely have spots open after the Match.)

Understand that the programs also feel oppressed by having to quickly attempt to fill their residency position with the best available person. In addition, unlike you, their program is listed on the NRMP's "Unmatched" website. This announces to the world that their program did not fill. They are not having good day either.

Another source of information about unfilled positions, both after SOAP and at other times during the year, is the AAMC's FindAResident website (www.aamc.org/findaresident). This subscription service is available to ERAS users for a nominal charge. Programs can post information about available positions for applicants to review. In addition, applicants can use their existing ERAS application to create an electronic résumé that can be easily downloaded and evaluated by the program directors.

Finally, remember that many originally unmatched applicants enter excellent residencies, some get into difficult-to-enter specialties, and, despite this very temporary setback, most go on to become excellent clinicians.

Figure 23.9
Applicants Participating in the 2010 "Scramble"

Seniors from U.S. M.D.-granting medical schools	1,078
Previous grads from U.S. M.D.-granting medical schools	747
Students/graduates of Osteopathic medical schools	601
U.S. citizen students/grads from international med schools	1,946
Non-U.S. citizen students/grads from international med schools	4,365
Total	8,794

Source: AMA Graduate Medical Education (GME) e-Letter, April 2010:2.

Supplemental Offer and Acceptance Program (SOAP)

While the percentage of U.S. seniors failing to match has remained steady, the number of positions unfilled after the PGY-1 Match decreased from 1,587 in 2006 to 1,246 in 2012. To address this increased competition for unfilled positions, in 2012 the NRMP began using the Supplemental Offer and Acceptance Program (SOAP). The process helps to automate, streamline, and equalize the process by which residency applicants acquire unfilled positions. Prior to this, applicants used "the Scramble," a term that describes exactly how it worked.

Of the 1,246 unfilled PGY-1 and PGY-2 positions after the 2012 NRMP Main Match, nearly half (607) were Preliminary Surgery and Preliminary Medicine PGY-1-only slots. Unfilled programs placed 1,131 positions into SOAP. By the end of the first day's two Offer rounds, 76% of SOAP positions had filled. By 5:00 P.M. Friday night when SOAP ended, 91% of the positions had been filled.

Eligibility

To participate in SOAP, applicants must be unmatched or partially matched and must be able to begin training on July 1 in the year of the Match. The applicant's medical school Dean or the ECFMG (for IMGs) must reconfirm that the applicant still meets eligibility requirements. The NRMP sends recertification requests to Deans and the ECFMG on Monday of the week prior to Match Week. Deans must recertify the status of their senior students and the ECFMG must recertify the status of their IMGs by Wednesday. *All applicants* are notified of their eligibility for SOAP at noon (ET) on the Friday before Match Week. (See Figure 23.5 for the schedule of events.)

To find out if you are SOAP "eligible," log onto the R3 system, using your AAMC ID and password, beginning at noon (ET) on the Friday before Match Week. The program will open your "Applicant Options" page. Your SOAP status will be displayed in the upper right corner of the screen. It should say that you are "eligible," and remain that way until Match Results are released on Match Day. You should also get an e-mail from the NRMP indicating your status.

Note that being declared "eligible" has nothing to do with whether you have matched. ALL applicants who can start their training on July 1 are initially listed as eligible. You will find out on Monday of Match Week if you have not matched or have only partially matched. If you have been declared "eligible" AND are unmatched or partially matched, you can participate in SOAP. "Partially matched" means that you matched either with an internship or with a residency, but not both, and that you will have to participate in SOAP for the other position.

On the left menu bar of your Applicant Options page, there are three SOAP links: the SOAP schedule, the List of Unfilled Programs, and SOAP offers. The Schedule contains detailed information concerning the events during Match Week and about SOAP.

Applicants are not notified if they have matched until noon (ET) on Monday of Match Week. Only those applicants who are unmatched or partially matched and are eligible for SOAP will be given access to the List of Unfilled Programs and allowed to participate in SOAP.

Finding Programs and Submitting Applications

The NRMP releases unmatched applicant and unfilled program information simultaneously at noon (ET) the Monday of Match Week. The "Unfilled Programs" link in R3 allows SOAP-eligible applicants access to Specialties with unfilled programs, and then to access a list of the individual programs with open slots to which the applicant may apply. ERAS opens at 1:00 P.M. (ET) on Monday for SOAP participants to create applications for unfilled positions. At 2:00 P.M. (ET), ERAS begins submitting applications to the programs. Both programs and applicants must use ERAS to send and receive applications; this replaces the logjam of phone calls, e-mails, and faxes of prior years.

During the SOAP period, applicants may transmit a varying number of applications (free of charge) to unfilled programs; normal ERAS fees apply before and during this time frame. Between noon (ET) on Monday and noon (ET) on Wednesday, you can submit 30 applications. From Wednesday at noon (ET) and to noon (ET) Thursday, you can submit 10 applications, and you can submit 5 applications from noon (ET) Thursday and to noon (ET) on Friday.

As in the initial Match, list the programs in the order that they interest you and enter that information on your ERAS SOAP list. ERAS will then submit your applications to the programs for downloading.

During Match Week, programs that participate in the NRMP Match must try to fill their unmatched positions only through SOAP and only with SOAP-eligible participants; the R3 System has been modified so that these positions are offered on the basis of the programs' preference lists. Programs are not, however, required to fill their positions during Match Week. Accepted positions are automatically deleted from the List of Unfilled Programs and no further applications for that position can be sent through ERAS. A program's unfilled positions will be offered in order of preference until all positions are filled or the preference list is finished.

Receiving and Accepting Offers

Programs must enter their SOAP preference list of applicants into the R3 system by 11:30 A.M. (ET) on Wednesday of Match Week. The first offers are released at noon, and the rounds continue through Friday (Match Day). Once the SOAP Offer rounds begin, check the R3 site and your e-mail often to see if you have received any offers.

At this stage of the game, both you and programs should be willing to make decisions based on the available information. The NRMP prohibits applicants (and others acting on their behalf) from contacting programs until after the program has contacted them and from using a method other than ERAS to apply for an unfilled position. This means you cannot e-mail, telephone, fax, or use any other method to initiate contact with a residency program. Unfilled programs cannot contact applicants prior to 2 P.M. (ET) on Monday of Match Week, which is when ERAS sends the SOAP applications to the programs.

Applicants can log into the R3 system to see if any offers have been extended to them during each round. Offers are shown in the main "SOAP Offers" screen, and the deadline to accept them is clearly stated, in large type. The NRMP will also notify you by e-mail about any outstanding offers. Be sure to have your Internet-capable phone available. *Check it frequently* to be certain that it is functioning.

To get information about the position being offered, click on "View Offer." You can also click on "Offers" on the left menu bar for additional details on each program.

There is a specific time frame within which applicants must accept or reject an offer before that offer expires; this is clearly stated on all materials. If you take too long to apply for a position, your chances of getting any reasonable PGY-1 slot are almost nonexistent. At this point, programs must rely on your ERAS application materials, and you must decide upon offers as they are submitted to you in each round of SOAP. You need a position, they need a resident—and you both need them *now*.

When you click on "View Offer" for information, you will also be given links to "Accept this offer," "Reject this offer," or "Return" to your SOAP Offers page.

When you click on "Accept" or "Reject" for an offer, the system will ask for your password to confirm that you understand the consequences of your choice: By accepting an offer, you enter into a binding contract. By rejecting an offer (or allowing the time to expire), you acknowledge that you will not receive another offer from that program.

Once you have made your choice, you must click "Submit" to return to your SOAP Offers page, where you will receive your confirmation letter. You will also get an e-mail from the NRMP confirming your acceptance. If you have received more than one offer in a round, the R3 system will automatically list other offers as Rejected after you have accepted an offer.

Before you hit the "Submit" button to accept an offer, be very sure that is what you want to do. *You will not be able to change your mind after you accept an offer!* All offers accepted during SOAP are considered binding and are subject to the Match Participation Agreement.

If you do nothing, the offer(s) will expire at the end of that round. *Once an offer expires, that program will not extend another offer to you.*

Keep copies of all SOAP-related emails.

SOAP's system works in real time, so once you accept a position, SOAP automatically removes you from other program's preference lists and no other offers for the same type of position will be extended to you. Of course, if you are applying for both Preliminary and Advanced positions, SOAP allows you to continue to seek the position with which you haven't matched yet. If, for example, you accept a Preliminary position, you will not be offered another Preliminary slot. However, you will still be sent offers for any Advanced positions to which you are applying.

The programs send you contracts and additional paperwork beginning the day after Match Day.

Other Training Opportunities

If you haven't matched, there is another avenue to consider. That is postponing your training at the PGY-1 level to pursue parallel training. You may have an interest in pursuing a graduate degree (for example, an M.P.H. or M.S.) or in doing research. This is a perfect opportunity. It gives you a chance to regroup and rethink both your decision about a specialty and your method of pursuing it. In addition, success in this year, if it is used to advantage, may even bolster your chance of getting the position you want. The bottom line is, don't waste this year, even if you decide not to do an internship immediately.

Matching In Advance (PGY-2 & Above)

One of the most confusing and frustrating aspects of the Match is that not all specialties participate. And even in some of those that do, not all programs participate. Although listed in the *NRMP Directory*, Neurology, Ophthalmology, Plastic Surgery (PGY-4 positions), and Urology essentially do not participate in the NRMP Match.

Most of these specialties use separate Matches, sponsored by one of their academic societies, to fill their PGY-2 positions. (See Figures 23.2 and 23.10.) The positions are predominantly filled one or two years ahead of time by senior medical students who will enter these programs after finishing preliminary training. These specialty Matches require that ROLs be submitted by early January, and they release their Match results in mid- to late January. Registration for Neurotology, Ophthalmology, and Plastic Surgery (PGY-4) is $100, which includes the set-up fee for the San Francisco Matching Program's Centralized Application Service (CAS). Most fellowship matches require either a $50 or $100 registration fee (2012).

Information and applications for Neurotology, Ophthalmology, and Plastic Surgery can be obtained by writing [Specialty] Matching Program, P.O. Box 45161, San Francisco, CA 94145-0161; www.sfmatch.org. The address *for overnight delivery only* is: SF Match, c/o Union Bank of California, Lockbox Dept-lockbox 45161, 460 Hegenberger Road, Oakland, CA 94621. The website also offers information about positions that have become available between the matches. Click on "Vacancies." These programs use the Centralized Application Service (CAS) rather than ERAS. Much of the information you need to provide is the same as that for ERAS, and includes your personal data, achievements, employment history, activities, personal statement, references, and supporting documents. In addition, both on-line and paper applications for the individual specialties are available on the CAS website.

Information about the Urology Match can be obtained online from the American Urological Association's Matching Program at www.auanet.org/content/residents/residency-match.cfm. The Urology Match cost $75 in 2012.

Anesthesiology, Dermatology, Emergency Medicine, Neurology, Physical Medicine & Rehabilitation, Plastic Surgery, Psychiatry, Radiation Oncology and Diagnostic Radiology offer both PGY-1 and PGY-2 (Advanced) positions through the NRMP Main Match. Nearly all programs in these specialties participate in the NRMP Match. The NRMP also runs many fellowship matches (Figure 23.10). Generally, ROLs must be submitted by early June. Most Match results are announced in late June, although it varies by specialty. Specific information is available by clicking "Fellowship Matches" at www.nrmp.org/.

Not Using A Match

Some residents get their positions without going through the NRMP or any specialty Matches. In recent years, nearly 20% of the residents in training programs had not gone through the NRMP Match to obtain their positions. Just how many of these individuals went through the specialty Matches, and exactly which positions (and their quality) were obtained, is unknown. There are opportunities outside the Match, though. And it is important to know about them.

Early Graduation

The NRMP PGY-1 Match is only for residency positions beginning in July. While not generally advertised, many programs (704 in 2012) have or can make positions available at other times. These are open for several reasons. For example, the program may not have been fully matched in previous years, it could be expanding, or a resident may have left voluntarily or been dropped from the program. Some programs have actually designed one or more positions to begin at midyear. Residency positions beginning in January, February, and March are not normally listed by the NRMP. However, there are not many of these positions (see "Programs offering multiple start dates" in each specialty's listing in Chapter 3).

Figure 23.10
Selected Specialties' Programs and Positions Available
through Other Non-NRMP PGY-1 Matches

Specialty Match	Total Programs (Programs in Match)	Total Positions (Positions in Match)[†]
Abdominal Transplant Surgery*	56 (55)	60 (71)
Cardiovascular Disease*	179 (169)	2,626 (718)
Child and Adolescent Psychiatry*	124 (105)	964 (327)
Child Neurology*	104 (71)	187 (99)
Colon & Rectal Surgery*	49 (43)	85 (78)
Critical Care (Surgery)*	95 (81)	214 (167)
Endocrin., Diab. & Metab. (IM)*	125 (112)	607 (213)
Gastroenterology (IM)*	155 (153)	1,482 (361)
Hand Surgery (All)*	77 (69)	161 (144)
Hematology-Oncology (IM)*	132 (123)	1,541 (449)
Infectious Disease (IM)*	145 (123)	783 (330)
Interventional Radiology*	90 (83)	261 (212)
Maternal-Fetal Medicine*	69 (68)	73 (84)
Neonatal-Perinatal Medicine*	91 (91)	711 (221)
Nephrology (IM)*	142 (142)	(374)
Neurological Surgery[‡]	99 (91)	1,266 (156)
Neuroradiology*	86 (75)	325 (199)
Ophthalmology	118 (117)	460 (458)
Ophthalmology Fellowships (Other)[‡]	275 (227)	618 (456)
Orthopaedic Spine	64 (64)	124 (124)
Pediatric Cardiology*	51 (45)	385 (118)
Pediatric Critical Care*	61 (47)	443 (93)
Pediatric Emergency Medicine*	48 (42)	328 (101)
Pediatric Hematology/Oncology*	68 (62)	487 (152)
Pediatric Radiology*	46 (17)	114 (34)
Pediatric Surgery*	43 (43)	76 (44)
Plastic Surgery (PGY-4)[‡,§]	87 (71)	448 (422)
Sports Medicine (FM)*	106 (95)	(146)
Pulmonary Dis. & Critical Care (IM)*	135 (124)	1,451 (410)
Radiology*	187 (158)	(411)
Rheumatology (IM)*	108 (97)	464 (179)

(Continued)

Figure 23.10 (continued)

Specialty Match	Total Programs (Programs in Match)	Total Positions (Positions in Match)†
Surgical Critical Care*	90 (81)	201 (167)
Urology**	120 (114)	251 (268)
Vascular Surgery*	96 (87)	262 (113)

*Match run by NRMP (Information from NRMP, January 2012).
†Many of the positions not in the Matches are offered through the U.S. Military.
‡Match run by the San Francisco Match (Information from www.sfmatch.com, 2011).
§Plastic Surgery also offers an "integrated" program beginning at the PGY-1 level.
**Match run by the American Urological Association.

One way to find positions that begin at times other than July is to use the AAMC's FindAResident system (described below). Another is to write to the programs and inquire. A list of programs that offer multiple start dates can be found on *FREIDA*. (Use the "Choose Optional Criteria" button to select "Start Dates other than June-July.") Your inquiry to the program should be specific. Tell them when you want to start and whether you will have officially graduated. If your diploma will not be granted early, indicate whether you will have a letter from your school certifying that you have completed all the requirements for graduation.

If you go outside the Match, there are some additional rules to follow. These revolve around actually obtaining the position. Unlike using the Match, you will need to decipher when you are actually being offered a position and how firm the offer is. Most programs do not have as rigid a structure for interviewing or selecting applicants for midyear positions as they have for those that are available in July. The selection process, in fact, may be a little sloppy.

Aside from the other rules listed for optimal interviewing, you must also nail down exactly when and how you will be notified of the program's decision. It is perfectly reasonable to let the interviewers know that you are applying to more than one program for a midyear slot and, though you would *really* like to go to their program, you will, of necessity, have to accept the first available position. This, of course, is not completely true. If your second-choice program offers you a position, ask for at least a 24-hour delay to consider the offer. Virtually all programs will give you that long. Then contact your first-choice program and press them for a decision. But don't bluff. While this may get you a position at your first-choice program, it might also leave you without *any* position if you force an early decision without having been offered a slot at another program.

Specifically, ask the residency director when you can expect to hear back from the program. Emphasize that an early decision is crucial. They will, undoubtedly, understand this. If you are a competitive candidate for the position, you will be seen as being even stronger at midyear. The program is not likely to wait for someone just a little bit better—that individual might not show up. So, be assertive. The day after you were supposed to hear a decision, assuming that you haven't, call the residency director's office and find out what is going on. In many cases, the program just will not have "gotten it together" enough to decide yet. Your demonstration of enthusiasm will be very effective. *For midyear matching, being assertive is the key to success.*

FindAResident™

FindAResident (www.aamc.org/findaresident) is available year-round to assist applicants seeking positions after the NRMP Match, those looking for advanced positions, and those wanting to transfer to a different program or specialty in mid-year. Some of the available slots are listed because they were unfilled in the Match and SOAP or because residents left the program.

FindAResident is a subscription service that, in addition to listing programs and their specific vacancies for applicants to review, allows applicants to create an electronic résumé for programs to view and evaluate. ERAS users may build their FindAResident résumé by downloading information from their existing ERAS application. Their Dean's and recommendation letters, however, cannot be posted. FindAResident services are available to ERAS users for $30 and to all other users for $75.

Applicants link their materials to one or more specialties so the programs in that specialty may access them. (If an applicant lists more than one specialty, the programs do not know: the list is confidential) Students who register with the service can also search for posted positions by specialty.

Programs participating in the Match that have vacancies cannot post PGY-1 positions on FindAResident until *after* NRMP Match results have been released. Otherwise, they can update their listing at any time, so the database contains the most current and accurate information. Once a position has been filled, programs remove the position from the FindAResident database.

New Programs

New programs, specifically those that have just recently been approved to offer training but are not yet in the NRMP Match, are potential gold mines for those with initiative. Not only will there be less competition for slots, but you also have the possibility of matching early, thus avoiding the hassle of sweating it out until March.

In addition, these programs offer you the unique opportunity to help shape a training program. The first residents through any program, though they encounter a lot of rough spots and often have no senior residents to act as role models, inevitably have closer contacts with the faculty than subsequent classes. They are frequently given more responsibility and obtain more intense training.

But how do you find out about these programs? There are a number of sources. Your mentor and the Dean of Students are the sources closest to home. Prominent individuals, especially other program directors and notable teachers in that specialty, often receive advance notification about new programs that have been approved to begin training residents.

Specialty societies are another source of information. Call and ask to talk to their Director of Educational Programs. New programs will often place advertisements in their specialty journals. Advertisements can also be found in general readership journals such as the *New England Journal of Medicine* and the *Journal of the American Medical Association*. Finally, search the Internet, especially *FindAResident*. Many new programs list themselves so potential applicants can find out about them before they are listed either on *FREIDA* or in the Green Book.

Once again, the student who puts forth a little extra effort will reap rewards from these opportunities. Also remember that new programs have fewer applicants. This is true not only for their first year, but also in the next few years. If you are not the most stellar of candidates, this source of training opportunities may be one of your best bets.

A warning, however. Every year, some new graduates begin internships with the promise that the residency program is "about to be accredited." It often isn't, and the intern is faced with the daunting task of finding a residency position during the most stressful year of her life. A newly accredited program often works out amazingly well; a "soon-to-be accredited" program is a recipe for disaster.

Following Other Training

Some people suggest that you might have better luck getting into a highly competitive specialty, such as Neurosurgery, Dermatology, or Orthopedic Surgery, if you first complete specialty training in another area, such as Internal Medicine. The theory is that with the greater emphasis on patient care in teaching centers, any trainee who is already competent in basic patient care will be prized. In some cases this might be true, but experience suggests otherwise.

Program directors ask the following questions: Why is someone who could go out and practice medicine applying for another training program? Are they unsure of themselves or their goals? Are they planning to become perpetual students? Are they even educable at this stage of their training? In addition, some federal rules restrict a program's reimbursement to training residents for their first completed specialty. So directors also ask, Do I want this applicant badly enough to reduce the Medicare payments we get for residents?

Obviously, training in a second specialty is a risky road to follow—not to mention a long one. Think hard before you take this path.

Specialties without Matching Programs

Preventive Medicine (General, Occupational, and Public Health), Medical Genetics, Nuclear Medicine, many Internal Medicine subspecialties, and many smaller specialties and subspecialties do not have matching programs and do not, for all intents and purposes, participate in the NRMP Match. If you are interested in these specialties, you must apply to the individual programs and make individual contracts.

Non-Approved Programs

Of all the non-Match methods for getting a residency training position, this definitely has the most risk. "Non-approved" means that the Residency Review Committee for that specialty has not certified a program. These committees send out surveyors to assess training programs using preset criteria. A program that does not gain approval was probably deficient in more than one area that was felt to be essential for an adequate training program. *Training at a Non-approved program may leave you unqualified to take the specialty's board examination.*

You should be aware of some other terms used to describe the accreditation of programs. Some programs have "Provisional" approval. This only means that a program is relatively new or has undergone significant changes. However, if the program is on "Probation," assess it carefully. It is in danger of falling into the "Non-approved" category. And, while provisions are usually made to accredit the training of the most senior residents in such programs, more junior residents may be in trouble.

Osteopathic Matching Program

Osteopathic medical students use the *Intern/Resident Registration Program* to match with American Osteopathic Association (AOA)-approved internships and residency programs (other than those in the Military). The Intern/Resident Registration Program is run under the AOA's auspices through National Matching Services (NMS). Their main office is in Canada, and all correspondence must end up there. So, if possible, call or send mail directly to that office at 20 Holly Street, Suite 301, Toronto, ON, Canada M4S 3B1; (416) 977-3431; fax, (416) 977-5020; e-mail, aoairp@natmatch.com; www.natmatch.com/aoairp. Their U.S. office is at P.O. Box 1208, Lewiston, NY 14092-8208; (716) 282-4013.

Program Types

Use the AOA's Intern/Resident Registration Program (the "Match"), the Military's matching program, or the NRMP (only for AOA-ACGME jointly approved programs) to get an AOA-approved residency or internship. There are three "Options" for AOA-approved first-year training, depending on the specialty involved. These are discussed in Chapter 14, and the Option required for each specialty is indicated in Figure 14.8.

Beginning in 2013, all programs offered in the AOA Match will provide OGME-1 training that meets the requirements for AOA-approved first-year training. These programs are one of two types:

Traditional Rotating Internship: a rotating internship (OGME-1T) for students who have not yet decided on a specialty, those who plan on going into an ACGME residency, or those who wish to enter a specialty that does not go through the Match and that requires a separate application (Option 3 specialty; currently, Dermatology and Preventive Medicine-Public Health). Beginning in July 2013, these programs involve a commitment for only one year of training. When interviewing for a traditional rotating internship position, you should discuss (and negotiate) the curriculum directly with the program.

Residency: These programs involve a two-year commitment. The student matches with both an OGME-1 position and an OGME-2 position (beginning the following year) in the specialty's residency program. Both Option 1 and Option 2 specialty programs are offered as residency programs (OGME-1R) in the Match.

Option 1 specialty programs will match graduating students directly into residency programs. This system parallels that used by most ACGME-approved specialties.

Option 2 specialty programs assure entry into both the preliminary year (AOA-approved internship) and the subsequent residency program. Applicants rank the two as a single program by using one Program Code Number. Both programs are normally at the same institution, but some may be at two affiliated institutions. In such instances, the specialty institution will be listed in the Match, while the institution providing the OGME-1 training will be identified in the program description.

Locating Programs

A list of available AOA-approved intern and residency positions can be found at http://opportunities.osteopathic.org/search. There are four types of searches you can do: Basic, Advanced, Program, and Hospital. Access these from the "Searches" box on the left side of the page. Generally, you will want to start with a Basic search, unless you have already completed your Must-Want Analysis and know which other criteria you want in a program. In that case, you should use the Advanced Search. The Program search is used to find information about a specific program: enter either the Program Name or Program Number in the box to obtain the information.

Both the Basic and Advanced Searches can find either intern or residency programs. The Basic Search uses the specialty and the location (state). However, you can search multiple specialties and multiple states simultaneously by holding down the "Ctrl" key as you make selections from the list. This method provides the maximum number of programs, since they are not eliminated by adding other selection criteria. Results appear as a list that includes the Program Number. A check box allows you to move any of the programs to your personal folder to review later. If you click on the Program Number, detailed information about the program appears.

If you need additional assistance on how to search, watch the 6-minute video located under "Help" on the left side of the main page. You can also contact the AOA at (800) 621-1773 or opportunities@osteopathic.org.

Program Information

The Advanced Search allows you to screen programs not only by specialty and location, but also by "Educational Features" and "Benefits" (Fig. 23.11). What each criterion means to each program is not always clear; carefully examine the detailed program description. A very important screening criterion that is hidden at the bottom of the page is a check box used to select only those programs that have dual AOA and ACGME accreditation.

There is an enormous amount of information available for listed programs. However, this information may not be current; most information is not verified by an outside source. The AOA does verify the number of filled and open

Figure 23.11
Advanced Search Criteria in AOA-NMS Internship/Residency Database

Educational Features	Benefits
ACLS certification provided	Childcare on-site
AOA & ACME accredited	CME allowance
Board review courses	Computer documentation of resident clinical logs
Components on Malpractice, Risk Management, Jurisprudence, and/or Physician-Patient Communication	Disability, Health, Life, and/or Malpractice insurance offered
Ethics curriculum/consultation	Housing
Formal Behavioral Medicine, Managed Care, and/or Osteopathic Manipulative curriculum	Leave for educational meetings & conferences
Journal club	Expenses paid for meetings/conferences
Procedures courses	Medical leave
Research opportunity	License paid
Structured End-of-life curriculum	Professional membership dues paid
Structured Practice Management experience	Salary
Written performance evaluation	Vacation duration
	Family, Maternity, and/or Paternity leave

positions: Programs' numbers often vary from this, but the AOA's numbers represent reality.

Useful information includes: Program Number, date the information was posted, number of filled/open positions in each year, number of faculty, ERAS participation, application requirements, interview dates/total number scheduled, residents' success on Board examinations, on-call frequency in each year, educational and other benefits (but often not in enough detail to be useful), salary, and contact information for hospitals/personnel involved with the program.

Fewer than three-fourths of all Osteopathic graduates choose Osteopathic internships. The number of new graduates choosing ACGME-approved (M.D.) programs ranges from 3% at some Osteopathic schools to 47% at others. In addition, nearly two-thirds of the Osteopaths taking specialty residencies do so in ACGME-approved programs. In 2012, Osteopathic applicants using the

NRMP Match for ACGME-approved programs had the highest match rates in Internal Medicine-Categorical (19.8%), Family Medicine (18.6%), Pediatrics-Categorical (14.5%), Emergency Medicine (11.3%), Psychiatry (7.3%), and OB/GYN (7.7%). These percentages have remained relatively constant for the last four years.

ERAS/Submitting Applications

As with the NRMP and other matching programs, applicants must still *apply* to the individual programs, usually through ERAS (see Chapter 13). Information about using ERAS to apply to Osteopathic programs is available at www.osteopathic.org/inside-aoa/education/students.

Applying for the Match

To be eligible to participate in the AOA Resident/Intern Registration Program (NMS Match), each student must register directly with the National Matching Service (NMS) by completing an Applicant Agreement. To do this, go to the NMS site at www.natmatch.com/aoairp/aoareg.htm, and download, print out, and sign the Applicant Agreement. Then send it with $60 (2012) paid by check, a money order drawn on a U.S. or Canadian bank, or an *international* postal money order. You must have your 6-digit AOA ID Number that you get from your Dean's office or from the AOA Member Services Center at 800-621-1773 (select option 1) to put on the form.

The AOA recommends registering for their Match by November 1 of your senior year. Once your Applicant Agreement is processed, you will receive a Match "Code Number" for the Registration Program (usually the same as your AOA ID Number). You must give that number to each program when you apply, so that they can list you on their rank-order list (ROL). To ensure that you don't miss vital messages from the NMS, be certain that any spam filter on your e-mail system accepts messages from "aoairp@natmatch.com," "matchinfo@natmatch.com," or any other address with "@natmatch.com."

Schedule: Interviews and Match

By the end of November, instructions for submitting ROLs (including special instructions for those participating in the Couples Match or the Military Match) and obtaining Match results will be available to students and programs registered to participate in the Match. (See Figure 23.12 for the Registration Program timeline.)

Students who wish to coordinate their Matches can enter as a "Couple." Each must register individually, then update their profile to indicate that they are part of a couple and provide their partner's Code Number before they submit their ROL. As with the NRMP, couples should submit "pairs" of program rankings.

Students with military commitments generally participate in the Military Match, which is completed prior to both the AOA and the NRMP Matches. Osteopathic medical students must notify the NMS if they match with a military program, so that they will be removed from the AOA Match. If students match through the AOA, the NRMP is notified automatically, and they are removed from the NRMP Match for those types of positions. For example, applicants that match through the AOA for an internship-only position (OGME-1) may not participate in the NRMP Main Match for a similar position that year. If they match with an Osteopathic combined internship/residency program (OGME-1 and OGME-2), they will be removed from the NRMP Match for both PGY-1 and PGY-2 positions.

AOA Registration Program Results

Matches between the programs and applicants are based on the ROL that each submits. The algorithm they use for the Match is applicant-optimal, i.e., it gives applicants' choices of programs a slight edge over the programs' choices of applicants. Additional information about the algorithm is at www.natmatch. com/aoairp/index.htm.

The Registration Program results are posted in mid-February at www. natmatch.com/aoairp/matres.htm. The results are binding. If an institution does not send a contract to a matched applicant within 10 working days after the Match, the applicant may be released from their obligation. If a matched participant does not sign a contract with that program within 30 days, he is banned from entering any other AOA-approved training program for one year. The only exception is if both the program and the applicant agree, in writing, to release each other from this obligation by signing the appropriate part of the intern contract.

If an applicant fails to match in the AOA Registration Program, they are provided with a list of unmatched programs, and should follow the procedures discussed under "What to Do If You Don't Match?" earlier in this chapter. Students who used ERAS when applying to programs may still use the service to send their information to unfilled programs.

Figure 23.12
Osteopathic Intern/Resident Registration Program Schedule

June: Students register at the National Matching Service (NMS) website: www. natmatch.com/aoairp. You need your 6-digit AOA ID Number that is assigned to you by the AOA. If you do not have it, contact your Dean's office or AOA Member Services at (800) 621-1773.

July–January: Students gather program information, submit applications to training programs (directly or through ERAS), and interview. Deadlines for submitting applications and interviewing vary: always ask each program for their deadline.

August–September: Institutions offering OGME-1 positions give their information to the NMS.

November 1: AOA recommends that students register for the AOA Match by this date. A list of participating programs is available at www.natmatch.com/ aoairp.

Late November: Instructions for submitting ROLs and obtaining Match results are posted on the NMS website.

Late January: Deadline for students and programs to submit their ROLs. *No ROLs or registrations for the Match will be accepted after this date.*

Mid-February: Match results are released to students, participating programs, Osteopathic schools, and OPTIs.

Institutions have 10 working days to send contracts for employment to matched students for their signature. Students must sign and return the contract to their institution within 30 days.

July 1: Internship or residency begins.

24

You've Matched–Now What?

Eureka! Eureka!
Archimedes

CONGRATULATIONS! YOU HAVE GOTTEN a residency position. You have matched! But you are still not through. As they say in tennis, it's the follow-through that makes winners. (I can't even hit the ball, but I know the rules.)

You will be firmly attached to this residency training program for the next several years. What you do in the next few hours and days will make a lasting impression on your new employers.

Contact The Program

By Telephone

As soon as you find out where you have matched and can calm down to a reasonable level of intelligibility, make a telephone call to your new residency director. The call should be brief and enthusiastic, even if the program was not your first choice. Tell him or her how glad you are to have matched with the program and how much you are looking forward to starting your residency training.

This also is a good time to ask if the program needs any additional information from you, their new resident. During this *short* telephone call, keep in mind that you want to establish a positive image of yourself in the residency director's mind. Now that you have an employer–employee relationship, doesn't that seem wise?

By E-mail and a Letter

Now that you have matched, you have to write some e-mails (immediately) and letters (in the next few days).

First, send an e-mail, and then a letter, to the program with which you have matched. Repeat your enthusiastic response to matching with them and starting your residency training. Ask again if they need any additional information. Also, of prime importance, *give them your e-mail address(es), mailing address(es) and telephone number(s) for the next several months* so they can contact you and send you any materials you might need. Every year some new interns fail to get their first few paychecks on time because they could not be reached in advance to fill out the necessary paperwork.

Your second e-mail and letter should be sent to your adviser or mentor. This is the individual who has probably done the most to help get you the position that you wanted. Of course, it is most appropriate to tell your adviser about your Match results in person, as soon as possible. But also send a note of thanks, saying how much you appreciate all his or her efforts on your behalf. It is also proper, if you so desire, to give a small gift as a token of your thanks. This, however, is purely optional and will depend upon the relationship you have developed.

Finally, send e-mails and letters to those individuals who wrote your reference letters. Thank them for writing the letters and tell them where you will be going for training. They will appreciate your thoughtfulness and this will, hopefully, help you to continue these valuable professional connections.

Post-Purchase Dissonance

Have you ever thought long and hard before buying a car, a home, or expensive electronic gear—only to finally buy it and then be fraught with uncertainty over whether you made the correct decision? Of course you have. It is normal human behavior. This behavior is called post-purchase dissonance.

You have just spent the past six months, and probably much longer, investigating specialties and residency programs before you "bought." You might now feel uncertain about that choice. You may, from some source, receive additional information about your program (no matter whether it is correct or not) or about your specialty (significant or not), and suddenly you are unsure about the life decision that you have made. Don't worry! This happens to almost everyone. If you have gone through the steps outlined in this book, you will be just fine. Now is the time to relax and enjoy yourself—you've earned it.

You might also wonder if the program's faculty does not also feel some post-purchase dissonance. They often do. But if you have contacted them as outlined above, their dissonance, if they have any, will not be directed toward you.

Contracting With The Program

After matching, you should soon receive a contract to sign from the program. The contract and accompanying information sent by the program should specify:
- the length of the residency program
- the duration of your appointment
- the conditions for your reappointment
- your responsibilities in the program
- the amount of your salary
- the amount of other stipends (meals, uniforms, laundry)
- the liability and disability insurance provided for you
- the health and life insurance coverage available for you and your family (and who pays for it)
- other benefits available to you
- vacation and leave (sick, maternal/parental/family, and professional) policies
- the effect of any leave(s) taken on completing the residency program
- disciplinary and grievance procedures
- duty-hours policies and procedures
- policies concerning sexual harassment
- policies on moonlighting
- policies regarding physician impairment and substance abuse
- policies regarding accommodations for disabled residents
- policies regarding reducing the size of or closing the residency program or institution
- the existence of non-competition or restrictive covenants (that prohibit you from working within a certain distance of the training institution or with a competing group for a specific time)

While no residency contract is perfect, programs should supply as much information as possible, in writing, before you start the residency. This will help eliminate confusion later on.

Occasionally, the information in a residency contract will vary from that provided when you were interviewing. It is not unusual for programs to slightly alter the benefit programs in concordance with their sponsoring institution. However, if there are important differences between this material and what you were initially told, immediately contact the program director to clarify the situation.

You might also want to look carefully for any pre-employment screening requirements, such as drug tests or infectious disease screens. The NRMP now takes the position that matching with the program is only part of the agreement, and that a prospective resident must pass any required screening before being hired. This is information that you should ideally know before you rank any program. Be certain that you look for it now, in case the program has a requirement you cannot pass.

Debt Management

As you begin your new career, you may not want to think about the medical school debt that you have acquired; but do it anyway. Before leaving your school, meet with the financial aid officer. She may be able to give you advice about how to best handle your debt burden. *Do it now.* State medical boards are increasingly withdrawing medical licenses and imposing other penalties for those who don't repay their student loans.

Several valuable tools exist to help residents manage their debts. The Association of American Medical Colleges (AAMC) has an excellent debt-management website titled "FIRST for Medical Education: Financial Information, Resources, Services, and Tools" (www.aamc.org/programs/first/). Medical school students and graduates can use the tools on the site to expand their financial literacy, make smarter decisions about student loans, and manage their student debt wisely. The site requires registration, but is free. The tools include several short modules addressing financial topics vital to medical students and residents: budgeting, managing bank accounts and credit card debt, using debit vs. credit cards, deciphering credit reports and scores, and understanding identity theft. There is a separate FIRST page for residents (www.aamc.org/programs/first/residents/start.htm). The FIRST site also contains automated budget worksheets and financial calculators.

The AAMC also has the *Layman's Guide to Educational Debt Management* (www.aamc.org/programs/first/laymansguide/start.htm), an excellent, detailed on-line publication. It discusses eight strategies for residents to use to manage their debt:
1. Know what you borrowed, from whom, and who services the loans.
2. Know the "relative cost" of your loans.
3. Know your grace periods and deferment and forbearance options.
4. Know your "decision points" and keep a calendar.
5. "Run the numbers" before choosing any repayment plan or consolidation option.

6. Keep good records.

7. Use a budget and know when you need outside professional help.

8. Know and use your support systems.

For more helpful information, especially about consolidating loans, see these websites:

- U.S. Department of Education, www.ed.gov/index.jhtml. Search for "Financial Aid" for how to obtain, pay for, and consolidate loans.
- Federal Direct Consolidation Loan Information Center, http://www.loanconsolidation.ed.gov/.
- Sallie Mae, www.salliemae.com.

Note that the federal Income-Based Repayment Plan took effect on July 1, 2009. Unlike prior plans, this plan *does not defer repayment*, but only decreases the amount paid each month. (This increases the length of time it will take for you to repay the debt.) Nearly all residents must still make a payment on their outstanding loans each month. Go to www.aamc.org/programs/first/students/assumptions.htm for more information.

Your New Home

A number of websites exist to help reduce the hassles of finding a new home. Some that seem to be good are:

- www.homepath.com
- www.bestplaces.net (cost of living, crime rates, climate, etc.)
- www.homefair.com (links to realtors, city and school reports, regional cost-of-living, and mortgage payment calculators)

More sites are popping up all the time. Use your search engine to find them, and then utilize them to eliminate a lot of aggravation.

Moving

If you have gotten a position far from where you now live or if you have just decided it is time to live in nicer quarters now that you will be getting paid (a little) for what you do, you need to move. Since this may be a new experience for you, and because many students have told me that they got "burned" when using movers, here are some helpful tips for hiring professional movers.

- *Call your local Better Business Bureau* before contacting any mover, to find out if there have been any complaints about them.
- *Contact, and get written estimates from, at least three movers.* Estimates come in three forms: Binding, where the price is fixed once the estimate

is signed by both parties; Non-binding, where you can be charged any price; and Not-to-exceed $X, which sets an upper limit on the cost.

- *Get details about what services are, and are not, included in the estimate.* These may include packing, unpacking, surcharges to go up or down stairs (on either end of the trip), packing materials, and insurance.
- *Carry irreplaceable items with you.* Do not entrust diplomas, legal documents, heirlooms, family photographs, jewelry, safe-deposit-box contents, or other highly valued, or easily broken, items to the movers. Take them with you.
- *Get adequate insurance for the possessions you will move.* First, check to see if your homeowners' insurance policy covers your possessions while the mover has them. If not, you can get Full-Value or Released-Value insurance from the moving company.
- Under *Full-Value Protection,* your mover is liable for the replacement value of lost or damaged goods in your shipment. If an article is lost, destroyed, or damaged by your mover, he will: (a) repair it, (b) replace it with a similar item, or (c) give you cash equal to the cost to repair or replacement the item. This insurance costs more, and usually limits the amount of the mover's liability for "articles of extraordinary value," such as jewelry or antiques. Unless you sign a request for Released-Value protection, your mover will automatically provide Full-Value protection (and charge you for it).
- *Released Value Protection* offers the least protection but is the cheapest, since it is usually offered at no additional charge. Under this option, the mover assumes liability for no more than *60 cents per pound per article. Note that this is valued by weight, so it is worthless for expensive items.*
- *Make a detailed list of all goods moved,* including a list of everything in each box. The mover will make his own list of items (and note whether furniture is "scratched," "dented," etc.) when they pack the boxes, or just before loading the van. Before anything is loaded, check that each item's condition is correctly stated, if not, tell them and note it on the list. They should place a number sticker on each item; this makes it easier to discover missing items when they unload. While it is a pain, it is most important that you account for each box or item at the end of the move and note any damaged items. Do this before the movers leave.
- *Take photographs* of any large or expensive items you must entrust to the movers, such as electronic equipment. Use your cell phone if you don't have a camera. Carry these photographs (or the memory card) with you.

- *Carry contact numbers* for your van's driver, and for the company's sales agent and dispatcher, so you can locate your truck when it is delayed. The Frequent-Mover's Law states: a moving truck will never arrive when scheduled.

The Federal Motor Carrier Safety Administration website (www. protectyourmove.gov) is a great place to get additional up-to-date information about moving. If you're moving within your state, there may be separate regulations governing moves within the State (www.protectyourmove.gov/related-sites/state-search.htm).

Conclusion

Now you are ready to begin residency training. Let me welcome you to what will undoubtedly be one of the most stimulating and exciting periods of your professional life. You have planned well and have used your own wants and needs to guide your selection of both a specialty and a training program.

Good luck in all your future endeavors. You deserve it!

A New Beginning

To an intern, personal time is always reckoned in minuses. It is the time remaining when work-ups, conferences, dictations, and clinic sessions are taken away or it equals the time left over after work, sleep and errand-running are subtracted from a day. Figured by whatever means, personal time often seems like a sum that is unaccounted for, the small amount that balances the ledger of hours. And in the tallying of hourly expenditures that every intern makes, it always lies on the debit side. Personal time is time still owed. . . .

Having spent the last two years of medical school rotating disaffectedly from one clinical service to another—with hardly any involvement in patient care and hardly any sense of continuity—I gladly forfeited any claim to private time in order to have greater responsibility for patients and a more permanent station in life.

Hoffmann SA: *Under the Ether Dome: A Physician's Apprenticeship at Massachusetts General Hospital.* New York: Scribner, 1986:209.

GLOSSARY

AAMC—*see* Association of American Medical Colleges.

ABMS—*see* American Board of Medical Specialties.

ACGME—Accreditation Council for Graduate Medical Education.

Advanced Positions—Residency positions obtained through a matching program at least eighteen months before the slot opens and training begins.

Adviser—One or more faculty members who gives you information about medical school, rotations, courses, specialties, and residency programs; may also be your mentor.

AHA—*see* American Hospital Association.

Allopathic Physicians—*Not* M.D.'s, but rather a therapeutic tradition believing that diseases are treated by producing a second condition that is incompatible with or antagonistic to the first.

AMA—*see* American Medical Association.

AMA-Fellowship and Residency Electronic Interactive Database Access—This AMA-produced computer program, popularly known as *FREIDA*, has in-depth information about nearly all residencies and many fellowship programs.

American Board of Medical Specialties—This group authorizes "official" medical (M.D.) specialties and subspecialties.

American Hospital Association—A professional organization of U.S. hospitals. It lobbies for and monitors hospitals, and has a large say (through the JCAHO) in the setting and enforcement of hospital standards.

American Medical Association—An association of physician members which establishes standards of care, monitors legal issues, and lobbies members of the U.S. Congress on issues important to physicians and their patients. It has special sections for IMGs, residents, students, and young physicians. The AMA publishes the *Journal of the American Medical Association (JAMA)* and other specialty journals, as well as reliable resources on many health-related issues.

American Medical Women's Association—An independent organization which represents the interests of women physicians and medical students.

American Osteopathic Association—An association of Osteopathic physicians which establishes standards of care, monitors legal issues, and lobbies members of the U.S. Congress on issues important to physicians and their patients. It also sponsors its own Intern/Resident Registration Program. All Osteopathic medical students must be AOA members.

AMWA—*see* American Medical Women's Association.

AOA—*see* American Osteopathic Association.

AOA (award)—Alpha Omega Alpha, the best-known and most prestigious medical student honorary society.

Association of American Medical Colleges—Association of U.S. and Canadian medical schools which accredits schools in the United States, Canada, and Puerto Rico. The AAMC also conducts an annual meeting, provides consultation, and publishes useful directories and educational materials.

Audition Elective—A senior clerkship taken to demonstrate your abilities to the faculty at residencies you wish to attend.

Canadian Resident Matching Service—The Canadian equivalent of the NRMP Match. Formerly called the Canadian Intern Matching Service (CIMS).

CaRMS—*see* Canadian Resident Matching Service.

CAS—*see* Centralized Application Service.

Categorical Internship—A first-year residency position in Internal Medicine or General Surgery designed for those who plan to complete a residency in that field.

Centralized Application Service—A system used to submit residency applications through the Dean's Office via the Internet. It is used by specialties participating in the San Francisco Matching Programs.

Certify—The term for approving a Rank-Order List submitted to the NRMP Match.

Clerkship—Structured clinical education provided to medical students.

Clinical Research Fellow—Designates either a U.S. physician or an IMG engaged primarily in research associated with patient care. Physicians in this category need full medical licensure if significant patient contact is involved, but no license if there is minimal patient contact under the supervision of a licensed physician.

Clinical Skills Assessment—A test formerly given by the Educational Commission for Foreign Medical Graduates to test clinical and communication skills. It has been supplanted by USMLE Step 2CS.

Clinical Years—The period of medical school when students "rotate" through the various clinical services. In a traditional four-year school, these are the third (junior) and fourth (senior) years.

Combined Programs—This training combines two to three non-surgical specialties into one program, making graduates eligible to take the Board examination in all of them upon completion.

COMLEX—*see* Comprehensive Osteopathic Medical Licensing Examination.

Comprehensive Osteopathic Medical Licensing Examination—A method of licensure that is available only to Osteopathic Physicians. It is a three-part written exam.

COTH—The Council of Teaching Hospitals, which publishes several references useful to residency applicants.

Couples Match—A method by which couples can rank their residency choices in program pairs for the NRMP Match so that they can stay in geographic proximity to one another.

CSA—*see* Clinical Skills Assessment.

Curriculum Vitae (C.V.)—A résumé.

Dean of Students—The key individual to ask for information about, and for assistance during, specialty selection and the matching process.

ECFMG—*see* Educational Commission for Foreign Medical Graduates.

Educational Commission for Foreign Medical Graduates—A nonprofit foundation sponsored by standard-setting associations and agencies to monitor the competency of graduates of foreign medical schools.

Electronic Residency Application Service—A method for residency applicants to submit applications through their Dean's Office via the Internet. Most M.D. specialties and Osteopathic internships use the system.

ERAS—*see* Electronic Residency Application Service.

EVIMG—*see* Exchange-Visitor International Medical Graduate.

Exchange-Visitor International Medical Graduate—A subset of foreign nationals applying for residency slots. These individuals are in the United States only temporarily as Exchange Visitors (with J-1 visas) to study, teach, or do research.

Externship—A clinical rotation taken at a location away from your primary teaching institutions.

FAIMER—Foundation for Advancement of International Medical Education and Research. They publish the book that lists all international medical schools acceptable to the ECFMG.

Federation Licensing Examination—A medical licensing exam which is no longer given. However, a passing score may still be used for licensure.

Federation of State Medical Boards of the United States—This organization maintains contact information for individual medical licensing authorities and responds to inquiries regarding medical licensure.

Fellow—An academic term used to designate one engaged in postgraduate training after completing a residency program. Also used for experienced scholars engaged in research, writing, or teaching.

Fifth Pathway—A now-defunct program that allowed U.S. citizens graduating from foreign medical schools that required a year of social service to work at U.S. hospitals instead. It has largely been replaced by a different program run by the New York Medical College. Those who completed Fifth Pathway can, however, still apply to residencies.

FLEX—*see* Federation Licensing Examination.

FMG—A term used by some organizations to indicate foreign-national physicians who are international medical graduates.

FMGEMS—*see* Foreign Medical Graduate Examination.

FNIMG—*see* Foreign-National International Medical Graduate.

Foreign Medical Graduate Examination—Examination once used to obtain an ECFMG Certificate, but not a medical license. It is no longer given.

Foreign-National International Medical Graduate—A non-U.S. citizen whose basic medical degree or qualification was conferred by a medical school not approved by the LCME. These schools are usually located outside of the United States, Canada, and Puerto Rico.

FREIDA—*see* AMA-Fellowship and Residency Electronic Interactive Database Access.

FSMB—*see* Federation of State Medical Boards of the United States.

Green Book—The AMA-produced *Graduate Medical Education Directory*. This book lists most residency and fellowship programs. It also contains the standards residency programs must meet and the requirements to take the specialty Board examinations.

Health Maintenance Organization—A managed-care plan under which medical treatment is prepaid through monthly premiums. HMO physicians are paid set salaries rather than collecting patient fees. Patients have a limited choice of physicians and, except in emergencies, must be admitted to HMO-designated hospitals.

Health Professions Scholarship Program—Military-sponsored scholarships for medical students.

HMO—*see* Health Maintenance Organization.

HPSP—*see* Health Professions Scholarship Program.

IAP-66—Visa document issued to a J-1 visa holder.

IMG—*see* International Medical Graduate.

Independent Applicant—Anyone in the NRMP Match who is neither a current student at nor a Sponsored Graduate of an LCME-approved medical school.

Individual Provider Association—The group contracting with independent physicians to provide services to an HMO's patients.

Integrated Program—Surgical programs which have residency and subspecialty training at one site following completion of medical school. It often shortens the time needed to complete subspecialty training.

Intern—The historical term for individuals in their first year of training after medical school. While not officially used except to designate specific positions (Transitional, Preliminary, and Categorical internships), clinicians still commonly use the term.

Intern/Resident Registration Program—A matching program for obtaining AOA-approved internships and some Osteopathic residency positions.

International Medical Graduate—Any individual whose basic medical degree or qualification was obtained from a medical school that is not approved by the LCME. These schools usually are located outside of the United States, Puerto Rico, and Canada. This includes U.S. or Canadian citizens who train in such a medical school and then return to the United States for residency training.

IPA—*see* Individual Provider Association.

LCME—*see* Liaison Committee on Medical Education.

Level 2CE—The COMLEX Cognitive Evaluation test, comparable to USMLE Step 2CK.

Level 2PE—The COMLEX Performance Evaluation test, comparable to USMLE Step 2CS.

Liaison Committee on Medical Education—This organization accredits U.S., Canadian, and some Puerto Rican medical schools. Foreign-national graduates of these schools do *not* have to obtain an ECFMG Certificate to continue training in the United States.

License—A state's permission to practice medicine. Each state has its own licensure requirements.

LOR—Letter of Reference or recommendation letter used to apply to residency programs.

Managed Care—Any type of health insurance that uses only specified physicians to see their patients. Examples include HMOs, IPAs, and PPOs.

Match Day—The day on which residency applicants participating in the NRMP or AOA Matches find out with which program they have matched.

Matching Program—One of the various methods by which students or physicians obtain a position in a residency or fellowship training program.

Medical Student Performance Evaluation—A Dean's letter.

Mentor—The faculty member who helps guide you through medical school and the residency-application process.

Moonlighting—Extra clinical work done for pay, usually not at the institution where one is a resident.

MSPE—*see* Medical Student Performance Evaluation.

Must/Want Analysis—The best method to determine what you want in a residency program and which programs meet those needs.

National Board of Medical Examiners—The organization that produces national physician licensing examinations, including the USMLE.

National Board of Osteopathic Medical Examiners—An organization which gives the COMLEX, a licensing examination for Osteopathic physicians.

National Residency Matching Program—A national program to match applicants with accredited U.S. residency programs.

NBME—*see* National Board of Medical Examiners.

NBOME—*see* National Board of Osteopathic Medical Examiners.

NRMP—*see* National Residency Matching Program.

OASIS—The ECFMG's Online Applicant Status and Information Service. It is the primary method that IMG applicants use to communicate with and get information from the ECFMG.

Objective Structured Clinical Examination—A patient-simulation examination used to test medical students' clinical skills.

OGME—Osteopathic Graduate Medical Education. Used with a numeral to designate the year of postgraduate training at an Osteopathic residency program. This system parallels that used for most ACGME-approved specialties.

OSCE—*see* Objective Structured Clinical Examination.

Participating Institution—One part of a multi-institutional graduate education program.

Part-Time Position—*see* Shared-Schedule Position.

PGY-1—Postgraduate Year-1. The internship year, otherwise known as the first year of residency.

PPO—*see* Preferred Provider Organization.

Preclinical Years—The period of medical school preceding clinical rotations, usually the first two years.

Preferred Provider Organization—A group of hospitals or physicians that contracts to provide comprehensive health coverage at a competitive rate. These networks combine aspects of a traditional health care system and an HMO.

Preliminary Internship—First-year positions in Internal Medicine or General Surgery designed for those who do not necessarily plan to complete a residency in that specialty. Many students who take these positions either are undecided about their career plans or intend to go into another field that requires prior clinical training.

Program—The designation for both a place and a curriculum to train residents.

R3 System—Stands for Registration, Ranking, and Results. This is the name of the system used by applicants to register, enter their rank-order lists, and obtain results for the NMRP Match.

Rank-Order List—The program rankings each applicant submits and the applicant rankings each residency program submits to matching programs.

Research Scholar—Term used to designate an individual holding a Ph.D., M.D., or equivalent degree who is in a research training program. The term implies that the training involves no patient contact.

Résumé—Also called a curriculum vitae or C.V., it briefly summarizes a person's accomplishments.

ROL—*see* Rank-Order List.

RRC—Residency Review Committee. The RRC for each specialty makes the rules that the residency programs must follow. It surveys the programs periodically to assure that they are following the guidelines.

San Francisco Matching Program—The organization which runs many of the "early" matches for specialties such as Neurology, Neurological Surgery, Plastic Surgery, and Ophthalmology.

Scramble—Former system by which unmatched applicants found unfilled positions at residencies. In 2012, the NRMP replaced this with a new program, called SOAP.

SFMP—*see* San Francisco Matching Program.

Shared-Schedule Position—One residency position shared by two individuals.

SOAP—Supplemental Offer and Acceptance Program. As of 2012, this is the NRMP's system to help unmatched residency applicants find positions.

Special Purpose Examination—A one-day examination to test the knowledge base of physicians who seek licensure in a new state or re-licensure in the same state at least five years after graduation from medical school.

Special Emphasis Internship—First-year training programs for Osteopathic physicians in Anesthesiology, Emergency Medicine, Family Practice, General Surgery, Psychiatry, and Diagnostic Radiology. Although these internships follow the curriculum of the specialty, they *do not* reduce the number of subsequent training years.

Specialty Track Internship—First-year training programs for Osteopathic physicians in Internal Medicine, Internal Med/Pediatrics, Obstetrics/Gynecology, Otolaryngology/Facial Plastic Surgery, Pediatrics, and Urological Surgery. These internships usually shorten specialty training by one year.

SPEX—*see* Special Purpose Examination.

Sponsoring Institution—The main hospital or clinic responsible for a residency training program. Often it is also the primary training site.

Step 2CK—USMLE Clinical Knowledge exam.

Step 2CS—USMLE Clinical Skills (simulated patient) exam.

Subinternship—A clinical rotation that gives a senior medical student added responsibility.

TOEFL—An examination called *Toward English As a Foreign Language*. Once used as the ECFMG's English examination, it has been supplanted by USMLE Step 2CS.

Token—The initial password used to access the ECFMG's OASIS system and obtain an AAMC Identification Number from the MyERAS website.

Transitional Internship—Also called a "rotating internship," it allows interns to rotate through a variety of clinical services, usually in most of the same specialties they went through during their third-year clerkships.

Unmatch Days—Starting two days before Match Day, the period of time when those who failed to match with a residency program may begin to receive offers for a residency position using SOAP.

USIMG—A U.S. citizen or permanent resident whose basic medical degree or qualification was conferred by a medical school not approved by the LCME. These schools are usually located outside the United States, Canada, and Puerto Rico.

United States Medical Licensing Examination—Primary examination required to practice medicine in the United States. This is the only exam that M.D. or equivalent physicians (without regard to their nationality or medical school) can use for licensing.

USMLE—*see* United States Medical Licensing Examination.

Annotated Bibliography

Knowledge is power.

Hobbes, *Leviathan*

References marked with a plus (+) can be obtained through Galen Press, Ltd., **www.galenpress.com**; P.O. Box 64400, Tucson, AZ 85728-4400; (800) 442-5369 or (520) 577-8363; fax: (520) 529-6459.

Medicine—The Big Picture

Bollet AJ. *Civil War Medicine: Challenges and Triumphs.* Tucson, AZ: Galen Press, Ltd., 2002. Forget what you thought you knew about medicine in the Civil War. Our forebears practiced cutting-edge medicine. Modern physicians' practices are based on methods and systems developed by these doctors on the battlefield. (+)

Bureau of Health Professions, Health Resources and Services Administration. *Changing Demographics: Implications for Physicians, Nurses and Other Health Workers.* Washington, DC: U.S. Dept. of Health and Human Services, 2003(Spring). This U.S. government report contains estimates of the need for physicians in the larger specialties under several scenarios through 2018. Look at this to see how your career plans might fit into the big picture. http://bhpr.hrsa.gov/healthworkforce/reports/changedemo/Content.htm.

Drayer J. *The Cost effective Use of Leeches and Other Musings of a Medical School Survivor.* Tucson, AZ: Galen Press, Ltd., 1998. One medical student's comic look at the trials and tribulations of medical school. A must read—but only if you don't take yourself too seriously. (+)

Iserson KV. *Death to Dust: What Happens to Dead Bodies?* Tucson, AZ: Galen Press, Ltd., 2001. An award-winning question-answer book describing, in detail, everything that has, does, or could occur to corpses. How were mummies and shrunken heads made? Why and how were graves robbed (by medical students, as well as others)? Why and how are bodies embalmed? Sky burials, cannibalism, and more are covered. Not exactly bedtime reading. (+)

Iserson KV. *Demon Doctors: Physicians as Serial Killers.* Tucson, AZ: Galen Press, Ltd., 2002. Okay, so it is the dark side of medical history. But it's my book, and it's a great read. Not one case of euthanasia among them, these are real (and really fiendish) physicians who intentionally killed—for power, money, sex, or nationalism. (+)

Iserson KV. *Grave Words: Notifying Survivors About Sudden Unexpected Deaths.* Galen Press, Ltd., Tucson, AZ, 1999. How to do the physician's toughest job—informing people that their loved one has suddenly and unexpectedly died. Poignant stories and relevant research results accompany the detailed protocols for a variety of situations (e.g., in the hospital, over the telephone, at home, or in school, the military, prisons, and after disasters). Also includes how to discuss organ-tissue donation, tell children the news, work with chaplains, and deal with the media. (+)

Iserson KV. *Pocket Protocols: Notifying Survivors About Sudden, Unexpected Deaths.* Galen Press, Ltd., Tucson, AZ, 1999. Contains all the charts and protocols from *Grave Words*, and fits in your shirt pocket! Also available in Spanish. (+)

Iserson KV, Sanders AB, Mathieu DR (eds.). *Ethics in Emergency Medicine*, 2nd edition. Galen Press, Ltd., Tucson, AZ, 1995. A classic case-based book describing common clinical ethical scenarios. Each has a commentary by a well-known bioethicist. (+)

Lewis S. *Arrowsmith*. New York: Harcourt Brace & Co., 1925. An inspiring classic that led many people to medicine as a career. It shows what physicians can do, as well as their limitations, in medical practice and in the laboratory. Although written in the pre-antibiotic era, the story remains relevant today. (+)

London O. *Kill as Few Patients as Possible: and Fifty-six Other Essays on How to be the World's Best Doctor*. Berkeley, CA: Ten Speed Press, 1987. Funny, short essays illustrate this practicing physician's rules about how to be a successful (and compassionate) physician. While the essays are tongue-in-cheek, much of the underlying advice really will make you an excellent physician. (+)

Reynolds R, Stone J. *On Doctoring: Stories, Poems, Essays*. 2nd edition. New York: Simon & Schuster, 1995. Classic and pithy descriptions of physicians, medical practice, diseases, and patients. Contributors include physicians (Sir Arthur Conan Doyle, William Carlos Williams, Richard Selzer, and others) and noted writers (Anton Chekhov, Ernest Hemingway, Kurt Vonnegut, and Alice Walker). A book to be read repeatedly throughout one's medical career. (+)

Schiedermayer DL. *House Calls, Rounds, and Healings: A Poetry Casebook*. Tucson, AZ: Galen Press, Ltd., 1996. Revealing the human vulnerabilities in doctor-patient relationships, these case studies in verse provide a glimpse of the strong bonds between first-rate clinicians and the patients. Written by a practicing Internist, the book will remind you of the reasons you became a physician—something we all occasionally forget. (+)

Selecting a Specialty

Cochran A, Melby S, Neumayer LA. An Internet-based survey of factors influencing medical student selection of a General Surgery career. *Am J Surg*. 2005;189(6):742-6. Interestingly, they concluded that medical students who choose surgical careers are not deterred by a negative perception of the lifestyle and workload, but are, instead, influenced by mentors and "personality fit."

Compton MT, Frank E, Elon L, Carrera J. Changes in U.S. medical students' specialty interests over the course of medical school. *J Gen Intern Med*. 2008 Jul;23(7):1095-1100. Think you know what specialty you want to enter? Think again, as most of these students did between their freshman and senior years.

Hauer KE, Durning SJ, Kernan WN, et al. Factors associated with medical students' career choices regarding Internal Medicine. *JAMA*. 2008;300(10):1154-64. This study found that students were more likely to pursue careers in Internal Medicine if they were male, attended a private school, were favorably impressed with their IM educational experience, enjoyed caring for IM patients, or had a favorable impression of the internist's lifestyle.

Ko CY, Escarce JJ, Baker l, Klein D, Guarino C. Predictors for medical students entering a General Surgery residency: national survey results. *Surgery*. 2004;136(3):567-72. This national survey of fourth-year medical students identifies factors related to the basic Surgery clerkship that are associated with the decision to enter a General Surgery residency.

Leigh JP, Tancredi DJ, Kravitz RL. Physician career satisfaction within specialties. *BMC Health Serv Res*. 2009;9:166. Which physicians are most satisfied with their specialty? Among the variables, career satisfaction correlated with income and working in a medical school, but was negatively associated with a work week longer than 50 hours, owning a practice, increased managed care involvement and an uncontrollable lifestyle. There were no differences between men and women or between whites and African-Americans.

McAlister RP, Andriole DA, Brotherton SE, Jeffe DB. Are entering Obstetrics/Gynecology residents more similar to the entering Primary Care or Surgery resident workforce? *Am J Obstet & Gynecol.* 2007;197(5):536.e1-6. Graduates of U.S. M.D. medical schools, women, and African-Americans were more likely to enter OB/GYN than Primary Care, while Asians were less likely. Women, African-Americans, and Hispanics were more likely to enter OB/GYN than Surgery; trainees who were Asian and "other" races/ethnicities were less likely to enter OB/GYN than Surgery.

McDonald FS, West CP, Popkave C, Kolars JC. Educational debt and reported career plans among Internal Medicine residents. *Ann Int Med.* 2008;149(6):416-20. Does debt influence IM residents' career choices? This study suggests it does: 54% of U.S. medical graduates had debts of $100,000 or greater, and were less likely than those with no debt (60% of IMGs) to choose a subspecialty career. U.S. medical graduates with debts of $50,000 to $99,999 were more likely than those with no debt to choose a Hospitalist career.

Newton DA, Grayson MS, Thompson LF. The variable influence of lifestyle and income on medical students' career specialty choices: data from two U.S. medical schools, 1998-2004. *Acad Med.* 2005;80(9):809-14. Lifestyle and income have become more important to medical students in their career choice, and the relative importance of these factors varies considerably among specialties. This study suggests that prior efforts to classify careers as those having an controllable or an uncontrollable lifestyle may ignore relevant complexities.

Pathway Evaluation Program for Medical Professionals. (http://medweb.usc.edu/pathways/intro. htm) Administered by Duke University School of Medicine in partnership with GlaxoSmithKline, this on-line course contains descriptions of the major medical specialties and subspecialties. Each one includes background material, profiles of individual practitioners, and anecdotes about why they entered the field. It then rates 17 aspects of practice in order of their importance to the physicians in that specialty. Factors include continuity of care, schedule, diversity, autonomy, manual activities, security, and income. It also contains an exercise to help you rate your interests against each specialty's typical profile.

Schlueter ME, Phan PH, Martin CS, Breece D, Boysen DA. Understanding Accreditation Council for Graduate Medical Education (ACGME) Guidelines: resident and program director interpretation of work-hour restrictions. *J Surg Educ.* 2009 Nov-Dec;66(6):374-8. This study found that residents and program directors from different specialties had various interpretations of the new guidelines, suggesting that ambiguities exist which will lead to different applications.

West CP, Drefahl MM, Popkave C, Kolars JC. Internal Medicine residents self-report of factors associated with career decisions. *J Gen Int Med.* 2009;24(8):946-9. Residents rated the importance of 9 factors in their career decisions. Overall, time with family was the factor most commonly reported as being of high or very high importance to career decisions, with women more likely to assign greatest importance to family time.

The Specialties

Alikhan A, Sivamani RK, Mutizwa MM, Aldabagh B. Advice for medical students interested in Dermatology: perspectives from fourth-year students who matched. *Derm Online J.* 2009;15(7):4. Four fourth-year medical students who matched into Dermatology highlight the factors they believed helped them the most in the areas of academics, extracurricular activities, research, and mentorship.

American Board of Medical Specialties. *Which Specialties Are Board Certified.* This frequently updated on-line list (www.abms.org/Who_We_Help/Consumers/specialties.aspx) provides short descriptions of all recognized medical specialties and subspecialties. But note that some subspecialties, such as Trauma Surgery and Hospitalist are not included, since they have not been officially sanctioned.

American Geriatrics Society, Core Writing Group of the Task Force on the Future of Geriatric Medicine. Caring for older Americans: the future of Geriatric Medicine. *J Am Geriat Soc.* 2005;53(6):S245-56. This paper describes how the discipline has defined its core values, as well as the knowledge base and clinical skills needed to provide acute and palliative care. It also discusses Geriatric Medicine's models of care and the treatment of common geriatric conditions. Most important, it describes their five goals for optimizing the health of older persons.

Anderson MR, Jewett EA, Cull WL, et al. Practice of Pediatric Critical Care medicine: results of the Future of Pediatric Education II survey of sections project. *Pediatr Crit Care Med.* 2003;4(4):412-7. This study summarizes the demographics and practice patterns of current Pediatric Critical Care physicians, and identifies issues that may affect future practice. Bottom line: More women are entering the field, and PCCM physicians work more than 65 hours/week. Of note, 34% of respondents planned on leaving the field of Critical Care before retiring from medicine completely.

Bagnall DL. Physiatry: what's the end game? *Am Acad Phys Med & Rehab.* 2010;2:3-5. A recent graduate assesses his mentor's impact on his practice.

Beaulieu MD, Dory V, Pestiaux D, et al. What does it mean to be a family physician: exploratory study with Family Medicine residents from 3 countries. *Can Fam Phys.* 2009;55(8):e14-20. This study reveals more similarities than differences in the vision of Family Medicine, including developing a "new general practice" versus a more traditional view. All respondents strongly believed that their profession was undervalued by their own medical schools.

Boyd JS, Clyne B, Reinert SE, Zink BJ. Emergency Medicine career choice: a profile of factors and influences from the Association of American Medical Colleges (AAMC) graduation questionnaires. *Acad Emerg Med.* 2009;16(6):544-9. Students choosing a career in Emergency Medicine have distinctly different priorities and influences than students entering primary care and surgical specialties. How do you compare with these students?

Chamberlain JK, Cull WL, Melgar T, Kaelber DC, Kan BD. The effect of dual training in Internal Medicine and Pediatrics on the career path and job search experience of pediatric graduates. *J Pediatrics.* 2007;151(4):419-24. This study found that Med-Peds-trained physicians had an easier job search and greater market valuation. Med-Peds residents were more likely to seek and accept generalist and Hospitalist positions, which had higher starting salaries, and to accept positions in rural areas/small towns, while Pediatric residents were more likely to be female or IMGs and to seek subspecialty careers and research opportunities. The groups were equally satisfied with their career choice and had equivalent debt.

Colen BD. *O.R.: The True Story of 24 Hours in a Hospital Operating Room.* New York: Signet (Penguin), 1994. A Pulitzer Prize-winning author's gripping minute-by-minute account of the operating room, as seen from several perspectives. Surgeries range from extraordinary surgical feats to the mundane. After reading this, you will either be certain you should be a surgeon or know why you don't want to enter this world. [+]

Ducatman BS. Be careful what you wish for. *JAMA*. 1997;278(14):1130. An insightful and beautifully written one-page piece on a student's experience with the consummate rural Family Practitioner—and reasons to rethink what seem to be idyllic career choices.

Freed GL, Dunham KM, Switalski KE, Jones MD Jr, McGuinness GA, & Research Advisory Committee of the American Board of Pediatrics. Recently trained general pediatricians: perspectives on residency training and scope of practice. *Pediatrics*. 2009;123(supp1):S38-43. One of several articles in this supplement on whether new pediatricians are happy with their training, in particular, whether General Pediatricians feel confident co-managing their patients with chronic disorders with subspecialists. A large proportion of generalists would have liked additional training in mental health, Sports Medicine, oral health, and Developmental/Behavioral Pediatrics.

Graham MM, Metter DF. Evolution of Nuclear Medicine training: past, present, and future. [review] *J Nuclear Med*. 2007;48(2):257-68. Nuclear Medicine and its training programs have undergone major changes since 1971, including a new CT training requirement in response to PET/CT. Nuclear Medicine is gradually evolving into molecular imaging.

Hanzlick R, Prahlow JA, Denton S, et al. Selecting Forensic Pathology as a career: a survey of the past with an eye on the future. *Am J Foren Med & Path*. 2008;29(2):114-22. Thirty to forty physicians become Board-certified each year in Forensic Pathology. What factors influenced them to choose this career path?

Harkin KE, Cushman JT (eds.). *Emergency Medicine: The Medical Student Survival Guide*, 2nd ed. Irving, TX: EMRA, 2007. Published by the Emergency Medicine Residents Association, this excellent resource endeavors to tell you everything you need to be successful in an Emergency Medicine residency and career.

Hoff TH, Whitcomb WF, Williams K, Nelson JR, Cheesman RA. Characteristics and work experiences of hospitalists in the United States. *Arch Intern Med*. 2001;161:851-8. Who are Hospitalists and what are they actually doing? Do they enjoy their work and how "burnt out" do they feel? This survey of Hospitalists answers those questions.

Huddle TS, Centor R, Heudebert GR. American internal medicine in the 21st century: can an Oslerian generalism survive? *J Gen Int Med*. 2003;18(9):764-7. American Internal Medicine suffers from an identity crisis, as managed care threatens what remains of the Oslerian ideal. Internists will have to adapt to continue to practice using the consultant-generalist model.

Jackson I, Bobbin M, Jordan M, Baker S. A survey of women urology residents regarding career choice and practice challenges. *J Women's Health*. 2009;18(11):1867-72. Urology has become an increasingly popular career choice for women. What challenges do they face during their training period?

Jazrawi LM, Egol KA, Zuckerman JD. *Orthopedic Residency & Fellowship: A Guide to Success*. Thorofare, NJ: SLACK, Inc., 2010. An excellent reference on Orthopedic Surgery for students applying to residency, fellowships, and, finally, jobs in this field.

Kheterpal S, Tremper KK, Shanks A, Morris M. A six-year follow-up on work force and finances of the United States anesthesiology training programs: 2000 to 2006. *Anesth & Analg*. 2009;108(1):263-72. This study finds a continuing need for institutional support for Anesthesiology training departments and a continuing, but decreasing, number of open Anesthesiologist faculty positions nationwide.

Kligler B, Eckert M, Cuadrado D, et al. The changing face of the general surgeon: national and local trends in resident operative experience. *Am J Surg*. 2010;199(5):652-6. Nationwide trends toward the increased use of nonoperative, minimally invasive, endoscopic, and endovascular techniques at the expense of traditional open surgery may radically change what it means to be a "General Surgeon.

Lebensohn P, Koithan M, et al. Measuring the 'whole system' outcomes of an educational innovation: experience from the integrative family medicine program. *Fam Med.* 2009;41(5):342-49. Integrative Medicine is increasingly used in Family Medicine residency programs. Six such U.S. programs developed a postgraduate Integrative Family Medicine (IFM) program; this paper looks at its implementation.

Lee JT, Teshome M, de Virgilio C, et al. A survey of demographics, motivations, and backgrounds among applicants to the integrated 0 + 5 Vascular Surgery residency. *J Vasc Surg.* 2010;51(2):496-502, discussion 502-3. This study found that applicants were older, were more likely to be from a non-U.S. medical school, had a higher number of publications (and more were cardiovascular-related) than the General Surgery applicants. Interviewees were nearly 40% female and more likely to have an additional degree. Those choosing Vascular Surgery as a career did so during the third and fourth years of medical school, and they were influenced in part by endovascular technologies/devices, challenging procedures, clinical rotations on Vascular Surgery, and the perceived need for Vascular Surgeons.

McAlearney AS. Hospitalists and Family physicians: understanding opportunities and risks. *J Fam Pract.* 2004:53(6):473-81. As Hospitalists take on more in-patient care, what impact will this have on Family Practitioners' careers?

McGaha AL, Schmittling GT, DeVilbiss AD, Pugno PA. Entry of U.S. medical school graduates into Family Medicine residencies: 2008-2009 and 3-year summary. *Fam Med.* 2009;41(8):555-66. Find out where Family Medicine residents come from in this report by the American Academy of Family Physicians (AAFP) detailing the percentage of each U.S. medical school's graduates entering Family Medicine residency programs.

O'Leary KJ, Williams MV. The evolution and future of hospital medicine. *Mount Sinai J Med.* 2008;75(5):418-23. Hospitalist Medicine, the fastest growing medical specialty in the history of American medicine, was initially fueled by research demonstrating reductions in lengths of stay and hospital costs. It continues to gather momentum in response to the reduction in residents' work hours, patient-flow challenges in hospitals, and a growing focus on patient safety.

Pawluch D. *The New Pediatrics: A Profession In Transition.* New Brunswick, NJ: Aldine Transaction, 2009. Written by a sociologist, this book highlights the negative aspects of Pediatric practice, especially the "dissatisfied Pediatrician syndrome." Since it is always best to know the negatives about a specialty as well as the positives, it is definitely worth a look for those contemplating Pediatrics.

Reed CE, Vaporciyan AA, Erikson C, et al. Factors dominating choice of surgical specialty. *J Am Coll Surg.* 2010;210(3):319-24. Most General Surgery residents plan to specialize—but what influences their decision? The three top factors are the type of procedures and techniques, exposure to a positive role model, and ability to balance work and personal life. The relative importance placed on these factors varied by gender and specialty. Work schedule was the most frequently selected shortcoming in every specialty except Plastics.

Richardson JD. Workforce and lifestyle issues in general surgery training and practice. *Arch Surg.* 2002;137(5):515-20. An experienced surgical educator speaks frankly about the problems with surgical education—and about possible solutions. Read this to learn the frustrations you will face.

Seelbach EB, Ottolini MC. Primary Care physicians and Hospitalists: two branches of the same tree. *Pediatr Ann*. 2010;39(2):84-8. Describes the evolution of Pediatric Hospitalist Medicine and ways the pediatric generalist can enhance their ambulatory and inpatient settings.

Sexson SB. Overview of training in the twenty-first century. *Child Adolesc Psychiatr Clin N Am*. 2007;16(1):1-16, vii. This article presents a history of Child and Adolescent Psychiatry and the development of training in the field. The author suggests that more training in basic core competencies is needed.

Tamaskar P, McGinnis RA. Declining student interest in psychiatry. *JAMA*. 2002;287(14):1859. So you want to be a Psychiatrist? This very short piece does a good job of describing why students are avoiding the field, and discusses the many misconceptions that lead students to make this decision.

Wu JJ, Davis KF, Ramirez CC, et al. Graduates of foreign Dermatology residencies and military Dermatology residencies and women in academic Dermatology. *Derm Online J*. 2009;15(5):2. Given the growing shortage of academic Dermatologists in the United States, this study found that their subjects comprise important proportions of full-time faculty members at U.S. Dermatology residency programs.

Weaver SP, Mills TL, Passmore C. Job satisfaction of Family Practice residents. *Fam Med*. 2001;33(9):678-82. This survey of Family Medicine residents demonstrated that they had relatively high job satisfaction that increased each year. Those in community-based programs were more satisfied than those in university-based programs.

Zussman R. *Intensive Care: Medical Ethics and the Medical Profession*. Chicago, IL: University of Chicago Press, 1992. An excellent book for those considering a specialty in which they may spend time in the ICU. This well-written book gives the real scoop on what practitioners do, rather than what they want you to think they do. (+)

The USMLE, Other Exams, and Licensure

American Medical Association. *State Medical Licensure Requirements and Statistics*. Chicago, IL: AMA, published annually. This is where to find details about state licensure for all physicians. It contains licensure requirements for every state and territory of the United States, including those for taking the USMLE and COMLEX, and the fees. All the permutations and combinations of licensing are included in easy-to-read charts. It has contact information for individual state boards to obtain additional information and updates, as well as hard-to-get information on IMG licensure requirements (including those for residents and for clinical clerkships by IMGs).

Dolinski LA. *Handbook of OMT Review*, 6th ed. Revere, PA: Pro-Medica, 2010. One of the texts used at Boards Bootcamp. Contains material for reviewing OMT and OMM fundamentals in preparation for the COMLEX.

Federation of State Medical Boards of the United States, Inc. www.fsmb.org. This website has information about the USMLE Step 3 administrative rules (including eligibility rules) for both M.D.'s and D.O.'s. Also has information about each state's medical board concerning requirements for initial licensure, licensure by endorsement, re-registration of one's license, licenses for postgraduate education, and special licenses. There are links to the state medical boards, the *USMLE Bulletin*, and the exam application.

Flauta V. *USMLE Step 2CS for the IMG*. Infinity, 2005. This book contains several USMLE Step 2CS mock exams and useful tips, including lists of questions to ask by body system and flashcard study materials. It also has a chart of the 35 most commonly seen cases, and a list of IMG-friendly hospitals to check out.

National Board of Medical Examiners and The Federation of State Medical Boards of the United States, Inc. *USMLE Bulletin of Information.* Published annually at www.usmle.org. This invaluable on-line booklet lists the current dates and eligibility requirements for the exams, as well as certification, registration, and testing procedures. Most important, there are subject/content outlines for each Step.

National Board of Osteopathic Medical Examiners. *[Annual] Bulletin of Information.* Contains all the necessary instructions to apply for, take, and interpret the COMLEX. Download from www.nbome.org.

Reteguiz J. *Mastering the USMLE Step 2 CS,* 3rd edition. New York: McGraw-Hill Medical, 2004. This interactive workbook prepares medical students for the USMLE Clinical Skills exam by simulating patient cases likely to be tested. In addition, it helps them to develop a checklist to better interact with SPs. It may also improve their performance on the OSCE.

Savarese RG, Fuoco GS, Bersen DG, Kaprow M. *OMT Review, 3rd edition.* Ft. Lauderdale, FL: Robert F. Savarese, 2003. A student-recommended text for reviewing OMT material for both Levels 1 and 2 of the COMLEX. Available from the American Academy of Osteopathy, www.academyofosteopathy.org/.

Swygert K, Muller ES, Swanson DB, Scott CL. The relationship between USMLE Step 2CS communication and interpersonal skills (CIS) ratings and the time spent by examinees interacting with standardized patients. *Acad Med.* 2009;84(10 suppl):S1-S4. This study suggests that spending more time interacting with standardized patients positively affects test scores. Examinee gender and spoken English proficiency also affect the results.

Selecting a Residency Program

American Academy of Family Physicians. *Directory of Family Medicine Residency Programs.* Kansas City, MO: AAFP, updated annually, available on-line and in print. This substantial directory   (www.aafp.org/online/en/home/membership/directories/residencyprograms.html) lists the currently approved Family Medicine residencies. Information includes: Number of positions at each level and who (U.S. or IMG) is filling them, salary and benefits, night-call frequency, faculty-to-resident ratio, and much more.

American Association for the Surgery of Trauma. *Trauma-Related Fellowships.* This on-line document (www.aast.org/fellowships/default.aspx) lists Trauma fellowships for clinical work and for research. It also notes whether they comply with AAST guidelines. Well worth a look for those interested in pursuing this specialty.

American Association of Academic Physiatrists. Directory of PM&R Residency Training Programs. (www.physiatry.org/Publications_Residency_Training_Directory.cfm). This on-line directory of PM&R programs allows applicants to search for programs by state and by how many slots are open. It also notes whether there are available positions at any level of the residency. It does not, however, provide more information than is available on *FREIDA.*

American College of Physicians/Internal Medicine. *Internal Medicine Programs.* Updated annually, this is an on-line (www.acponline.org/medical_students/residency) listing of U.S. and Canadian Internal Medicine programs by state, by the track and combination residencies offered, and by hospital type. Each program's individual pass rates on the Board examinations can also be accessed through this site.

American College of Preventive Medicine. *Resident Directory At-a-Glance.* A detailed listing of all subspecialty programs (www.acpm.org/education/residency/ataglance.htm). It often contains information that *FREIDA* does not provide.

American Medical Association. *Fellowship and Residency Electronic Interactive Database Access* (known as "*FREIDA*"). For most residency applicants, this system has replaced the "Green Book." Hundreds of items of information are available on-line about training programs and their parent institutions. However, the information that the programs provide is not validated by any outside source; always verify that the information is correct. Applicants can access the system at the AMA's Resident homepage or directly at www.ama-assn.org/ama/pub/education-careers/graduate-medical-education/freida-online.shtml.

———*Graduate Medical Education Directory.* Chicago, IL: AMA, published annually. Known as the "Green Book," the *Directory* includes information on nearly all ACGME-accredited and combined specialty programs. Also includes the institutional and program requirements for all approved M.D. specialties/subspecialties and the requirements for medical specialty Board certification. It is also available on CD-ROM. The *FREIDA* system has mostly replaced this book.

American Osteopathic Association. *Yearbook and Directory.* Accessed through the AOA's website at www.osteopathic.org/index.cfm?PageID=ps_yearbook. Everything that an Osteopathic medical student, resident, or practitioner needs to know about the field is on this site. Under the section "Postdoctoral Education," there is a current listing of all AOA-approved internships and residency programs, the procedures for entering the Intern/Resident Registration Program (Match), and the requirements for getting non-AOA training approved.

American Psychiatric Association. *Clearinghouse of Psychiatry Residency Training Program Vacancies.* This Psychiatry database is searchable by state, program, and date of vacancy, or by "all vacancies." (http://archive.psych.org/career_corner/careers_psych/clearinghouse/CHsearch.cfm).

American Urological Association. *Accredited Urology Training Programs.* This on-line directory (www.auanet.org/content/residency/residency-program.cfm) of accredited Urology residencies can be searched by state or be printed intact. While the listings duplicate much of the information in *FREIDA*, they do state how many applicants each program interviews, whether the 2-year "pre-Urology" training must be at the same institution as the residency, and how much time is devoted solely to research. It also includes each program's unique AUA Match Number.

Council of Teaching Hospitals and Health Systems Membership Directory. Available on the AAMC's website (www.aamc.org/members/coth/), the "Member Teaching Hospitals and Health Systems" link leads to both an alphabetical and a geographical list of all teaching hospitals. Contains links to some hospitals' websites, which, even when they don't contain much solid information, can give you a sense of the hospital's milieu.

Intersociety Council for Pathology Information, Inc. *The Directory of Pathology Training Programs* (annual). Online at www.pathologytraining.org. This non-profit organization's list includes Pathology residencies and fellowships in the United States and Canada; each section can be printed on demand.

Raff MJ, Schwartz IS. An applicant's evaluation of a medical house-officership. *NEJM.* 1974;291(12):601-5. An extensive list of questions that can be used to supplement the "Must/Want" Analysis list. Although the paper is almost forty years old, virtually all the questions are still pertinent.

Society of Academic Emergency Medicine. *SAEM Residency Catalog.* Continually updated (http://saem.org/Home/Communities/MedicalStudents/ResidencyCatalog/tabid/680/Default.aspx). Click on a State or type in a specific Emergency Medicine residency to find a myriad of details about each program. More detailed than the *FREIDA* listings, it categorizes programs by state, by length, if M.D. or D.O., and whether they are a PGY 1-4, PGY 2-4, or PGY 1-3 program.

Society of Critical Care Medicine. *Fellowship Programs.* On line at (www.sccm.org/Professional_Development/Fellowship_Programs/Pages/default.aspx.) A list of available Critical Care Medicine fellowships in Internal Medicine, Internal Medicine–Pulmonary Disease, Pediatrics, Anesthesiology, and Surgery, including fellowship director, contact information, and a link to their website.

Society of General Internal Medicine. *Primary Care Residency Directory and General Internal Medicine Fellowship Directory.* (www.sgim.org/residencydir.cfm). Two lists: the Primary Care IM residencies and General IM Fellowships. Both contain information similar to that found in *FREIDA*, and can be searched by geographic region.

Yorke RF. Informed evaluation of Pathology residency programs—a guide for Pathology resident candidates. *Arch Pathol Lab Med.* 2000;124(6):853-8. What those seeking a Pathology residency should look for in a program, and what they should expect from their training.

International Medical Graduates

Alguire PC, Whelan GP, Rajput V. *The International Medical Graduate's Guide to U.S. Medicine & Residency Training.* Philadelphia: ACP Press, 2009. Written in cooperation with the ECFMG and the American College of Physicians, this comprehensive guide features information on the application process, residency training in America, American medical culture, certification, and more. The ACP has posted "Appendix B: Internet Web Sites" on their website at wwws.acponline.org/acp_press/img_guide/.

Boulet JR, Cooper RA, Seeling SS, Norcini JJ, McKinley DW. U.S. citizens who obtain their medical degrees abroad: an overview, 1992-2006. *Health Affairs.* 2009;28(1):226-33. A closer look at U.S. citizens trained abroad, who typically do not perform as well as other IMGs or U.S. graduates. They are also more likely than non-U.S. citizens to be engaged in primary care activities.

Cohen JJ. The role and contribution of IMGs: a U.S. perspective. *Acad Med.* 2006;86(12):S17-S21. An overview of the role IMGs play in U.S. medicine.

Desbiens NA, Vidaillet HJ Jr. Discrimination against international medical graduates in the United States residency program selection process. *BMC Med Ed.* 2010;10:5. Do residency directors discriminate against IMGs? This survey of research about Family Practice, Psychiatry and Surgery programs suggests they do.

Eckhert NL. Perspective: private schools of the Caribbean: outsourcing medical education. *Acad Med.* 2010;85(4):622-30. This comparative study looks at the offshore medical schools that supply an increasing number of U.S. physicians.

Educational Commission for Foreign Medical Graduates' website (www.ecfmg.org) provides all the necessary information for IMGs about the USMLE, ECFMG-sponsored visas, applications and ERAS, and getting credentials verified.

Foundation for Advancement of International Medical Education and Research (FAIMER). *International Medical Education Directory* (www.faimer.org/resources/imed.html). An on-line list of international medical schools approved by the ECFMG. It is searchable by region, city, country, or medical school. Graduates of the listed schools are allowed to obtain ECFMG Certification. You cannot practice medicine in the United States unless your school is on this list.

Shah MM, Summerhill EM, Manthous CA. Medical professionalism in the new millennium: are there intercultural differences? Brief report and commentary. *Connecticut Med.* 2009;73(5):289-94. The authors were surprised to find no demonstrable differences in notions of medical professionalism among USIMGs and IMGs.

Women in Medicine

American Medical Women's Association. Their website (www.amwa-doc.org) has both a student newsletter and *Connections* newsletter, as well as links to professional organizations.

Andrews NC. Climbing through medicine's glass ceiling. *N Engl J Med.* 2007;357:1793-5. The first female dean of Duke's medical school reflects on the state of women in academic medicine.

Conley FK. *Walking Out on the Boys.* New York: Farrar, Strauss & Giroux, 1998. An interesting book written by the first female tenured Neurosurgery professor at Stanford University School of Medicine, who resigned her position to protest sexual harassment and gender-based discrimination. She has since regained her position and continues to be active in the movement against gender-based discrimination.

DesRoches CM, Zinner DE, Rao SR, Iezzoni LI, Campbell EG. Activities, productivity, and compensation of men and women in the life sciences. *Academic Med.* 2010;85(4):631-9. This extensive study found that despite comparable qualifications, women in academic medicine earn significantly less than do men. They also publish fewer articles and work fewer hours as assistant professors; do less research; and work longer hours as full professors, mostly on administrative tasks.

Gautam M. Women in medicine: stresses and solutions. *West J Med.* 2001;174(1):37-41. A list of specific, practical steps that women physicians can use to decrease the stress in their professional and personal lives.

Langelan MJ. *Back Off! How to Confront and Stop Sexual Harassment and Harassers.* New York: Simon & Schuster, 1993. The title pretty much describes it, and the book delivers. (+)

Magliato K. *Healing Hearts: A Memoir of a Female Heart Surgeon.* New York: Broadway Books, 2010. With occasional black humor, this book chronicles Magliato's journey to become one of the world's few female heart surgeons, while learning to balance career and motherhood. (Her husband is also a surgeon.)

McFarland FK, Smith AJ, West CA, Rhoades DR. African-American female physicians in South Carolina: role models and career satisfaction. *Southern Med J.* 2000;93(10):982-5. Why do women go into medicine? For the same altruism and role modeling that influences most male medical students. Their frustrations also stem from the same sources as those of their male colleagues.

McMurray JE, Linzer M, Konrad TR, et al. The work lives of women physicians—results from the physician work life study. The SGIM Career Satisfaction Study Group. *J Gen Intern Med.* 2000;15(6):372-80. This is what is really happening in the lives of women physicians.

Mobilos S, Chan M, Brown JB. Women in medicine: the challenge of finding balance. *Can Fam Phys.* 2008;54(9):1285-6. This discussion with women physicians about lifestyle challenges concludes that more on-site daycare centers and flexible scheduling, the option of job sharing, and replacement staff for when they are on maternity leave are needed.

More AS, Fee E, Manon P, eds. *Women Physicians and the Cultures of Medicine*. Baltimore: Johns Hopkins University Press, 2009. Leading scholars cover 150 years of women struggling for equality, accomplishment, and happiness in medicine.

Oancia T, Bohm C, Carry T, Cujec B, Johnson D. The influence of gender and specialty on reporting of abusive and discriminatory behavior by medical students, residents and physician teachers. *Med Educ.* 2000;34(4):250-6. Not surprisingly, this study found that female surgical residents adopt the prevailing culture during training, but after residency revert to behavior and attitudes more akin to their non-surgical peers. Good insights into how women "go along to get along" in surgical residencies.

Reed V, Buddeberg-Fischer B. Career obstacles for women in medicine: an overview. *Med Educ.* 2001;35(2):139-47. An international review of women in medicine. Looks at women's access to medical school, the specialties they enter, promotion rates, frequency of part-time work, and salary inequities. Also reviews the obstacles women physicians face and what can be or is being done about them.

Roubidoux MA, Packer MM., Applegate KE, Aben G. Female medical students' interest in Radiology careers. *J Am Coll Radiology.* 2009;6(4):246-53. Women continue to be underrepresented in Radiology. The authors found that early interest in Radiology did not differ by gender but that the opportunities for flexible hours, intellectual challenge, patient care, and mentoring should be promoted to female students to maintain their interest.

Marriage and Parenting

American Academy of Pediatrics. *Children's Health Topics/Child Care.* An excellent web-based (www.aap.org/healthtopics/childcare.cfm) guide to childcare services for families and professionals, including the types of childcare services, what to look for, the questions to ask, and the different childcare needs of children as they grow and when they are ill.

Cole S, Arnold M, Sanderson A, Cupp C. Pregnancy during Otolaryngology residency: experience and recommendations. *Am Surgeon.* 2009;75(5):411-5. Surgical training programs have unique challenges and stressors for all trainees. But, how does pregnancy affect women surgical residents? Overall, long hours, unpredictable work demands, and guilt over colleagues' increased workloads and altered schedules were significant sources of stress, as were high personal expectations and doubts over balancing pregnancy with career demands.

Cujec B, Oancia T, Bohm C, et al. Career and parenting satisfaction among medical students, residents, and physician teachers at a Canadian medical school. *Can Med Assoc J.* 2000;162(5):637-40. Should you have children? While the more common question is "when?", this study suggests that medical students and residents are much more displeased with the time they have to spend parenting than are their colleagues in practice.

Fabre J. Fatherhood and medicine. *Clin Med.* 2010;10(2):138-40. A doctor whose physician–wife's career was affected by childcare (his was not) looks at how to create a working environment that optimizes a mother's career progression.

Jagsi R, Tarbell NJ, Weinstein DF. Becoming a doctor, starting a family leaves of absence from graduate medical education. *NEJM.* 2007;357(19):1889-91. Both men and women are affected by parental leave policies.

McNichol B. Babies on board. *New Phys.* March 2005, on-line. A variety of women talk about their experiences of balancing motherhood and medical school.

McPhillips HA, Burke AE, Sheppard K, et al. Toward creating family-friendly work environments in Pediatrics: baseline data from Pediatric department chairs and Pediatric program directors. *Pediatrics.* 2007;119(3):e596-e602. Do pediatric residency programs and academic departments create family-friendly work environments as outlined in the Report of the Task Force on Women in Pediatrics? Despite some progress, changes are still needed, including better accessibility to quality childcare, improved lactation facilities, clearly written parental leave policies, and flexible work schedules.

National Network for Child Care. The Learn section of their website (www.nncc.org) provides up-to-date links to many articles dealing with childcare. Click on "Childcare Evaluation and Assessment," then "Parental Assessment" to access a checklist of factors to consider when selecting a childcare option. There is also a listing of childcare information (including regulations and licensing by state) at "Tools/Resources."

Schrier DK, Shrier LA, Rich M, Greenberg L. Pediatricians leading the way: integrating a career and a family/personal life over the life cycle. *Pediatrics.* 2006;117:519-22. Practical suggestions for physicians to integrate their careers and family lives as expectations shift for younger physicians entering the field.

Sobecks NW, Justice AC, Hinze S, et al. When doctors marry doctors: a survey exploring the professional and family lives of young physicians. *Ann Intern Med.* 1999;130(4)Pt.1:312-9. A useful survey of physician–physician marriages and their effect on the participants' professional and personal lives.

Disabled Students and Residents

Essex-Sorlie D. The Americans with Disabilities Act: I. History, summary, and key components. *Acad Med.* 1994;69(7):519-24. Excellent overview of the Americans with Disabilities Act, and how it relates to medical schools. While the article does not address questions of residency application directly, it gives enough information from which to extrapolate. Clear, concise, and free of legal mumbo-jumbo.

Harris Family Center for Disability and Health Policy. This website (www.cdihp.org/) from the Western University of the Health Sciences has excellent links to up-to-date information for disabled medical students and residents.

Schroeder R, Brazeau C, Zackin F, et al. Do state medical board applications violate the Americans with Disabilities Act? *Acad Med.* 2009;84(6):776-81. The authors look at whether detailed questions about physicians' health on licensure exams, which often require follow-up documentation, may discourage physicians from seeking treatment.

Takakuwa KM, Ernst AA, Weiss SJ. Residents with disabilities: a national survey of directors of emergency medicine residency programs. *Southern Med J.* 2002;95(4):436-40. Discusses the prevalence of known and suspected disabilities among physicians in residency, and the willingness of residency directors to provide resources to assist these residents.

Special Situations

Beagan B. Micro inequities and everyday inequalities: race, gender, sexuality and class in medical school. *Can J Sociology.* 2001;26(4):583-610. It's not just the overt discrimination that medical students and residents encounter, but also the "every day practices of inclusion and exclusion that cumulatively convey messages about who does and who does not belong." Worth reading.

Burke BP, White JC. Well-being of gay, lesbian and bisexual doctors. *West J Med*. 2001;174(1):59-62. This article reviews the problems faced by these physician groups. Also discusses the questions they need to ask themselves about how their lifestyle may affect their choice of career and the discrimination they may face. Worth reading before "coming out."

Council on Graduate Medical Education. *Minorities in Medicine: An Ethnic and Cultural Challenge for Physician Training, an Update*. Washington, DC: Health Resources & Services Administration, U.S. Dept. of Health & Human Services, April 2005. This online (www.hrsa.gov/advisorycommittees/bhpradvisory/cogme/Reports/seventeenthrpt.pdf) document looks at progress since their 1998 report. It also makes recommendations for increasing underrepresented minorities in the education pipeline.

Croasdale M. Clinical retraining programs hard to find. *Am Med News*, June 4, 2007. Only a few programs exist to help physicians wishing to reenter the workforce. This article discusses the need for greater system flexibility as physicians, who take time off for a variety of reasons, wish to return to work.

Cronin WA, Morgan JA, Weeks WB. The cost of pursuing a medical career in the military: a tale of five specialties. *Acad Med*. 2010;85(8):1316-20. This study finds that choosing a military career in Internal Medicine or Psychiatry returns a larger cumulative net-present-value on the educational investment, while civilian careers in Gastroenterology, General Surgery, or Orthopedics offer much greater returns on their educational investments.

Kamei RK, Chen HC, Loeser H. Residency is not a race: our ten-year experience with a flexible schedule residency training option. *Acad Med*. 2004;79(5):447-52. Participants in the Flexible Option residency training schedule offered by the University of California at San Francisco Pediatric Residency Program believe that the advantages outweigh the disadvantages.

Lesko S. Women in medicine: challenges in part-time residencies. *Am Fam Phys*. 2002;65(1):31. This very personal letter discusses the difficulties of actually finding a part-time residency position and advocates for them to be made available.

Mullan F. The journey back: a physician retrains. *JAMA*. 1997;278(4):281-3. An old, but excellent, description of an experienced (older) physician-administrator retraining to enter clinical practice.

Nunez-Smith M, Curry LA, Bigby J, et al. Impact of race on the professional lives of physicians of African descent. *Ann Int Med*. 2007;146(1):45-51. A look at how African-American physicians in six New England states experience race in the workplace.

Peterson NB, Friedman RH, Ash AS, et al. Faculty self-reported experience with racial and ethnic discrimination in academic medicine. *J Gen Intern Med*. 2004;19(3):259-65. While no updated information exists for residents, this study involves minority faculty. They report experiencing racial or ethnic bias in academic medicine and have lower career satisfaction than other faculty. Despite this, minority faculty who reported experiencing discrimination achieved academic productivity similar to that of other faculty.

Osteopathic Medicine

American Osteopathic Association. *Yearbook and Directory of Members*. This compendium (online at www.osteopathic.org/index.cfm?PageID=ps_yearbook) contains virtually everything anyone needs to know about Osteopathic medicine, including current information on

Osteopathic residency programs, medical schools, and state-by-state or international licensure requirements.

————Division of Postdoctoral Training: Osteopathic graduate medical education. *J Am Osteopath Assoc.* (Usually the November issue.) This annual article gives an overview of the number of AOA-approved and funded residency positions, the number of graduates, how many D.O.'s are taking ACGME-approved training, and the rules for specialty certification.

Cummings M, Sefcik DJ. The impact of Osteopathic physicians' participation in ACGME-accredited postdoctoral programs, 1985-2006. *Acad Med.* 2009;84(6):733-6. In this time span, D.O. participation grew 400%, and by 2006, two out of three D.O.'s in postdoctoral training were enrolled in an ACGME program. The authors anticipate that the increase in Osteopathic medical schools and the limited capacity of AOA postdoctoral programs will cause a decline in opportunities for Osteopaths in the future.

Gevitz N: *The D.O.'s—Osteopathic Medicine in America,* 2nd ed. Baltimore, MD: Johns Hopkins University Press, 2004. An entertaining and enlightening look at the development of Osteopathic medicine in the United States. It is required reading for all D.O.'s and anyone else interested in Osteopathy. (+)

Rogers FJ, D'Alonzo GE Jr, Glover JC, et al. Proposed tenets of Osteopathic medicine and principles for patient care. *J Am Osteo Assoc.* 2002;102(2):63-5. This is the updated philosophy of Osteopathic medicine.

Shannon SC, Teitelbaum HS. The status and future of Osteopathic medical education in the United States. *Acad Med.* 2009;84(6):707-11. In 2010, 25% of all U.S. medical graduates were D.O.'s. The authors look at where the profession began and the challenges it faces.

Criteria for Selecting Residents

Edmond MB, Deschenes JL, Eckler M, Wenzel RP. Racial bias in using USMLE Step 1 scores to grant Internal Medicine residency interviews. *Acad Med.* 2001;76(12):1253-6. This study shows that when USMLE Step 1 scores are used as a criterion for residency interviews, Black students suffer disproportionately.

Gilbart MK, Cusimano MD, Regehr G. Evaluating surgical resident selection procedures. *Am J Surg.* 2001;181(3):221-5. Contains inside information on what Orthopedic Surgery residencies seek in candidates: work ethic, interpersonal qualities, orthopedic experience, and enthusiasm.

Green M, Jones P, Thomas JX. Selection criteria for residency: results of a national program directors survey. *Acad Med.* 2009;84(3):362-67. Factors program directors in twenty-one specialties use to choose their residents: Excellence in clinical performance, reference letters and audition electives rank highly, as do USMLE results. In fact, the authors advise students to take both Step 1 and Step 2 in time for the residency application.

LaGrasso JR, Kennedy DA, Hoehn JG, Ashruf S, Przybyla AM. Selection criteria for the integrated model of Plastic Surgery residency. *Plas Recon Surg.* 2008;121(3):121e-125e. What qualities make a successful Plastic Surgery resident? Program directors cited membership in the AOA Honor Society as the most important objective criterion, followed by publications in peer-reviewed journals and letters of recommendation from plastic surgeons known to the director. Leadership capabilities were considered the most important subjective criterion, followed by maturity and interest in academics.

Lotfipour S, Luu R, Hayden SR, et al. Becoming an emergency medicine resident: a practical guide for medical students. *J Emerg Med.* 2008; 35(3):339-44. Acceptance into Emergency Medicine residencies is competitive. This article explains what factors residency directors value, from the pre-clinical years to the interview.

Melendez MM, Xu X, Sexton TR, Shapiro MJ, Mohan EP. The importance of basic science and clinical research as a selection criterion for General Surgery residency programs. *J Surg Ed.* 2008;65(2):151-4. What criteria do Surgery program directors use when selecting residents? The primary factors were the interview, demonstrated interest in Surgery and AOA membership; basic science and clinical research were important but secondary criteria.

Nallasamy S, Uhler T, Nallasamy N, Tapino PJ, Volpe NJ. Ophthalmology resident selection: current trends in selection criteria and improving the process. *Ophthalmology.* 2010;117(5):1041-7. This study found the following factors most important in Ophthalmology resident selection: interviews, clinical course grades, recommendation letters, and board scores.

Taylor CA, Weinstein L, Mayhew HE. The process of resident selection: a view from the residency director's desk. *Obstet Gynecol.* 1995;85(2):299-303. This article contains the results of a survey of Family Practice and Obstetrics & Gynecology residency directors. The results reflect the decision-making processes used by residency directors in Internal Medicine, Pediatrics, Psychiatry, and the surgical specialties. Old, but still interesting.

Villanueva AM, Kaye D, Abdelhak SS, Morahan PS. Comparing selection criteria of residency directors and physicians' employers. *Acad Med.* 1995;70(4):261-71. This article lays out what residency directors in Pediatrics, Surgery, Family Medicine, and Internal Medicine seek in residency candidates' applications. It then compares the personal qualities they desire in residents with the qualities that academic medical centers, private practices, managed care organizations, hospitals, and other health care systems look for when hiring new physicians. While this article is old, it contains valuable information.

Yudkowsky R, Elliott R, Schwartz A. Two perspectives on the indicators of quality in Psychiatry residencies: program directors' and residents'. *Acad Med.* 2002;77(1):57-64. What makes a "good" Psychiatry residency? Program directors and residents have different views, and both are included in this paper.

Application Materials and Interviewing

Biegeleisen JI. *Make Your Job Interview a Success*, 4th ed. New York: Prentice-Hall, 1994. The chapter, "63 Guaranteed Ways to Muff a Job Interview," is enlightening reading. It is also funny. Well worth the time, it may prevent you from making a serious faux pas. (+)

Girzadas DV, Harwood RC, Delis SN, et al. Emergency medicine standardized letter of recommendation: predictors of guaranteed match. *Acad Emerg Med.* 2001;8(6):648-53. This study confirms the factors that go into a strong recommendation letter. You may want to forward a copy of the article to your letter writers.

Hunt DD, MacLaren C, Scott C, et al. A follow-up study of the characteristics of dean's letters. *Acad Med.* 2001;76(7):727-33. An excellent review of what is contained in Dean's letters. It should give you a good idea of information that might be included in a Dean's letter but that is not in yours, or what information you may want to suggest *not* be included in your own letter.

Keim SM, Rein JA, Chisholm C, et al. A standardized letter of recommendation for residency application. *Acad Emerg Med.* 1999;6(11):1141-6. Describes the standardized recommendation letter used by Emergency Medicine programs. This letter probably will show up, in some form, in other specialties.

Shea JA, O'Grady E, Morrison G, Wagner BR, Morris JB. Medical School Performance Evaluations in 2005: an improvement over the former dean's letter? *Acad Med.* 2008;83(3):284-91. The "Dean's Letters" name was changed to encourage evaluation over recommendation, but what are Deans actually putting in your MSPE? This study found that comparative data is still not consistently included, and MSPEs within a school did not distinguish significantly between top-, middle-, and lower-tier students.

Tysinger JW. *Résumés and Personal Statements for Health Professionals*, 2nd ed. Tucson, AZ: Galen Press, Ltd., 1998. A classic, this book guides you through the arduous process of describing your accomplishments in the best possible way to develop unique résumés and personal statements that reflect who you really are. Describes how to build a personal inventory and then use the inventory items to write a professional-looking document that will impress residency directors. Written by an educator with years of experience, the book includes lots of examples to help you. Also discusses cover and thank-you letters. A must for all applicants. (+)

Venolia J. *Write Right! A Desktop Digest of Punctuation, Grammar, and Style*, 4th ed. Berkeley, CA: Ten Speed Press, 2001. A powerful and easy-to-understand pocket guide on how to avoid making mistakes on résumés, personal statements, and other important documents. (+)

The Match

American Osteopathic Association. *AOA Intern/Resident Registration Program*. Results for the current and past years' matches are posted at www.natmatch.com/aoairp/, organized by specialty and by medical school.

Englander R, Carraccio C, Zalneraitis E, Sarkin R, Morgenstern B. Guiding medical students through the match: perspectives from recent graduates. *Pediatrics.* 2003;112(3 Pt 1):502-5. Survey results of PGY-1 Pediatrics residents' satisfaction with their pre-match counseling and match results. Residents were very satisfied with where they matched, and less satisfied with the advice received. The top three resources were *FREIDA*, their adviser, and resident-to-student counseling. Only the Green Book was rated unhelpful.

National Resident Matching Program. *Results and Data [Annual] Main Residency Match*. Washington, DC: NRMP. This on-line report, available for free as a pdf file, details the outcome of the annual NRMP Match by specialty and institution. Additional data that compares past years of the Match and that lists Match results by state, specialty, and applicant type is posted on-line under "Data and Reports."

Medical Practice

American Medical Association. *Physician Characteristics and Distribution in the United States*. Chicago: AMA, published biannually. This book contains an extensive breakdown, by specialty and by county, of the characteristics of physicians practicing in each specialty in the United States. It goes into the specifics of who, what, and where the physicians are.

Association of American Medical Colleges. *AAMC Data Book: Medical Schools and Teaching Hospitals by the Numbers*. Washington, DC: AAMC, published annually. Contains current and historical statistical information related to medical schools and teaching hospitals. Available at all medical school libraries.

Urman RD, Ehrenfeld JM (eds.). *Physicians' Pathways to Non-Traditional Careers and Leadership Opportunities*. New York: Springer, 2012. It's no secret that many physicians, after some time in practice, find that they prefer not to be at the bedside, but rather in the lab, board-room, lecture hall, or other venue. This book's chapters, each written by a physician who followed that particular path, explore several non-traditional career alternatives (there are many more). It offers common sense advice for readers at any point in their careers.

Scheurer D, McKean S, Miller J, Wetterneck T. U.S. physician satisfaction: a systematic review. *J Hosp Med*. 2009;4(9):560-8. These authors found that physician satisfaction was relatively stable over time, with a slight decline for Primary Care physicians. Factors most associated with satisfaction include the physician's specialty and job features, such as control over their work, colleague support, and income.

General Information

American Medical Association. *GME e-letter*. This free monthly newsletter covers the latest news in graduate medical education (GME), such as resident duty hours and physician workforce concerns. Also contains updates on GME accreditation activities. Subscribe to this and other AMA newsletters at www.ama-assn.org/ama/pub/news/subscribe-newsletters.shtml.

American Medical Student Association. *The New Physician*. Published monthly in print and on-line, and free with AMSA membership. Contains articles on medical specialties and practice, interviewing, the Match, international medical graduates, and other topics of vital interest to medical students.

Medical Organizations' Contact Information & Websites

American Academy of Family Physicians (AAFP), P.O. Box 11210, Shawnee Mission, KS 662207-1210; (800) 274-2237 or (913) 906-6000; www.aafp.org.

American Hospital Association (AHA), 155 N. Wacker Dr., Chicago, IL 60606; (312) 422-3000; www.aha.org.

American Medical Association (AMA), 515 N. State St., Chicago, IL 60654; (800) 621-8335; www.ama-assn.org.
- AMA Medical Student Section, www.ama-assn.org/ama/pub/about-ama/our-people/member-groups-sections/medical-student-section.shtml.
- *FREIDA Online*, www.ama-assn.org/ama/pub/education-careers/graduate-medical-education/freida-online.page.

American Medical Student Association (AMSA), 1902 Association Dr., Reston, VA 20191; (800) 767-2266 or (703) 620-6600; www.amsa.org.

American Medical Women's Association (AMWA), 100 N. 20th St., 4th Floor, Philadelphia, PA 19103; (215) 320-3716; www.amwa-doc.org.

American Osteopathic Association (AOA), 142 E. Ontario St., Chicago, IL 60611; (800) 621-1773 or (312) 202-8000; www.osteopathic.org.
- Opportunities, http://opportunities.osteopathic.org/.

American Urological Association Residency Matching Program, 1000 Corporate Blvd., Linthicum, MD 21090; (866) 746-4282, ext. 3919; e-mail: resmatch@auanet.org; **www.auanet.org/content/residency/residency-match.cfm.**

Association of American Medical Colleges (AAMC), 2450 N Street NW, Washington, DC 20037-1126; (202) 828-0400; www.aamc.org.
- Careers in Medicine, www.aamc.org/students/medstudents/cim/.
- Electronic Residency Application Services (ERAS), www.aamc.org/students/medstudents/eras/.

— Send technical questions to the MyERAS Help Section at myeras@aamc.org.
- FindAResident, www.aamc.org/students/residents/findaresident/70050/findaresident.html.

Canadian Resident Matching Service (CaRMS), 171 Nepean St., Suite 300, Ottawa, ON K2P 0B4, Canada; (877) 227-6742 or (613) 237-0075; email: **help@carms.ca**; www.carms.ca.

Council of Medical Specialty Societies (CMSS), 230 E. Ohio St., Suite 400, Chicago, IL 60611; (312) 224-2585; e-mail: mailbox@cmss.org; www.cmss.org.

Educational Commission for Foreign Medical Graduates (ECFMG), www.ecfmg.org.
- ERAS/ECFMG, 3624 Market St., Philadelphia, PA 19104-2685 USA; (215) 386-5900; e-mail: eras-support@ecfmg.org; www.ecfmg.org/eras/index.html.

— Send completed documents by mail: ECFMG-ERAS Program, P.O. Box 11746, Philadelphia, PA 19101-0746 USA.

— Send completed documents by courier delivery: ERAS, ECFMG, 3624 Market St., Philadelphia, PA 19104-2685 USA.

- ECFMG/USMLE Information, 3624 Market St., Philadelphia, PA 19104-2685; (215) 386-5900; www.ecfmg.org.

Federation of State Medical Boards of the U.S., Inc. (FSMB), P.O. Box 619850, Dallas, TX 75261-9850; (817) 868-4000; www.fsmb.org.
  - For USMLE Step 3 questions, (817) 868-4041; e-mail: usmle@fsmb.org; www.fsmb.org/m_usmlestep3.html.
  - For questions regarding test accommodations for USMLE examinees with disabilities, www.fsmb.org/usmle_testaccommodationrequest.html.

Foundation for Advancement of International Medical Education and Research (FAIMER), 3624 Market St., Philadelphia, PA 19104-2685, USA; e-mail: inquiry@faimer.org; www.faimer.org/contact.html.

Gay and Lesbian Medical Association (GLMA), 1326 18th Street NW, Suite 22, Washington, DC 20036; (202) 600-8037; www.glma.org.

National Board of Medical Examiners (NBME), 3750 Market St., Philadelphia, PA 19104-3102; (215) 590-9700; www.nbme.org.

National Board of Osteopathic Medical Examiners (NBOME), 8765 W. Higgins Rd., Suite 200, Chicago, IL 60631-4174; (773) 714-0622; e-mail: candidateservices@nbome.org; www.nbome.org.

National Health Service Corps (NHSC), (800) 221-9393; http://nhsc.hrsa.gov/.

National Medical Association (NMA), 8403 Colesville Rd., Suite 920, Silver Spring, MD 20910; (202) 347-1895; www.nmanet.org.

National Resident Matching Program (NRMP), 2450 N Street NW, Washington, DC 20037-1127; (866) 617-5838 or (202) 828-0566 (8:30 A.M. to 5:30 P.M. Eastern time); e-mail: NRMP@aamc.org; www.nrmp.org.

San Francisco Matching Programs (SFMP), 655 Beach St., San Francisco, CA 94109; (415) 447-0350 [including Vacancy Line]; e-mail: help@sfmatch.org; www.sfmatch.org.
  - For check payments only: SF Match, c/o Wells Fargo Lockbox Services, SF Matching Program Dept #34059, 3440 Walnut Ave., Bldg A, 2nd Floor, Fremont, CA 94538.

Medical Organizations' Websites

Organization Name	Website
Aerospace Medical Assoc. (ASMA)	www.asma.org
Alpha Omega Alpha Student Research Fellowships	www.alphaomegaalpha.org/ student_research.html
Amer. Acad. of Allergy, Asthma & Immunology (AAAAI)	www.aaaai.org
Amer. Acad. of Child & Adolescent Psychiatry (AACAP)	www.aacap.org
Amer. Acad. of Clinical Psychiatrists (AACP)	www.aacp.com/
Amer. Acad. of Dermatology (AAD)	www.aad.org
Amer. Acad. of Emergency Medicine (AAEM)	www.aaem.org
Amer. Acad. of Facial Plastic & Reconstructive Surgery (AAFPRS)	www.aafprs.org
Amer. Acad. of Neurology (AAN)	www.aan.com
Amer. Acad. of Ophthalmology (AAO)	www.aao.org
Amer. Acad. of Orthopedic Surgeons (AAOS)	www.aaos.org
Amer. Acad. of Osteopathy	www.academyofosteopathy.org
Amer. Acad. of Otolaryngology (AAO-HNS)	www.entnet.org
Amer. Acad. of Pain Medicine (AAPM)	www.painmed.org
Amer. Acad. of Pediatrics (AAP)	www.aap.org
Amer. Acad. of Physical Medicine & Rehabilitation (AAPMR)	www.aapmr.org
Amer. Assoc. for Geriatric Psychiatry (AAGP)	www.aagpgpa.org
Amer. Assoc. for Hand Surgery	www.handsurgery.org
Amer. Assoc. for the Surgery of Trauma (AAST)	www.aast.org/
Amer. Assoc. for Thoracic Surgery (AATS)	www.aats.org/
Amer. Assoc. of Clinical Urologists, Inc. (AACU)	www.aacuweb.org
Amer. Assoc. of Immunologists (AAI)	www.aai.org/
Amer. Assoc. of Neurological Surgeons (AANS)	www.aans.org
Amer. Assoc. of Neuromuscular & Electrodiagnostic Medicine (AANEM)	www.aanem.org/
Amer. Assoc. of Public Health Physicians (AAPHP)	www.aaphp.org
Amer. Board of Medical Specialties (ABMS)	www.abms.org
Amer. Coll. of Allergy, Asthma & Immunology (ACAAI)	www.acaai.org/
Amer. Coll. of Cardiology (ACC)	www.acc.org
Amer. Coll. of Chest Physicians	www.chestnet.org

Amer. Coll. of Emergency Physicians (ACEP)	www.acep.org
Amer. Coll. of Gastroenterology (ACG)	www.acg.gi.org
Amer. Coll. of Medical Genetics (ACMG)	www.acmg.net/
Amer. Coll. of Nuclear Medicine	www.acnmonline.org/
Amer. Coll. of Obstetricians & Gynecologists (ACOG)	www.acog.org
Amer. Coll. of Occupational & Environmental Medicine (ACOEM)	www.acoem.org
Amer. Coll. of Osteopathic Emergency Physicians (ACOEP)	www.acoep.org
Amer. Coll. of Osteopathic Family Physicians (ACOFP)	www.acofp.org
Amer. Coll. of Osteopathic Internists (ACOI)	www.acoi.org
Amer. Coll. of Osteopathic Obstetricians & Gynecologists (ACOOG)	www.acoog.org/
Amer. Coll. of Osteopathic Pediatricians	www.acopeds.org
Amer. Coll. of Osteopathic Prolotherapy Integrative Pain Management	www.acopms.com
Amer. Coll. of Physician Executives (ACPE)	www.acpe.org
Amer. Coll. of Physicians (ACP)	www.acponline.org
Amer. Coll. of Preventive Medicine (ACPM)	www.acpm.org
Amer. Coll. of Radiology (ACR)	www.acr.org
Amer. Coll. of Rheumatology	www.rheumatology.org
Amer. Coll. of Sports Medicine (ACSM)	www.acsm.org
Amer. Coll. of Surgeons (ACS)	www.facs.org
Amer. Congress of Rehabilitation (ACRM)	www.acrm.org
Amer. Federation for Aging Research (AFAR)	www.afar.org
Amer. Gastroenterological Assoc.	www.gastro.org
Amer. Geriatrics Society	www.americangeriatrics.org
Amer. Medical Directors Assoc. (AMDA)	www.amda.com
Amer. Neurological Assoc. (ANA)	www.aneuroa.org
Amer. Nuclear Society (ANS)	www.ans.org/
Amer. Orthopedic Assoc. (AOA)	www.aoassn.org
Amer. Orthopedic Soc. for Sports Medicine	www.sportsmed.org
Amer. Osteopathic Acad. of Orthopedics (AOAO)	www.aoao.org
Amer. Osteopathic Acad. of Sports Medicine (AOASM)	www.aoasm.org
Amer. Osteopathic Coll. of Dermatology (AOCD)	www.aocd.org
Amer. Osteopathic Coll. of Occupational & Preventive Medicine (AOCOPM)	www.aocopm.org

Amer. Osteopathic Coll. of Physical Medicine & Rehabilitation (AOCPMR)	www.aocpmr.org
Amer. Osteopathic Coll. of Radiology	www.aocr.org
Amer. Osteopathic Coll. of Ophthalmology & Otolaryngology (AOCOOHNS)	www.aocoohns.org
Amer. Pain Society	www.ampainsoc.org/
Amer. Pediatric Soc.-Soc. for Pediatric Research (APS-SPR)	www.aps-spr.org
Amer. Pediatric Surgical Assoc. (APSA)	www.eapsa.org
Amer. Psychiatric Assoc. (APA)	www.psych.org/
Amer. Roentgen Ray Soc. (ARRS)	www.arrs.org
Amer. Soc. for Clinical Pathology (ASCP)	www.ascp.org
Amer. Soc. for Dermatologic Surgery (ASDS)	www.asds.net/
Amer. Soc. for Investigative Pathology (ASIP)	www.asip.org
Amer. Soc. for Reproductive Medicine (ASRM)	www.asrm.org
Amer. Soc. for Surgery of the Hand	www.hand-surg.org
Amer. Soc. for Therapeutic Radiology & Oncology (ASTRO)	www.astro.org
Amer. Soc. of Anesthesiologists (ASA)	www.asahq.org
Amer. Soc. of Clinical Oncology (ASCO)	www.asco.org
Amer. Soc. of Colon & Rectal Surgeons (ASCRS)	www.fascrs.org
Amer. Soc. of Dermatology (ASD)	www.asd.org/
Amer. Soc. of General Surgeons (ASGS)	www.theasgs.org
Amer. Soc. of Hematology (ASH)	www.hematology.org
Amer. Soc. of Nephrology (ASN)	www.asn-online.org
Amer. Soc. of Plastic Surgeons	www.plasticsurgery.org
Assoc. for Research in Otolaryngology (ARO)	www.aro.org
Assoc. of Academic Physiatrists	www.physiatry.org
Assoc. of American Indian Physicians (AAIP)	www.aaip.org
Assoc. of Military Surgeons of the U.S. (AMSUS)	www.amsus.org
Assoc. of Teachers of Preventive Medicine (ATPM)	www.atpm.org
Cardiothoracic Surgery Network	www.vascsurg.org
Child Neurology Society	www.childneurologysociety.org
Coll. of Amer. Pathologists (CAP)	www.cap.org
Congress of Neurological Surgeons	www.neurosurgeon.org/
Emergency Medical Residents' Assoc. (EMRA)	www.emra.org
Endocrine Society	www.endo-society.org
Federal Direct Consolidation Loan Information Center	www.loanconsolidation.ed.gov/

Federal Student Aid (FSA)	http://studentaid.ed.gov/ PORTALSWebApp/ students/english/repaying. jsp?tab=repaying
Foundation for Reconstructive Plastic Surgery	www.frps.org
Genetics Society of America	www.genetics-gsa.org/
Infectious Diseases Soc. of Amer. (IDSA)	www.idsociety.org
International Medical Education Directory (IMED)	http://imed.ecfmg.org
Gay and Lesbian Medical Association	www.glma.org/
Marshall Univ. Medical H.E.L.P. Program	www.marshall.edu/medicalhelp/
National Association of Managed Care Physicians (NAMCP)	www.namcp.com/
National Hispanic Medical Assoc. (NHMA)	www.nhmamd.org/
National Institutes of Health Clin. Rsch. Training Prog.	www.cc.nih.gov/training/crtp/crtp.html
National Matching Services (NMS)	www.natmatch.com
Pathway Evaluation Prog. for Medical Professionals	medweb.usc.edu/pathways/intro. htm
Radiological Soc. of North America, Inc. (RSNA)	www.rsna.org
Renal Physicians Assoc.	www.renalmd.org
Sarnoff Endowment	www.sarnoffendowment.org
Soc. for Academic Emergency Medicine (SAEM)	www.saem.org
Soc. of Critical Care Medicine (SCCM)	www.sccm.org
Soc. of General Internal Medicine (SGIM)	www.sgim.org
Soc. of Hospital Medicine (SHM)	www.hospitalmedicine.org
Soc. of Nuclear Medicine (SNM)	www.snm.org
Soc. of Thoracic Surgeons (STS)	www.sts.org
Soc. of Toxicology	www.toxicology.org
Student Doctor Network	www.studentdoctor.net/
Thomson Prometric Testing	www.prometric.com
U.S. Equal Employment Opportunity Comm. (EEOC)	www.eeoc.gov
U.S. Medical Licensing Exam (USMLE)	www.usmle.org
Univ. of Kansas School of Med.	www.kumc.edu/som/medsos/opp. html
Univ. Missouri-Kansas City, Institute for Professional Preparation	www.umkc.edu/ipp/
Women Physicians Congress (WPC)	www.ama-assn.org/ama/pub/ about-ama/our-people/ member-groups-sections/ women-physicians-congress. shtml
Women's Health.gov	www.4women.gov/index.htm

About the Author

KENNETH V. ISERSON, M.D., MBA, FACEP, FAAEM, FIFEM, is Professor Emeritus of Emergency Medicine at The University of Arizona, Medical Director (Emeritus) of the Southern Arizona Rescue Association (search & rescue), a Supervisory Physician with Arizona's Disaster Medical Assistance Team (AZ-1), and a member of the American Red Cross disaster response team. He is also a past president of the Society of Teachers of Emergency Medicine.

He directed the residency program in Emergency Medicine at The University of Arizona College of Medicine in Tucson for ten years. A noted clinician and medical educator, Dr. Iserson frequently speaks to medical students, advisers, and residents on how best to navigate the complex process of selecting a specialty; choosing a residency program; and applying to, interviewing for, and obtaining a position at a desired residency program.

Dr. Iserson now limits his medical practice to global and disaster medicine. In the past few years, he has practiced or taught on all seven continents, including 6 months as Lead Physician for the US Antarctic Program and work with NGOs in rural areas of Central and South America, Zambia, Bhutan, Ghana, and South Sudan. He also runs the www.REEME.arizona.edu Project that freely distributes more than 700 Spanish-language PowerPoint presentations on Emergency Medicine.

The author of hundreds of scientific articles on emergency medicine and biomedical ethics, he has also written several other books published by Galen Press Ltd. Tucson, AZ (www.galenpress.com), including:

Death to Dust: What Happens to Dead Bodies? 2nd ed.
Ethics in Emergency Medicine (Senoir editor), 2nd ed.
Get Into Medical School: A Guide for the Perplexed, 2nd ed.
Grave Words: Notifying Survivors about Unexpected Deaths
Pocket Protocols: Notifying Survivors About Sudden, Unexpected Death (in English and in Spanish)
Demon Doctors: Physicians as Serial Killers
The Autopsy: More Than You Ever Wanted to Know (e-book)

The following book, published in 2011 by McGraw-Hill Medical:
Improvised Medicine: Providing Care in Extreme Environments

Index

T